DISEASE

AS A SYMBOL

Psychosomatics–
The Messages behind Your
Symptoms

DISEASE

AS A SYMBOL

Psychosomatics–
The Messages behind Your
Symptoms

RUEDIGER DAHLKE, M.D.

Translated by Simone Duxbery

*In co-operation with Margit Dahlke,
Christine Stecher, Vera Kaesemann, Dr. med. Robert Hößl
and Prof. Dr. med. Volker Zahn
Translated by Simone Duxbury-Ziemer in co-operation with Rita Fasel*

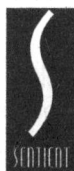

SENTIENT PUBLICATIONS

First Sentient Publications edition 2025

A paperback original

Book design by Laura Waltje
Cover Design by Laura Waltje
Cover Illustration by Benjavisa Ruangvaree Art

Library of Congress Control Number: 2024948528
Publisher's Cataloging-in-Publication Data

Names: Dahlke, Ruediger, author. | Duxbery, Simone, translator.
Title: Disease as a symbol : psychosomatics - the messages behind your symptoms / Ruediger Dahlke, MD; translated by Simone Duxbery.
Description: Includes index. | Boulder, CO: Sentient Publications, 2025.
Identifiers: LCCN: 2024948528 | ISBN: 978-1-59181-340-8 (print) | 978-1-59181-341-5 (epub)
Subjects: LCSH Medicine, Psychosomatic. | Medicine and psychology. | Mind and body. | Mind and body therapies. | BISAC BODY, MIND & SPIRIT / Healing / General | HEALTH & FITNESS / Healing | HEALTH & FITNESS / Diseases & Conditions / General | MEDICAL / Holistic Medicine
Classification: LCC RC49 .D3415 2025 | DDC 616.08--dc23

SENTIENT PUBLICATIONS
A Limited Liability Company
PO Box 1851
Boulder, CO 80306
www.sentientpublications.com

Heilkundeinstitut Dahlke GmbH & Co KG

I would like to express my thanks to the employees of the "Heil-Kunde-Zentrums Johanniskirchen" for corrections, additions and suggestions to the original German version of this text.

Freda Jeske, Christa Maleri, Josef Hien, Elisabeth Mitteregger and Sybille Schlüpen.

Publisher E-Book version Heilkundeinstitut Dahlke GmbH & Co KG
Oberberg 92, A-8151 Hitzendorf
www.dahlke.at
© 2012

Translated from the 15th completely revised and extended edition
© 2007 by Bertelsmann Verlag GmbH, Munich,
member of the Publishers Random House GmbH

Table of Contents

Introduction

*"The best medicine for man is man himself. The highest
form of medicine is love."*
—*Paracelsus*

The idea of using disease patterns and symptoms as opportunities for growth on the path of development dates from time immemorial, and its essence can be found in the holy scriptures of many religions. In modern times, due to the decline of religion and the triumphal progress of natural scientific medicine, it has been pushed into the background and largely forgotten, although admittedly it has experienced a revival since the first publication in 1983 of *Krankheit als Weg* (which was later translated into English with the title *The Healing Power of Illness*)[1]. In the meantime, this approach – which has since been continually broadened and more widely developed – has even begun making the breakthrough into traditionally-accepted medical practice, and since 2005, I have been holding further training courses for a German medical association. Amongst naturopathic and psychologically-orientated therapists, the approach had long ago secured its rightful place. For the most part, however, the popularity of this old, rediscovered art of the interpretation of disease patterns has not come about through professional therapists,

---

1   Titles marked with (*) have been translated into English, but may be currently out of print. Titles marked with (**) have not yet been translated into English. The various titles in question, however, may be available in other languages. A list of the 200 translations in 23 languages that are currently available can be found at [www.dahlke.at] by clicking on the respective national flags in the Dahlke International category.

as originally hoped, but through the people affected. Patients have brought the method to their therapists, the majority of whom were originally unwilling to follow such a simple and plausible path. This despite the fact that there had long been indications about the importance of the meaning and interpretation of diseases, such as when Viktor Frankl emphasised: "The 'desire for meaning' is inherent to life. If the meaning can be successfully interpreted, the disease will be more easily overcome."

At the physical level, anyone can indicate, at least by pointing (hence the term index finger), to where the problem lies - to where the shoe is pinching or where the pain is causing suffering. In an extended, figurative sense, too, it is only a matter of putting one's finger on the (symbolic) wound and asking the right question – the question that, even as far back as the legend of Parsifal and the Holy Grail, could have relieved the wounded Grail King Amfortas of his suffering. This healing question concerns the shadow which is embodied in every wound and every disease pattern – this "Dear Uncle, what is troubling you?" – a question Parsifal initially fails to ask because ignorance of his own pain and woundedness renders him incapable of empathy. The body is the stage for unconscious spiritual experience, or as expressed in negative terms by the author Peter Altenberg: "Disease is the outcry of an offended soul." Accordingly, it is necessary to find out what has offended the soul, and the body indicates its needs for this process.

The language of the body, of which the language of symbols is just one subcategory, albeit a particularly important one, is the most widely-spoken language on this Earth. All people speak it, even if they are not always aware of this fact and many no longer understand the language of their own body. Nevertheless, most people, even those of today's modern world, still have a latent awareness of this language of the body and can therefore re-learn it amazingly quickly. Seemingly, it is part of the great and mysterious wealth of knowledge which has slumbered within us since ancient times, simply waiting to be reawakened.

Through the understanding of the language of our body, we are able to regain access to our roots, both in our own culture and in the wider human family. At the same time, we can experience how immaculate this means of expression of the body truly is and return to that original state of existence before the Babylonian confusion, when all people got by with one and the same language. When tears are shed, we interpret them from the context spontaneously and correctly as tears of joy, of sorrow or of pain. The more archaic the person, the more primal his or her means of expression, and so we can learn from ancient times and thereby notice that we still carry within us the experiences of those times. It is for this reason, as well as by popular request, that in this supplement to the 15th edition, completely normal and healthy aspects of the language of the body have also been included in the *Directory of the body regions and organs*, such as the shape of the eyebrows or the chin. Part 1 therefore provides an even more reliable analysis of this original state. This allows us to recognise that the form of our body always provides information, both with regard to the life tasks carried along into this life, and also those which are to emerge later. These can fundamentally be interpreted identically – in line with the recognition that everything which has form must also have sense and meaning. The language of the body therefore leads all people to one and the same stage of honesty with regard to their own self.

Building on the interpretations of disease patterns in general that have been covered in many of my previous books and my books on specific health issues such as heart problems, digestive problems, weight problems and the psychology of smoking, the purpose of the present reference work is to approach the sum of disease patterns with a claim to comprehensiveness. After 30 years of work based on these interpretations, the time seemed ripe to close the few remaining gaps. To this end, the interpretation results of my more recent books on aggression and depression as opportunities for growth, and the importance of sleep for our general well-being have also been included, together with those of my latest book describing how our body acts as a mirror for the soul. I have also received important suggestions over the course of the years from many letter and email writers, to whom I would like to express my thanks at this point.

This new edition therefore provides interpretations of many hundreds of disease patterns, with thousands of individual symptoms, enabling users easy and rapid access to the corresponding symbolism of a particular disease pattern.

Although in *The Healing Power of Illness we chose to follow the traditionally-accepted medical procedure of arrangement by organs, and for example, grouped together all liver and kidney diseases, ten years later, in the 'sequel' *Krankheit als Sprache der Seele* (**Disease as a Language of the Soul)*, I opted instead for a head-to-foot model in order to enable better reference to the relevant adjoining areas of the disease pattern. For the current reference work, alphabetical arrangement was the only possibility for the purposes of better and more reliable orientation. Of course, all arrangement systems have their advantages and disadvantages, and the best strategy when dealing with these is a sound knowledge of the systems in question, in particular, their disadvantages. The arrangement by organs, for example, can tempt us towards very restricted viewpoints which run counter to a more holistic perspective and which thus lead to distortions of the type the "Kidney in Room 12", as is well-known from traditionally-accepted medicine. Although the head-to-foot model gets around this problem, it is not clear enough for orientation purposes, since many disease patterns, such as blood or nerve diseases, cannot be clearly assigned to a particular bodily region. The alphabetical arrangement, on the other hand, offers the quickest overview and – by means of numerous cross-references – the most reliable orientation, although with the obvious disadvantage of thereby completely ignoring the sense and function relationships.

In view of this disadvantage, the best method with respect to the interpretation of disease patterns is the combination of different levels in accordance with the following approach: First of all, find the meaning and interpretation of the affected region in the first part of the manual – such as the neck in the case of inflammation of the tonsils – in order to discover the overall symbolic meaning of the problem area. The next step – again in the first part of the manual – leads to the affected organ or body part, with its more specific symbolism and function; in our case therefore, to the tonsils, and thus to the superordinate level at which the problem is occurring: the immune system as a line of defense. The next step leads to the second and main part of the manual: the basic problem and its interpretation; in our case therefore, to the inflammation and its symbolism. Only then is it recommended as the last step to refer to "Tonsillitis".

The second part of the manual - the directory of symptoms - also gives advice on the handling and resolution possibilities of the subject for every basic and special problem. In our example, ideas are offered on the handling of the inflammation problem in general, and how one might be able to come to terms with its deeper meaning. Only then does it make sense to take the step to the specific problem (the tonsillitis). However tempting it might appear to refer straight to the end point first, the less this is advisable. Only the groundwork of the preceding steps makes it possible to to do justice to the subject in its full depth and complexity. In this particular case, an essential contribution can be made by intensive exploration of the subject of aggression, such as in the book *Aggression als Chance*[2] (**Aggression as an Opportunity*). This path from the general to the more specific also represents a tried-and-tested archetypal pattern.

The references to the archetypal principles can also be used as important aids, particularly with regard to the handling and resolution of the problem. These are given both for the body regions and organs in Part 1 and in the disease patterns and symptoms described in Part 2 so that, in addition to the special task, the "model example" that is provided by the archetypal environment also becomes perfectly clear. Even with little knowledge of this system of archetypes, it is possible to develop deeper understanding in this respect through the use of this reference work. In the case of unclear correlations, explanatory keywords are occasionally given in brackets behind the archetypal principles. In all cases, the archetypal principle of the affected region is given first, i.e. the level at which the problem is occurring, followed by the archetypal principle of the symptomatology, joined by a hyphen. These will frequently be mixtures of the relevant archetypal principles, and this is indicated by a forward slash (/).

The system of incorporating different levels in combination with the archetypal principles makes it possible for the dangers which would otherwise be presented by a formulaic translation of symptoms into interpretations (i.e. premature conclusions which bypass the essential and overly-simplified equivalencies) to be restricted to acceptable limits. By placing the different levels within a hierarchy, the overall relationship to the complete organism, in which every disease pattern is embedded, can also be identified more clearly. In every case, the whole person is ill, and must also be treated as such; the alternative would be an inappropriate and relatively random interpretation or treatment of symptoms. By means of the hierarchical placement, the crucial and pivotal point of the problem can be found, without neglecting the overall context. Even if the word "hierarchy" nowadays does not really carry positive connotations

---

2   ** Note: currently not available in English but potentially available in other languages, see www.dahlke.at

– literally translated it actually means "rule by the holy/sacred one", or "rule by a single one" – it can still help us to progress, because this is precisely what must be our prime concern - finding the one decisive point that the patient is stuck on or "ruled by".

Anyone who can no longer see the wood for the trees will find it difficult, if not impossible, to come to terms with the topic of disease. Ultimately, a person's connection to the environment, even at the societal level as reflected in family and community issues and in the social domain of their living and working environment, belong to this topic as well – even if these can only be touched on peripherally. Such references are comprehensively illustrated in the book *Woran krankt die Welt? (**What is making our world sick?)*. The broader and more varied the pattern becomes, the better the resultant indications derived from it are, and thus the more likely they are to lead towards recovery. Paracelsus believed that a doctor should be able to recognise from the environment what disease the patient was suffering from, and vice versa, should also be capable of drawing conclusions about the environment from the disease pattern. A therapist who understood nothing of these archetypal principles (here, Paracelsus used the word "astrology", which in his time clearly referred to the archetypal principles) was, in his eyes, flatly disqualified from being a doctor. We now live in a time in which the understanding of archetypes or archetypal principles is more the exception than the rule amongst doctors, although somewhat encouragingly, a noticeable increase in interest is being demonstrated in our training seminars.

In many cases, I have observed that doctors have also embraced this point of view of the involvement of patients in their diseases and the associated learning tasks, particularly because this in no way hinders, but instead supports their other therapy approaches. In essence, the interpretation of disease patterns is intended not to diminish the co-operation between doctor and patient, but on the contrary, to strengthen it. Patients who take responsibility for themselves make the doctor's work easier. The more the patients contribute their thoughts, feelings and commitment to the process, the more effective the therapy will be. To this extent, this reference work is meant more as a stimulus to enhance the relationship between the therapist and patient, although admittedly with the long-term aim of enabling patients to discover their own inner doctor. Assisting this development is as much the noblest task of every doctor as it is of this book. In this respect, full use should be made of the opportunities offered by disease pattern interpretation, especially the great possibilities that it offers in the area of prevention.

In an era which, in actual fact, can no longer afford its high-tech medicine, prevention has become somewhat of a magic word. This is all the more alarming, since hardly anybody, from the officials in the Ministry of Health to the doctors responsible for administering their policies, really knows what this actually involves. Caught in this dilemma, traditional medical practitioners resort to a deceptive labelling trick, which in the meantime has almost become socially acceptable. What in actual fact amount to mere early detection measures are somewhat cheekily referred to as "prevention". Although early detection is certainly better than late detection, it still has nothing to do with prevention. The German word for "prevention" is *Vorbeugung* (literally: 'bending first'). In keeping with the underlying metaphor of the German equivalent, prevention in this sense would involve getting to know the essence of a disease or disease pattern in order to discover what needs to be done to "bend first" - perhaps simply by kneeling or bowing down with respect and humility – and doing this voluntarily while there is still time, rather than waiting for Fate to finally "bend" us by forcing us to our knees.

Nevertheless, in its struggle against the disease, which takes the form of a flood of medications (antibiotics, antihypertonics, antihistamines, etc.), inhibitors (acid-, ACE-inhibitors, etc.) and (beta-) blockers, traditional medicine hardly gets to know the essence of the disease patterns in question and is therefore incapable of preventing them. In sometimes appalling campaigns, its representatives attempt to cover up this shocking failure. Even the campaigns of destruction against wombs – embarrassing for the whole medical profession – of recent decades have been marketed as preventive measures against cancer. Using the same deplorable form of "argument", gynaecologists could just as well have their ears amputated as part of an equally crazy method for preventing skin cancer. In fact, we have now arrived once again at the beginning of a similar medical grotesqueness. Following the discovery of the connection between breast cancer and a particular combination of genes, the fear of hereditary cancer has grown enormously. Lamentably, it is not only in the USA that women who are carriers of this gene have healthy breasts amputated out of fear. However shocking this may be, we should not overlook the helplessness on both sides that is expressed in this fact.

Women whose mothers and grandmothers suffered from breast cancer are naturally and justifiably afraid of contracting the disease themselves. They make intensive use of the possibilities of our so-called "cancer prevention", and sometimes request several mammograms every year. Since this all takes place within the framework of so-called prevention, they feel themselves medically safe. After 10 years, such a woman will have undergone dozens of mammograms, thereby significantly increasing her risk of breast cancer. In such a case, we clearly cannot talk of prevention; instead, we are dealing with a false understanding of early detection. What this example clearly shows, however, is just how dangerous deceptive labels can be in this area.

A further compelling argument against the simplistic model of causality that underlies this form of "prevention" is provided by a Danish study which revealed the following: when researchers traced the biological parents of 1,000 adopted children and investigated what connection might exist between the incidence of cancer prior to the age of 50 in at least one of the adoptive parents and the probability of cancer in their biological child, none was found. In contrast, when they examined the incidence of cancer in at least one of the adoptive parents prior to the age of 50 and the probability of cancer in the adopted child, there was a five-fold increase in the rate of cancer. This thus speaks clearly for the absence of genetic factors and the predominance of other causes.

In any case, the idea of reducing risks by timely amputation is in itself a lamentable notion of medicine, which lives from the fact that prevention does not work. If one takes such considerations to their ultimate conclusion, as increasingly threatens to be the case coming from the USA, everything ends with nothing more than a brain in a nutrient solution. This brain however will have a morbid fear of developing a brain tumour. The future of medicine clearly cannot lie in such a macabre outlook.

It is certainly possible to provide sensible prevention on the basis of interpretation of the disease pattern in combination with an understanding of the original archetypal principles behind it. As soon as the essence or pattern of the breast cancer is understood, the people who are affected can voluntarily "bend first" in the direction of the forthcoming tasks, accept the challenge and break out of the dangerous family pattern underlying the disease – a pattern which, as the Danish study of adopted children strongly suggests, is more likely to be behavioural than genetic. Of course, this is not intended to create the impression that this will be easy – although it is nevertheless possible. Provided that this interpretation process is successful, the idea of prevention can be applied to any instance of illness, and medicine could finally fulfil one of its noblest tasks.

Prevention is a consideration which forms a continuous thread throughout my work, and thus also throughout this book. In keeping with this, the book also includes a number of individual interpretations which are obviously pointless in an acute situation, perhaps because the patient is not even conscious. These are then aimed at the preventive aspect, which becomes important as soon as the patient has recovered from the immediate threat. After getting over an acute illness – irrespective of by what means – the following question should actually automatically force its way to the surface: "What have I learned from this, and how can I find other, and above all, better planes of experience for my learning in future?" In addition, using the benefit of hindsight, the standard questions in interpreting disease patterns are also useful: "Why me in particular? Why this and in this way? Why right now at this time of my life? What is the disease pattern compelling me to do, and what is it preventing me from doing?"

There is a further lesson to be learned from the example of the fear of breast cancer that has been promoted by genetic discoveries. It is a characteristic feature of traditionally-accepted medicine that, as soon as some physical causative component has been found, the disease pattern is immediately stripped of all spiritual components. This may be due to the fact that traditional medical practitioners are very reluctant to surrender anything to the "competition from psychosomatics" and are delighted if it can be brought back into their area of influence. This narrow and limited departmentalised thinking is, however, very obstructive for the whole field of medicine. We will in the future find more and more genetic relationships in disease patterns, simply because the field of genetics is making such progress, and the human genotype has now been almost completely decoded. Similar progress will be made in immunology. This should not, however, become a reason to take a one-sided view, as has already happened in the case of stomach ulcers, which in recent times have come to be attributed entirely to the bacterium Helicobacter. The simple fact alone that half of the population carry Helicobacter in their stomachs, without developing stomach ulcers, and fortunately not all patients with the relevant gene develop breast cancer, should suffice to show us the way in this case, before we again throw out the baby with the bathwater. The discovery of the breast cancer gene is a scientific advance, which should be welcomed as such. If, however, it comes to be understood as an argument against psycho-oncology (the teaching of the psychological components involved in the development of cancer), then far too much is being interpreted into it, and above all, the wrong things. Some time ago, American researchers also successfully isolated particular compounds which circulate in our bloodstream when we are in love. Now that we finally have a reason to consider it a purely physical phenomenon, we would certainly not now claim to have for centuries falsely believed love to be a mental or spiritual state. Despite this interesting discovery, being in love remains a spiritual phenomenon, which simultaneously finds a physical correlation in the body. This is indeed the very meaning of psychosomatics: synchronicity between the psyche and the body.

Just as it is advisable to familiarise oneself at the very beginning with the limitations of the selected method, it also seems appropriate to get to know the philosophy of life that underlies it in order to be able to openly acknowledge and deal with its opportunities and risks. In our case, this basis is formed by the world view of archetypal medicine based on spiritual philosophy, although due to space considerations it is not possible to convey this here in detail. For this − at least as far as the interpretation of disease patterns is concerned − the reading of *Krankheit als Sprache der Seele (**Disease as a Language of the Soul)* is recommended. A self-evident component of the spiritual world view is the teaching of reincarnation. Although this is not necessary for the interpretation of disease patterns and in itself has no inner connection with the symbolism of diseases, it nevertheless represents an important aid and source of alleviation in the case of difficult interpretations which go beyond the standard sensory framework of a normal lifetime. In this respect, a few special remarks are warranted: Congenital deformities, for example, which will be interpreted here just as consistently as symptoms occurring in later life, are seen as life tasks we bring with us, which within the framework of the teaching of reincarnation are much easier to acknowledge and accept. From this understanding of the world also follows further consistency with regard to interpretations concerning children or even newborn infants, which do not differ in principle from those of adults. People have tasks, and already bring the bulk of these with them at birth. For our modern understanding, the sophisticated findings of genetics make this clear, even without the teachings of reincarnation or karma; however, with the aid of these teachings, there is much that can be better and more deeply understood. Interpretations of disease patterns which are typically fatal lose much of their harshness and apparent senselessness if one keeps the greater chain of different lives in mind. In fact, we know today from thanatology – without wanting to push the idea of reincarnation too strongly – that people still learn much when dying, as for example, when their life flashes like a film before their inner eye. Reincarnation therapy based on the spiritual world view also generates many interpretations and realisations which more scientifically-orientated users might find more difficult to grasp, such as the certainty that suicide does not help, because it does not really end the life in question, but merely leads to the re-taking of the particular class that was rejected in the general school of life, and often also under more difficult conditions.

The interpretations in this book originate from the direct translation of the language used by the body and its symptoms into the level of symbolic language used by our spiritual reality. Whereas previous books gave preference to major and very common disease patterns, for which there is naturally more existing experience with patients, in this manual, for the sake of completeness, we also examine many so-called minor or rarer disease patterns, even though less therapeutic experience on these was available.

For those affected, their disease pattern is naturally always the most important, and the distinction between major and minor, common and rare, and therefore supposedly less important, leaves a bitter "medicynical" aftertaste. We have therefore dispensed with such distinctions in this book; it should, however, be mentioned that some of the rarer disease patterns have, for this reason, been interpreted more according to the tried-and-tested rules, with sometimes little or no corresponding psycho-therapeutic experience to support these interpretations. Nevertheless, in line with the sense of assurance and confidence in the coherence of the body's means of expression that has developed out of 30 years of work with this approach, this methodology seemed justifiable. In any case, it is the task of the user to remain alert and to be clear in general about the fact that there can be no two identical stomach ulcers, but always only individual patients, who have to come to terms with similar disease patterns. Keeping these individual components in mind is extremely important in order to avoid measuring all patients who have the same diagnosis by means of the same yardstick. On the other hand, disease patterns often act as excellent "model" examples. The description of these is the primary aim of this reference work, which in some respects can be compared with a repertorium for homeopathy. If in doubt, it is advisable to consult a doctor or therapist who is familiar with this approach in order to work together to identify the individual components within the overall binding pattern.

The differences in the range of experience with various disease patterns explain the differences in the level of detail in coverage. The length of the discourse on a symptom in the book therefore has less to do with any assessment with regard to its importance, and far more to do with the experience that is available with regard to it, although the prevalence of a disease pattern naturally reflects, on the one hand, its importance for the society concerned, and on the other hand, results in greater experience on the therapeutic side. In this respect, malaria, which overall claims by far the greatest number of human lives, comes off relatively badly in comparison to anorexia in puberty, which is much more widespread in our society, and therefore underpinned by a great deal of therapeutic experience. Epidemics and widespread disease patterns reflect the conditions in their distribution area. We can therefore interpret such diseases as cardiac infarction, cancer and depression, and also tooth decay and colds as typical of our situation, time and society. This manual should thus be understood on the basis of the author's present situation living in a highly-industrialised meritocracy in central Europe of the third millennium, and makes no claim to provide any objective measure of the importance of a symptom by means of the length of its coverage, quite apart from the fact that every symptom is, in any event, the most important (subjectively) for the person who has it. In the same way that this new edition has been greatly expanded, there are also plans in future to revise the manual at extended intervals in order to take further insights into account, for example, with regard to rare disease patterns or newer developments, such as depression or hyperactivity.

As far as interpretation work is concerned, it is also worth keeping in mind that when dealing with living subjects, there can be no one hundred percent correct conclusions, and therefore also no interpretations which apply to everybody and in every case. Interpretations can generally only be accurate if the corresponding symptoms are also present. A diagnosis by itself often means very little and may in fact have no relevance to a disease and thus also be of no value for an interpretation. Low blood pressure which produces no symptoms, for example, does not need to be interpreted.

Since every individual has a share in the collective world of imagery, while simultaneously possessing their own unique inner world of imagery, only a truly individual interpretation will be fitting, and pre-defined interpretations can only be general indications, albeit valuable ones, which provide the overall frame and often also the colours and essential structures of the image. Mood and atmosphere – decisive for the effect of the image – are and remain something highly individual, which can only be discovered through one's own personal struggle with the individual disease pattern.

Such limitations may result in precisely the unpleasant truths in the interpretations not being accepted as such, which would be a pity. In actual fact, the hardest interpretations are frequently the most important, because there is always shadow concealed in the manifestation of a disease. The form of expression used in colloquial language with regard to disease patterns is often very unflattering and honest. Fate also frequently chooses hard paths with its intervention and proverbial blows. After almost 30 years of reincarnation therapy, I know from experience that Fate is not inimical, but is simply dedicated with all its available means to our development. I therefore ask all users to believe me when I say that any interpretations provided that might be perceived as hurtful are intended only in the sense of promoting awareness and self-development.

In general, interpretations are always without value judgements to the extent that one can never know exactly on what level somebody experiences something. Where colloquial language might associate the expression "as crooked as a dog's hind leg" with a hunchbacked person, this is without doubt (de)valuing. In this book, such an association is mentioned because it points out the subject in a hard but clear way: moral uprightness or lack thereof, and above and beyond this, humiliation, but also (in the resolved sense) humility. The hunched back "embodies" these topics, and colloquial language expresses them disrespectfully. From the purely physical manifestation, however, it is never apparent from which of these two poles the patient experiences the topic involved. A hunchbacked person will frequently suffer humiliation at the hands of those around him or her and may feel humiliated by Fate. Nonetheless, it is, of course, possible that the task concealed in this, namely of getting down (off one's high horse) and bowing down with humility (to Mother Earth) has already been mastered, and the humiliation transformed into genuine humility. We cannot see this externally from the body, but we can notice it from the person, provided that we first get to know him or her well.

From all of this, it should become clear that it never makes any sense to misuse interpretations of disease patterns for the purpose of making value judgments. Interpreting patterns enables progress in the development towards greater awareness, judging them – whether in others or oneself – will only cause harm. The misuse of interpretations for value judgements, or even worse, condemnation instead says more about the character of the person making the judgement and shows that he or she has not (yet) understood the essence of the approach advocated here. Disease reveals our shadow, and that shadow is then rejected: there are very few who are willing to face up to it. Those who give others an ear-bashing with unwanted interpretations do not genuinely want to help but instead want to put others down, and they will generally, and justifiably, meet with strong resistance. The interpretation of disease patterns can be a wonderful aid in helping people along their path – but only if they request such aid, and only with the necessary respect and in acknowledgement of the fact that one can never be quite certain when making such interpretations from the outside.

The great desire to apportion guilt is so closely linked with the history of Christian culture that one cannot caution against this strongly enough. Blame is a topic in religion, and the Christian churches already handle this so clumsily that it should definitely not be introduced into medicine as well. The problem is not the Bible itself, but the policies that the "ground crew" have developed from it. Christ himself does not engage in the sort of sin-mongering which his professional representatives on Earth have developed to such perfection. It seems highly unlikely he would have wanted the Our Father – the only prayer which he passed down to us – to be understood as a punishment following confession. Five Our Fathers for masturbating 10 times is a common Christian misunderstanding, which has nothing at all to do with Christ. In fact, the Gospels tend more toward advocating the complete opposite: Christ devoted his efforts above all to the tax collectors and prostitutes, the scum of the Jewish society of the time, and he was extremely critical in his dealings with the scribes. In the parable of the adulteress, he prevents her from being stoned to death by making clear to the Jews that they are all guilty of adultery; he prevents, in effect, the projection of this "guilt" onto the adulteress. The same applies to his interpretation of the Commandments in the Sermon on the Mount. If just one envious thought is enough to have broken the Seventh Commandment, who here would not soon have sinned. According to his interpretation of Mosaic Law, we are all guilty of everything, and it is this "collective guilt" that is also meant by the concept of original sin. Banished from the unity of Paradise, we, as the descendants of the first man and woman, are all sinners, which in its original sense simply meant "isolated". Our isolation from this unity, however, does not require punishment, but instead dedication to the lifelong task of regaining the unity of Paradise. On this point, the various traditions, if we return to their original sources, are all in agreement. All the guilt projections come later when the religions become politicised and acquire worldly power in the course of their "development" or perhaps "entanglement" is a better word. Quite apart from whether the concept of guilt really belongs in religion, we should definitely keep it out of medicine at all costs; otherwise it simply leads to terrible stigmatisations.

Using this apportionment of guilt, unjustifiably derived from the Gospels, the churches had found a means of bringing people under their control, and by associated means – ranging from the sale of indulgences to the creation of feelings of sexual guilt – of making them compliant. Over the centuries, guilt has developed into a powerful field of consciousness, which to this day even people who have moved away from the church obviously find difficult to elude. In the meantime, this desire to apportion guilt has more or less become a trademark of Western civilization and has a particularly disturbing effect in the therapeutic field. Feelings of guilt demonstrably make people ill, and their conveyance by the world of medicine is a dangerous form of malpractice; in contrast, bringing such feelings to our awareness and pointing out ways to handle them is an important therapeutic task.

In relation to the interpretation of the disease pattern, this issue of guilt brings us to the most serious misunderstanding in this respect. If a person already has a difficult task in the form of a disease pattern, and then also starts to feel guilty about it, the situation naturally becomes even more difficult. The American author Joan Borysenko aptly refers to this as "New-Age guilt", which is just as inimical to development and life as the "Old-Age guilt" that religions dumped upon their followers in order to make them more compliant.

This deeply-rooted need in us for guilt affects wide areas of our social and interpersonal life. As far as medicine is concerned, it turns the potential opportunities of the disease pattern interpretation into their complete opposite. All of this has now advanced to the point where hardly anyone in our society wants to apologise or admit "mea culpa" for anything, because this would allow them to be "ex-culpated" (Latin: 'free of guilt/ blame') or "exonerated" (Latin: 'unburdened'). Instead, each individual attempts to place the guilt on other people, which makes the lives of those people difficult, and causes the individual even greater feelings of "guilt". Such rewarding guilt transactions flourish everywhere from politics to our partnerships. On the path to development, we need to dissociate ourselves from all of this, and could start straightaway with the interpretation of disease patterns.

If we believe the Bible, we are all tainted by original sin, as evidenced by our transgression of the unity of Paradise, and by the fact of our mortal existence here on Earth; we are responsible, so to speak, for the realisation of this unity on a more conscious level. Above and beyond this, we have no guilt, but "only" the responsibility to develop ourselves towards unity. Since this is actually where we come from, our task in fact lies in returning, which is most clearly demonstrated to us in the mandala as the universal pattern of life (see relevant section in *Lebenskrisen als Entwicklungschancen (**Life Crises as an Opportunity for Development)*). The doctor, psychotherapist and philosopher Georg Groddeck is merely expressing this same connection in a different way when he sees in every illness a longing for the mother and an attempted return to childhood. As was the case back then, the ill person receives love and care without having to do anything in return. Even our modern healthcare provision joins in the process here. The continued payment of salary in the event of illness is an attempt to return to the original land of milk and honey, where everything was provided without having to give anything in return. Of course, this also harbours certain dangers, namely the potential for misusing illness as an attempt to run away from responsibility. Taking refuge in illness as an unconscious and failed attempt to achieve unity is one of the most effective means of repression in our society, and one of the last socially-acceptable alibis. It requires great courage to dispense with it.

Returning to the mandala, we can see that it presents us with a wonderful timetable and roadmap for our life, with all archetypal transition points, and the starting and endpoint in the centre. Coming from the centre, we reach the outer edge of the circle in the turnaround period midway through our lives; at this point, we change direction and return home to find our (re)solution in the unity of the centre. The basic requirement for reaching a "holy" or "healed" state - both words which are related to the concept of "wholeness" - which can only be found in the centre of the mandala, is the realisation that we are not, and can never be, completely safe and secure on our way through the polar world. It is impossible to keep all evil away from us. Despite healthy eating, sufficient exercise and positive thoughts that promote development, we cannot force Fate in any way, even though all three of these factors obviously make a decisive contribution towards our well-being. Fate is greater, broader, and above all, extends over greater time spans than even our most sophisticated attempts to bypass or even deceive it are able to. There is no cosmic life insurance available – not even through exemplary conduct.

Reconciling ourselves with death as the (re)solution of our life is therefore the best basis for healing. Even the saints and sages died, sometimes at an early age. We need to learn to overcome our Western system of values, which reaches its peak in the notion that life is good, and death is bad. There is little to support the idea that a life is all the better the longer it lasts. If we regard life – as proposed by spiritual philosophy – as a school, the weightings immediately change. Remaining in school as long as possible is not a particularly outstanding achievement. We should ideally stay as long as necessary and as long as there is something still to be learnt, quite apart from the joy of life and pleasure that life can bring us. The attempt to compel Fate to grant a long life by living a life "pleasing to God" harks back to the old puritanical misconception that God particularly loves the ambitious, diligent, healthy and successful, and therefore rewards them with a long life. Most saints, for example, do not fall into this category, and certainly not Christ himself.

Disease patterns represent learning tasks to be completed, and not punishments. The French philosopher Blaise Pascal formulated it very simply and clearly in the sentence: "Disease is the place where one learns." If life is a type of school, then disease patterns are part of the curriculum. The report card for one class may indicate future learning tasks by giving bad grades, and while this is certainly a consequence of the previous school year, it is not a punishment for it. Disease patterns also clarify tasks that have yet to be resolved. They do not intend to punish or condemn us. We must, however, interpret the marks of the report card in the correct way, and also accept responsibility for them in order to be able to reach the necessary conclusions for the future. The question of whether all disease patterns represent learning tasks can also be easily determined by this analogy: Those who are still in school clearly still have tasks to deal with, and all those who live on Earth likewise.

In the same way that, in school, we do not speak of guilt when one is faced by a significant test such as the school-leaving examination, we should also refrain from doing so in the case of the tests that disease patterns present us with. The same applies accordingly for other problems and crises in life. After the oceanic experiences of vastness and weightlessness in the womb, the child will nevertheless have to leave this infant paradise as birth inevitably approaches, and nobody is to blame for this. When a playful and carefree childhood reaches its natural end in puberty, we also do not speak of guilt, and this is also the case when, after its first half, life leads us to the catastrophe (Greek: *he katastrophe* = 'turning point') of change. Even if many today interpret this turning point in life only as a catastrophe in the negative sense, there should at least still be no talk of guilt. Such (life) crises are just as able to be interpreted as disease patterns are and are also frequently associated with symptoms. Since these are comprehensively described in another of my books that deals with the developmental opportunities inherent in crises – *Lebenskrisen als Entwicklungschancen (**Life Crises as an Opportunity for Development)* – they are only referred to in this manual with regard to their symptomatology visible in the body.

Recognising the tasks which life presents us with in the form of disease patterns, crises and other tests and accepting them as such is difficult enough in itself. Telling somebody else what their learning tasks consist of is also difficult, and if one has not been asked to do so, presumptuous to boot. Therapists claim this right for themselves, but this in turn can only be justified if they are able to refrain totally from making value judgements. As has already been emphasised several times, the concept of guilt has no place in the therapeutic context. Interestingly, the German word for "guilt" (*Schuld*) also carries the meaning of "debt".

Anyone who finds they cannot dissociate themselves from the concept of guilt could at least restrict themselves to this alternative sense of the German equivalent and instead ask the question: "What debt do I owe to the future?"

As a sincere and straightforward teacher, the body can provide the answer to this question. If we allow it to communicate with us and teach us, we have the most honest therapist, who accompanies our every step through life, and keeps an accurate account of all shortfalls and slip-ups. What we are missing (both in the sense of lacking or not reaching an aim) is something we can read from the body, and provided that we learn to ask the body when necessary, it will tell us how we can help both it and ourselves to "heal" in the sense of returning to "wholeness". The question "What am I missing?" is also worthwhile in the school of life and can also be understood as the question of "Where I have missed the sense of my life, and thus the central point of the life mandala". "Missing the point" is one possible translation of the Greek word for "to sin": *hamartanein*. In this context, everything which removes us further from the centre is a sin. Every step in the direction of the centre, however, would be the opposite: the redemption of sin, and this is, in fact, the path that Christ shows us. In this extended sense, there are then no more mistakes or bad moves in the absolute, objective sense so to speak, but only relative ones, as measured against the personal life sense and objective.

By no means does everything in this book have to apply in every case, but experience has shown that most things about the body are in harmony with the corresponding spiritual and psychological topics. In order to discover this parallelism, it is necessary to immerse oneself deeply enough in the subject matter. A book can only offer guidance and suggestions. Every individual is required to find out for themselves what the priority is in their own individual "case", although anyone who simply picks out what bests suits their particular viewpoint will throw away the best opportunities of interpretation, because shadow reveals itself above all in those aspects about ourselves which do not suit us at all.

In the last 30 years, during which 5 million of my books have found readers, and above all users in the German-speaking world alone, we have received a great many letters and mails, the majority of which follow a striking pattern. In the introductory sentence, the writers express their praise, because they have recognised everyone in their family in the symptom descriptions given in the book, particularly also difficult family members such as the mother-in-law or partner. However, they then complain that, in their own particular case, the interpretations given are not accurate. They know this perfectly well since they have had this disease pattern for so and so many years. Overall, these letters express broad agreement to the great majority of the interpretations and sharp criticism of certain individual ones. The broad agreement refers to the disease patterns of others and the individual criticism almost without exception to their own case. It can therefore certainly do no harm to recall the biblical wisdom which says - "First take the beam out of your own eye, and then you will see clearly how to remove the splinter from your brother's eye" - for it is, above all, those splinters and beams which we remove from ourselves which are critical for our own development.

This step in the direction of acknowledging our own failings can become all the easier to take when viewed in light of the fact that it is precisely these failings which offer the greatest opportunities for growth. Only when we are ill are we asked what is wrong – a question which implies a deficiency and prompts us to consider what we have been overlooking. Only then can we track down the missing elements, and if we find them, integrate them into our life. For this very reason, disease becomes an opportunity. With the aid of this manual, the user can set out in search of what he or she is missing in order to return to a state of wholeness. And every failing which leads to the integration of a missing piece of the spirit or soul is a step on the way to returning to a (w)hol(i)er or healed state.

The disease pattern embodies an archetypal principle or a pattern of archetypal principles in unresolved form which has sunk down into the unconscious. This topic from the shadows allows us to recognise the archetypal principles involved and also to find possibilities for deriving positive development steps from these. The subcategory "Resolution" in the main section is directed at the possibility of finding another, more redeeming level, on which the same archetypal energy can be lived out without disturbing physical functioning – and hopefully even with the opportunity of coming closer to one's own main life theme. The subcategory "Handling" provides advice on how one can best approach the underlying topic(s) concealed in the disease pattern. Concrete therapy suggestions have only been included where they contribute something to the interpretation.

The advice on handling and resolution generally follows the homeopathic approach, and only as an exception makes reference to the opposite allopathic pole. Both directions set the tone in medicine and superfluously polarise therapists and patients, who in this respect both have their tasks, and like all opposing poles, are in actual fact dependent on each other rather than mutually exclusive. Allopathy is capable of saving life, and therefore of fulfilling one of the noblest tasks of medicine, but unfortunately it cannot heal in the sense of returning to an original whole state. Homeopathy, in contrast, can heal, and even in the case of chronic disease patterns, can still at least offer opportunities for improvement. In acute cases, on the other hand, it is often not capable of saving life.

This became clear to me personally by way of a striking example at the beginning of my work as a doctor. At a meeting of naturopathically-minded therapists, one participant suffered an allergic shock as a result of an insect bite. Although homeopathic and naturopathic remedies such as Apis and Rescue Remedy (Bach flower essences) were soon dripping out of his ears, the circulatory collapse persisted, and the patient was well on his way to the next world. Through the drastic use of allopathic medications, it then proved possible to stabilise his circulation surprisingly quickly, and after only an hour, the man was again taking part in the seminar. Nevertheless, he was not healed of his allergy. Nor is this possible with the aid of noradrenalin and cortisone. Using the homeopathic approach, both in the interpretation and the administration of the corresponding remedies, it is, in contrast, possible to get to the roots of the allergy, and even to eventually be done with it once and for all. Both approaches are therefore absolutely essential: without the allopathic treatment, the patient would no longer be alive, but without the homeopathic treatment, no "healing" would be possible, because the mere suppression of the symptoms by means of allopathic medications is not worthy of this designation. Freedom from symptoms and healing have in essence nothing to do with each other; in fact, it is quite the contrary, since suppression actually reduces the chances of healing.

For the method of disease pattern interpretation, it is fortunately not necessary to choose between the two major directions of medicine, particularly since they are in fact pulling on the same rope, albeit as a tug-of-war in opposite directions. When patients are afraid, they long for the allopathic opposing pole of vastness and openness, which they are missing in the constricting state of their fear. If they are in danger of harming themselves in the course of a panic attack, it may make sense to provide the corresponding openness by means of allopathic medication. This will not, however, solve the fear problem in the long term. This is once again only possible by being willing to enter the constricting state of fear, pass through it, and find vastness and openness beyond it. Only by passing through this constricting state can one reach a lasting expansive state. It may therefore be necessary in the acute situation to resort to allopathic means to preserve life, but for healing we must rely on homeopathic means. As in the example of fear, the opposing pole often comes naturally almost of its own accord if one delves deeply enough (homeopathically) into the principle which is causing the suffering. From this, it also follows naturally that, in spite of the possibilities of disease pattern interpretation, in threatening and acute situations, we remain dependent on traditional medical aid.

The interplay between interpretative and invasive medicine also has obvious advantages in the area of remedial medicine. It is, for example, advisable to figure out the deeper sense of an intestinal fistula, although this may not cause it to disappear. If it is later closed surgically, there is, however, a much better chance that it will not re-form. Interpreting disease patterns does not mean neglecting all additional options, quite the contrary: if the sense and learning task have been understood, surgical correction will in any case have a better chance of proceeding without complications and relapses.

Furthermore, the difference should also be considered between the application of medication-based allopathy in order to suppress symptoms versus its application in the spiritual area in order to get closer to the centre by way of the opposing pole. In a homeopathic sense, depressive patients will have to be willing to face their anxiety topics – darkness, death and aggression – but experiences with light which reveal the other side of the coin will also help them further. It is therefore understandable that both shadow therapy, as well as exposure to light and the sun, and in particular encounters with one's own inner light can work together in a meaningful way on the path back to the centre, which indeed is the aim of all therapy.

Being ill ultimately means that one has fallen out of the centre (of the life mandala), and thus represents an imbalance, or respectively the attempt to compensate for an imbalance on the physical plane. Healing must strive towards the centre, and this lies by definition between the poles, which is why therapy must always work along this axis in an effort to restore the centre. The fastest (acute) way there often leads via the opposing pole (allopathically). The homeopathic approach on the other hand will, with its first step, actually increase this one-sidedness, which sometimes exacerbates the problems in the form of an initial worsening of the condition. Its longer-term aim, however, is to stimulate the self-healing powers of the organism so that movement in the direction of the centre gets going using the patient's own resources. In all cases, both sides work along the same axis on the same topic.

We can therefore already regard disease in itself (as expressed in the symptom) as a correction of the imbalance on the physical level, which is necessary in order not to tip the scales too much to one side. And to continue this analogy, the aim in the process of recovery is to ensure this balance not by involuntary and painful steps, but by voluntary and consciously-chosen advances. On the scales of life, the body and the soul have equal weight, whether we (and traditional medicine) like it or not. If we do not overcome something on the spiritual level, the body steps in and does the job in its own physical way. Seemingly, it is only in this manner that the beam of the scales can be held horizontal. If we now also begin to deal with the spiritual topic, the body can ease up in its symptomatic efforts again, the scales remain in balance, and we speak of recovery. The soul returns to its responsibility and consciously experiences the topic which the body previously had to unconsciously manifest in the form of the disease pattern. It is therefore incomparably better to open and expand one's heart to love (and loving one's neighbour) than to leave this to the physical level, which then achieves this – within the framework of cardiac insufficiency – in the form of cardiac dilation. Nevertheless, even patients already suffering from heart insufficiency can still relieve the strain on the physical pump organ by lovingly opening their heart. In contrast, with regard to the biblical advice that we should "become as children again", we should definitely keep the figurative level in our sights from the very beginning because if this takes place in the body in the form of Alzheimer's disease, only very little help is possible. The focus in this case must be placed on genuine prevention.

The standard doctor's question "What's wrong with you?" implies deficiency and is directed first and foremost at the allopathic approach; not surprisingly, it is from this that the superficially more obvious main path of medicine has developed. The homeopathic direction is interested in the question: "How do I best achieve a balance in the long term?" It proceeds indirectly, but in return leads to genuinely stable balances because it relies on the self-healing powers of the body instead of assisting it with foreign troops (such as antibiotics). The latter makes the organism permanently dependent on outside aid, while the former allows it to become increasingly autonomous and self-reliant.

The symptomatology brought out by the medical question "What's wrong with you?" reveals both what we do and don't have, and thus the archetypal principle in question. Allergy-sufferers suffer from the conflicts being waged by their immune system against supposedly hostile allergens. The principle of the conflict is symbolised in the archetypal principle of Mars, and so it is the Mars theme which is lacking here. What they long for is peace, which is represented by Venus. If, however, Mars expresses itself in the disease pattern, and is consequently lacking in their consciousness, Mars must also be learnt as a priority. i.e. such patients must learn to deploy their energies openly and offensively, to *tackle* life in order to *get to grips* with it and to *grasp the nettle*. When they have done this, the opposing pole – Venus – will fall into their hands just like a ripe fruit.

Only when the essence of allopathy and homeopathy have been understood can both directions be properly attuned and complement each other. A pragmatic path, which has proven itself effective within the tense field of conflict between traditional medical science and complementary methods, is to mentally separate diagnosis and therapy. The former should be made, or at least confirmed, on the basis of traditional medicine. Whatever can be established by laboratory examinations of the blood should always be confirmed in this way and not, for example, divined using a pendulum. This does not argue on principle against the use of a divining pendulum by a naturopath or dowser; however, in general, this method involves an enormous uncertainty factor and depends largely on the relevant naturopath or dowser and his/her skills, which is not the case to any comparable extent in laboratory examinations and most other traditional medical diagnosis methods. In spite of the dangers of the effects and side effects of allopathic medicine, it should not be overlooked that its diagnosis procedures are often harmless and very illuminating. For the interpretations given in this manual, I have therefore also drawn on the results of traditional medical science as often as possible. In diagnosis, the tried-and-tested rule is to proceed as far as (safely) possible using traditional medical methods, and in treatment, to use these as little as reasonably possible. Even gruesome-looking examination methods such as computer and nuclear spin tomography are largely physically harmless, at least compared to the routine x-ray examinations which we were subjected to as children without a second thought. Obviously, the same does not apply to examination by means of injection of radioactive materials or the removal of tissue samples.

Even though I advise using traditional, i.e. in practice allopathic medications, as little as humanly possible, acutely life-threatening disease patterns must be treated immediately in an allopathic sense, typically with medications which avert the danger by means of suppression. In such a situation, even affirmations, which almost without exception cover over spiritual problems, would also be reasonable. Both methods can preserve life through suppression, but cannot heal. Nor should they be allowed to make this claim, because they then hinder development. Those who use affirmations should in any event know that, in this case, they are not on the spiritual path, but on the contrary, are attempting in their hour of need to ignore problems and the resulting tasks. The success of such measures always has a time limit even if the timeframe may sometimes be long. It is precisely then that it becomes particularly dangerous since the connection to the original problem disappears *over time*. Once the acute danger has been averted, it would be a good time to once again turn one's thoughts to healing and therefore to the homeopathic path. This route can be taken both via known medications as well as the corresponding interpretations and the resolution of the resulting life tasks. The best solution is to pursue both types of homeopathic therapy in parallel, which by their very nature, complement each other wonderfully.

The treatment of acutely life-threatening situations by homeopathic means can have fatal consequences, because these often do not take effect quickly enough. This would require nothing less than complete mastery of the art of homeopathy. Equally inappropriate and frequently dangerous, however, is allopathic treatment (traditional medicine or affirmations from the field of "positive thinking") of non-acute, chronic disease patterns in the hope of thereby achieving healing. However well-meant this procedure might be, it can only conceal and suppress symptoms, and therefore drive them further into the shadows. Therapies which promise healing, however, must in contrast reveal, process and ultimately resolve the problem.

The interpretation of disease patterns can often render other treatment methods superfluous; it can, however, just as easily be combined in whatever way is desired with both directions of medicine, allopathy and homeopathy, and does not in principle exclude any particular form of treatment. Naturally, it is advisable to apply allopathically-suppressive methods as sparingly as possible, and instead to reserve these for genuine emergencies. Should one want to make use of additional physical treatment methods, it is advisable, in addition to the exercises and meditations resulting from the interpretations, to first and foremost make use of natural healing procedures, although it is worth keeping in mind that these have largely gone hopelessly astray in the tangled thicket between homeopathy and allopathy. Even though comparatively harmless agents are generally used in naturopathy, this is still done all too often with the intention of suppression. Many naturopaths even use homeopathic agents on an allopathic basis (such as many so-called complex remedies). Even more incomprehensible is the combative antagonism between traditional medicine and the so-called "alternative" directions. It would in any case be better to use the term "complementary methods", since this emphasises their supplementary nature rather than an intention to fully replace something. We do not need any alternative medicine, but rather a synthesis in medicine, which on the basis of a common philosophy of disease and health, manages to combine the different methods to whatever extent this is advisable in the relevant situation.

In any event, the artificially-created trenches between traditionally-accepted medicine and naturopathy do not really withstand rational examination. Many medications used in traditional medicine originate from nature, such as the digitalis preparations for the heart, which come from the foxglove plant, or penicillin, which is produced by the mould Aspergillus penicillium; even the much-criticised cortisone, as one of the body's own stress hormones, should actually be attributed to naturopathy. If administered over an extended period, it does, however, have major side-effects. Not everything which originates from naturopathy is inherently harmless. Much of traditional medicine, on the other hand, is based on experience and is not backed up by scientific knowledge of the exact mechanisms causing the effect. Classical homeopathy, in turn, is frequently considered part of naturopathy, although its potentised remedies are never to be found in nature. The elimination of these senseless opposing fronts would benefit the whole of medicine and clear the way for a synthesis. The interpretation of disease patterns in the sense of the psychosomatics described here could in this case assume a bridging function, because it harmonises with both basic directions of medicine, and can very well point out their mutual reliance on each other.

In addition, it opens up the opportunity to bring body and soul back together again. This happens in a more basic sense than is the case with the psychosomatics derived from psychoanalysis. In my understanding, which underlies what is presented here, everything which takes shape in the body also has, without exception, a spiritual side. Where there is form, there must also be content, or as Plato already formulated this concept thousands of years ago: "Behind everything in nature, there must be an idea." As soon as the content leaves the form, this disintegrates, as can easily be observed from a corpse. If consciousness is withdrawn from a region or an organ, the abandoned structure becomes diseased, even if this withdrawal of awareness is not intentional and does not even take place consciously. This part of the body is, of course, not immediately dead; in fact, precisely the topic which consciously has not been addressed continues to live on here in an unconsciously vital but troubled form. Fortunately, the times are now past when traditional medical practitioners could take great pleasure in pointing out, to the sound of enthusiastic applause from their public, that in thousands of operations, they had never ever come across a single soul. Incidentally, this argument was in any case an expression of arrogance and sheer stupidity. We would see through this immediately in the analogy of a TV technician if he were to claim that, despite opening thousands of TV sets, he had never yet found a programme, and therefore drew the conclusion that no programmes existed. Luckily, TV technicians have never sunk to such a terrifyingly low mental level.

The emergence of psychosomatic medicine as part of traditionally-accepted medicine may, on the one hand, appear to be an encouraging development, but on the other hand, is also a questionable symptom in itself. The shadow side that is hidden in this after all is the implication that some disease patterns are not psychosomatic. Even though the number of disease patterns which have been recognised or acknowledged by traditional medicine as psychosomatic has grown over recent years, there still remain some which supposedly have nothing to do with the soul. At the same time, any holistic dentist knows that each tooth is intrinsically linked to different aspects of the soul, and that apart from in the mental constructions of scientists, it is impossible anywhere in life to make such a separation between the body and the soul.

The fact that everything is psychosomatic does not, on the other hand, imply that everything is purely psychological. The body naturally also has its part to play. In this respect, however, the traditionally-accepted medical perception is peculiarly absolutist. Once it has acknowledged or recognised the psychosomatic character of a disease pattern, it leaves this "bones and all" to the specialists for the soul. Even when the latter emphasise the connection between body and soul, as is clear in the term "psychosomatics" itself, traditional medicine and the medical science that is taught at universities immediately insist in practice on their separation again. Their "psychosomatic practitioners" are, as analysts, entirely specialised on the soul. If, as a psychosomatic practitioner, one makes the, in actual fact, self-evident claim of taking care of both, this is still frequently met with rejection – which shows how far the *universi*ties have drifted away from their original claim of finding *uni*ty in everything.

Whether the spiritual or physical side predominates in the development history of a disease pattern has to be clarified in the individual situation, whereby both aspects will always be identifiable, provided that the framework of understanding is laid out broadly enough. The fact that one cannot see something says little about its existence. Those who claim that things that they cannot find do not exist are on the level of children who shut their eyes in order not to be seen. This attitude unfortunately characterises almost all of our psychiatry, which, for example, denies the (admittedly very difficult to understand) spiritual content of all so-called endogenous psychoses. If only psychiatrists would make the effort to lay out the observation framework as broadly as described by the American psychiatrist Edward Podvoll in his book *Recovering Sanity*, they too could probably find sense and meaning in their main field of activity.

Frequently, a primarily spiritual problem may become embodied, but there are also situations in which the physical aspect carries far more weight. The workers in the Chernobyl reactor who were exposed to radiation and later developed cancer did not need any particularly pronounced spiritual cancer pattern due to this radiation dose. Yet even here, there is still a spiritual component, although it plays a relatively subordinate role in comparison to the radiation exposure. Ultimately, there can be any mixture of spiritual and physical components. It therefore makes obvious sense to always include both sides in the treatment from the very beginning.

Understanding disease as a symbol opens up the opportunity to track down the relevant life tasks. In this respect, the physical aspect of disease is of crucial importance because it is only by this means that we can arrive at the meaning of symptoms. In ancient times, the "symbolon" was an earthenware ring that enabled friends to recognise each other even after many years. On parting, the ring was broken into two pieces so that, by fitting them together again, the connection between friends could be confirmed after any length of time.

Even today, symbols have remained an expression of how form and content belong together, and still help us to recognise *interrelationships* and connections. Without content, the physical symbol is meaningless; without form, the symbol continues to exist, and is therefore not completely meaningless, but it is not able to be grasped. Only physical disease patterns enable us to get close to the spiritual contents that are encrypted within them. Physical form without content cannot exist (see the example of the corpse); content without physical form, on the other hand, can certainly exist – we need think only of ideas or of the immortal soul. Spiritual contents are brought to our awareness by their embodied form as disease patterns amongst other things. So-called mental illnesses provide examples of disease patterns which, without assuming concrete physical forms, nevertheless make themselves very clearly apparent.

In the Christian Book of Genesis, but similarly almost every other account of creation, we can follow this sequence in exemplary form. First comes the idea, the thought, the word or the sound, and only then does it come to the point of embodiment. The statement from the gospel of John "In the beginning was the Word, and the Word was with God" and later "the Word became flesh" leaves no doubt as to this sequence. All Creation comes from unity or oneness, and becomes embodied upon entering into polarity. Every step towards embodiment leads deeper into polarity. Disease belongs along the pathway to polarity. If we think in terms of hierarchies, it would certainly make sense to concede the first place to the mental-spiritual aspect, ahead of the body; nevertheless, in this approach to disease, it has proven helpful to regard both as being equally important, and not to give preference, or even complete priority,

to the subordinate physical level, as still happens in the case of traditionally-accepted medicine.

Tips on practical application

We cannot force freedom from disease patterns by means of any
therapy, but we can do and bring about everything possible in
order to switch the tracks in the direction of development. In my
experience, the essential criteria for healing are:
- the belief in recovery, and thus in one's own powers and
  possibilities,
- the step towards authenticity and
- experiences of spiritual unity.

Although I have become aware of these points most particularly
in the therapy of cancer patients, they apply in principle to all disease patterns. If we understand the message of a symptom, it
can become superfluous and disappear. Nevertheless, this is not
necessarily the case, and it is also possible that the task of tolerating a limitation or bearing pain remains. However, if the meaning
behind it is understood and accepted, the suffering will cease. Understanding and acceptance are always necessary although they
do not compel recovery in the physical sense. Disease should
definitely be understood *as a path*.

Re-habilitation of disease means, literally-speaking, "re-housing".
Taking back possession of the house of the body, reviving all rooms,
limbs and organs with awareness – this is the great opportunity offered
by every disease pattern. Already in the late sixties, the analyst Alex-
ander Mitscherlich spoke in *Krankheit als Konflikt (Disease as Conflict)*
of how diseases developed through the withdrawal of awareness from
certain parts of the body. Convalescence and recovery are consequently
steps back into the rightful home of one's body, and this manual of psychosomatics is an invitation for re-entry to one's own birthright. The expression "to put one's house in order" could have its roots here, and in
any case, certainly its meaning. In addition, the external building, which
in turn accommodates the house of the body, can be interpreted as a
reflection of the current life situation. Nobody would doubt that occupying a spacious villa makes a different statement than inhabiting a poky

basement flat does. Visitors spontaneously interpret the condition of a dwelling, the prevailing atmosphere, the presence or absence of cosiness, etc. Above and beyond this, we also make the distinction between good and expensive or not so good and therefore cheaper areas to live. We can approach our bodily housing in a similar, and in fact, even more differentiated way, gradually making this step-by-step into a suitable temple for our immortal soul.

When it comes to understanding (the meaning of disease patterns) we, or rather the left, archetypally-male half of our brain, thinks above all of itself. Intellectual understanding alone, however, cannot solve problems of this type; otherwise, the simple reading of a book of interpretations would lead to recovery. On the path to healing in the sense of returning to "wholeness/holiness", making use of our other side – symbolised in the right, archetypally-female half of the brain – is simultaneously a task and an aid. As a bridge to this side, it is advisable, in addition to reading and carefully considering the interpretation of the disease pattern, to have it read out by somebody else, while paying careful attention to which points they accentuate and their own emotional reactions. Heartbeat and changes in breathing rhythm can often provide useful indications. In keeping with this, it would make sense to invite one's counterpart to talk about what they have just read and how what resulted from it bears a relationship to oneself. These interpretations should best be listened to without any response, while in turn paying close attention to one's own emotional reactions. This could be followed by a dialogue on what has been read and discussed.

A further tried-and-tested aid is also to formulate questions on the topic of the disease, analogous to those provided in *Krankheit als Sprache der Seele (**Disease As a Language of the Soul)*, and to then thoroughly consider, discuss and meditate with regard to each question.

Further help can be provided by exercises and rituals relating directly to those learning tasks which are *sign*-ificant for the disease pattern. With regard to one's own rituals, attention is drawn to the book *Lebenskrisen als Entwicklungschancen (**Life Crises as an Opportunity for Development)* which contains instructions on the creation of individual rituals. Periods of intensive searching for the sense of one's own problems can often also be deepened by fasting. Fasting has the additional advantage that it is an excellent means of general prevention.

Painting or drawing therapies, in which one can give form to the disease pattern and express its various dimensions in colours and emotions, also provide useful assistance on the way to one's essential self. As with guided meditation and different forms of psychotherapy, the crucial aspect is the very first thought that must be given expression immediately with no ifs and buts.

If no progress can be achieved without outside aid, or if the disease pattern is too threatening, there is of course always the possibility of psychotherapy. A tried-and-tested approach in this respect is "disease-pattern therapy", which works with the tools of reincarnation therapy, such as regressions and breathing exercises, and which can be mastered in the short time of one to two weeks (For more information, see Heil-Kunde-Zentrum Johanniskirchen; address details in the appendix). In the case of major disease patterns, however, we still recommend taking a complete moon cycle, respectively 40 days or 20 days time.

This manual cannot and does not intend to take away any responsibility; on the contrary, it is aimed at providing people with possibilities to take on full responsibility for their own life with all its learning tasks. It aims to help them see through disease as an alibi and means of escape, and to recognise the underlying challenge. Those who show the courage to meet the challenge will be *encouraged* – by Fate.

As a reference work, it is naturally no substitute for a necessary visit to the doctor, even if in the long term, there is always the chance that people will get better and better in dealing with disease patterns and other challenges of Fate by themselves using their own resources, and, above all, in setting out on the path of prevention. Fortunately, more and more therapists are also beginning to obtain training in this type of comprehensive psychosomatic understanding of disease and its corresponding form of consultation, with the result that the chances of being able to find one's own "external" doctor in this area are increasing. The work with the inner doctor has always been the central focus of attention and will always remain so, since ultimately, it is only with the help of this power that healing is at all possible. In serious cases, the external doctor can only reasonably ally him or herself with the inner doctor, and in this endeavour, this book hopes to be a useful aid for both sides.

In conclusion, I would like to once again express my sincere thanks to all those readers and users of this interpretative approach, who with questions and suggestions in letters and mails, at presentations, seminars and training sessions, have contributed to the continual further development of the manual, which in the 15th edition has now undergone its second thorough revision and extension.

Montegrotto, December 2006,

Ruediger Dahlke

Part 1

Directory of the body regions and organs

Directory of the body regions and organs

A

Abdomen

see Stomach

Abdominal cavity

Symbolic meaning: Security, focus, nest of the organs.
Task/subject: Bowel cavity: warmth, protection; providing the organs with a home.
Archetypal principle: Moon.

Abdominal wall

Symbolic meaning: Protection; outer protective cover of the soft body parts (the internal organs).
Task/subject: Covering the abdominal cavity, protective cover of the abdominal organs, covers the front side of the body made more vulnerable by walking upright; fat storage between the outer skin and muscle layer.
Archetypal principle: Saturn, Moon.

Achilles tendon

Symbolic meaning: Spiritual take-off power, forward movement/progress, ascendance; strongest cord of the body (àtendon), that the ankle musculature used for jumping is attached to; enables the great leap forward and every take-off (relationship to great, high-flying dreams and expansive objectives); classical weak point: although the tendon can withstand 400 to 800 kgs, it can tear, but only if we "reach the end of our tether", lose our "foothold" in a situation, or if we stretch something too far; it happens suddenly with a loud crack, which dramatically emphasises the seriousness of the situation, just as we can also "crack" under pressure; vulnerability of the Achilles tendon: Achilles was held by his heel when he was immersed in the River Styx (the river of immortality), with the result that this remained his only vulnerable point.
Task/subject: Giving somebody a leg up, enabling progress and advancement.
Archetypal principle: Mercury-Uranus.

Acoustic nerve

see Nervus statoacusticus

Adamantine

see Teeth (enamel)

Adrenal glands

(hormone glands, consisting of the cortex, which is capable of producing over 40 different steroids and the medulla, which produces the stress hormones adrenalin and noradrenalin, see also Hormones, Neurotransmitters)
Symbolic meaning: Centre for stress regulation, water balance and sex life that is subordinate to the pituitary gland; real physical implementation of commands coming from above.
Task/subject: Handling of stress (cortisone and noradrenalin/adrenalin secretion); regulation of the water balance: mineral corticoid secretion such as aldosterone; sex hormone production; active intervention in the flow of life.
Archetypal principle: Mercury (transport by hormones)-Mars (stress hormones)/Moon (water balance)/Pluto (sex hormones).

Ankle joint

(Fetlock; see also Joints)
Symbolic meaning: Articulation on the ground, basis of smooth, easy locomotion; showing how one approaches one's life; anyone who has problems here is chained: "to put somebody in chains"; dynamism of

one's own stance and standpoints in life, one's path through life; origin of standing erect on the hind legs; take-off point for all (large and small) leaps: "to be always on the hop".
Task/subject: Enables the rolling movement of the foot when walking, and thereby smooth locomotion; elasticity, elegant progress; rearing up on one's hind legs: leaping to the plateau of the gods.
Archetypal principle: Mercury-Neptune, Uranus.

Antibodies

Symbolic meaning: Specialised guided weapons of the àimmune system, which like military cruise missiles direct themselves specifically against known enemies.
Task/subject: Conducting warfare kamikaze-style: launching oneself on one's enemies in line with a special programme and perishing together with them.
Archetypal principle: Mars.

Anus

Symbolic meaning: Entrance and exit of the underworld, rear exit, exhaust; regulating channel between the inner and outer world.
Task/subject: Guarding the exit, guardian of the last threshold (the sphincter muscle is consciously controllable from the last anal phase); ensuring a clean closure, taking leave, letting go; valve for relieving aggressive pressure from behind (kicking up a stink); forms the first product, the first gift of the child to the world; the meconium thus becomes the forerunner for all later gifts.
Archetypal principle: Pluto.

Aorta

Symbolic meaning: Main traffic route of the life flow; alertness and presence for the outer world.

Task/subject: Energy transport from the centre to the periphery, energetic connection between top and bottom, auxiliary motor for upholding the even pressure gradient of the blood pressure (air chamber function).
Archetypal principle: Sun-Mercury.

Appendix

(Caecum)/Vermiform appendix
Symbolic meaning: Dead end (vestigial organ) from the early period of evolution, defensive bastion of the intestines (lymphatic defense centre), defensive facility of the underworld: police station of the shadow kingdom.
Task/subject: Unconsciously ensuring order, defence against foreign intruders into the underworld.
Archetypal principle: Mars-Pluto.

Arms

(see also Upper arms, Forearms)
Symbolic meaning: Force, strength, power (Latin arma = 'weapons, arms'): "arms race", "armed and dangerous"; struggle: "up in arms", "taking to arms"; perseverance: "a shot in the arm", exerting influence: "using strong arm tactics", "the long arm of the law", "twisting someone's arm"; to express love and devotion: "receiving/welcoming with open arms", "arm in arm", "giving one's right arm for something"; to maintain distance: "keeping at arm's length", "crossing one's arms"
Task/subject: Contact with the outer world; bringing the (physical) world closer, lovingly embracing it, dealing with it or consciously keeping it at arm's length.
Archetypal principle: Mars-Mercury.

Arm (type)

Symbolic meaning: 1. Strong, muscular: able to lift/bear a great deal; to give protection and security, "a bear hug"; danger of musclemen becoming "high-handed" or "overbearing";

2. Thick-set: feigning strength with fat; belligerence, "puffing oneself up", "throwing one's weight around"; (quarrelling);

3. Weak: feebleness in the struggle of life; not being able to hold on to anything or anybody, not being able to lift or move much; long considered elegant in women, but has always been a problem with men.

Task/subject: 1. Grabbing hold of life, forcefully pushing through one's own interests and holding things out (persevering), clearing obstacles out of the way;

2. Maintaining a firm grip on life and giving oneself a good hold;

3. Trusting in life, going along with the flow of life, taking part.

Archetypal principle: 1. Mars; 2. Jupiter-Mars; 3. Moon.

Arteries

(see also Blood vessels)
Symbolic meaning: Energy pathways, (power) supply system, first half of our circulation (=type of circle)
Task/subject: Energy distribution, energy transport.
Archetypal principle: Mercury (connection), Mars (energy).

Athletic type

see Constitution

Atlas

(the first cervical vertebra, see also Axis and Cervical vertebrae)
Symbolic meaning: Pivot point of the head, feeling of self-esteem.
Task/subject: Bearing the weight of the heavenly firmament (the myth of Atlas, who carries "the weight of the world" on his shoulders as a punishment); mobility in the sense of a lighthouse platform open on all sides; enabling overview and circumspection, guaranteeing far-sightedness; responsibility.
Archetypal principle: Saturn (bearing the load), Mercury (pivot point).

Auditory canal

Symbolic meaning: Sound funnel, hearing tube.
Task/subject: Picking up sound and information and directing it inside; conveying the world of sounds.
Archetypal principle: Mercury.

AV nodes

Symbolic meaning: Second, subordinate centre in the hierarchy of the heart, reserve centre in the hierarchy.
Task/subject: Lifelong readiness to spring into action in an emergency (e.g. AV blockage).
Archetypal principle: Sun-Uranus-Saturn.

Axillary glands

(Secondary sexual glands)
Symbolic meaning: Personal scent.
Task/subject: Secretion of one's own distinctive scent ensuring a trademark odour, territory marking; recognising who passes the "sniff test" or who we "turn our nose up at" perhaps because they "get up our nose"; in earlier times, young women would draw a handkerchief through the axilla (the armpit) and throw it to their hero.
Archetypal principle: Venus-Pluto.

Axis

(the second cervical vertebra)
Symbolic meaning: Highpoint of the world axis; axis around which everything turns; aspiration and ambition.
Task/subject: Providing mobility and leadership.
Archetypal principle: Mercury-Jupiter.

B

Back

(see also Spinal column)
Symbolic meaning: Reveals one's
age ("up and coming" or "stooped
with age"); load-carrier of life: the
burden of life, strenuous exertion
("bending over backwards for someone"); strength, having good backing;
beauty, grace ("a beautiful back can
also delight"); honesty and uprightness, straightforwardness: "being
upstanding", "standing up for something", "standing behind someone or
something".
Task/subject: Raising up; carrying
and bearing, the ability to bear something (a yield).
Archetypal principle: Saturn.

Backbone

see Spinal column

Balance nerve

see Nervus statoacusticus

Balance organ

(in the inner ear)
Symbolic meaning: Balance sensor.
Task/subject: Keeping the body and
life in harmony/balance; reporting the
list and roll of the ship of life; perception of gravity; finding the physical
(spiritual) centre.
Archetypal principle:
Venus-Mercury.

Bartholin's glands

Symbolic meaning: These produce
the female juices of pleasure and life.
Task/subject: Moistening the vaginal
vestibular area; "lubricating" the entrance to the temple of pleasure and
reproduction.

Archetypal principle: Moon-Venus.

Beard

Symbolic meaning: Primitiveness,
primordial forest of the (male) face
(the barbarian is bearded); masculinity; in unresolved form, it becomes a
hiding place (àPart 2, Female facial
hair); attempt to conceal highly symbolic elements, e.g. (un)sensuous
lips, receding or very prominent jaw;
image cultivation, demonstrating
membership of a class; political, religious or fashion statement, making
an impression; emphasising power
and authority.
Task/subject: Being able to deal with
the inner barbarian, e.g. cultivating
him out of existence (completely
clearing the primordial forest), showing him off or cutting him back (every
reduction of body hair, and therefore
also the beard, is a cultural act);
primitiveness in the sense of atavism
(Latin atavus = 'ancestor, forebear';
recurrence of anatomical features
which were actually typical of our
forebears); consciously concerning
oneself with one's own origin and
ancestors.
Archetypal principle: Mars-Venus.

Beard (shape)

Symbolic meaning: 1. Long, full
beard: archaic character, nature
instead of culture, ideal concealment
for wrinkles and messages conveyed
by the mouth, chin and cheeks;
one does not truly manifest oneself,
lack of openness to the point of
dishonesty, (pseudo-) masculinity; a
seaman's beard is nowadays associated with a country bumpkin image;
convenience to the point of laziness
(unkempt "shaggy bear" look); short,
neat full beard: artificially-cultivated
grimness, domesticated wildness;
2. Moustache: concealing one's sensuality (upper lip), playing the great
macho (a theme of entire cultural

groups, e.g. the Islamic culture), snapping at others ("Schnauzer", "whiskers"), unapproachable, prickly defence, being bristly ("walrus beard.");
3. Chin beard: emphasis of claim to power (chin) and willpower; emphasising the intellect, pedantic (pointed beard) to mischievous ("goatee beard"); obsessive tendencies (Lenin beard);
4. Designer stubble: fashionable beard of the modern macho, demonstrative "coolness", unconventionality and bristly masculinity; time-consuming cultivation of the unkempt image;
5. Artistically-shaped beards: demonstration of special programmes, e.g. wanting to be the (little) emperor in one's own kingdom (muttonchops and upturned handlebar moustache = "Kaiser Wilhelm beard"); eccentricity, snobbishness (upturned, twisted moustache like Dalí; thin, trimmed pencil moustache like David Niven); authoritarian pretentions, dictatorial allure (toothbrush moustache like Hitler);
6. Strongly emphasised, particularly large sideburns: broadening the face, making an impression, making oneself important ("puffing oneself up").
Task/subject: 1. Sticking to one's archaic, primordial aspirations; conscious rejection of culture; naturalness, letting everything just grow, not only the beard;
2. Development of a genuine male self-image;
3. Achieving true inner power, cultivating a sharp, calm and incisive intellect;
4. Demonstrating true masculinity, developing the animus with regard to being honest about one's own problems;
5. Becoming aware of the issue being expressed, trimming one's life into shape so that it is truly fitting;
6. Taking up more space, making a greater impression.

Archetypal principle: 1. Mars-Pluto; 2. Mars-Mars; 3. Mars-Mars/Mercury; 4. Mars-Venus; 5. Uranus; 6. Jupiter.

Belly

Symbolic meaning: Feeling, instinct (gut feeling); enjoyment; the abdominal cavity as our "cave of origin", seat of child-like emotions; the navel as the centre of the world and source of (original) nourishment and care, feeling "well-rounded"; in earlier times, it was protected between the extremities (in four-legged creatures facing towards the ground); today, the "paunch of prosperity" is proudly thrust forward.
Task/subject: Protection, security, digestion; expression of existential fears/threats, a storage cupboard for stockpiling reserves; expression of confidence in the material future.
Archetypal principle: Moon.

Belly (shape)

(see also in Part 2: Drooping belly, Roemheld's syndrome, Drum belly)
Symbolic meaning: 1. Flat: fashionable shape (preference for a depression rather than a hill); danger of making little of one's own spiritual centre and instead emphasising the body excessively; being fit, steeled in the centre, in itself a masculine shape; for women, an unnatural ideal, which has to be earned the hard way through fasting and training; preferring to suffer instead of wallowing in excess;
2. Large: the paunch of prosperity, material wealth; struggling under the weight of one's possessions; having a "burdensome life" or "a heavy weight to bear"; dissolving the clear outlines of the front view or facade; placing soft barriers between oneself and life; cushioning oneself; digestion (of life) is "outsourced"; the digestive tract is pushed outwards and lugged in front of oneself, consuming the

world (Buddism. Bhoga = consuming karmic fruits) becomes problematic; bursting one's banks to the front and running off into boundlessness;
3. Pot belly: appearing pregnant, feigned fertility, "phantom pregnancy", not producing anything significant, but trying to "conceive" something: something wants to get out into the light;
4. Beer belly: round feminisation in the direction of pregnancy (beer contains ingredients similar to oestrogen), impotence;
5. Washboard stomach/six-pack: masculine ideal, achievable through training and abstinence; frontal view/ facade armoured down to below the belt line, soft parts protected ("hard shell – possibly a soft core?").
Task/subject: 1. Passing in streamlined fashion through life without creating a great wake; not overvaluing the body; not accumulating any treasures (at the material level);
2. Building up reserves; placing the focus on "digesting" life;
3. Identifying what one is trying to "conceive" in a spiritual sense; ensuring the corresponding births; turning one's own life into a "well-rounded" affair;
4. Finding out what is to be drowned by drinking; realising one's own feminine aspects in the sense of the anima; becoming gentle and emotional at the spiritual level;
5. Bracing oneself, ensuring safe surroundings and security, in which feelings can flourish and be expressed.
Archetypal principle: 1. Moon-Mars; 2. Moon-Jupiter; 3. Moon-Moon; 4. Moon-Neptune; 5. Moon-Mars.

Belly button

Symbolic meaning: Physical centre, Hara = world centre of mankind (Dürckheim).
Task/subject: Connection to the origin, to the mother, to the paradise of the first land of milk and honey.
Archetypal principle: Moon.

Bile

see Urinary bladder

Bladder

see Gall bladder

Blood

(see also Erythrocytes [red blood corpuscles], Granulocytes/ Leukocytes [white blood corpuscles], Thrombocytes [blood platelets])
Symbolic meaning: Life force, life flow; connection of the four elements: Blood serum (from Latin: '(water)y fluid, whey') as the basis, electrolytes = salts (earth), oxygen (air) and the red colour = haemoglobin (fire).
Task/subject: Material bearer of life ("being of flesh and blood", "sucking/ bleeding somebody dry"); expression of individual dynamism (Faust must sign his pact with the devil in blood because it "is a juice of very special kind", being hot-blooded, cold-blooded or calm and cool-blooded, "it is in my blood", "one's own flesh and blood" = relatives who belong completely to the clan by virtue of blood); energisation, nourishment; basic pillar of religious mysteries; blood (Hebrew: dam) also meant mother and woman; found in Indo-Germanic with the meanings: madam, dame, but also curse, damnation: the old designations often included the opposite pole as an expression of the eternal truth of polarity.
Archetypal principle: Mars (energy)-Sun (individual self).

Blood circulation

Symbolic meaning: Life energy circuit which completes itself at every moment; dispensing and disposing.

Task/subject: Connecting, convey-ing, supplying, dynamising, nourish-ing, circling around the centre.
Archetypal principle: Sun/Mars-Mercury.

Blood pressure

Symbolic meaning: Energy (blood)-resistance (vessel walls) phenomenon; harmony between human beings and the world; indica-tor of one's spiritual state of tension and one's presence: high pressure = struggle, high tension; low pressure = easing of tension to the point of blackout/total powerlessness.
Task/subject: Supplying the organ-ism (with energy, nutrients, messen-ger substances), ensuring dynamism; balance between driving force and acceptance of the circumstances.
Archetypal principle: Mars-Saturn.

Blood vessels

(see also Arteries and Veins)
Symbolic meaning: Transport routes of the life force, energy pathways; transport, communication.
Task/subject: Supplying, nourishing; dispensing and disposing, transport-ing (to and away from).
Archetypal principle: Sun/Mars-Mercury.

Body (form)

see Constitution

Body (sides)

Symbolic meaning:

1. Left: Female – emotional side (Yin);
2. Right: Male – side of strong will (Yang).

Task/subject:

1. Receptive, sensitive side; the re-ceiving hand, which forms itself into a bowl;

2. The side of doing and giving, in contrast to the left, receptive side; rational activity, forceful assertion, power: the sword of power is held in the right hand; the clenched right fist shows the will for power.
Archetypal principle: 1. Moon; 2. Sun.

Body (size)

Symbolic meaning: 1. Very tall: standing out (being outstanding), standing/walking tall, towering above others, being prominent, head and shoulders above the rest; size matters more, greater things are attributed to the great; being tall and well-built, also popular today amongst women (model figure); shadow as-pect: looking down on others, being arrogant; the beanstalk shoots for the stars (ambition); women in particular tend to play down their size;
2. Very small: looking up to others, feeling oneself put down, feeling small; former feminine ideal ("my little woman"), men in particular tend to compensate for their small stature by great deeds and a "big mouth" (collo-quially: "big-noting oneself").
Task/subject: 1. Standing proud with regard to one's height; inwardly matching the external size, walking tall, standing out, becoming the great-est, striving to become the number one at the highest level, realising unity; maintaining an overview;
2. Standing proud with regard to one's height/small stature ("small, but effective"), practising humility, taking oneself less seriously, finding one's place; deliberately fostering consider-ation, making oneself notable.
Archetypal principle: 1. Sun; 2. Moon.

Body hair

Symbolic meaning: Primitive, un-tamed animal power; very hairy manly chest: emphasis of our animalistic, instinctive origins; very hairy female legs: reminiscent of our animalistic origins.

Task/subject: Demonstrating "animal" strength; protection (in the past against cold): a thick hide.

Archetypal principle: Mars (strength, instinctive power), Saturn (protection).

Bones

(see also Skeleton)

Symbolic meaning: Inner stability, constancy (of the personality structure), compliance with standards.

Task/subject: Providing stability and structure, framework function, conveying a feeling of inner constancy; enables upright locomotion and our overall size: "standing up for something"; ossification is essential for survival at the beginning of life, but later in life is a hindrance.

Archetypal principle: Saturn.

Bone marrow

Symbolic meaning: Generation site of the life force (blood formation, particularly at the beginning of life), weapons forge of the body, essence ("something penetrates/chills or grips us to the marrow").

Task/subject: Regenerating vitality; recognising and defending the uniqueness of the organism; preserving our essence deep within.

Archetypal principle: Saturn-Moon.

Bosom

see Breast, female

Brachial joint

see Elbow

Brain

(see also Cerebellum, Cerebrum)

Symbolic meaning: Communication; logistics, central administration, archive and library (memory); (seat of) central government.

Task/subject: Co-ordination of communication both internally and with the external world, central control switchboard of the head - the capital city of the body; planning, controlling, processing, co-ordinating, archiving.

Archetypal principle: Mercury, Uranus (flashes of inspiration).

Brain hemispheres

Symbolic meaning:

1. Left half: the "male" brain;
2. Right half: the "female" brain.

Task/subject:

1. Intellectual control, understanding, reason (ratio), analysis; recognition, naming;
2. Holistic thinking, perception of patterns and shapes, conveyance of creativity and intuition.

Archetypal principle: 1. Mercury-Sun; 2. Moon-Venus.

Brain stem

(see also Limbic system, which makes up the major part of the brain stem)

Symbolic meaning: Earliest co-ordination, first computer model; (in evolutionary terms) the old brain, which controls the primitive survival functions (such as respiration); the stem of the brain, from which all other branches (including the cerebrum) were able to develop.

Task/subject: Processing and co-ordinating signals from within the body with those from the outside world; regulating the bodily functions necessary for survival.

Archetypal principle: Pluto.

Breast, female

Symbolic meaning: Motherliness, nourishment, security, second only to the umbilical cord as the most important connection to the maternal; desire, sex appeal, seduction; feminine power/charisma (breasts: in various cultures the symbol of womanhood); female feeling of self-esteem; swapping of the gender roles: the breast becomes an offensive intruder (corresponding to the penis) with the mouth of the partner as the recipient; in patriarchal society: pert, evenly formed breasts of medium size = ideal; very small breasts = deficiency; very large breasts = provocation; only organ which only develops in parallel with reaching womanhood (only in humans permanently present, irrespective of breast-feeding); most frequently "corrected" organ (ahead of the nose) with resultant scarring at all levels; closeness: "in the bosom of nature" (close to nature), "cherishing a serpent in one's bosom" (allowing an enemy to get very close), "bosom buddies" (close friends).

Task/subject: Nourishment, relationship (nourishment), providing; sexual attraction: indulging, tempting, seducing; holding one's own in the modern-day tense relationship between providing (care) and seducing.

Archetypal principle: Moon (the maternal), Venus (the seductive).

Breast, female (shape)

Symbolic meaning: 1. Large, full: demonstrative womanliness, motherliness and nourishment, sensuality and eroticism, female fullness and over-the-top abundance, overflowing excess, softness, a "well-rounded" affair;

2. Hanging, full: having fully experienced womanliness and motherliness;

3. Hanging, sagging: leached dry by life, exhausted vitality; the result of draining, weakening provision of nourishment; having been sucked dry, having given everything to the children, having nothing left over for oneself; in modern societies (like almost everything female) defamed instead of honoured; putting oneself down, lowering oneself, letting everything slide;

4. Girlishly small: youthfully immature charisma (less commonly, Lolita-style character), very popular amongst immature men; masculine type, sporty figure, Amazonian; ideal for "being the man"; ·

5. Pointed: usually firm, young, unused breasts; perky, ("phallic") challenging, coquettish, pert-looking; pushing forward, wanting to show oneself, "pricked and at the ready" in the sense of sexually teasing, a "hot dish" that one would like to sink one's teeth into; youthfully fresh charisma.

Task/subject: 1. Doing justice to one's ample gifts and both sides of the feminine: the nourishing (Moon) and the seductive (Venus); nourishing life and living love;

2. Letting oneself flow gently in the positive sense with respect to the major female themes of seduction (Venus) and nourishment (Moon), the latter also in the figurative sense of mental-spiritual nourishment; becoming "well-rounded", the breasts as regions of orgiastic desire in flowing and experiences of oneness;

3. Consciously letting oneself hang loose; leaving things in peace, letting go of tension, putting one's feet up, regenerating; with respect to the principal themes of femininity, letting go of further children's wishes;

4. Coming to terms with the modern ideal; calmly going one's own archetypally masculine way; not allowing oneself to be hindered by femininity and female themes and arguments;

5. Challenging; combining femininity with masculine behaviour patterns and living offensively.
Archetypal principle: 1. Moon-Venus; 2. Venus-Moon; 3. Moon-Saturn; 4. Moon-Venus-Mars; 5. Venus-Mars.

Breastbone

(Sternum)
Symbolic meaning: Protective shield, centre of the Self: self-awareness and Ego (point where one beats oneself to drum up courage and to demonstrate claims to dominance/strength); frontal closure of the rib cage.
Task/subject: Protection, breastplate, marking the centre of the chest.
Archetypal principle: Sun-Saturn.

Bronchia

Symbolic meaning: Connecting channels between the inner and outer world; pathways for energy and waste gases; the bronchial *branches* form the inner *tree* of the lungs.
Task/subject: Conducting the current of breath (Prana), connection between inside and outside; energy supply and disposal; communication, rhythm.
Archetypal principle: Mercury.

Buttocks

Symbolic meaning: Passive perseverance, sitting something out (ability to sit tight); strength to kick *butt*; the posterior, consisting of the largest muscle is jokingly referred to as the seat of wisdom; the most important thing in coining this term seems to have been the ability to sit tight (patience) and relax; weight(iness), wealth; sexual signal ("tight buns").
Task/subject: Sitting things out, kicking butt; taking one's rightful place, making an impression; acting as a turn-on, sitting on possessions.
Archetypal principle: Jupiter.

Buttocks (shape)

Symbolic meaning: 1. Large, fat: "fast-food" or "lard arse" as a result of incorrect diet (too many refined carbohydrates) and lack of exercise, also a sign of lethargy and convenience, sluggishness and ungainliness; complacency; lack of inner strength to kick butt; stuck sitting on one's backside;
2. Small: boyish, modern ideal of women, androgynous;
3. Taut, muscular, round: expression of powerful thighs; modern ideal for both sexes; looks young and youthful, manly; firm, curvaceous "tight, sexy ass", strong enough to crack even hard nuts; sex appeal, "tight pants"; seductive, "sweet peaches";
4. Flabby: powerless, "unable to get off one's backside", a "saggy" behind, "a hung game", letting everything slide with regard to kicking butt; overripe fruit that is past its prime in contrast to "sweet peaches";
5. Pear-shaped: being drawn downwards into the female domain, broadened basis.
Task/subject: 1. Kicking butt, developing the ability to sit tight, sitting out serious problems; forcefully applying oneself; allopathic approach: getting moving again;
2. Looking for, accepting and enjoying the inner child; integrating a childlike basis into the hard patriarchal world;
3. Using the strength from behind for one's own pleasure and that of others;
4. Staying relaxed, allowing oneself to yield instead of one's flesh;
5. Finding one's place, spreading oneself out and putting down roots.
Archetypal principle: 1. Jupiter; 2. Jupiter-Moon; 3. Jupiter-Mars; 4. Jupiter-Saturn; 5. Venus/Moon-Jupiter.

C

Calf

see Lower leg

Cardiovascular arteries

Symbolic meaning: Supply channels for the heart.
Task/subject: Energy supply of the heart: with the aid of these, the heart must provide itself with fresh life energy (blood).
Archetypal principle: Sun-Mercury.

Cartilage tissue

Symbolic meaning: Elasticity, bridge-building substance, binding ability (commitment); tissue of youth (elastic stretching capacity, bendability of the young tree).
Task/subject: As the surface coating for joints, guarantees connections (àJoints), bridging function; precursor of the bone: from the very beginning of life and at all new beginnings, paves the way for the element that gives structure and stability.
Archetypal principle: Moon-Saturn.

Celiac plexus

see Solar plexus

Cerebellum

(see also Brain)
Symbolic meaning: Co-ordination centre for involuntary movement and fine motor control in the lower back part of the head, subordinate to the central government.
Task/subject: Fine co-ordination of movements; provides the finishing touch to co-ordination so that everything runs in a well-rounded way.
Archetypal principle: Mercury-Venus.

Cerebral fluid

(Liquor cerebrospinalis)
Symbolic meaning: Aqueous (spiritual) protective cushion around the central control switchboard and its outlying outposts.
Task/subject: Encasing the control centres of the organism, protecting (against impacts and concussions), insulating, flowing around and supplying.
Archetypal principle: Moon.

Cerebral membranes

(Outermost layer: Dura mater, middle layer: Arachnoid mater, directly on the brain: Pia mater)
Symbolic meaning: Packaging, protective covering of the central control switchboard by the 'hard' mother (Dura mater); this mothers the central control switchboard from the outside (and is simultaneously the periosteum to the roof of the cranium); the 'tender/pious' mother (Pia mater) lies directly on the brain as a metabolic membrane and mothers it in a gentler way; between the Pia mater and the Arachnoid (from Greek meaning "cobweb-like) mater, the cerebral fluid circulates as a buffer zone so that the more male-like central control switchboard is surrounded on all sides by a (female-spiritual) cushion of water.
Task/subject: Protecting, partitioning off, nestling in a water-bed, shock-absorber function, buffering, insulating; supplying, enveloping with the spiritual; conveying the cranio-sacral rhythm.
Archetypal principle: Saturn, Moon.

Cerebrum

(see also Brain)
Symbolic meaning: The latest big thing in evolutionary development (the newest computer version); basis of a cool head; supraordinate centre

for co-ordination of life, especially the female and male poles.

Task/subject: The hardware for the intellect: rationality (left hemisphere) and at the same time for holistic thinking (right hemisphere); representation of polarity at the highest level: Schizophrenia (literally: splitting of the brain) is actually our basic situation, since the left and right hemispheres are completely separated, and only connected at a deeper level by the Corpus callosum.

Archetypal principle: Mercury-Uranus.

Cervical vertebra (column)

(see also Atlas, Axis, Spinal column)

Symbolic meaning: Emphasis of the dynamic and flexible aspect of the vertebrae (Latin: vert(ere) = 'to turn') as opposed to the static aspect of the spinal column; mobility of the head, a spineless person easily changes sides and opinions.

Task/subject: Enabling overview and circumspection for the head; holding the head up high or above water, expressing acute problems.

Archetypal principle: Mercury(-Saturn).

Cervix

(Cervix uteri)

Symbolic meaning: Fertility, gateway to the primordial cave of all beginnings (womb), to the female underworld.

Task/subject: Protection; transport, communication (formation of cervical mucus in line with the female cycle).

Archetypal principle: Moon-Saturn.

Chakras

(7 higher-level energy centres along the spinal column; various subsidiary centres, e.g. in hands and feet; in Hindu mythology: the energy or Kundalini serpent that initially lies dormant in the first chakra, ascending in the course of development to the highest chakra)

Symbolic meaning: Energetic vortices in the body, which on the one hand, establish connections with the Cosmos, and on the other, control the organs.

Task/subject: Co-ordination of human development on the level of the aura (anima); mediator between the soul and the physical level; absorption of cosmic energy (Prana = life force); in particular:

1. Root chakra at the end of the coccyx ("Muladhara"): Centre for energy, vitality;

Subject: Deep-rootedness, basic trust, stability, will to live, death and rebirth processes; Activates: Blood, spinal column; in the case of energy overload: egoism, avarice; in the case of energy shortage: weak constitution, lack of self-awareness; Element: earth; Colour: red;

Archetypal principle: Pluto.

2. Sacral chakra below the navel ("Svadhishthana"): Centre for emotions;

Subject: Eroticism, sexuality, erotic power of attraction, womanly feeling, creativity, inspiration; Activates: spleen, kidneys, female sexual organs, mammary glands; in the case of energy overload: aggression, sexual obsession, manipulation; in the case of energy shortage: frigidity (of both sexes), feelings of guilt, anxiety, timidity; Element: water; Colour: orange;

Archetypal principle: Venus, Moon.

3. Solar plexus chakra ("Manipura"): centre for the vegetative nervous system;

Subject: joy for life, self-confidence, intelligence, spiritual order; Activates: pancreas and digestive organs, diaphragm, skin, adrenal gland; in the case of energy overload: perfectionism, workaholism, over-taxing; in

17

the case of energy shortage: envy, mistrust, lack of concentration and self-awareness; Element: fire; Colour: yellow;
Archetypal principle: **Mercury.**
4. Heart chakra ("Anahata"): Centre for sympathy;
Subject: love, sympathy, humanity; Activates: thymus, immune system; in the case of energy overload: moody, critical, demanding, judgemental; in the case of energy shortage: desire for confirmation, self-pity; anxiety about being abandoned or rejected; Element: air; Colour: green;
Archetypal principle: **Sun.**
5. Neck/throat chakra ("Vishuddi"): Centre for motor function, activity, will to lead;
Subject: communication, openness, expression, self-responsibility; Activates: motor nervous system, muscles, ears, parathyroid gland; in the case of energy overload: arrogance, bossiness, talking too much, macho behaviour; in the case of energy shortage: intimidated; inability to express one's own thoughts; concealed manipulations; Element: ether; Colour: turquoise;
Archetypal principle: **Mercury.**
6. Forehead chakra (third eye, "Ajna"): centre for sensitivity;
Subject: recognition, charisma, intuition; Activates: pituitary gland and brain stem; in the case of energy overload: egocentric, authoritarian, dogmatic; in the case of energy shortage: over-sensitive, undisciplined, lacking self-awareness, fear of success; Element: –; Colour: indigo;
Archetypal principle: **Jupiter.**
7. Crown chakra on the head ("Sahasrara"): centre for universal awareness, spirituality;
Subject: being one with the divine; Activates: cerebrum, pineal gland, nervous system; in the case of energy overload: depression, frustration, psychosis, migraine; in the case of energy shortage: lack of joy for life,

inability to make decisions; Element: –; Colour: violet;
Archetypal principle: **Saturn, Uranus.** Archetypal principle: (Chakras overall) **Neptune-Sun.**

Cheeks

Symbolic meaning: 1. General: reveal one's method of biting one's way through life since they are made up of the chewing muscles; points of particular receptiveness to tenderness (Venus), but also predestined for the exchange of aggression e.g. in the form of a slap across the face (Mars);
2. Full cheeks ("hamster cheeks"): problems with taking; being downcast, innocent expression;
3. Hollow cheeks: suffering, stern expression; not getting (having) enough; looking old, haggard, ill, emaciated; nowadays considered to be attractive (almost all models have hollow cheeks with high cheekbones).
Task/subject: 1. Exchanging tenderness, demonstrating potential for aggression; developing real bite and sinking one's teeth into things;
2. Turning one's attention more to one's own basis, taking what one needs, consciously letting things hang loose in the sense of regeneration;
3. Developing contours; learning to be stern with oneself; finding a positive connection to suffering; understanding ascesis as an art of living.
Archetypal principle: 1. **Venus-Mars**; 2. **Jupiter**; 3. **Saturn.**

Chest

(see also Breast, female)
Symbolic meaning: Sense of self ("I am"), personality ("puffing up one's chest", "having a weak chest"; when weighed down by problems, it helps "to get a load off one's chest"); body armour (Wilhelm Reich): "chest swollen with pride", "chesty as a peacock"; bony cage for the winglike lobes of the lungs and the heart;

powerfulness, importance, protection and safety for the heart (feeling) and lungs (communication).

Task/subject: Demonstrating the sense of self; taking up space, impressing (a deep, chesty voice is more convincing), stretching oneself; protection of the internal organs and thus the world of feeling and emotion of the heart and the communication location of the lungs; integration of everything rational which comes down from above, everything intuitive and archaic which comes up from below and everything emotional which comes from within.

Archetypal principle: Saturn (protection, "cage")-Sun (centre).

Chin

(see also lower jaw)

Symbolic meaning: Will (power), capacity to push oneself forward (self-assertion), "gritting one's teeth and biting one's way through life" with strength and power, self-expression, determination (the chin beard emphasises this aspect in men).

Task/subject: Pushing one's way through, forceful self-assertion.

Archetypal principle: Mars-Saturn.

Chin (shape)

Symbolic meaning: 1. Projecting, prominent: wanting to show oneself as self-assured, seeking the foreground; sense of honour, honesty, generosity, dominance (àPart 2, Double chin);

2. Receding: the spiritual outweighs the will; lack of willpower, drawing back from life, giving power interests a back seat; apparent harmlessness, considered to be backward, underestimated;

3. Small: reserved, shy; fear of making mistakes, often leads to doing nothing at all;

4. Shapeless, round: lack of contours, having worn oneself down, tendency to nag;

5. Wide, angular: masculine impression, physical strength and ability to apply it; prepared to take risks, good feeling of self-esteem, strong ability to forcefully assert oneself;

6. Cleft, dimpled: striking, emphasised masculinity, pronounced aspect of will, good relationship to polarity and to the world, willingness to forcefully assert oneself;

7. Pointed: intellectual inclination, often sharply critical about getting to the point of everything; frequent lack of emotionality, not wanting to become emotionally involved.

Task/subject: 1. Consciously stepping forward, exerting one's will over oneself and others;

2. Practising polite reserve; becoming aware of one's defensive life situation, consciously holding oneself back, shifting the focus of life inwards;

3. Looking for a good hold oneself;

4. Preferring to round off corners and edges more in the figurative sense instead; letting one's will become well-rounded and harmonious so that it fits one's character;

5. Deliberately applying masculine strength, handling the strikingly masculine animus responsibly; in women: indication of concern for the animus, the masculine side of the soul, and the desire to develop this, in particular with regard to the aspect of the will;

6. Understanding polarity as a task and facing the world and its demands (challenges); 7. Using the outstanding, sharp intellect to obtain access to other worlds.

Archetypal principle: 1. Mars; 2. 3. and 4. Moon; 5. and 6. Mars; 7. Mars-Mars.

Cholesterol

(basic material of the sex hormones, the bile acids [fat digestion] and the myelin sheaths of the nerves formed in the àliver; divided into "benign" HDL which protects the cell walls and "malignant" LDL which damages the cell walls)

Symbolic meaning: Polar material, in which good and evil lie close together; sealing, stabilising, protecting ("emergency helper"); (cell) sealing material and bandage material of the organism (is administered in Latin America in cases of haemolysing snake and spider bites for sealing blood vessels); material basis of sexuality, protection of the 'cables' in the body's landscape (myelin); transformation of the greasy lipids and fats into usable energy.

Task/subject: Mending holes, sealing; therefore high concentration in the blood in the event of ruptures of the vessel inner walls (intima) due to stress and blood pressure peaks (high blood pressure) for sealing purposes; anyone who is "a little cracked" (crazy) needs it in higher doses; preserving life: preventing the lifeblood from running away; enabling and protecting connections (myelin).

Archetypal principle: Mercury-Saturn.

Clitoris / clit

Symbolic meaning: Desire, sensibility, thrill of the erotic.

Task/subject: Excitement and stimulation; basis of the clitoral orgasm, the "penis" of the woman (also from an evolutionary point of view).

Archetypal principle: Venus-Mars.

Coccyx

(Os coccygis, see also Spinal column)

Symbolic meaning: Vestige of evolution, last remnant of the tail of vertebrates; in humans, now simply acts as bony marker of the floor of the pelvis, like a bony spur in the soft tissue; lowest point of the pelvis, connection to the Earth (root chakra, àchakras); at risk in the event of falling backwards, (pain-)sensitive shock-absorber: falling on one's rear = symbol for a crash landing, which indicates that something fundamental in life is not in order.

Task/subject: Protecting the contents of the pelvic bowl; marking the end of the spinal column.

Archetypal principle: Pluto.

Connective tissue

Symbolic meaning: Connection, stability, binding nature in contrast to the specific functional tissue of the organs; basic system (of vegetative regulation).

Task/subject: Giving form (to the organs, the face, the body), ensuring interconnectedness; fatty and bone tissue also form part of the connective tissue: storing energy (fat), providing a good hold (bones).

Archetypal principle: Mercury-Saturn.

Constitution

Symbolic meaning: 1. General: material framework of life, basic endowment with which one is sent into life; 2. Leptosome (asthenic): taut, tough, emaciated, capable of holding out, resilient, ascetic, hard; modern figure ideal; can eat without putting on weight; constitution which makes one "look old", "bean-pole"; 3. Athletic: sporty, strong, sleek, fit, powerful, attractive, manly, broad shoulders for leaning on, strong legs for a firm stand in life, hands-on approach, broad back which can carry (bear) a great deal; 4. Endomorphic: small, roundish, "having things pretty cushy"; efficient food utiliser, can build up plenty of (flesh) from a few (calories); "pot-belly", "Buddha belly", earlier an advantage in times of scarcity, today a disadvantage in times of abundance;

agile, nimble (good dancer), cosy and comfortable.

Task/subject: 1. Making the best out of the given potentials that one has brought along into life, grasping the opportunities; giving form and stature to one's plans, ideas and objectives; 2. Giving up everything superfluous, casting off ballast, gaining structure, getting to the core of one's own being, concentration on the essential, realising the art of life (ascesis from Greek askein = 'to do something conscientiously'); 3. Facing life, bearing the burden of life, mastering great tasks, grasping life firmly, giving those weaker than oneself a leg up, protecting them; 4. Becoming inwardly well-rounded, turning life into a well-rounded affair; showing level-headedness, deriving strength from calmness.
Archetypal principle: 1. and 2. Saturn; 3. Mars; 4. Sun, Moon.

Costal pleura

(Pleura)
Symbolic meaning: Outer lining of the lungs; the cloth in which the lobes of the lung are wrapped, and which lines the inner surface of the rib cage; simultaneously a tensioning framework and envelope; support and boundary for our wing-like lobes.
Task/subject: Enveloping and keeping open the contact organ of the lungs by means of low pressure in the pleural cavity between the lungs and ribs; ability to glide smoothly, adaptability in the area of communication.
Archetypal principle: Mercury.

Cruciate ligaments

(see also Knee, Knee joint)
Symbolic meaning: Bands (àLigaments) which keep the knee in order by holding the structures in their correct place; they guide the bones, thereby enabling them to work together properly; securing the

connection between the past, tradition (thigh) and one's own path, individuation (calf).
Task/subject: Stabilising and guiding the knee; mediation between the strongest structures of the body.
Archetypal principle: Mercury.

D

Diaphragm

(Greek: 'partition, barrier')
Symbolic meaning: Bellows (of the lungs), border (between the upper and middle world), mediation between conscious exchange (upper body) and unconscious processing (lower body); (in earlier times:) seat of the soul; home of the breath.
Task/subject: Executive rhythm organ; separation of the upper male (air, fire) and lower female half of the body (water, digestive juices); mediation between anima and animus.
Archetypal principle: Mercury (connection) Sun (centre), Moon (resonance).

Digestive organs

Symbolic meaning: Consuming and digesting the world (Buddhism: Bhoga).
Task/subject: Absorbing and processing the material world; processing the karmic fruits, which ripen in our consciousness.
Archetypal principle: Moon (stomach)-Mercury (small intestine)-Pluto (large intestine and rectum).

Dreams

Symbolic meaning: Worlds of spiritual imagery as a balancing factor to rational, waking imagery.

Duodenum

Task/subject: Balance between Archetypal masculine and feminine forces; keeping life in balance; giving time and space to the mystical essence of the shadow kingdom and its themes, e.g. Nemesis (retribution) and the Furies (revenge), the Muses (Fate and Shadow in the form of nightmares) and Cupris (desire, longing).
Archetypal principle:
Moon-Neptune.

Duodenum

see Small intestine

E

Ears

Symbolic meaning: Hearing – paying attention – listening to (obeying) commands; more important than eyes/vision (deafness is more difficult to bear than blindness); the outer ears are passive receiving organs that are always at the ready; telescopic antennae for the external environment, our showpiece feature; the outer ear acts as a mandala and is the external manifestation of the inner mandala - the cochlea; carrier of reflex zones which reflect the whole person, and in this way, enable therapeutic access to him or her; size as an indication of the orientation of the person towards the outside (large ears) or the inside (small ears).
Task/subject: Letting in; hearing, paying attention, integrating the outside world at the vibrational level, listening to (obeying) commands; humility; listening in-depth to the roots of life; resonating in synch, empathy; "There are none so deaf as those who will not hear"; combining the inner and the outer, the microcosm and the macrocosm (reflex zones) and bringing them into balance; bringing the inner and outer worlds into harmony with each other and making them resonate in synch; given that it is closely connected with the àorgan of equilibrium, the ear possesses the same function.
Archetypal principle: Moon-Saturn.

Ear (shape)

Symbolic meaning: 1. Large, sticking out: strong orientation towards the outside world, eager to receive signals; large reflex zone maps; healthy self-confidence, which is put to the test by the symptom ("bat ears", "jug ears" or "Dumbo ears" as a reason for teasing); well-developed logical thinking, imagination and self-control; low level of access to feelings; good stamina and forceful self-assertion, measuring up well to the world;
2. Small: attention directed inwards, less interest in the outside world, introverted; tendency towards simple, less differentiated views of the world, uncomplicated conceptions of life;
3. Angular, pointed: having sharp contours, being on one's guard with pricked ears (suspecting evil), difficult relationship with God and the world (Mephisto's ears are normally depicted as pointed); sharp and angular, being hard on oneself and the world, quick to take offence, objectionable, finding rough edges and sharp corners everywhere;
4. Extremely rounded: rich inner life, attractive aura (anima), well-rounded personality;
5. Large earlobes: sign of advanced development and maturity (see Buddha illustrations, ears of old people); idealistic attitude with the tendency towards being visionary, but often an unrealistic view of the world; thinking in pictures, transcendental experience;

6. Small earlobes: rationality-based, well-connected to reality, interested in the things of this world, level-headed, objective, results-orientated, geared towards control;

7. Attached earlobes: intensification of small ear lobes, extremely rational level-headedness, control, protection, straightforwardness, mechanical thinking and experience.

Task/subject: 1. Being open to everything, growing and showing that one is able to measure up to the world;

2. Making the most of one's talents, exploring the inner world and finding a home in it; experiencing calm and fulfilment in oneself; starting off small in the outside world;

3. Getting to know and accept one's own "snags and catches"; helping oneself in order to be able to help others later; being careful and attentive ("pricking up one's ears"); airing secrets;

4. Using the mandala in the ear as a signpost towards the realisation of completeness;

5. Developing one's personality in the spiritual sense; taking one's own visions for real and sign-ificant, bringing illuminating (transfiguring) magic into the cold, rational world;

6. Getting closer to the world by objective means, natural science as a task and opportunity;

7. Learning to truly understand the physical world, then using objective methods to turn one's attention to what cannot be truly grasped.

Archetypal principle: 1. Jupiter; 2. Moon; 3. Saturn-Pluto; 4. Sun; 5. Neptune; 6. Mercury; 7. Virgo-Mercury.

Elbow

(see also Joints)
Symbolic meaning: Willingness to be assertive: "elbowing one's way through life", capacity for perseverance: "using elbow grease", ability to put up a fight: "using one's elbows", "making some elbow-room", "giving and getting the elbow" in a dog-eat-dog society.

Task/subject: Setting all levers in motion; forceful assertion, making room and space for oneself, helping to push through one's own ideas, demonstration of power.

Archetypal principle: Mars.

Elbow (crook of)

Symbolic meaning: Flipside of the à elbow: Region of great sensitivity.

Task/subject: Signalling openness and receptiveness/devotion; offers the opportunity for taking blood, since the blood vessels in this region lie gently embedded directly below the surface.

Archetypal principle: Venus.

Electrolyte

see Salt

Endomorphic type

see Constitution

Epididymis

(Greek: 'on the testicles')
Symbolic meaning: Reservoir of male fertility; masculine maturity.

Task/subject: Storing the semen before it begins its journey.

Archetypal principle: Pluto.

Epiglottis

(Greek: upon the tongue)
Symbolic meaning: The switching point between the respiratory and alimentary tracts.

Task/subject: Prevents us taking things the wrong way; keeps food well awayfrom the passageways of the lungs (otherwise danger of àaspiration pneumonia)

Archetypal principle:
Mercury-Saturn

Epiphysis

see Pineal gland

Epithelium corpuscles

see Parathyroid glands

Erogenous zones

(Clit/clitoris, labia, glans, back of the penis, nipples, perineum region, neck, inner sides of the upper thighs and upper arms)
Symbolic meaning: Desire; erotic playgrounds and fields, pleasure gardens of the body, arousal zones.
Task/subject: Conveying and feeling desire, ensuring procreation.
Archetypal principle: Venus.

Erythrocytes

(red blood corpuscles; see also Blood)
Symbolic meaning: Energy-carrier of the life flow.
Task/subject: Conveyance/transport of oxygen and Prana (life force).
Archetypal principle: Mars.

Extremities

see Limbs

Eyes

Symbolic meaning: Insight, perspective: "a real eyeopener", "seeing through something", "seeing the light"; outlook, windows; mirrors and lights of the soul; entrance and exit of the spiritual world: "a soulful look"; starry eyes (sparkling vitality): "a gleam/twinkle in one's eye"; determining the field of view: "a bird's eye view", "a worm's eye view", "out of the corner of one's eye", "eyes in the back of one's head"; active sense, making eye contact: "giving someone the eye", "catching someone's eye", "making eyes at someone"; the evil eye: "if looks could kill", "looking daggers at someone"; fixing one's eyes on something; eyeing someone up and down: "feasting one's eyes upon something", "to only have eyes for", "eyes glued on something"; overlooking something (an oversight): "being blinded by something", "having the wool pulled over one's eyes"; being alert: "keeping one's eyes open", "keeping an eye on/out for something", "all eyes on something"; rejection: "turning a blind eye to something", "being blinkered"; third eye = sixth chakra ("Ajna"): the second face.
Task/subject: Allowing in impressions, letting out feelings and moods, reflecting feelings, expressing spiritual proximity and distance; perceiving the world; practising intensive, close eye contact: looking each other in the eye, looking deep into someone's eyes as the windows of the soul; seeing in the sense of gathering information; looking in the sense of looking inward in order to obtain visions (the outer sight and the inner insight).
Archetypal principle: Sun (Goethe: "If the eye were not Sun-like, it could not see the sun ..."); Moon (mirror of the soul) – in women: right eye = Moon; left eye = Sun; the reverse in men.

Eyebrows

Symbolic meaning: The headline for the eyes; expression.
Task/subject: Essential "performance organs" of the intuitive, natural and consciously-used facial expressions, emotional expression; protection of the look-out point (the eyes) against wetness or too much light; frames the eyes.

24

Archetypal principle: Saturn-Venus.

Eyebrow (shape)

Symbolic meaning: 1. Highly-arched curve: astonishment, surprise, amazement; childlike openness, sensitive, vulnerable;
2. Straight lines: neutrality, patient and careful, hesitant, often sluggish;
3. Double curve: torn to and fro, up and down mood swings, restless, fickle, unbalanced; often exaggerated, violent reactions;
4. Deep-set: primitive power; overshadowing, sad; lurking, intense, sinister expression
5. Joined in the middle: here "there is something brewing" (danger of a fit of temper), great concentration, creative thinking, impressive, intensive;
6. Long curves, well-formed: buoyant spirit, cheerful disposition, successful balance between body and soul, inner joyfulness;
7. Short: good self-confidence, great vitality, decisive, proceeding by the most direct route;
8. Thick: powerful, vital, resilient; overshadowed view with the danger of being blind to one's own faults;
9. Bushy: resilient, robust constitution; wild, uncultivated growth of thoughts, creativity; danger of losing perspective in the jungle;
10. Thin, only hinted at: dispassionate, lacking self-assertion, "not having the hang of something", unable to get into the swing, often in the case of severe candidamycosis, frequently with leprosy;
11. Steeply sloping: often direct access to intuition, tendency towards unreasonableness;
12. Sharply angled: vital, hungry for experience, not wanting to miss anything, interested in everything; danger of a lopsided, rough-edged life.
Task/subject: 1. Transforming vulnerability into sensitivity, learning self-criticism, "getting the hang of things", successfully negotiating a difficult bend in the road, preserving the wonderment of childhood;
2. Finding the direct, straight path;
3. Getting into the swing of things, consciously integrating the ups and downs into the flow of life, finding a balance;
4. Coming to terms with one's own dark aspects, living intensely, waiting for favourable opportunities;
5. Concentration on essential things such as the centre of life;
6. Achieving harmony, "getting the hang of things", getting into the swing of life;
7. finding a close connection to oneself, using self-confidence for self-realisation;
8. Remaining true to oneself, finding one's own way and following it with perseverance and strength;
9. Developing one's own views, going one's own way, striving for creative points of view and solutions; sticking to one's own primitiveness in the sense of atavism (Latin atavus = 'ancestor, forebear'; recurrence of anatomical features which were typical of forebears): staying in touch with one's own past (with one's ancestors);
10. Beginning in a small way, taking small steps ("less is more"), finding the way back into one's own life;
11. Developing gut feelings and turning them into a constructive force for oneself;
12. Devoting oneself consciously to life; omitting nothing, but addressing everything.
Archetypal principle: 1. Moon; 2. Saturn; 3. Uranus; 4. Pluto; 5. Saturn; 6. Jupiter; 7. Mars; 8. Saturn, Mars; 9. Uranus; 10. Moon-Saturn; 11. Neptune; 12. Jupiter-Uranus.

Eye colour

Symbolic meaning: 1. Brown: Great unfathomable depth; mysterious and inscrutable, and therefore unpredictable; hidden passion, emotional outbursts; introverted, withdrawn, often strongly connected to nature, down-to-earth with a rich emotional world; genetically dominant over the other colours;

2. Blue: rare and precious, baby-blue eyes; blue-eyed innocence, naivety, credibility; open and expansive, looking deep (into the windows of the soul); open-minded, generous and happy-go-lucky like "Hans in Luck" from the Brothers Grimm fairytale, "The Fool" of the Tarot; colour of loyalty (true-blue) and the sky, devoted love and chastity;

3. Green: rare, fascinating, "cat's-eyes"; reflect the green force Viriditas; sensual, passionate, capable of inspiration and rapid transformation, tendency to mood fluctuations, distance from prosaic reason and logic; the colour of faith, belief and fertility;

4. Grey: rare; the colour of age ("old and grey"); colourless, undifferentiated ("all cats are grey in the dark"), condition between life (white) and death (black); shy of contact, distanced (grey eminence); depression, sadness: "seeing everything as grey and drab".

Task/subject: 1. Exploring the unfathomed depths of one's own soul, reconciling oneself with one's own feelings and passions;

2. Awakening the inner child, seeing the world with the wondering eyes of childhood;

3. Actively pursuing openness for development and transformation; exploiting the possibilities of one's own sensuality and passion;

4. Simply becoming, learning to be al(l)-one, recognising the state of being alone as an opportunity to be a(l)l -one with oneself, transforming knowledge into wisdom.

Archetypal principle: 1. Pluto; 2. Moon; 3. Pluto; 4. Saturn.

Eyelids

Symbolic meaning: 1. General: the curtains of the soul;

2. Drooping: concealing oneself behind curtains, avoiding eye contact, blocking the view into the soul, sleepy or introverted "droopy eyes", isolation; expression of immersion (in Buddha); as a disease symptom of myasthenia gravis;

3. Puffy: tear-stained look, something is making one want to cry;

Task/subject: 1. Protection for the eyes against drying out, external force or injury and too much light (dimming or darkening effect), regulation of the amount of light and information that is let in depending on the state of consciousness; closed eyelids indicate withdrawal into the inner world, open eyelids indicate openness and receptiveness;

2. Granting oneself times of withdrawal, clarifying and enjoying one's own inner life, regeneration, navel-gazing, meditative immersion;

3. Examining why one is holding back the tears; crying one's eyes out, bringing one's emotional life into flow.

Archetypal principle: 1. Sun/Moon-Saturn; 2. Neptune; 3. Moon.

Eye teeth

see Teeth

F

Face

Symbolic meaning: Identifying mark, calling card, self-expression (direct or feigned mimicry), individuality; stage for non-verbal communication; barometer for moods (from the "honest face" to the "poker-face"); honesty, showplace for emotions; façade, mask; centre of perception; open eyes indicate openness, closed eyes the opposite, drooping eyelids reveal fatigue (sleepy, let-me-go-back-to-bed look or bedroom eyes can tempt in that direction), squinting eyes stand for exertion and self-denial; a high forehead reveals intellectuality (receding hairline); the size of the mouth reveals the degree of maturity , i.e. ability to speak for oneself or the "big mouth"; the lips express sensuality, the teeth vitality; the nose reveals the phallic powers, the chin willpower; the lines and wrinkles are honest markings of the passage of time.

Task/subject: Image, reputation and appearance: "saving face" or "losing face"; making contact, expression/ masking of moods: pulling faces; "showing one's true face", "grinning and bearing things", "having a face like a wet weekend", "making/pulling a long face", "getting a slap in the face", "saying something to someone's face"; taking for real (perception): spotting, sniffing out, catching wind of.

Archetypal principle: Sun (self-expression), Moon (moods), Venus (beauty, façade).

Face (shape)

Symbolic meaning: 1. Round(ish): Friendly, fetching, "all-round satisfaction", granting oneself things; honesty, empathy and sympathy; rich sensual life, often with mood swings; "Moon-faced": indistinct, soft contours, harmless and unaggressive-looking; childlike-female Moonlike radiant auru; a "Moon-face" as the extreme, tendency to smile and bring a smile to others

2. Angular: self-control, decisiveness, harshness; energetic, uncompromising and without frills, reserved, cool;
3. Broad: open, soft aura (anima); material dominance, (sometimes

clumsy) realistic, practical, successful, enthusiastic;
4. Narrow, long: wistful, fragile; "steeple face", distance from life, danger of a life spent in the ivory tower;
5. High cheekbones: typical of faces concealing a soul looking outwards that tends more towards melancholy; hard contours reflect hardships suffered, expression full of suffering: common beauty ideal today (in trying times?).

Task/subject: 1. Making one's own life more complete and harmonious; allowing the inner woman (anima) to blossom, letting the inner child live freely;
2. Giving life (sharp) contours and a clear profile; acting consistently, developing directness, deliberately setting limits, asserting oneself energetically;
3. Building on the broad foundations of one's own possibilities, developing a fruitful relationship between rationality and emotions;
4. Consciously maintaining distance from detrimental things;
5. Standing by what one has undergone, and facing up to the moment; facing up to hardship and suffering as an opportunity to grow in general and grow beyond one's boundaries.

Archetypal principle: 1. Moon, Sun; Moon-Venus (Moon-faced); 2. Mars; 3. Jupiter; 4. Uranus; 5. Saturn.

Facial nerve

see Nervus facialis

Fallopian tubes

Symbolic meaning: Fertility; as the muscular connection between the ovaries (depot) and womb (nest), an active "message in a bottle" system; the first slide in life.

Task/subject: Transport (peristalsis) of the egg under its own muscle power, conveyance of fertility.

Archetypal principle: Mercury
(transport) Moon (fertility).

Fascia

Symbolic meaning: The sensitive
outer lining of the muscles.
Task/subject: Protection and cohesion of the mechanical power gener-
ators of the body; giving stability and
elasticity and ensuring that the muscles glide smoothly when functioning
together
Archetypal principle: Saturn.

Fatty tissue

Symbolic meaning: Excess, reserve;
storage form with the highest calorific
value of all energy-providers, today
due to excess availability has fallen
significantly in estimation.
Task/subject: Soft shaping (e.g.
in the face), cushioning, (heat)
insulation, being overweight as a
modern-day social isolation topic;
protective layer; carrying weight
(importance).
Archetypal principle:
Jupiter-Venus-Moon.

Fetlock

see Ankle joint

Fingers

(see also the individual fingers)
Symbolic meaning: Dexterity, getting a grip on the world, grasping, the
subtle touch in relation to feelings.
Task/subject: Grabbing hold:
"twisting someone around one's little
finger", "having a finger in every pie",
"touching on a sore point", "getting
one's hands dirty for someone";
manual work (from writing to sewing
and shaking hands) but also: "keeping one's fingers out of something",
"not lifting a finger", "getting a rap
across the knuckles", "getting one's
fingers burnt"; cheating in the sense

of manipulating: "having someone in
the palm of one's hand", "playing into
somebody's hands", "sleight of hand"
Archetypal principle: Mercury.

Finger (shape)

(see also Hand shape)
Symbolic meaning: 1. Long:
elegant, fine, graceful, beautiful;
"long-fingered" is however also associated with thieving, being artful and
capable of manipulation: "twisting
someone around one's little finger";
2. Short, thick: pragmatic, direct,
uncomplicated; "stubby fingers" are
considered inelegant and clumsy;
3. Bent: one-sided use of the hands,
wanting too much, letting go of too
little, "getting one's hooks into something", "being involved in crooked
dealings".
Task/subject: 1. Getting to grips with
life with elegance and skill, expressing gracefulness, beauty and meaningful topics (mudras);
2. Letting things function "like clock-
work"with emphasis and energy,
generosity and smoothness;
3. Taking what one needs; finding the
right balance between tension and
release.
Archetypal principle: 1. Mercury-Mercury; 2. Mercury-Jupiter; 3.
Mercury-Saturn.

Fingernails

(see also Toenails)
Symbolic meaning: Claws, our aggressive legacy, tools of aggression
("showing one's claws", wildcat);
bringing out the animal in ourselves;
our origins.
Task/subject: The struggle of life
("clawing one's way to the top");
expressing aggression ("showing
one's claws", "sharpening one's
claws"); greed ("getting one's claws
into something"); red (polished) claws
reveal vitality and enthusiasm (blood
still staining the claws?): such wild

(or predatory) cats scare off those with an anxious disposition, but magically attract courageous partners (for the battle of the sexes); setting boundaries.
Archetypal principle: Mars (Aggression) / Saturn (Halt).

Fingertips

Symbolic meaning: Antenna tips, the subtle touch (instinctive feeling).
Task/subject: Feeling one's way through the world, or not ("keeping one's fingers out of something"); finding one's bearings in sensitive areas; gathering erotic experiences: caressing, perceiving, stimulating.
Archetypal principle: Mercury (finding one's bearings)-Neptune (perceiving by means of instinctive feeling).

Foot / feet

Symbolic meaning: Own standpoints, understanding; standing firm, steadfastness, steadiness, withstanding; humility; roots, deep-rootedness, basis of life, being down-to-earth, contact to Mother Earth or the opposite: having no vibrant contact to the ground, becoming anxious, being unable to defend one's standpoint or maintain one's position ("pulling the rug out from under somebody's feet", "trampling all over someone or something", "getting cold feet", "getting one's feet wet").
Task/subject: walking the Earth, getting a foothold in life: "standing on one's own two feet", "stepping out in style"; sense of reality, putting forward standpoints, "landing on one's feet"; working from the opposite pole: "lying at someone's feet"; defining social hierarchy by the feet: being a "boot-licker" or "trampling" on others, "fighting tooth and nail"; hen-pecked husbands are right at the bottom, the victor who places his foot on the neck of the vanquished right at the top; trophy-hunters strike a pose by placing

their foot on their quarry; but also gestures of humility: "throwing oneself at somebody's feet", foot-washing; allowing in the love of the mother (Earth).
Archetypal principle: Neptune (our "fins").

Foot (arch)

Symbolic meaning: Being human, double arch (lengthwise and transverse arch), on which our being human is based; unique in Creation (in contrast to the cerebrum); basis of orientation upwards to the heavens, longing for greater overcoming of gravity (rising up into free space towards spiritual freedom); take-off point for all (large and small) leaps.
Task/subject: Has enabled (since time immemorial) the standing erect on our hind legs and walking upright; orientation from above to below: man between Heaven and Earth; provides elasticity when walking: basis for harmonious steps forward (progress).
Archetypal principle: Uranus (leap)-Jupiter (arch, bridge).

Foot (shape)

Symbolic meaning: 1. Broad: broad standpoints, realistic stance, down-to-earth;
2. Small, narrow: considered decorative (in women), are more like "fins", and thus more suitable for swimming than for deep-rootedness; in dreamers with high-flying fantasies (i.e. in those with more connection to water and air than to the Earth), tendency to lift off, becoming "rooted" in transcendental areas; lacking grounding, nimble and agile; often as a compensation for energetically putting oneself forward; in men an expression of too little staying power;
3. Large: good staying power, being wasteful: "stepping out in style", the grand entrance, making broad tracks, archetypally more fitting for men;

danger of "getting too big for one's boots" and "overstepping the mark"
4. Unkempt: having too little respect for one's own roots, neglect of one's own origins; no cultivated basis for life.
Task/subject: 1. Striving to broaden standpoints, be grounded and deeply-rooted;
2. Putting down roots in the heavens, focusing on the spiritual way;
3. Standing firmly on one's own two feet, developing standpoints and stability, learning to make a good entrance, doing great things, making an impression; keeping pace with spiritual development; stepping in for oneself and stepping forward; becoming magnanimous;
4. Becoming more easy-going (reconciling oneself) with issues such as homeland, deep-rootedness, being down-to-earth.
Archetypal principle: 1. Neptune; 2. Neptune-Moon; 3. Neptune-Jupiter; 4. Neptune.

Forearms

(see also Arms)
Symbolic meaning: Leverage power, "levering someone out of the running"; "forcing the world closer"
Task/subject: Holding (tight); bringing the world closer; facilitating; capacity to act.
Archetypal principle: Mercury.

Forehead

Symbolic meaning: Target surface which we offer to life for any attacks, the battlefront and forefront; confrontation (Latin frons = 'forehead'), "affronting somebody", "having the front to do or say something", "ramming one's head against the wall"; "putting on a brave front"; spiritual strength.
Task/subject: Heading, confronting, being at the forefront; protective shield behind which the process of thought takes place.

Archetypal principle: Mars (front)-Uranus (connection to Heaven).

Forehead (shape)

Symbolic meaning: 1. High: "lofty brow", guided by reason, objective, unprejudiced; thought and action guided by clear understanding;
2. Narrow: single-minded thinking, narrowly-defined view of the world, danger of one-sidedness and fanaticism;
3. Domed: Thinking needs a great deal of space (that is quite over the top); extremely good imaginative powers, grand (overflowing) imagination;
4. Sloping: archaic visage, the original man, "primitive" aura (anima), intellectually "challenged", but in return more in connection with the world of emotions and feelings (middle brain) and basic survival instincts (brain stem);
5. Smooth, unlined: happy, carefree, youthful appearance, life has left no marks behind, smooth mask (as if "putting on a front" and "acting the innocent"), an unlived life, not allowing anything to get close and affect one , lack of life experiences;
6. Vertical lines: "worry lines", the seriousness of life is "written on one's face";
7. Vertical and horizontal lines: bearing the cross of life on one's forehead, being cross with oneself; feeling crushed and crumpled, dissatisfaction, thwarted hopes, marked by life.
Task/subject: 1. Taking thought to a high level, allowing the spirit to dominate over matter, philosophy as the love of wisdom;
2. Going about things in a concentrated way; thinking through narrow, restricted domains exhaustively (specialisation)

3. Allowing room for the imagination, letting it grow; giving expression to the world of spiritual imagery;
4. Living out primal themes, e.g. feelings and emotions; developing a survival personality;
5. Cultivating straightforward, clear thinking, enjoying the youthful aura (anima), allowing oneself to be touched emotionally, getting in contact with the inner child;
6. Facing the responsibility of life consistently and seriously;
7. Taking up one's cross; making one's mark.
Archetypal principle: 1. Mercury-Jupiter; 2. Virgo-Mercury; 3. Mercury; 4. Pluto; 5. Moon; 6. and 7. Saturn.

Foreskin

Symbolic meaning: Curtain in front of the spear-point.
Task/subject: Protecting, maintaining sensitivity.
Archetypal principle: Mars-Saturn.

Frontal sinuses

see Sinuses

G

Gall bladder

Symbolic meaning: Refined aggression (bile acids): "feeling the bile rising", congealed bitterness: "spitting poison and bile", "bilious humour"; transformation; in Traditional Chinese Medicine: the "Official of Decision Making"; origin of the courage to make decisions; Assignments: Yang, element - wood, complementary to the liver (Yin).
Task/subject: Aggressive breakdown, separation from each other, deciding (from Latin dēcīdere to

cut off); aggression not as a frontal attack, but as soft soaping; digestion of fat: taming, soft soaping, absorbing the fat; taming of the lavish and excessive; getting excess under control; smooth refinement and transformation that is hidden in the background; enjoying the abundance, spice and luxury of life with gusto; pouring turbulent, wild aggression into cultivated forms. For cholerics (Greek. cholé = bile, aírein = rising up): letting the life energy flow in a fiery and spontaneous manner, letting enthusiasm run free; for melancholics (Greek. mélas = black, cholé = bile): extolling the beauty of human life and suffering.
Archetypal principle: Pluto-Mars.

Ganglia

(Nerves)
Symbolic meaning: Local communication node points.
Task/subject: Gathering local information, bundling it and passing it on according to the principle of "all or nothing".
Archetypal principle: Mercury-Uranus.

Glands

(see also the individual glands)
Symbolic meaning: Control, information.
Task/subject: Self-regulation, adapting one's own performance to the needs of the complete organism; production of messenger substances.
Archetypal principle: Mercury.

Glans

Symbolic meaning: Warhead of the male weapon, spearhead of masculinity; point of maximum male sensuality and stimulation.
Task/subject: Piercing, penetrating, forcing one's way through; sensing, feeling, conveying desire.
Archetypal principle: Mars (spearhead) Venus (sensuality).

Granulocytes

(fraction of the white blood corpuscles; see also Leukocytes, Blood)
Symbolic meaning: Non-specific defensive troops, general military units and stand-by police force of the body.
Task/subject: Standing up to, hindering and containing intruders, preventing them from multiplying and eventually destroying them.
Archetypal principle: Mars.

Groin

Symbolic meaning: Inner courtyard of the intimate sexual region; softness; vulnerability (large blood vessels directly under the surface), sensitivity.
Task/subject: Connection of the lower body and lower extremities; limitation of physical load-bearing capacities.
Archetypal principle: Moon-Venus.

Gullet

(Pharynx)
Symbolic meaning: Incorporating (possession), swallowing (a company); being tight, miserly; biting off more than one can chew (choking); (lymphatic) defensive ring.
Task/subject: Taking in, embodying; fending off (enemies).
Archetypal principle: Venus-Pluto.

Gums

Symbolic meaning: Cradle of the weapons, bed of the teeth; basic trust.
Task/subject: Ensuring stability and supply; regeneration of the aggression tools.
Archetypal principle: Moon.

H

Hair

see also Beard, Body hair
Symbolic meaning: Power of representation, freedom (hippies, Musical Hair); vitality, carefreeness: "not letting things give you grey hair", "letting one's hair down", "a hair-raising adventure" that "stretches" the truth; primeval, untamed strength (Samson); beauty, grace, charisma; outward perception: antennae; power: "getting in each other's hair", "having someone by the short hairs", "losing fur in the fray"; fear: "one's hair stands on end", "tearing one's hair out", "one's hair bristles"; wishes that are continually growing, but which can also be cut back down to size; women tend to conceal their ears (the organs of listening carefully and obeying) under their hair, hippies also did the same intentionally; for soldiers, it is forbidden: they must keep their ears and chin (will, assertion) free, and can at most conceal their sensuality (lips) behind a beard (moustache); over-refined perception: "splitting hairs", "finding a hair in one's soup".
Task/subject: Reflecting strength and radiance; representing the right to freedom; demonstrating power, dignity and strength; expressing one's rights; conveying beauty; antennae towards the outside.
Archetypal principle: Uranus (freedom), Sun (strength [Samson]), Venus (beauty).

Hair (colour)

Symbolic meaning: 1. Blond: easily impressed, sensitive, sympathetic, childlike, naive ("dumb blondes" and "blond jokes"), innocent and pure; "bright" (clever, alert), hair colour of heroes and princesses; for genetic reasons, blonde hair will become rarer and rarer;

2. Red: signal colour, indicator of danger, the fiery redhead (e.g. Anne of Green Gables); in the Middle Ages, especially in Germanic culture, red hair was seen as the mark of a witch; passionate, emotional, impressionable, often unforgiving, seductive, extrasensory abilities energetic, adventurous, hot-headed ("Irish") temperament;

3. Black: racy, southern, passionate temperament ("Latin lover"), "femme fatale", high capacity for enthusiasm, often with a tendency to the fanatical and lyrical; exotic beauty, dark secrets;

4. Brown, brunette: flexibility, adaptability and versatility; active, energetic and enterprising; closeness to nature;

5. Grey: loss of vitality, regeneration capacity and differentiation ("all cats are grey in the dark"), "looking old", "being colourless"; growing old gracefully, silver hair;

6. White: gleaming wreath which crowns the head; distinction, wisdom of old age, experience of life, at peace with oneself, closeness to God (white is the colour which contains everything, which has integrated all else – this is also the claim on old age).

Task/subject: 1. Turning impressionability into sensibility and cultivating this (to the point of sensitivity); experiencing the exceptional, distinguishing oneself;

2. Experiencing emotion passionately and passion emotionally, allowing oneself to be impressed by life, standing out positively and strikingly, accepting the distinction and living up to it;

3. Inspiring and thrilling, standing up for one's ideals, experiencing and enjoying passion;

4. Finding one's momentum and living it; choosing activities which promote life; engaging in undertakings that are worthwhile in the long term;

5. Addressing the themes of old age and death and reconciling oneself with them; maturing, becoming wise, incorporating (life) experience, earning respect for oneself, taking advantage of the charm of greying temples (in the "mature man");

6. Unfolding the golden halo of the thousand-leafed lotus (supreme "Sahasrara" or Crown chakra) and finding self-actualisation, being one with the divine, becoming wise, coming to rest, following the higher will.

Archetypal principle: 1. Moon; 2. Mars; 3. Pluto; 4. Mercury; 5. and 6. Saturn.

Hair (texture/form)

Symbolic meaning: 1. Smooth: directness, predictability; in combination with a parting: love of order; in the case of a central parting: balance;

2. Curly: enticing wildness, confusing diversity; desire to go one's own way, to slip into other roles; creative spiritual life, rousing feelings and emotions; twirling and whirling of many things, unconventional, crazy ideas ("woolly hair – woolly thinking");

3. Thick: vitality, "wild (lion's) mane", power, passion, beauty, spiritual connection;

4. Thin: weakness, reserve, deficiency, "plucked chicken", stage of building up or breaking down processes (in young children and old people).

Task/subject: 1. Ensuring clear relationships, taking the direct route, putting one's own world in order;

2. Following the winding paths of one's own vitality, giving in to temptation (entanglements); being tempted/entangled (by life) and roping others in to live out their own originality;

3. Using one's strength sensibly, being productive, solving "hairy matters";

4. Homeopathic approach: withdrawing oneself, drawing in the antennae,

thinking carefully about oneself, withholding oneself with regard to the anima; allopathic approach: gradually and cautiously trusting oneself to develop one's anima; becoming grown up, connecting oneself to the divine energy, taking up one's place, asserting oneself.

Archetypal principle: 1. Virgo-Mercury, Saturn; 2. Venus-Mars; 3. Sun; 4. Saturn.

Hands

Symbolic meaning: 1. General: taking possession and grasping: "laying one's hands on something", "holding out one's hands", "being left empty-handed"; tenderness: "by a fair hand", "asking for someone's hand in marriage", "hand in hand for life", "being in good hands", "eating out of the palm of someone's hand"; protection and assistance: "offering a helping hand", "many hands make light work", "working hand in glove"; manipulation (Latin manus = 'hand'): "one hand washes the other", "underhanded", "having one's hands in the till" (being corrupt); intellectual abilities: "having all the trumps in one's hand", picking up on suggestions and ideas, "knowing something like the back of one's hand", "with a steady hand"; grasping and letting go; "first-hand knowledge", "tangible information" that is readily "at hand"; ability to handle things; hands as the most important tools (giving and taking): "taking something in hand", goods "change hands" as part of a business deal; basis for communication by gestures, gesticulation; conciliatory welcoming gestures: giving someone one's hand; to express deference: kissing the hand or back of someone's hand; honesty: "open-handed", "at first hand", "washing one's hands of something", "sealing a promise with a handshake"; expressing aggression: "coming to blows" (taking

the law into one's own hands), "mishandling (someone or something)"; demonstration of force: clenched fist, losing control and "raising one's hand against someone", "having the upper hand", "having a hand in something"; the hands carry out what the head has decided to do; activity: "coming to grips" with life, "not sitting on one's hands", handling things.

2. Left hand: allocated to the female archetype; the more passive hand, often associated with greater creativity and non-conformity, thus producing success more easily and with less effort, the left comes from the heart (from the domain of feeling); left-handedness.

3. Right hand: allocated to the male archetype; the more powerful, more active; here everything "goes right" and follows the right path, although in a more strenuous, laborious, time-consuming and less inspiring way than something done in the more creative and non-conformist left-handed way; right-handedness.

Task/subject: 1. Recognition, learning; communication, contact; dexterity, manipulation; giving signs and devotion; focussing on and questioning how one handles things;

2. Taking things on board, getting things flowing;

3. Exercising power, dedicating oneself to the "right" path, being righteous.

Archetypal principle: 1. Mercury; 2. Moon; 3. Sun.

Hand (shape)

(see also Finger shape)

Symbolic meaning: 1. Delicate, slim: elegance, empathy, the fine touch (sensitivity), hands "of the finer folk" (hands of a lady), attractive, enchanting;

2. Large, powerful: paws for grasping and holding firm (men's hands),

taking life "in one's hands", having "a grip on things";

3. Hairy: archaic, animalistic, masculine, "a hairy affair";

4. Unkempt: uncultivated handling of the world, "impurities".

Task/subject: 1. Realising beauty, acting with cautiousness, cultivating sensitivity;

2. Getting a grip on life, steering the ship of life with confidence, putting one's own stamp on life;

3. Keeping the archaic, primordial demands of life in mind, acting straightforwardly and directly, reflecting on one's origins and instincts, trusting in one's own primitive strength;

4. Becoming aware of the dirt in other essential (mercurial) areas of life, such as the intellectual world rather than the domain of hygiene and becoming calmer and more relaxed about it.

Archetypal principle: 1. Venus; 2. Mars; 3. Pluto; 4. Mercury-Pluto.

Hand surfaces

Symbolic meaning: Sense of touch; honesty, openness; bowl of neediness (one cups one's hands to receive); readiness to offer and to give gifts (outstretched hands form a kind of offering plate).

Task/subject: Handling things: healing with the hands and dispensing blessing; expression; communication coming from the heart: "extending the hand of friendship to someone", "holding someone's hand"; map of life in the lines of the hand.

Archetypal principle: Mercury-Moon (map of the soul).

Head

Symbolic meaning: Capital city of the body, the head or chief aspect, personal globe of the microcosm, supreme authority for the bodily institutions (also at the highest point outwardly), opposing pole of the body (top – bottom); home of mind, reason and thought: "a mastermind", "a brilliant mind", "keeping a cool head", "turning somebody's head"; the neck and sometimes the (passionate) heart determine in what way the (cool) head sits on the shoulders; (self-)expression; arrogance: "striding with one's head held high", "being stuck up" (in earlier times, it was considered impolite to look one's betters directly in the face); the bearing of the head reveals the person who is straightforward; the slightly-inclined head is a request for indulgence and lenience, fawning favour.

Task/subject: Control of life; expression of mood: "hanging one's head", "burying one's head in the sand", "pulling in one's head", "ducking"; (self-)assertion: "keeping one's head held high", "Chin up!", "not letting others bring one down"; forceful assertion: facing things "head-on" and being "headstrong" or even "pigheaded", "having a mind of one's own", "being in over one's head" or "unable to keep one's head above water", "putting someone's nose out of joint", "giving someone a piece of one's mind", "leading someone around by the nose"; overview, orientation: "not knowing where one's head is"; "not having one's head screwed on right", "not getting one's head around something"; command and control; sensitive warning of problematic attitudes ("ramming one's head into a brick wall") and dangerously one-sided thinking ("racking one's brains", "my head is throbbing") due to high pain sensitivity, but also in the case of mental underachievement and blockage (a dull headache, being a "blockhead").

Archetypal principle: Mars (Lancepoint of the body)-Sun (head)-Uranus (close to Heaven)-Mercury (function).

Head (shape)

Symbolic meaning:
1. Accentuation of the forehead and the rear area of the skull: spiritual tendencies in the foreground;
2. Accentuation of the front facial area: worldly ambitions such as enjoyment and the striving for power in the foreground;
3. Large: personality, leadership strength, forward thinker ("a great mind"), superiority, power, inflated importance ("big-headed"), forceful assertion ("having a thick skull");
4. Small: in this case, although a small head still occupies the top position, the body aspect is more in the foreground; a smaller housing ("marble") and correspondingly smaller brain, the world of ideas takes a back seat to the physical sphere; reduction; concentration on the essential with regard to the spiritual sphere;
5. Round: a well-rounded affair, sociable, unselfish, altruistic, helpful, able to make decisions;
6. Square: burly, "blockhead", off-centre in life, rigid thinking, having "rough edges and sharp corners", mentally stonewalling, strong-willed, having strong assertiveness and decisiveness;
7. Triangular: accentuation of the brain part of the skull and thus thinking ability, common sense, diplomatic aptitude;
8. Oval: good balance, well-rounded personality; flexible, creative spirit, enjoys life; often finds it difficult to take criticism;
9. Trapezoid (more angular at the top, with broad head becoming even broader at the bottom, often with "hamster cheeks"): material considerations in the foreground; hands-on, assimilating; practical, results-orientated thinking, very little reference to theory, often successful;
10. Pronounced back of the head: caput musicalis –believed to indicate 'a head for music', ideal of the Egyptians (Nefertiti), "high-minded"(aesthetically and spiritually), intelligence, connection to higher things, fashionable profile (in older times, the back of the head was accentuated by bun hairstyles; nowadays by teasing, beehive hairstyles, etc.);
11. Flat back of the head: shallow thinking, pragmatism.

Task/subject: 1. Developing spirituality and intellectuality;
2. Knowing one's own mind in creating material abundance;
3. Developing expansive thoughts, making headway mentally and spiritually in a broad and dignified way, attributing importance to oneself;
4. Being selective ("small, but effective"), self-effacing;
5. Letting one's own life become well-rounded, making the mandala form into a symbol for one's life; becoming the sun for oneself and others;
6. Giving life contours and a clear profile, becoming a liberated, lateral thinker, bringing one's own will into harmony with the will of God;
7. Giving precedence to reason, developing aptitude; think first, then act;
8. Bringing the poles together, finding balance in life, learning to understand criticism as an opportunity to become even more well-rounded;
9. Experiencing external demands from the inside out as well; incorporating fulfilment in fullness, finding meaning and content in the form;
10. Fostering musical talents, training fine-matter perception, looking across into the other dimension;
11. Meaningfully shaping what is close at hand.

Archetypal principle: 1. Mercury; 2. Mars; 3. Sun; 4. Moon; 5. Sun; 6. Saturn; 7. Mercury; 8. Venus; 9. Jupiter; 10. Venus-Neptune; 11. Mercury.

Hearing

see Ears

Heart

Symbolic meaning: Seat of the soul, source of the life energy; centre of the human being, energetic focal point (of life); cardinal point which represents the unity/the divinity in us; centre of our existence, gateway out of polarity into unity; centre and starting point of (capacity for) love and emotions, home of feelings and fears: "one's heart skips a beat, stands still or sinks like a stone and is in one's boots" or "one feels one's heart in one's mouth", place of the deepest feelings, barometer of the emotions: "not taking things to heart", "opening one's heart", "wearing one's heart on one's sleeve", "doing something with a heavy heart"; highest sensory organ: "the heart rules the head", "a heart-to-heart conversation", "listening to one's heart", "following one's heart", "having one's heart in the right place"; heart tissue as prime example for co-operative behaviour, resonance; bravery, generosity, courage (lion-heart); I-identity; in Traditional Chinese Medicine: the "Emperor"; the heart exercises the directing, controlling effect on all the other organs ("Minister" and "Official"); Assignments: Yang, element - fire, emotion – joy, complementary to the small intestine (Yin).
Task/subject: Love and unity; expressing matters of the heart: "opening/giving one's heart freely"; perceiving and allowing in the central themes of life ("taking something to heart"); willingness to absorb: "being all heart" and approaching life "whole-heartedly"; to develop oneself; to pass from duality to unity; keeping the life energy (blood) in flow; controlling the rhythm of life.
Archetypal principle: Sun.

Heart valves

Symbolic meaning: Outlets of the life flow and stream of energy.
Task/subject: Giving direction and order to the flow of the life energy, making connections between the different chambers of the heart.
Archetypal principle: Sun-Mercury.

Heel

(see also Achilles tendon)
Symbolic meaning: Classical weak point (Achilles heel); most vulnerable point for seduction (snake-bite), and in keeping with this, represents the bond to Earth and a greater distance from spirit and spirituality (man is drawn back to Earth, although he wants to enter Heaven): Point of conflict between upward-striving consciousness and the downward pull of unconsciousness (high heels as an attempt - at least outwardly - to elevate oneself above polarity with elegance).
Task/subject: Most intensive connection with Mother Earth, point of contact and conflict between the unity of Paradise and earthly polarity, entry portal for unhappiness as an expression of polarity (the serpent is said to have followed on the heels of Eve and her daughters; at Christ's crucifixion, one of the nails went through the heel bone).
Archetypal principle: Neptune-Saturn.

Hips / hip joints

(see also Pelvis, Joints)
Symbolic meaning: Stepping out, taking the first steps, moving forward; radius of action, range; the swing of life (swing of the hips).
Task/subject: Basis of stepping out; home of our steps, both the steps forward and upward in small and large matters, in good just as in evil; basis of the outer and inner journeys; stepping out and overstepping (exaggeration, over-indulgence); ensuring that things run smoothly.
Archetypal principle: Jupiter.

Hormones

(see also Neurotransmitters)
Symbolic meaning: Messenger(substances) of the body, mediators.
Task/subject: General: mediation between the various entities of the organism, between control and execution levels; Special: Melatonin: the chief of the hormones, is produced at night by the pineal gland (epiphysis) (when it is dark and the digestive tract is at rest; is therefore disturbed by late eating, light in the bedroom and electro-smog); is responsible for the day-night rhythm; promotes the production of growth hormone (HGH) and the neurotransmitter serotonin; inhibits the sex hormones. Growth hormone (HGH = Human Growth Hormone): stimulates all growth processes, feels as wonderful as growth naturally does; disturbed by everything which inhibits melatonin production (light, late meals, electro-smog). Thyroid gland hormones: bring the metabolism up to speed, "firing up". Female sex hormones (Oestrogen [the most female of the female hormones], gestagen [opposing substance for oestrogen: the "male" amongst the female hormones], oxytocin [the bonding hormone, which is stimulated through breast-feeding/ sucking]): such hormones promote gender-specific female behaviour, control all "female" bodily processes from menstruation to pregnancy. Male sex hormones (Androgens, e.g. testosterone): promote gender-specific male behaviour, control the "male" bodily processes from erection to semen production.
Archetypal principle: (Hormones in general) Mercury.

Hypophysis

see Pituitary gland

Hypothalamus

Symbolic meaning: Subordinate seat of government in the upper house (centre of the vegetative nervous system, supraordinate to the hormone brain of the pituitary gland, directly subordinate to the central government).
Task/subject: Co-ordination of the visceral nervous system and involuntary processes, the nerve impulses and the hormone levels.
Archetypal principle: Mercury.

I

Ileum

see Small intestine

Immune system

Symbolic meaning: Defence, resistance.
Task/subject: Defence against external "enemies", handling conflicts using militant measures (àantibodies).
Archetypal principle: Mars.

Incisor teeth

see Teeth

Index finger

(see also Finger)
Symbolic meaning: Pointer (shows the direction and the way to go); finger for giving instructions, but also for attributing guilt or blame, know-it-all finger (putting one's hand up in school); the Jupiter finger.
Task/subject: Orientation (the raised index finger loves lecturing, but pointing at others with the index finger is poor manners, and is correctly interpreted by others in an Archetypal sense, namely as aggressive [Mars]).

Archetypal principle: Mercury-Jupiter.

Intervertebral discs

Symbolic meaning: Female pole of the spinal column (soft discs between hard vertebrae).
Task/subject: Cushioning of stresses ("soft landing"), shock-absorbers; flexibility.
Archetypal principle: Moon-Saturn.

Intestines

(Intestinum; see also Large intestine; Small intestine)
Symbolic meaning: Labyrinth system of the body for the processing of material impressions (in contrast to the brain labyrinth of the head for the processing of immaterial impressions).
Task/subject: Absorption, breakdown and assimilation (acceptance) of the material world as a requirement for its transformation into the body's own tissue and energy; ability to make something out of it for oneself; absorbing what is essential for life, letting go of what is superfluous.
Archetypal principle: Mercury (small intestine), Pluto (large intestine).

Iris

(Iris = In Greek mythology, the personification of the rainbow and goddess of mediation and peace, who like Hermes has access to all kingdoms: the underworld [Hades], the human world, the water world [Poseidon], and the divine world [Olympus]).
Symbolic meaning: Shutter of our camera - the eye; Ring mandala, which gives the eye its colour and adds depth to the mirror of the soul; Atlas of the organs (iris diagnosis).
Task/subject: Regulating the amount of (en)light(enment) which reaches our inner being.

Archetypal principle: Mercury-Sun/Moon.

J

Jaw

(see also Upper jaw, Lower jaw, Chin)
Symbolic meaning: The upper jaw stands for the higher instincts that drive mankind, but also for one's (family) origin, the lower jaw for the lower instincts and the individual; in this respect, often unconscious conflicts between tradition and individuation; jaw problems often correspond to generation problems.
Task/subject: Mediation between the higher and lower instincts/drives of mankind and also between the generations.
Archetypal principle: Mars.

Jejunum

see Small intestine

Joints

(see also Elbow, Ankle joint, Wrist joint, Hips/hip joints, Mandibular joint, Knee joint, Shoulder joint)
Symbolic meaning: Mobility, articulation, standing for connections in life (from the earliest connections to those with other family members and on to those of later life, e.g. professional and social), expression of togetherness in life.
Task/subject: Ensuring connections (to God and the world, to family members and other members of society); mediation between the inner and outer world; bringing in the world, and bringing people into the world; conveying flexibility in dealing with one's own environment, enabling dexterity; expression.

Archetypal principle: Mercury.

Joints (inner sides)

Symbolic meaning: When shown (outwards) they reveal openness, the feeling of security and trust, the need for contact, but also vulnerability (the armpit, crook of the elbow, for example, are only offered in situations of trust).
Task/subject: Attracting, using one's own vulnerability as a form of appeal, defencelessness.

Joints (outer sides)

Symbolic meaning: When shown (outwards) they reveal uncommunicativeness, withdrawal into oneself, lack of need for contact (e.g. folded arms).
Task/subject: Protection (e.g. knee-cap), distancing.

K

Kidneys

Symbolic meaning: Balance and partner(ship) organs.
Task/subject: Preserving the balance between acidic (male) and basic (female) forces, thereby creating harmony between the male and female poles; level control between the extremes in order to find the centre between the poles; balancing out differences, harmonising differences/contrasts; contact with other people as a confrontation with the unconscious spiritual aspect = shadow; filtering; wholeness; in Traditional Chinese Medicine: responsible for the first potentialisation of strength and willpower; governing birth and growth, reproduction and development in general; seat of the inborn Qi, material basis, constitution; Assignments:

Yin, element - water, emotion - fear/fright, complementary to the àurinary bladder.
Archetypal principle: Venus.

Knee

Symbolic meaning: Humility, knees as a worldwide gesture of humility: the curtsey to royalty, genuflecting in church, "falling to one's knees"; humiliation: "bringing someone to their knees", "putting somebody over one's knees", "a knee-jerk reaction" is one that does not pay the respect of devoting enough time or thought to the affair at hand; expression of fear: going weak at the knees, shaky knees; defence: pointed knees as if on guard; meeting point of inherent (hereditary) powers in the shape of the upper thigh and self-developed powers in the lower leg (knee joint, cruciate ligaments, meniscus).
Task/subject: By kneeling, one shows one's superiors the honour due to them, by making oneself smaller; expressing honour and reverence (towards God and previously the [divine] King); lowering oneself to Mother Earth; expressing acknowledgement of the hierarchy with regard to God; learning humility (prominent life task in the case of protruding, thick knees); pointed knees: developing the ability to defend oneself.
Archetypal principle: Saturn.

Knee joint

(see also Joints, Meniscus, Cruciate ligaments)
Symbolic meaning: Meeting point of the strongest bones/structures in our life: the thigh bone (femur), the shin bone (tibia) and the calf bone (fibula) (àlegs are responsible for one's path in life, the subject is successfully moving forward); sensitive point of contact optimised by means of padded discs (menisci); the family bonds and one's own path to individuation

correspond at the symbolic level to these strongest structures and forces in life; they meet in concrete terms at the knee, and make it a critical, often neuralgic point: the knee joint as the connection between the traditional way of one's forebears and one's own attitude to life, which must both be in harmony in order to support us along our path in life; establishing the ideal connection between both of these demands amongst other things a great deal of humility, and can bring one to one's knees or force one to one's knees.

Task/subject: Creating connections, bridging the generations, finding one's (own) path between the present and one's ancestors.

Archetypal principle: Saturn.

L

Labia

(see also Vulva)

Symbolic meaning: The outer gates to the sexual inner world.

Task/subject: Outer labia: outer shutters of the sexual world; inner labia: inner shutters.

Archetypal principle: Pluto-Venus.

Large intestine

Symbolic meaning: Unconscious; underworld, kingdom of shadows and of the dead, the dark, nocturnal side, Hades (Greek: "shameful secretiveness" but also "shameless exposure") of the body; treasure chamber of matter; greed; in Traditional Chinese Medicine: "Minister of Excretion"; Assignments: Yin, element - metal, complementary to the lungs (Yang).

Task/subject: Giving and presenting (excrement = money); creating life (vitamin production by means of the

intestinal flora); letting go of the old (both in material and unconscious terms) and of matter in general; overall handling of material things: generosity and greed; conversion and transformation (metamorphosis): "Death and rebirth" (Goethe); the mysteries of waste removal; Blind gut (caecum) = cul-de-sac of the past (from the early days of evolution); Vermiform (from Latin:worm-shaped) appendix = the cul-de-sac of the cul-de-sac.

Archetypal principle: Pluto.

Larynx

Symbolic meaning: Expression; home of speech and song; musical instrument of the body, conveys the vibe (tone/mood) through its vibrations (voice); male accessory in the form of the Adam's apple; breathing.

Task/subject: Creation of tone (mood) and expression.

Archetypal principle: Venus-Mercury.

Legs

Symbolic meaning: (Path of) movement, mobility; development and progress in life: "getting a leg on", "being knocked/run off one's feet", "being on one's last legs", "standing or falling on something" (=being a success or failure); getting ahead: "getting a leg up"; standing firm: "standing one's ground", "standing up to/up for/by something or someone"; self-reliance: "standing on one's own two feet"; stability: "long-standing"; upright attitude: a man of good "standing" "having high standards", "not having a leg to stand on"; power to stand up and stand out: "standing tall", "standing head and shoulders above the rest"; being hindered "standing in the way of", "a ball and chain" (= a hindrance to one's progress from the practice of tying these to the legs of prisoners to prevent escape)

Task/subject: Showing "how things stand"; contact with the ground, demonstrating staying power; carrying on through life, getting ahead, progressing; standing firm; withstanding: standing the test of time, understanding, standing behind someone/something, standing out; taking the path of necessary changes; demonstrating the ability to stand alone and know what you stand for.

Archetypal principle: Mars-Jupiter.

Leg (shape)

Symbolic meaning: 1. Thick: firm, supporting columns, demonstration of stability and strength, plodding attitude to life, problems with one's position/stance; clumsy, ungainly impression;

2. Thin: weak position, unsteady standpoints, weak, poorly-supported position/stance;

3. Muscular: self-assured position, strong stance, steadfast and well-founded standpoints;

4. Knock-knees: tangled, unable and/or unwilling to get one's knees apart; closed lap, protecting and concealing the intimate areas, making them unreachable;

5. Bow legs: Open stance, cocky; stalking in boldly like a rider who still appears to be straddling a horse when walking; looking for stability.

Task/subject: 1. Generating greater internal stability, steadfastness and security; devoting energy to determining one's position; taking a stance and defending one's standpoints, finding one's life focus, becoming more down-to-earth;

2. Relying on agility, striving for flexibility, staying in the flow;

3. Standing behind one's own standpoints and putting them forward enthusiastically, upholding one's positions, withstanding stresses, being

able to stand on one's own two feet, stepping out boldly;

4. ensuring a self-contained, closed personality in the extended sense of complete and coherent; giving oneself time and space to develop inner balance;

5. Finding a good foothold, being able to actually fill the "cowboy boots", letting life in, proactively providing substance to back up the flaunted openness.

Archetypal principle: 1. Jupiter; 2. Mercury; 3. Mars; 4. Saturn; 5. Jupiter.

Leptosome type

see Constitution

Leukocytes

see Granulocytes

Ligaments

(see also Cruciate ligaments, Tendons)

Symbolic meaning: Connections, anchoring cords, cohesion.

Task/subject: Holding up (supporting) and holding out (bearing), holding together the structures of the body; conversion of one's own powers and energies into practical form; prevention of physical desires that are too extreme.

Archetypal principle: Mercury.

Limbs

(Extremities; see also Arms, Legs)

Symbolic meaning: Mobility, activity; extensions towards the outside.

Task/subject: the upper extremities bring the world closer or help us to set out limits from it; the lower extremities bring people into the world or keep them out of it; Extremities bring the extreme within reach.

Archetypal principle: Mercury, Mars.

Limbic system

(Main component of the brain stem controlling the thalamus, hypothalamus and pituitary gland)

Symbolic meaning: emotional brain (in animals, the largest and most important part of the brain; in humans, exceeded by the cerebrum, although not actually sub-ordinate to it, and instead more co-ordinate with it).

Task/subject: Supraordinate centre of the entire vegetative-nervous and hormonal regulation systems; monitoring and control of the so-called primitive bodily functions (such as breathing, digestion, etc.), which nevertheless form the basis of life; processing and co-ordination of signals from within the body with those of the outer world.

Archetypal principle: Mercury-Moon.

Lips

Symbolic meaning: Sensuality (tasting, caressing and kissing); turning the inner apects to the outside (the "inner" mucous membrane becomes visible to the outside world); upper lip = mental and spiritual disposition, the characteristics inherited from one's ancestors; lower lip = sensuality, the self-created situation; full lips = vital sensuality; thin lips = calculating intellect; hard lips = hard, demanding character; soft, moist lips = capacity for giving oneself completely, soft and gentle character.

Task/subject: Forming speech ("giving someone lip" or "risking a fat lip"); sensual communication; sensual contact with food (tasting) and other lips (kissing).

Archetypal principle: Moon-Venus.

Liquor cerebrospinalis

see Cerebral fluid

Little finger

(see also Finger)

Symbolic meaning: Benjamin (son of joy) amongst the fingers; its relative position shows how one feels about oneself; the "cocked" little finger stands for coquetry/affectation, the expression of a particularly demanding and high-handed/pretentious nature; a long nail on one's little finger in China reveals a person who does not need to work.

Task/subject: Sensing, conveying; the outer and most sensitive antenna of the hand; completes the hand.

Archetypal principle: Mercury-Mercury.

Liver

Symbolic meaning: Closely connected with life (as reflected in the name liver), the condition of the liver answers the question: "How do I handle my life?"; rebirth of new life; the immortal liver in mythology: the eagle eats it every day, and during the night, it grows back again (Prometheus, Loki), reflected medically in the liver's ability to recover even after long toxic excesses; the liver also re-grows completely when parts have been removed by operation; evaluation, philosophy of life, (re-) connection downwards (to the beginning, origin) and upwards (meaningfulness); laboratory; substance abuse as the eternal search for substance in life; in Traditional Chinese Medicine: the "Commander", who is responsible for deliberations and plans; Assignments: Yang, element - wood, emotion - anger/rage (colloquially "having a shitty liver"), complementary to the gall bladder (Yin).

Task/subject: Differentiation and evaluation; re-connection to the source, the original form of life - re-ligio(n); finding the right measure and the sense in life; spiritual synthesis: breaking down foreign protein

43

and building up one's own ("being constructive"), making the fatty (excessively rich) digestible; detoxifying; producer/barometer of moods, whereby this does not so much refer to one's personal mood, but instead to whether there is an overall sense and purpose in one's life, and to its basic characteristics and temperament (choleric, melancholic, sanguine, phlegmatic; the 14th Tarot card "Temperance" embodies the most essential liver subject – moderation): the melancholic has more than just "a shitty liver", the choleric tends to spit "poison and bile"; bile (Latin chola) = digestive juice produced in the laboratory of the liver; as the producer of bile, the liver is also involved in the expression of aggression "having the gall to do something"; seat of resentment and revulsion: "looking a little green around the gills".
Archetypal principle: Jupiter.

Lower jaw

(see also Chin)
Symbolic meaning: Weapons store, movable home and base for our lower weapons (the teeth); as the basis for the chin, expression of will (to power) and (power of) forcful assertion.
Task/subject: Makes chewing possible since the upper jaw is fixed; gives us bite: "biting off something", "gritting one's teeth and biting one's way through life"; also facilitates digestion by means of chewing; holding on to what has been captured and allowing the trap to finally snap shut.
Archetypal principle: Mars-Saturn.

Lower leg

Symbolic meaning: Take-off power; tensioning force, elasticity; one's own strength on the (development) path; spontaneity ("always ready to spring into action"); security vault for emotional over-tension; connection of the ankle muscles to the heel via the Achilles tendon; calf muscles connect the second-strongest muscles via the strongest ligament to the most sensitive point (bite of the snake, Achilles heel); thick calves: always ready to make the leap, waiting for the right moment for take-off, trudging through life with many emotions.
Task/subject: Getting the (right) boost, demonstrating readiness to make the leap; expressing unacknowledged overloading; bringing about (sudden) changes; storing up emotions; thick "stompers" (thick calves and ankles): stepping out boldly, pushing through one's own will, assuming firm standpoints.
Archetypal principle: Uranus-Mars.

Lumbar vertebrae

(see also Spinal column)
Symbolic meaning: Carrying (bearing) the main burden of life; double burden: stability and mobility, which simultaneously emphasises the dynamic and flexible aspect of the vertebrae (Latin vert(ere) = 'to turn') as opposed to the static aspect of the spinal column; problem zone of the world axis (over 95% of all slipped/herniated discs occur in this area), where conflicts between the lower pelvic impulses (urges) and upper impulses (heart, head) manifest themselves.
Task/subject: Carrying and bearing: bearing weight and (existential) responsibility, carrying one's cross; carrying the upper body through life; connection of the sacred basis (àSacrum/Os sacrum)
Archetypal principle: Jupiter.

Lung

Symbolic meaning: Connection of the inner tree of the lungs with the external trees that we are connected to as part of the cycle of respiration; contact, communication, exchange (speech = modulation of the flow of breath); breathing in: inviting life into oneself; breathing out: giving something back to life (carbon dioxide as nutrition for green vegetation); freedom, being able to breathe (deeply) and freely; lightness: the wing-like lobes of the lungs turn us into winged beings, allowing us to resemble the angels (life was breathed into us by the divine breath); in Traditional Chinese Medicine: the "Minister" subordinate to the "Emperor" (heart), which is responsible for rhythmic order and respiration, and which rules the Qi; also referred to as the "Father"; Assignments: Yin, element - metal, emotion - sadness/resignation, complementary to the à large intestine (Yang).

Task/subject: Establishing and maintaining contact with the outside world, gas exchange: harmonising giving and taking; connecting the "Self" to the non-"Self", relationship; the second most important contact organ after the skin; breathing as the umbilical cord to life; connection between all living beings: we all breathe the same air.

Archetypal principle: Mercury.

Lymph nodes

(formerly: Lymph glands; see also Axillary glands)

Symbolic meaning: Police stations of the body.

Task/subject: Stationed within the lymph flow, they filter (monitor) the flow, constantly on the lookout for unauthorised intruders; maintaining order at the regional level: first line of defence against enemies; the àlymphocytes formed in these nodes attack all foreign bodies: follow-up care and differentiation of the impressions which were allowed in too deeply and too quickly.

Archetypal principle: Mars-Saturn.

Lymph system

Symbolic meaning: Third vascular system of the organism; return transport to the heart; cleansing of the tissue by flushing things out: àlymphocytes (= policemen) are swept along with the flow to the lymph stations (Latin lympha = 'water').

Task/subject: In combination with the veins, functions as the return flow system for larger molecules (fat, protein); the main vessel: the thoracic duct is the largest lymph vessel and the main return transport route for fat and blood plasma.

Archetypal principle: Mercury-Moon.

Lymphocytes

(fraction of the white blood corpuscles; see also Granulocytes, Blood) Interpretation: Elite troops, special units for combatting enemies.

Task/subject: Combatting and elimination of specific, identified enemies in kamikaze style; principle of self-sacrifice.

Archetypal principle: Mars-Pluto.

M

Mammary glands

see Breast, female

Mandibular joint

(see also Upper jaw, Lower jaw, Chin, Joints)

Symbolic meaning: Here the claims to power of our ancestors meet with our own, the past and present come together, clash of the generations.

Task/subject: Mediation between the higher and lower instincts/drives of mankind and also between the generations; bringing both into harmony with each other.

Archetypal principle: Mercury-Mars.

Maxillary sinus

(see also Sinuses)

Symbolic meaning: Lightness and airiness of the head; shaping element.

Task/subject: Lightening the load of the head (physically and mentally); loosening up the hard, fixed bone structure; bringing the air element into the earth element; making it easier to bear the load of the head; it is only the lightness of being that enables us to buoyantly strive towards higher spiritual planes (for anthroposophists the maxillary sinus, is associated with the seat of consciousness); moistening and warming the breath in preparation for communication with the outer world; resonance base for the voice (nasal voice if the sinuses or nose are blocked); shaping of the individual face.

Archetypal principle: Uranus.

Member

see Penis

Meninges

see Cerebral membranes; Spinal cord membranes

Meniscus

Symbolic meaning: Padded disc in the àknee joint; buffer between the thigh (family tradition) and the calf (one's own path), often worn down by over-exertion.

Task/subject: producing a binding connection; cushioning against impacts, balancing, enabling easy, gliding motion.

Archetypal principle: Mercury.

Meridians

(Network of pathways or fine-matter energy vessels, known as nadis in Indian medicine, which connect together all parts of the body; basis of Chinese energy medicine, particularly acupuncture. This network consists of 12 main channels, which are assigned to and correspond to the 6 Yin functional circuits [lung, spleen, heart, kidneys, liver, pericardial sac/pericardium] and the 6 Yang functional circuits [large intestine, stomach, small intestine, bladder, gall bladder, triple heater]. There are also 8 extraordinary pathways, as well as many small auxiliary pathways in net formation.

Symbolic meaning: Fine-matter energy pathways which ensure continual circulation and make the body into an integrated whole instead of a series of independent structures.

Task/subject: Energy co-ordination and control of the body and its organs; maintenance of the energy balance; according to the traditional Taoist concept, man stands between Heaven and Earth: his physical structure with all its functions is (similar to the Hermetic philosophy) a reflection of the macrocosm.

Archetypal principle: Neptune-Mercury.

Middle finger

(see also Finger)

Symbolic meaning: Amongst the four fingers, the finger that stands out, the central column; shows one's own personality and its objectives, but is also the finger we stick up to make rude gestures, thus indicating boundaries.

Task/subject: Leadership of the four fingers.

Archetypal principle: Mercury-Saturn.

Molars

see Teeth

Mound of Venus

Symbolic meaning: Sexuality; gentle mound of desire, which rises up over the pubic bone and is covered by the triangle of pubic hair.
Task/subject: Protecting and concealing the entrance to the "palaces of one's sexual energies (animus and anima)"; veiling yet enticing: the mound wants to be climbed and conquered.
Archetypal principle: Venus.

Mouth

Symbolic meaning: Sphere of enjoyment (orality of psychoanalysis): assimilation; communication; central organ for the expression of body language: kissing and pouting; a straight or crooked mouth reveals "straight" or "crooked" intentions; sexuality (parallels between top and bottom in colloquial language): lips as a symbol of sensuality, the object of one's "all consuming" passion is "dishy" or "good enough to eat"; maturity, i.e. ability to speak for oneself;: "having a quick tongue", "opening one's big mouth", "keeping one's mouth shut" or "running off at the mouth about others", "getting a smack in the mouth", "standing around gawking with one's mouth agape"; gateway for speech; entrance (and exit) to the world of the body.
Task/subject: Absorption and expression.
Archetypal principle: Moon (absorption), Mercury (articulation), Venus (form, function).

Mouth (shape)

Symbolic meaning: 1. Large: broad, expansive emotional life, enables seductive laughing; full, curvaceous lips: luxuriant sensuality; friendliness, lovableness, empathy, understanding; but also being a "big mouth", "biting off more than one can chew", ("giving someone lip" or "risking a fat lip"), "talking big" or "shooting one's mouth off";
2. Small: expressing oneself very little, holding back feelings; rational, often shy, reserved and withdrawn; lack of enjoyment of life; with small creases and as if sewn shut: suppressing self-expression, forbidding oneself the right to speak; small, pursed, heart-shaped lips like those on a china doll: in keeping with their sweet, feminine-childlike nature, popular with women but frowned upon by men; little claim to verbal expression; in contrast to the "big mouth", has a discreet, modest, rather amiable aura; even today, still the make-up model/ideal of many (generally more conservative) women; in the past, when women were not allowed to have their say and for the most part had to keep their mouth shut, it was the ultimate ideal (e.g. the geisha); the small, kissable mouth, which was intended to reduce women to this aspect; this is, however, going out of fashion; today female mouths are made larger with the aid of lipstick, collagen and tattooing;
3. Downturned corners of the mouth: seriousness, mistrust, resignation, depression, being a sourpuss; result of experiences dragging them down, unresolved issues; fending off the world arrogantly, scornfully, and haughtily or letting it simply run off "like water off a duck's back";
4. Upturned corners of the mouth: uplifted mood, cheerfulness, joy, love of life, permanent optimism (dolphin's grin), grinning and bearing things; inviting in and accommodating the world.
Task/subject: 1. Expressing, thinking, feeling and achieving great things; celebrating feasts of the senses;
2. Expressing oneself with care; keeping oneself withdrawn, exercising caution when opening one's mouth;

consciously becoming a more expressive person;

3. Honestly taking stock, accepting the status quo; coming to terms with unresolved sadness, unacknowledged disappointments; confronting and questioning one's own arrogance;

4. Letting the smile also spread to the eyes and heart; passing on the uplifted mood.

Archetypal principle: 1. Venus-Jupiter; 2. Moon-Venus; 3. Saturn; 4. Jupiter.

Mucous membranes

Symbolic meaning: Protective lining, inner boundary, second threshold to the inside: barrier between the inner world that we show the outside world and our real inner world; absorption membrane; mucous as a symbol of fertility.

Task/subject: Protection of the organs, producing lubricant (mucous); conveying inner exchange, regulating the flow, absorbing; creating a viable environment for life.

Archetypal principle: Moon.

Musculature

Symbolic meaning: Dynamism, life force, the body's motors (development of power); polarity: building up and releasing tension.

Task/subject: Conquering the outside world by means of an antagonistic mode of operation; activity, mobility, flexibility (adaptation to the outside world); defence in the physical and spiritual area (muscle-based armour, armouring of one's personality in the chest area also created through muscle mass).

Archetypal principle: Mars.

N

Nails

see Fingernails, Toenails

Navel

see Bellybutton

Neck

Symbolic meaning: Assimilation of possessions; connection, communication and passageway between top and bottom, between rationality (head) and feeling/emotion (stomach/chest); rotation and pivot point (basis) of the "head" (=main) issues; elegance (of the swan-neck); location of fear/anxiety in the body (fear causes the throat to constrict).

Task/subject: Assimilation: the insatiable greed of the miser who can never seem to get his fill; cut-throat (= profiteer), "being up to one's neck in debt", "forcing something down someone's throat"; expression of (mortal) fear, fear = tightness: "feeling one's heart in one's throat", "being up to one's neck in problems", "having one's neck on the line", "having someone breathing down your neck", or "a millstone around one's neck"; "going for someone's throat" or "wringing someone's neck"; creating clarity and overview through the possibility of different viewpoints, expanding the spiritual horizon, being able to observe something from all sides, "putting someone's head straight"; pride; grace; obstinacy, stubbornness; infatuation: "turning someone's head (and thus also the neck)", "throwing oneself around someone's neck"; the inside of the neck as a place of defence (Waldeyer's tonsillar ring, tonsils): "screaming one's tonsils

out", "being fed up to the back teeth with something".
Archetypal principle: Venus (assimilation, beauty, connection), Saturn (restricting fear/tightness), Mercury (mobility).

Neck (back of)

Symbolic meaning: Connection between top and bottom; place of power and iron will: this is where the yoke (of the ox) rests; place for breaking somebody's will: serfs wore a heavy ring around their neck; the rabbit punch (so-called because hunters use a similar technique to kill rabbits) involves a quick, sharp blow to the back of the neck as do the executioner's axe and the guillotine, which are both intended to break the will of the condemned forever; if someone is "breathing down our neck", it becomes threatening; place of hard-headedness: always keeping one's head up is tiring, both for the will and also for the neck muscles; anyone who lets their head droop, however, becomes hard-headed, because this also overtaxes the neck muscles; at the same time, a place of great sensibility, sensuality and tenderness: neck massage (caressing someone's neck), necking; being bothered by someone who is "a pain in the neck"; bull-neck (combination of strong, broad and short neck): being rigid, strong-willed and stubborn in order to "ram one's head through the wall"; possessing great strength; cushioning the most sensitive point and protecting oneself against further blows to the neck and back.
Task/subject: Upholding one's head (main) focus; protecting the data highway (spinal column); in the case of bull-necks: "dragging the cart out of the mire" (sorting out the mess).
Archetypal principle: Venus-Saturn.

Neck (shape)

Symbolic meaning: 1. Thick: greed, "insatiability"- never being able to get one's fill (àPart 2, double chin);
2. Scrawny: bottleneck, neediness, deficiency; highly vulnerable, sensitive, often even spiritually endangered (bad connection between centre and torso);
3. Wrinkly: "old-looking", haggard, exhausted, used-up;
4. Long: grace, elegance ("swan-neck"); outstanding position, but also pride and arrogance, "ivory tower", "long pipeline".
Task/subject: 1. Taking what one needs; looking after oneself well, ensuring reliable, stable connections between the centre and the body;
2. Applying wise restrictions, making a choice, no longer letting everything in;
3. Reducing spiritual demands and material needs;
4. Regarding one's own assets as gifts and coming to terms with them inwardly; in the case of a long pipeline, taking the necessary time and carefully and considerately creating harmony with oneself and the demands on one, allowing development to take place gradually (at one's own pace); in the case of low day-to-day suitability, carefully making the daily routine into a ritual, raising oneself above it; however, not arrogantly, but with modesty and humility.
Archetypal principle: 1. Mars (assertion)-Jupiter (abundance); 2. and 3. Saturn; 4. Venus.

Nervous system (general)

Symbolic meaning: Telecommunications system of the body, news service.
Task/subject: Communication in a multi-dimensional system: conveying, controlling, regulating, checking;

creating electro-chemical connections, passing on news; connection between awareness and the body; voluntary nervous system: agent for fulfilling the requirements of conscious will and sensation (the new, "human" nervous system); involuntary nervous system (visceral nervous system, parasympathicus, sympathicus): executive organ of unconscious action, reflexes (the old, "animal" nervous system).
Archetypal principle: Mercury.

Nervus facialis

(facial nerve)
Symbolic meaning: Expression of mood and identity, stages the world of emotions on the face; individuality.
Task/subject: Facial expressions which show different faces.

Nervus opticus

(optic nerve)
Symbolic meaning: interactive light channel, insight, clear-sightedness; vulnerable to attack in the context of a destructive world view/destructive thoughts with regard to one's own world, which are frequently based on fear.
Task/subject: Mediation between light stimulation and inner images, which we then think of as outer images; perception (taking for real) of the outer, visible world.

Nervus statoacusticus

(acoustic and balance nerve)
Symbolic meaning: Interactive telephone line, cable of the balance sensor.
Task/subject: Conveying balance and hearing, finding the physical (spiritual) centre; enabling the hearing of commands (obedience).

Neurotransmitters

Symbolic meaning: General: messenger substances between the structures of the nervous system; conveyance of news within the body's terrain; more specifically: Adrenalin (also epinephrine): hormone formed in the adrenal medulla and secreted in stress situations; causes the organism to "step on the gas" so that it can survive in dangerous situations. Noradrenalin: hormone that is (chemically) similar to adrenalin, formed in the adrenal medulla and in the sympathetic nervous system; acts primarily on the arteries of the body circulation, increases the blood pressure by raising the peripheral resistance (without increasing the volume per minute), reduction of the pulse rate. Serotonin: is built up in the central nervous system, in the lungs, spleen and intestinal mucous membranes from the amino-acid L-tryptophan and stored in the nerves and in blood platelets (thrombocytes) and mast cells; a balanced or slightly-elevated serotonin level creates well-being and a feeling of satisfaction to the point of ecstasy and rapture ("the happy hormone"); is also actively reabsorbed into the nerve cells (membrane transport) and reused (modern anti-depressants, the selective serotonin resorption inhibitors, such as Prozac/ Fluctin, inhibit this active resorption); acts in the lungs and kidneys to restrict the vessels, but also, on the other hand, to enlarge them in the skeletal musculature; has a polarising and therefore inhibiting effect on the membranes of nerve cells; depression, bipolar and anxiety disorders are probably accompanied by a lack of serotonin in the brain; the symptoms of these disorders are relieved by an increased serotonin level; influences sexuality by conveyance of ecstatic sensations; an increased dose brings about a "protective plastic

bubble effect": one has the sensation of being in another, better world, filled with love (anti-depressants, ecstasy effect). Dopamine: so-called dopaminergic neurones responding to dopamine are found in the central nervous system, above all in the middle brain; from the middle brain, dopaminergic systems rise into the telencephelon (end brain) and the interbrain; dopamine is also active in some systems of the vegetative-nervous system, where it helps to regulate the blood circulation of internal organs; important for a number of vital control and regulation processes (including the overall hormone balance); the dopamine balance has a relationship with aspects of psychoses and various disorders; in accordance with the so-called "dopamine hypothesis", an excessively high dopamine level in certain areas of the brain is linked with schizophrenia (psychoses); it also probably plays a decisively important role in addictive disorders: with various addictive drugs, this results in the secretion of endorphines, dopamine and serotonin; disturbance of the dopamine level could be responsible for some of the associated withdrawal symptoms; abuse of highly dopaminergic substances (amphetamines such as Ecstasy, Ritalin) can also manifest itself in corresponding symptoms amongst healthy people.
Task/subject: Mediation between the different neuronal elements of the organism, between control and implementation levels; changed states of awareness.
Archetypal principle: Mercury.

Nipple

Symbolic meaning: The German word for nipple "Brustwarze" (literally: breast wart) evokes the disparaging and disgusting shadow realm (who would want to put a wart in their mouth?); new words coined by the German Women's Liberation Movement have included "Brustperle" (breast pearl) and "Brustknospe" (breast bud); desire, erotic attraction; point of sensuality and maximum arousal; indicator of arousal; stimulation of the nipples increases secretion of the hormone oxytocin, which is also referred to as the "bonding hormone", i.e. a bond is created between the mother and child or between two partners either by breast-feeding or erotic stimulation respectively; nourishing, demonstrating devotion; drinking nozzle for the suckling baby, today frequently replaced by rubber dummies/pacifiers.
Task/subject: Offensive measurement and display instrument for sensual desire, "unambiguous" and "honest" messages, seduction, radiating sexual attraction: erection of the nipples in the state of erotic arousal; the greater the stimulation on the part of the child and/or man, the greater the sensibility and feeling of desire to the point of orgastic experiences and genuine orgasms; conveying orgasms; nourishing, indulging, feeding (children) and soothing, satisfying the partner.
Archetypal principle: Moon (the maternal), Venus (the seductive).

Nipple (shape)

Symbolic meaning: 1. Large: pronounced sensibility and sensual pleasure; large drinking nozzle, mouth-sized offering which makes things easier for nursing babies; phallic form symbolises aggressive components;
2. Small: more difficult for babies and partners to come to grips with; granting less to oneself and others, not giving oneself away so easily; girlish sensuality;
3. Inverted nipples (left refers to Moon-maternal subjects, right to Venus-partnership subjects à Part 2:

Nipples, inverted): shy buds, unsuitable mouthpieces; negative buds due to introversion, crawling back inside instead of blossoming out, rejecting instead of inviting; boycotting one's own femininity.

Task/subject: 1. Making it enjoyable, easy and sensual for oneself and others; giving gifts gladly and unconditionally;

2. Not making it too easy for oneself and others, setting high standards; unfolding and blossoming;

3. Turning oneself inwards, giving gifts to oneself first before others; enjoying one's own life energy, nourishing oneself; keeping everything male and phallic out of the game of love; allowing oneself to be conquered; deliberately setting the bar (very) high.

Archetypal principle: 1. and 2. Moon (the maternal), Venus (the seductive); 3. Saturn-Moon, Saturn-Venus.

Nose

Symbolic meaning: Power ("looking down one's nose at someone"), pride ("sticking one's nose up in the air"); expression of personality; organ for making contact: "sniffing someone up and down" or "turning one's nose up at them"; sexuality (the size/ shape of a man's nose has long been believed to indicate the size/ shape of his penis); the inside of the nose accommodates reflex zones for many organs of the body; those of the sexual organs are particularly easily accessible, and are preferably activated by picking the nose and taking snuff; self-expression; second only to the breast, the most common organ for cosmetic operations; otherwise, the nose is preferably concealed or toned down with make-up, because as a sexual and power symbol, it is perceived as too sign-ificant – it must never be allowed to shine for example, or protrude too far into the foreground; instead it is discreetly powdered; the bluish-red "brandy-blossom" nose is also both honest and embarrassing; the wart-covered nose of the witch, on the other hand, is proverbial, and represents her evil, monstrous essence.

Task/subject: Sensual perception: "the nose knows", "nosing around in something" in order to find out more about it; creating confidence by "sniffing each other up and down" to see who "passes the sniff test"; testing meals in advance with the nose; general taste: life is tasted with the nose; instinct ("having a good nose for something", "scenting or smelling danger"), curiosity (being "nosy", "a stickybeak"); cleaning: filtering the air we breathe; attunement and attitude to the outside world: warming the air we breathe; looking for surroundings that don't "get up our nose"; channelling of the life energy Prana (according to Indian belief, the dominance of the nostrils, and thus the polarity of the Prana flow, changes every 20 minutes); recognition of scent markings: territory marking (original lock-and-key principle of perception); getting wind of things, plumbing the emotional spectrum; signpost in the material/physical world ("following one's nose") as well as in the intuitive domain ("having a nose for something"); an honest mirror: reading the character/truth from the tip of the nose ("as plain as the nose on one's face").

Archetypal principle: Mars-Mercury.

Nose (shape)

Symbolic meaning: 1. Long: good forceful assertiveness and stamina ("enough breath to go the distance"), often having better leverage; independent, selfless, generous; always a nose-length in front; able to stick one's nose into everything, passing on knowledge;

2. Broad, flat: having apparently survived many battles, "boxer's nose", "getting a punch on the nose"; good and close connection to the body; stepping back, projecting little of oneself outwards, not wanting to lean onself too far out of the window (face); hands-on, pragmatic, often less intellectually orientated;
3. Thick, fleshy, round: the themes of power and pride (nose) are concealed behind a jovial, harmless-looking "clown's nose"; rich, spirited life, sensual-erotic orientation; frequently amongst emotional, tolerant and open people who tend to the irrational; red: "red light" (rhinophyma);
4. Snub nose: comical to meddlesome; nosy, cute and sweet, corresponds to small child pattern (Konrad Lorenz), evokes sympathy and the protective instinct; street-wise, always "having one's nose to the wind"; "healthy commonsense"; in the case of a highly-pronounced turned-up nose, danger of self-complacency, being stuck-up, rejection of unity;
5. Hook or beak nose: boldness, courage, combat strength, nobility (Hapsburg nose).
Task/subject: 1. Living and thinking in broad strokes, allowing others to participate, sharing (one's views);
2. Striving for a broad basis, living in line with the body;
3. Developing one's emotional life, fulfilling sensual needs, tolerantly and openly "sniffing out" life and its opportunities, making the art of love and culture into a life theme (tantra);
4. Becoming like children again, developing the inner child;
5. Bravely venturing far forward, accepting leadership responsibility.
Archetypal principle: 1. Jupiter; 2. Saturn; 3. Jupiter-Venus; 4. Moon; 5. Mars.

O

Oesophagus

(Greek: 'channel for eating')
Symbolic meaning: Nutrition supply.
Task/subject: Transport of nutrition by rhythmic wave movements; onward transport of everything swallowed.
Archetypal principle: Mercury.

Optic nerve

see Nervus opticus

Organ of equilibrium

see Balance organ

Os sacrum

see Sacrum

Ostium uteri

see Womb, external orifice of the

Ovaries

Symbolic meaning: Supply chambers for fertility; treasure chambers of evolution, evolutionary memory; wellspring of creativity, i.e. of the primordial female potential.
Task/subject: Giving life; passing on one's own (genetic material); guaranteeing the cyclical female rhythm.
Archetypal principle: Pluto, Moon.

P

Palate

Symbolic meaning: Taste sensor, place of palatory pleasures; roof of the oral cavity, anchoring point for the tongue and therefore important for the ingestion of food.

Task/subject: Tasting, testing, determining good taste, evaluation of meals: taste perception and orientation, deciding what one wants to take in or take on as one's own.

Archetypal principle: Venus-Jupiter.

Pancreas

Symbolic meaning: Production of explosive substances for the breakdown of nutrition: aggressive, energetic analysis (pancreatic juice); self-discovery: getting to the essence of things; sweet enjoyment (insulin-producing islet cells); war and peace.

Task/subject: Digestion, breakdown of nutrition into small individual parts; absorption of the sweetness of life (insulin); making energy available.

Archetypal principle: Mercury (analysis), Mars (breakdown), Venus (enabling absorption of the sweetness of life).

Parasympathicus

Symbolic meaning: One half of the visceral nervous system: the female opposite pole to the (male) sympathicus.

Task/subject: Regeneration and calm, rest and relaxation and all inwardly-directed activities which belong more to the feminine pole and are aimed at conservation of the species ("Serenity is the source of strength").

Archetypal principle: Moon-Venus.

Parathyroid glands

(Epithelium corpuscles, Glandula parathyreoidea)

Symbolic meaning: Creates balance between ossification and instability, between cramping and slackening (between calcium and phosphate levels); responsibility for stability of the scaffolding and the motoric elements.

Task/subject: Giving structure, enabling good hold, keeping ossification within the necessary limits (regulation of the bone metabolism by parathyroid hormone production); stability, strength; regulating states of tension (strain).

Archetypal principle: Mercury-Saturn.

Parotid gland

(Greek: parōtís 'near the ear')

Symbolic meaning: Largest salivary gland of the mouth; moistener of the mouth, which is activated by chewing.

Task/subject: Producing saliva, which causes the mouth "to water"; ensuring that nourishment slides down well.

Archetypal principle: Moon.

Pelvis

(see also Hips/hip joints)

Symbolic meaning: Bedrock of life, basis; sounding board, musical instrument for the deep tones of existence, sensual resonance with Mother Earth; catchment basin (pelvis = 'basin' in Latin); birthing bowl, vessel of fertility; pelvic bowl, home of the "palaces of one's sexual energies (animus and anima)"; basis of the life axis (spinal column) = foundation for standing upright; contains the portals of life and death: the life-giving sexual organs and the entrance and exit to the kingdom of the dead of the large intestine; source of life energy and desire, the Kundalini (energy) serpent rests in the pelvis (lowest "Muladhara" chakra, coccyx, sacrum); narrow pelvis: expression of the masculine archetype; broad, expansive pelvis: expression of the fertility of the feminine archetype; broad hips used to be popular, but are nowadays despised; modern "problem zone" for women;

the childishly-narrow pelvis of today as a new (problematic) ideal for both sexes.

Task/subject: Resonating in synch; showing how things currently stand or are progressing; providing stability, acting as a "catchall", enabling forward movement/progress; knowing what one stands for; developing a stable personality; creating a broad basis for (one's own) life, resting firmly and securely in life.

Archetypal principle: Saturn-Moon, Jupiter.

Penis

Symbolic meaning: The 'member' (although the term 'member' can refer to any limb, it is most readily associated with this one, which may indicate its importance); phallus: masculine power ("manhood"); organ of conceiving (putting a seed into the womb) and convincing (putting a seed into the mind), copulation organ; magic wand (gives life); thrusting force, gSun-barrel for the sperm (= guided weapons); sword which longs for the sheath in order to find rest (and desire); exercise of power: penetrating, deflowering ("spear"), injuring; having one's way (domineering) and giving away (donating) lie close together; the importance of its size is overestimated; (for most women) the skill in using it is more important; the organ for gaining entry to a woman; admission can be forced with dominance, or obtained playfully, requested and received as a gift.

Task/subject: Channelling (new) life, giving desire; serves as the launching ramp for semen; on the one hand, exercising the craving for power, and on the other, becoming involved with the world of the female; coupled with the female counterpart, the vagina, allows the possibility of overcoming the dichotomy of humankind for a moment:

conveying experiences of unity in the moment of orgasm.

Archetypal principle: Mars.

Pericardial sac

(pericardium)

Symbolic meaning: Nourishing and protecting sack for the heart, like the pouch of the female kangaroo for its young; protection and security for the capital city of the body's terrain; double protective wall around the heart; in Traditional Chinese Medicine: the "Dependent Envoy" that desire and joy are derived from; Assignments: Yin, element - fire, complementary to the triple heater (Yang).

Task/subject: Screening of the heart against diseases from the surrounding area (mediastinum); prevention of acute over-expansion of the heart by means of fixed boundaries.

Archetypal principle: Sun-Saturn.

Peritoneum

Symbolic meaning: Nourishment and warning, gut perceptions; inner skin, lining of the abdominal cavity.

Task/subject: Lining of the abdominal cavity, covering of the "innards" or "guts" (the abdominal organs are enveloped in it as if in a cloth) for the supply of energy (blood) and information (nerves); warning system "gut feelings" (the only part of the abdominal cavity provided with nerves, and therefore sensitive to pain): source of stomach pains sensing when something is drawing on one's last reserves

Archetypal principle: Moon-Mercury.

Pineal gland

(epiphysis)

Symbolic meaning: Produces melatonin, the "boss" of the àhormones; dictator of the inner rhythm (of life), the inner clock; according to occult anatomy, has a relationship to the third eye (àchakras) and thus to insight.

Task/subject: Regulating the day-night rhythm.

Archetypal principle: Chronos-Saturn (quantity of time), Kairos (quality of time: the best time for an undertaking), Moon (rhythm).

Pituitary gland

(Hypophysis)

Symbolic meaning: the brain for the glandular system, seat of government of the hormones: harmony and adaptation at the highest level.

Task/subject: Control of the inner world, adaptation of the inner world to the outer world; maintenance of the metabolic balances (homoeostasis) by means of feedback loops: control and regulation (cybernetic system).

Archetypal principle: Mercury.

Placenta

Symbolic meaning: Nourishment; Latin placenta = 'flat cake' - the first cake that the mother bakes for her child: symbolic model for all the later ones; feeding new life with one's own life force (blood) (like the pelican as a religious symbol, which tears open its own breast for its young in order to nourish them with its blood).

Task/subject: Nourishment, taking care of new life.

Archetypal principle: Moon.

Pleura

see Costal pleura

Prostate

(prostate gland)

Symbolic meaning: Thumb-sized gland which surrounds the urethra and contributes the main volume of the ejaculate (the seminal fluid); "lubricates" the male spearpoint (penis)

and is responsible for its moistness and slipperiness; confidence in (male) sexuality, vitality, masculine self-esteem and love of life; guardian at the threshold to the second half of life.

Task/subject: By means of the prostatic secretions ensures the right environment and nutrition of the sperm on their way to the egg cell; enables the sensually-competent man to become just as moist as the vagina in non-frigid women (a fact which in the Western-male style of rapid-fire eroticism has been more or less forgotten, or putting it another way: almost all men now remain dry, and are therefore frigid in the true sense of the word); if men were to make their contribution (via the prostate) in the original, natural sense to the slippery success of the sexual act, there would be no frigid women.

Archetypal principle: Moon-Mars.

Pubic bone

Symbolic meaning: Bony base of the mound of Venus or pubic mound; protection of the sexual region.

Task/subject: Closing and stabilising the pelvic ring.

Archetypal principle: Saturn-Venus.

R

Rectum

(intestinum rectum = 'straight intestine')

Symbolic meaning: Exit from (entrance to) the underworld; place where faeces are held back (related to stinginess - "tight-arsed"); last station of the production line before release of the end product; exhaust pipe.

Task/subject: Collecting and excreting of waste (faeces), disposing of

waste gases: "shitting" (money) like the gold-ass in the Brothers Grimm fairytale, "pecunia non olet – money doesn't stink" but "stinking rich", "not giving a crap/shit about anything".
Archetypal principle: Pluto.

Renal pelvis

(see also Kidneys)
Symbolic meaning: Catchment basin for waste overflow; popular place for unresolved partnership and shadow matters to turn to stone.
Task/subject: Collecting the flow of (spiritual) waste, before it descends; unresolved task: giving room to larger stones on the rocky road of life.
Archetypal principle: Venus-Moon.

Respiratory tract

(see also Nose, Trachea, Bronchia, Lungs)
Symbolic meaning: Transport channels of the air we inhale (oxygen) and the waste gases we exhale (carbon dioxide), communication (gas exchange) and speech (= modulation of the breathing flow), giving and taking.
Task/subject: Energy production and exchange, communication with other people and with all other beings on this Earth, including with the plant kingdom.
Archetypal principle: Mercury (connection), Mars (energy).

Retina

(see also Eyes)
Symbolic meaning: Conversion membrane, self-regenerating photographic plate of the eye.
Task/subject: Converting light stimuli into electrical stimuli, intermediary step in the creation of inner images as a reflection of outer images.
Archetypal principle: Mercury/Uranus-Sun/Moon.

Rhinencephalon

Symbolic meaning: The nose connects "getting wind of something" with the world of feelings and sense/instinct with intuition.
Task/subject: As the phylogenetically-oldest part of the telencephalon (end brain), it connects us with our beginnings, i.e. the world of instinct and feelings; processing scents.
Archetypal principle: Pluto (the primordial brain)-Neptune (scents, sensation).

Ribs

Symbolic meaning: Basic construction elements of the rib cage, which contribute to its density and strength; safety and protection; flexibility and adaptation (to the rhythm of respiration – to polarity).
Task/subject: Protecting, adapting, functioning.
Archetypal principle: Saturn-Mercury.

Rib cage

see Chest

Ring finger

(Gold finger; see also Finger)
Symbolic meaning: Status symbol; shows amongst other things one's marital status; illustrates one's relationships (above all with the opposite sex).
Task/subject: Shining, revealing one's social position.
Archetypal principle: Mercury-Sun.

S

Sacrum

Symbolic meaning: Rear section and termination point of the pelvic bowl; area on which the àspinal column (our world axis) rests; consequently, it bears the full burden of our existence; home of the Kundalini serpent, which lies in the depths of the pelvis rolled together in 3 ½ coils in front of the "sacred bone" (Latin Os sacrum), waiting for its awakening; starting point of spiritual development (àchakras).

Task/subject: Foundation of the world axis, home of the life energy; holding the pelvis together; giving the bowl of life a good hold.

Archetypal principle: Pluto.

Salivary glands

Symbolic meaning: Appetite, desire ("something makes one's mouth water"); closeness, saliva as an intimate fluid of desire: kissing and licking saliva.

Task/subject: Mixing together (of food and people): when we want to devour or sink our teeth into someone or something, we first try to break them/it down with saliva; spitting into one's hands when one wants to stimulate the desire or courage to do something; in many cultures, spitting on or near someone is a way of wishing good luck.

Archetypal principle: Venus-Moon.

Salt

(electrolyte)

Symbolic meaning: Salt of life: the essence of life, the essential (those who use a lot of salt reveal that they are lacking salt in their soup (of life) and that their life has become bland and tasteless); sal(t) has the same linguistic route as healing/whole/holy.

Task/subject: Maintenance of the voltage potentials at the cell membrane (battery); bonding of the water: salt is the spice that binds the interest of the spiritual element; in alchemy, salt corresponds to the body.

Archetypal principle: Saturn.

Scent glands

(see also Axillary glands)

Symbolic meaning: Personal scent, perfumeries (in the domain of the secondary sexual organs).

Task/subject: Enticement, attraction; exclusion, rejection; secondary, more intimate level of partner selection.

Archetypal principle: Venus/Mars-Saturn.

Sensory organs

Symbolic meaning: Bridges between the inner and outer world: vision as both sight and insight, having "a good nose" for smells or "catching wind" of things, hearing and obeying (from Latin: ob "to" + audire "listen, hear"), taste in the dual sense of flavor and personal preference; sensing (physically touching) and the sixth sense (intuition).

Task/subject: Enabling us to recognise the world; helping us to find "sense" in it, conveying sensuality and sensual pleasure.

Archetypal principle: Mercury-Jupiter (from the senses to the sense).

Septum of the heart

(from Latin "saeptum" meaning a "dividing wall or enclosure")

Symbolic meaning: Demarcation line of the polarity in the heart; threshold between this world and the next in our centre.

Task/subject: the initially single chamber of the unborn, which is still closely connected with unity, is

completely separated into two sides (the left and the right heart) with the first breath.
Archetypal principle: **Sun-Saturn.**

Sexual organs

(Genitalia)
Symbolic meaning: **Sexuality; polarity, Yin and Yang, Lingam and Yoni (Ind. for the [male] sword and the [female] sheath); organs of regeneration in the extended sense: ensuring the survival of mankind, are already in the service of the next generation; new life always springs from the lower, archetypally female pole; the sexual act, in which an egg is fertilised, draws the soul of the child into the body in a spiral undertow; analogy to the temple as the place where the spiritual sinks into the material (Latin mater = 'mother') and fertilises it; (in the East: "palace of one's sexual energies (animus and anima)":**
In women: The àlabia correspond to the curtains of the temple courtyard, with the àvagina itself as the temple courtyard, the àexternal opening to the womb represents the temple entrance and the àwomb the temple itself; female sexual organs have generally been denigrated in the patriarchate: "the Bermuda triangle", the shame cave, i.e. the female genitals as something to be ashamed of, "bad girl – stop that at once" (when young girls touch themselves in this area in public);
In men: The àpenis corresponds to the tower; the àtesticles, which symbolise the eyes, bring into play the aspect of sensual perception, which ultimately should lead to the ability to make sense of things and the final sense of sensuality; also as the member corresponding to the nose; male sexual organs have generally been glorified and over-valued in the patriarchate, as demonstrated by names given in colloquial language: "pride

and joy", "the little man", "the spear", "the sword", "the magic wand".
Task/subject: **Continuing life; bestowing sexual desire; overcoming polarity and experiencing the ecstasy of unity; allowing the death of polarity (orgasm as a momentary death, disappearance of the I-You boundary) in order to make way for new life.**
Archetypal principle: **Venus/Mars-Pluto (procreation).**

Shoulders

Symbolic meaning: **One of the most mobile parts of the body (àshoulder joint); right shoulder: problems imposed on one by others, left shoulder: problems imposed by oneself; in general: load-bearing capacity ("shouldering a burden") and the willingness to accept responsibility; bearing towards life (àshoulder shape); padding out one's shoulders: acting as if one had broad shoulders and could carry (bear) a great deal; bearing towards other people ("giving someone the cold shoulder", "rubbing shoulders with someone"); closing ranks: standing together (with and) for others (shoulder-to-shoulder), "resting one's head on someone's shoulders"; coming to terms with the world: drooping shoulders (resignation, feelings of inferiority), "shrugging something off lightly", "looking over someone's shoulder", "beefed-up shoulders" (being overbearing), "tapping/patting someone on the shoulder" (praising someone and thereby physically putting them down?), "shrugging one's shoulders" (perplexity, ignorance).**
Task/subject: **Carrying and bearing, dragging around (emotional and physical) burdens; reflecting one's inner bearing outwardly; connection between the expressiveness of the hands and arms with the chest as the place of the centre and integration; giving the arms freedom of action.**
Archetypal principle: **Saturn-Jupiter.**

Shoulder (shape)

Symbolic meaning: 1. Broad: shouldering life, being able to take on a great deal, giving protection and security, conveying safety; archetypally masculine silhouette;
2. Narrow: No broad backing available, low ability to bear heavy loads; need for help; in men: sign of weakness, lack of strength and resilience, unmanly; in women: fragility and need for protection, archetypally feminine silhouette;
3. Drooping: depressed, resigned impression, unable to bear heavy loads, overstrained, unbearable feelings of guilt, lack of energy, exhausted, shrugging everything off and letting it slide;
4. Hunched: rigidity, fear, shock, need for protection.
Task/subject: 1. Demonstrating courage and energy; carrying responsibility for others;
2. Caring for oneself;
3. Not taking on more than one can carry (bear); less is more; reviewing the stresses and burdens that are weighing one down; consciously allowing oneself to be taken down into the depths of one's own unconscious and shadowy realms; shrugging off the superfluous and letting it slide; drifting unburdened with the flow of life;
4. Protecting oneself, placing the central headquarters in safety, learning to "pull one's head in" at the right time; gathering together all one's strength and courage; becoming capable of acting, not just being a puppet for others.
Archetypal principle: 1. Mars; 2. Moon; 3. and 4. Saturn.

Shoulder blades

Symbolic meaning: Bony wings, similar to the lobes of the lungs as inner wings; their condition indicates the lightness with which we swing through life
Task/subject: Providing good hold and bearing (as part of the shoulder girdle).
Archetypal principle: Mercury-Uranus.

Shoulder joint

(see also Joints)
Symbolic meaning: Extremely mobile, but therefore less stable ball joint; compromise between the greatest possible freedom of movement on the one hand and stability and safety on the other; flexibility on the upper level; basis of one's own way of doing things, starting point of abilities; mediation of the world: while the hip joints enable us to move towards the world, the shoulder joints enable us to draw the world to us.
Task/subject: Creating access to the world on the physical level, acting and articulating; grants us great freedom with only minor restrictions, but prevents extremes of articulation, by becoming disjointed; animates us to bold (spiritual) agility and to taking the risk of throwing our energy into the greater (life) plan and thus growing beyond ourselves; basis of all our hand-tools; enables us stretch the range of manual activities over a wide span; reacts sensitively, however, if over-stretched; enables us to create a broad circle of influence, but punishes any over-straining of the articulation capacities; shows when manual work is being over-exaggerated in relation to spiritual work.
Archetypal principle: Mercury-Mars.

Sinuses

(see also Maxillary sinus)
Symbolic meaning: Lightness and airiness of the head; the lightness of being has its basis in the air cushions of the skull bones; with clear sinuses, one's awareness of life is free, light

and airy with a tendency towards cheerful bouyancy in contrast to the heavy-headed and totally blocked feeling of the sinuses when somebody is up to their ears or eyeballs in something and thus sick to the back teeth of it all; shaping element. Task/subject: Airing; lightening the head by relieving the hard, fixed bone structure (bringing the air element into the earth element); moistening and warming the breath in preparation for communication with the outer world; resonance base for the voice (nasal-sounding voice as soon as the sinuses or nose are blocked); with a cold, the lightness of being is immediately lost; with a chronically-blocked nose (blocked sinuses), it is lost gradually; shaping of the individual face. Archetypal principle: Uranus.

Sinus nodes

Symbolic meaning: Centre in the heart which dictates the beat and the rhythm; the top of the hierarchy: Primus inter pares (the first among equals), since all other heart cells are also rhythm-producing organs, only at a lower frequency level. Task/subject: Running the heart off its feet, driving it on with every electrical impulse, and at the same time disempowering all other centres (electrical depolarisation) in order to preserve the hierarchy. Archetypal principle: Sun-Uranus.

Skeleton

(see also Bones) Symbolic meaning: The element which gives structure to the body, the support. Task/subject: Marking out the individual structure, which keeps us upright and enables us to walk upright; giving life a framework and thus stability and firmness. Archetypal principle: Saturn.

Skin

Symbolic meaning: Map of the soul; anyone who has experienced great sorrow shows this in corresponding traces: their "hide has been tanned", they carry their scars as signs of the ravages of life, these signs are a distinction, or they feel themselves specially marked by them; boundary (to the outside), border fortification; conveyance of contact and tenderness; (skin) breathing. Brown (tanned) skin: more robust, thicker, less sensitive, protected by more pigment; looks vital and dynamic and is the current fashion, was previously regarded as the complexion of the lower classes because it was associated with working in the fields; tanning is the sun protection reaction of white skin; signalises active, successful people, and also slackers, who know how to have a good time on the sunny side of life. White skin: less protected, more sensitive and sentimental, more easily irritated, "more sensually appealing", white skin (under the underclothes) and a seamless tan compete with each other for favour (white skin/ genteel paleness is preferred by more conservative people and appears more secretive; a seamless tan is today the ideal amongst the masses). Rosy, light, reddish complexion: even more sensitive than white skin, minimal pigment protection, reacts sensitively to sunlight; indicates sensitive, easily hurt people, who are thin-skinned and easily affected (insulted), and who have no "thick hide"; the "red face" of quick-tempered cholerics who immediately allow everything to get under their skin and burst correspondingly quickly. Yellowish complexion: considered amongst white-skinned people as unhealthy since it indicates liver problems (jaundice); amongst Asians, on the other hand, a yellow complexion was considered the traditional ideal, just as a tan is to white people; today, the Chinese prefer an olive complexion, which develops in the sun, something that was traditionally unpopular just as a suntan used to be in Europe. Black skin: the thickest and most resistant, the best sun protection; ideal for life in the southern hemisphere and in the sun, the "thick hide" par excellence, belongs to people with a good sense of rhythm, who stand robustly on the earth and as a rule are more sensually-gifted than people with white skin.

Task/subject: Protective shield, forming an insulating layer, which can become a prison for the soul: "being close to bursting" but "unable to shed one's skin"; contact: conveying human warmth and devotion; touch; perception: sense of touch, communication, "having nothing to hide"; expression: mirror of the spiritual inner world (face colour, etc.); indicator of psychic processes and reactions: "thin-skinned", "thick-skinned", "baring all", "putting one's skin on the line", "being highly strung and easily offended", "not feeling comfortable in one's own skin", blushing with shame; projection surface for the internal organs (reflex zones).

Archetypal principle: Venus (contact), Saturn (border, protection, insulation), Mercury (touch, communication, breathing).

Sleep

Symbolic meaning: The dark side of life, female half of existence, nightmare journey of the soul.

Task/subject: Regeneration, processing of day-to-day and life conflicts; balancing out the archetypally male day.

Archetypal principle: Moon.

Small intestine

Symbolic meaning: Analysis (breakdown); assimilation (absorption) of material messages; in Traditional Chinese Medicine: the right hand of the "Emperor" (heart), responsible for the power of judgement, distinguishing the important from the unimportant; Assignments: Yang, element - fire, complementary to the heart (Yin).

Task/subject: Conscious, analytical processing; digestion of material impressions; assessment of what is to be integrated; existential fears; critical faculties (duodenum from Latin "intestīnum duodēnum digitōrum" = intestine of twelve finger-widths); making foreign matter one's own; absorption into one's innermost world. Duodenum = analysis; Jejunum (from Latin: "empty" because usually found empty in dissections) = absorption of selected matter (assimilation, integration); Ileum (from Latin "groin, flank") = balancing, "catchment basin" when overloaded with impressions.

Archetypal principle: Mercury.

Solar plexus

(Latin: solar 'sun' and plexus 'interwoven network', so-called due to the raylike pattern of the nerve fibers)

Symbolic meaning: self-confidence, joy for life (corresponds to the "Manipura" chakra, àchakras).

Task/subject: Control of the stomach and intestinal tract.

Archetypal principle: Sun-Mercury.

Sperm duct

Symbolic meaning: Racetrack for the sperm, path of life.

Task/subject: Giving and guiding new life.

Archetypal principle: Mercury.

Spinal column

(backbone; see also Back, Atlas, Axis, Thoracic vertebrae, Lumbar vertebrae, Sacrum, Coccyx)

Symbolic meaning: Stability and dynamism: spinal column = dynamism and simultaneous structural stability (Latin vert(ere) = 'to turn') and bearing [column]); polar life axis and shock-absorber; measure of uprightness: the upright posture, "standing up for something"; connecting axis between the upper and the lower; place of incarnation, human ascendance: home of the Kundalini (energy) serpent; like the spinal column, it is only the (biblical) serpent which makes man human; mirror of human evolutionary history; reflection of primordial symbolism = interchange between male and female elements (vertebral body – intervertebral disc); world axis that all life revolves around, just as in earlier times everything used to revolve around the Marian column in Catholic villages, around the Omphalos stele in settlements of the megalithic culture, around the Obelisk in Ancient Egypt and today still around the Totem-pole amongst Indian peoples.

Task/subject: Giving good hold, ensuring mobility and flexibility; cushioning the blows of life: double-S shape; carrying (bearing) the weight of existence: intervertebral discs as padded discs; carrying the chief authority: the proudly-poised head; organ of expression: "standing up straight", "showing backbone"; disclosure and demonstration of inner stances: "with head held high"; "crooked as a dog's hind leg", "adopting a position"; connecting the upper and lower domains: the roots in Mother Earth, the head with the Holy Father in Heaven; rising up (an uprising): ascending from the community of living beings: becoming like God.

Archetypal principle: Saturn.
Assignments of the vertebrae to spiritual problems and disease symptoms (according to Dieter Dorn et al.)
1. Cervical vertebra (Atlas): Anxiety versus self-awareness – blood pressure problems (low/high pressure), headaches, migraines, chronic fatigue, insomnia, dizziness, signs of unilateral paralysis, forgetfulness.
2. Cervical vertebra: Self-denial and ambition – eye and ear problems, allergies, sinus afflictions, speech problems.
3. Cervical vertebra: Feelings of guilt and need for freedom – problems with teeth and ears (also tinnitus), acne, eczema.
4. Cervical vertebra: Ambivalence towards life – allergies (e.g. hay fever), colds, deafness, teeth problems.
5. Cervical vertebra: Lack of self-assurance, dissociation problems – neck pains, hoarseness, laryngeal inflammations.
6. Cervical vertebra: Lack of flexibility – tonsillar inflammations, arm and shoulder pains, coughing, croup, stiff neck.
7. Cervical vertebra: Helplessness and problems with letting go: thyroid gland problems, depression, anxieties, catarrh.

1. Thoracic vertebra: Status problems – lower arm pains (tennis elbow, tendon sheath inflammation), respiratory problems (coughing, asthma).
2. Thoracic vertebra: Taciturnity, disappointments – heart complaints, anxieties, blood pressure problems, chest pains.
3. Thoracic vertebra: Communication problems, self-abandonment – bronchitis, lung inflammation, respiratory complaints, dry coughing.
4. Thoracic vertebra: Embitterment – Gall bladder complaints, jaundice, headaches, shingles.
5. Thoracic vertebra: Emotional blockage – Liver problems, low blood pressure, anaemia, circulatory deficiency, shingles, tiredness, anaemia.
6. Thoracic vertebra: Worries and anxieties, repressed matters – digestion problems, heartburn, stomach complaints.
7. Thoracic vertebra: Problems with enjoyment – diabetes, digestive complaints, gastritis, hiccuping.

8. Thoracic vertebra: Self-disparage-ment, frustration – spleen problems, immune deficiency.
9. Thoracic vertebra: Victim role, self-deception – allergies, urticaria, disturbed hormone production of the adrenal glands.
10.Thoracic vertebra: Projection tendency – kidney, skin problems, arteriosclerosis.
11.Thoracic vertebra: Low feeling of self-esteem – skin complaints, bed-wetting.
12. Thoracic vertebra: Lack of (self-) assurance – flatulence, growth disor-ders, rheumatism.

1. Lumbar vertebrae: Separation problems – intestinal problems (constipation, diarrhoea), ruptures (hernias).
2. Lumbar vertebrae: Hopelessness – excess acidity, (stomach) cramps, varicose veins, appendix problems.
3. Lumbar vertebrae: Guilt and abuse– pregnancy disorders, men-struation problems, impotence, blad-der pains, knee pains.
4. Lumbar vertebrae: Compulsions, control – sciatica, lumbago, prostate problems.
5. Lumbar vertebrae: Inability to enjoy things – circulation disorders, swellings and cramps in the feet and lower legs.

1. Sacrum: Revenge – pains in the legs and feet, sciatica, chronic consti-pation, abdominal problems.

1. Coccyx: Balance problems – hae-morrhoids, anal itching (pruritus ani), pain when sitting.

Spinal cord

Symbolic meaning: Data highway of the body (between top and bottom); regional administration.
Task/subject: Controlling things on-site (at the horizontal level), passing on important things upwards and from top to bottom.
Archetypal principle: Mercury.

Spinal cord membranes

(Meninges)
Symbolic meaning: Rhythm; pack-aging of the main nerve channels.
Task/subject: Isolation, protection and rhythm (rhythmic pulsing of the cranio-sacral flow).
Archetypal principle: Saturn-Moon.

Spleen

Symbolic meaning: Source of joy for life, entrance gate for ethereal forces, responsible for the control of the pranic vital forces, vitalises the ethe-real body - the energy body; also reg-ulates the intake of energy so that the body is not overloaded: in the case of an excess supply, it gives off the excess energy again; filter of the life force, vitality (blood) store; both grave and cradle for red and white blood corpuscles (womb and cemetery – compare the great goddesses Hekate and Kali, who also give and take life); lymphatic tissue in the service of the immune system; fixed ideas, rigid adherence to the point of obstinacy can reside here; for this reason, it can be useful to "vent one's spleen" to clear it; in Traditional Chinese Medi-cine: the "Official" responsible to the "Emperor" (heart) who is responsible for defence and controls reason, also referred to as the "Mother"; controls clarification processes with regard to nutrition, bodily fluids and ener-getic influences; Assignments: Yin, element - earth, emotion - brooding/worrying, complementary to the stom-ach (Yang).
Task/subject: Cleansing of the life force; in spiritual medicine: organ important for the aural body; amongst theosophists, having the status of a

chakra; in anthroposophic medicine, relationship to the subject of death.
Archetypal principle: Mars-Moon-Saturn.

Sternum

see Breastbone

Stomach

Symbolic meaning: Feeling; absorption capacity, storage place for everything swallowed; the sickle shape is reminiscent of the moon (see Archetypal principle); nest of one's feelings, nest of one's childhood, place of preparation and security; in Traditional Chinese Medicine: "Official of the State Granaries", receives the nutrition and makes it fruitful; Assignments: Yang, element - earth, complementary to the spleen (Yin).
Task/subject: Absorption, reception, impressionability, passivity, willingness, being open; female pole: feeling, "the way to a man's heart is through his stomach", "having an upset stomach", "being (un)able to stomach something", unwanted padding as the result of comfort eating; male pole: aggressive breaking down of things (stomach acid), "an acerbic/acrimonious/caustic wit", "being eaten up by something"; retention of repressed emotions "bottling things up"; hunger for fulfilment, longing.
Archetypal principle: Moon/Mars.

Straight intestine

see Rectum

Sweat glands

Symbolic meaning: Regulating channels (from inside to outside); skin regulators.
Task/subject: Stabilising the skin environment: protecting (against drying out), defending (creating the acidic coating of the skin), cooling (in situations of over-heating), cleaning (through perspiration); marking out one's territory.
Archetypal principle: Mercury-Moon.

Sympathicus

Symbolic meaning: One side of the visceral nervous system: the "male" counterpart to the "female" àparasympathicus; brings us into the "on-guard mode".
Task/subject: Responsible for fight or flight, for confrontations, storming ahead and all outwardly-directed activities which belong more to the masculine pole and which are aimed at furthering the species.
Archetypal principle: Sun/Mars.

T

Tailbone

see Coccyx

Taste buds

(on tongue and palate)
Symbolic meaning: Taste sensors, preliminary food tasters.
Task/subject: Protecting against dangers; repelling unpleasant tastes; affording pleasure; organs of selection: pre-tasting and deciding whether Life is to one's taste or not.
Archetypal principle: Venus-Jupiter (sense of taste).

Tear glands

Symbolic meaning: Expression of emotions and feelings, overflowing spiritual energy; Tears = symbol of pain, sorrow and joy.
Task/subject: Washing the windows of the soul; expressing intense

feelings, which exceed our capacity to absorb them.
Archetypal principle: Moon.

Teeth

Symbolic meaning: 1. General: (hard) weapons in the mouth, aggression; vitality, potency, reduction; overcoming problems (breaking down large chunks into smaller pieces), willingness to integrate;
2. Incisor teeth (1, 2): upper left (1) stands for anima, the female principle, mother; upper right (2) for animus, the male principle, father; lower left shows how the female pole has been integrated into life and experienced; the lower right how the male pole is faring in this respect;
3. Eye teeth (3; Canini = 'dog teeth', tearing teeth): capturing prey ("sinking one's teeth into someone or something"), "giving one's eye teeth for something"; the right upper (3) shows how one presents oneself to the world; the left upper how one reacts to transformation and change; the right lower provides information on bodily growth and aspirations in life; the left lower on how spiritual changes are overcome;
4. Back teeth (molars): grinding down, re-hashing, handling problems ("ruminating", "having something to chew on").
Task/subject: 1. Seizing, grasping, attacking: "chewing someone out", "biting someone's head off", having a "razor-sharp wit", fighting tooth and nail to defend oneself: "getting a grip on life"; robbing someone of an illusion: "giving someone a kick in the teeth"; deeply-rooted convictions; letting out (expressing) aggression and putting it to use: "baring/showing one's teeth"; forceful assertion: "gritting one's teeth and biting one's way through life"; showing life force and potency: "having bite", being "long in the tooth", a "hot dish" that one would like to sink one's teeth into moves men to "manly" thoughts; assuring oneself of one's share: biting off (more than one can chew), overcoming problems: "cracking tough nuts", breaking down large chunks into smaller pieces; aggression blockage: being "hard-bitten" like a dog with a bone, being contrite (Latin: 'crushed');
2. Biting off one's share, getting one's own piece of the action;
3. Giving life an edge, marking out one's field;
4. Sorting out impressions, putting solutions into motion.
Archetypal principle: 1. Mars, Saturn; 2. and 3. Mars; 4. Saturn.

Teeth (enamel)

(adamantine)
Symbolic meaning: Hardness pole: steel for weapons, diamond substance of the body; enamel (originally derived from a word meaning "something melted"): its hardness and brilliant vitality makes the partner melt.
Task/subject: Steeling the weapons, arming the teeth for the rigour of life's struggle; cutting (sharp-edged) and grinding down (meal).
Archetypal principle: Saturn.

Teeth (roots)

Symbolic meaning: The roots of our weapons in the mouth.
Task/subject: Giving the weapons stability and strength and adequate nourishment.
Archetypal principle: Saturn.

Teeth (shape/position)

Well cared-for teeth: One's own weapons are in good condition and ready to rip into action.
Gleaming white: Fresh, dazzling situation, vitality.

Regular teeth: Ordered relationships in the domain of vitality, harmony in the domain of energy.

Irregular teeth: Lacking battle formation, chaos in the aggressive domain, lone fighters who step out of line need much more attention at all levels (from individual treatment with floss through to the spiritual equivalent); Task: More courageous, wilder handling and application of aggressive energy, trusting oneself to do things and daring to step out of line, fighting for one's own way; taking unusual, original paths of forceful self-assertion; learning to stand behind even crazy ways of expressing one's vitality.

Noticeably large and protruding: Great strength and energy (as strong as a horse, "horsey teeth"), vitality and potency so that one can really get stuck into things, dangerous; Task: Proving oneself worthy of such good weapons, living courageously.

Small ("mousy teeth"): Harmless, kind, not wishing to harm anyone, powerless, needy, making oneself small; refined, small but effective; Task: Economising on one's strengths.

Gap between the upper middle incisors (diastema): mother and father, anima (the inner woman) and animus (the inner man), the goddess and god distance themselves from each other; the female (left 1) and male (right 1) side cannot be brought together easily, lack of integration of these two aspects of the soul: women like to call (their) men into question as a matter of principle; men often feel themselves both attracted and rejected by (their) women at the same time; Task: Consciously increasing inner distance from the opposite pole.

Large 1, which dominates or overlays the 2 ("Rabbit teeth", "buck teeth"): Dominance of the male principle and the parents; parents extend their rule intrusively into the life of the children; strong aggressive energy.

Small 1 ("mousy teeth"): anxiety.

Overlaying of one upper 1 by the other 1: The particular parental and corresponding aspect of one's being that has been displaced out of the first row plays a subordinate role, or the one pushing forward dominates (left 1: Anima, mother image, right 1: Animus, father image); Task: Taking for real (perceiving) and taking seriously the displaced part of the spirit once again without weakening the other part.

2 projecting further forward than 1: Desire to overtake, (wanting) to go one's own way in freedom); bypassing the parents, placing oneself above them, early independence.

Noticeably small 2 (to the point of "mousy teeth"): lovable, friendly, often allowing oneself to come up too short, firstly in relation to one's parents and then later in relation to their representatives.

Backward right or left 2: Subjecting oneself to male authority (right 2) or female authority (left 2).

Prominent eye teeth (3): "Vampire teeth", tearaway predator aspect, phallic power.

Lower 3 projecting beyond upper 3: In women, indicates that the male part of the soul is repressed, and in men that the female part of the soul is repressed.

Assignment of the teeth to the meridians

1 and 2 upper and lower: Urogenital system: kidneys/urinary bladder and pharyngeal tonsils, frontal sinus, ears.

3 upper and lower: Liver/gall bladder and eyes (hence "eye-teeth"); palatine tonsils, cuneiform sinus, hips, knees.

Premolars (4 = first back teeth and 5 = second back teeth): top: lungs/large intestine, paranasal sinuses, bronchia, ethmoid bone cells; bottom: larynx, maxillary sinus, mammary glands; left: spleen and stomach; right: pancreas and stomach; 5 bottom: lymph vessels.

Molars (grinding teeth; 6 = first grinding teeth and 7 = second grinding teeth): larynx, sinus maxillaris; top right: pancreas and stomach; top left: spleen and stomach; bottom: large intestine and lungs, bronchia, paranasal sinuses, ethmoid bone cells. Wisdom teeth (8): Heart, small intestine, middle ear, shoulders and elbows; top: central nervous system; bottom: peripheral nerves; right: duodenum; left: ileum, jejunum.

Tendons

(see also Achilles tendon, Ligaments)

Symbolic meaning: Binding cords that everything hinges on; transmission belts of the musculoskeletal system and thus the impulses of the will; attachment cables (for the muscles), transmission of the movement dynamics to structural elements (bones); making the connections between bones and muscles; if these are lacking, neither the bones nor muscles make any sense (of the commands of the will); similarly, if the connection/contact between two people is lacking, there is the longing to stretch oneself to reestablish the bond (tendon from Latin *tendere* 'to stretch').

Task/subject: Conversion of one's own strengths and energies into practice (transmission of the muscle power to the bones); giving tensile force like the string of a bow, which must be stretched, but not overstretched (this is also why a marathon is best run over a firm surface, and not on sand).

Archetypal principle: Mars-Mercury (transmission of power)-Saturn (Mercury connects Mars and Saturn).

Testicles

Symbolic meaning: Fertility (the testicles are colloquially referred to as "nuts": a nut carries the seed of new life), fitness for life, vitality, creativity, excess production; going one's own masculine way, using one's talents, exploiting one's potential; the most sensitive part of a man: "grabbing someone by the balls"; symbol of power, male strength (castration = disempowerment, emasculation).

Task/subject: Giving life; safety policy of nature (overflow/excess), wasteful use of resources for the benefit of preserving life; teeming with vitality and power; organs of desire.

Archetypal principle: Pluto.

Thigh

Symbolic meaning: The strongest muscles, the greatest strength of the organism, operated by the largest muscle (Gluteus maximus); the strength of forward and upward movement; stands for the strength which one has brought along (inherited) as an aid on one's (development) path; family tradition; the desire to conquer everything that one can wrap one's legs around.

Task/subject: Stepping out (of line), striding forward = getting ahead.

Archetypal principle: Jupiter (Dionysius, the God of ecstasy and intemperance, sprang from Jupiter's thigh).

Thigh (shape)

Symbolic meaning: 1. Strong, muscular: in women female power of the great goddess; mighty power in order to protect the "palaces of one's sexual energies (animus and anima);" vanquishing the man between them (Brunhilde); in an age of male-based ideals of femininity, tends to be frowned on, except in female athletes; in men, great (thrusting) power; conquering everything they can wrap their legs around, having everything under control, "staying in the saddle" (rodeo, cowboy); gaining access to a woman and being able to assert oneself between her thighs

2. Thick, soft: in women - soft, female aura (anima); in earlier times, fleshy thighs with little strength were a beauty ideal, but today are frowned on as shapeless and flabby cellulite landscapes; in men - in every respect, but above all archetypally, unfitting, powerless and weak in structure; unsuitable for staying in the saddle and getting a good foothold in life;

3. Thin, slim: desired by women as the modern, female ideal of beauty; preferring elegance over strength, although slim thighs can produce a wiry, forceful aura (anima); in men: expression of powerlessness, not being able to forcefully assert one's masculinity, not being able to easily maintain one's grip in the saddle, losing one's foothold and power.

Task/subject: 1. Conveying a convincing stance, forceful self-assertion, bringing strength into life; standing with both feet firmly on the ground; improving one's standing; knowing what one stands for;

2. in women: developing the capacity for gentle yielding, cultivating flowing surrender (soft water wears away even the hardest stone); appreciating and learning to love one's own feminine archetype; in men: looking after the anima, the female aspect of one's soul;

3. in women: opening oneself willingly, offering life permission to enter, being quick and agile rather than defensive; withdrawing elegantly from the affair rather than offering massive resistance; in men: giving way, beating a hasty retreat rather than fighting; learning to give way and be adaptable in sexual matters; being flexible instead of strong.

Archetypal principle: 1. Jupiter-Mars; 2. Jupiter-Jupiter; 3. Jupiter-Venus.

Thoracic vertebrae

(see also Spinal column)
Symbolic meaning: Stability; supporting column of the upper body.
Task/subject: Stability for the world of feeling of the heart region; providing backing for the feelings and emotions; mirrors one's stance towards life: "bending over backwards", "bowing to the will of others", "bowing and scraping through life", but also "straightening up" and being upright and honest.
Archetypal principle: Saturn-Sun.

Throat

see Gullet

Thrombocytes

(blood platelets formed in the àbone marrow; see also Blood)
Symbolic meaning: Agents of blood coagulation.
Task/subject: Stopping bleeding, trapping the blood corpuscles in (fibrin) nets, sealing wounds.
Archetypal principle: Mars-Saturn.

Thumb

(see also Finger)
Symbolic meaning: Unity; antagonist of the four fingers, enables grasping due to its opposition, just as the polarity of concepts enables them to be grasped mentally; polarity symbol (also has only two joints) in the gesture of the "thumb's up" or "thumb's down" signal; guarantees fine motor control, the basis of culture (writing) and technology; expression of the will and forceful self-assertion ("putting the thumbscrews on somebody"); weakest point of a grasp; in spiritual medicine: the connection of the other

fingers with the thumb in special mudras (symbolic finger positions in Indian tradition) brings the Archetypal subjects related to the corresponding fingers into contact with unity.
Task/subject: Getting a grip on life, taking hold.
Archetypal principle: Mercury-Sun (symbol of the unity of the spirit: distinguishes man from animals).

Thymus gland

Symbolic meaning: Defense headquarters and training centre of the body's own armies for internal self-defence; development of immunity; original base of the T(hymus)-lymphocytes; (place of) maturation of the personality (identifying what is one's own and keeping out the foreign); intensification of the life energy (gorillas beat their chests before a fight, as do kinesiologists nowadays); relationship to faith in God, which is very pronounced in childhood as long as the thymus gland is still fully active; it atrophies increasingly over the course of life or becomes fatty.
Task/subject: The teaching of how to unmask and attack enemies; inner self-defence.
Archetypal principle: Mars-Sun-Jupiter.

Thyroid gland

(see also Hormones)
Symbolic meaning: Regulation point of the metabolism, determines the metabolic rate (the gross national product of the body); development, evolution, maturity; temperature regulator; authority that sets the measures for vitality, activity, motivation and self-determination.
Task/subject: Regulation of one's temperament and mood; further development, growth.
Archetypal principle: Mercury-Uranus.

Toes

Symbolic meaning: The lower fingers, grasping the earth; a stable foothold.
Task/subject: Good grip, steady footing, ensuring balance, guaranteeing the dynamism of progress, laying the groundwork for the future ("treading on someone's toes" = slowing them down, hindering their progress); mobility of the feet; finer roots: the end of the body; connection via the reflex zones to the head (as above so below).
Archetypal principle: Mercury-Neptune.

Toenails

Symbolic meaning: Lower (rear) claws.
Task/subject: Digging in one's claws, finding a good foothold.
Archetypal principle: Mars.

Tongue

Symbolic meaning: Forming speech: "speaking in many tongues" and "speaking in tongues" (biblical) as an expression of higher guidance; directness of verbal expression, weapon: "a pointed tongue", "sharp-tongued"; honesty: "speaking with a forked tongue"; chewing aid: pushing food between the grinding teeth; sensuality: licking and lapping up, tongue kissing.
Task/subject: Determining taste: differentiation; communication; facilitation, transport, assimilation; (aggressive) expression: "sticking one's tongue out at someone".
Archetypal principle: Mercury, Venus.

Tonsils

(palatine tonsils)
Symbolic meaning: Strongest police stations in the immune defence area

of the so-called Waldeyer's tonsillar ring, guard posts to the outer world, defensive bastions of the inner world against invasive pathogens from outside.
Task/subject: Guarding the entrance gates; if necessary, blocking the passage to the inner world if things have been swallowed which are indigestible.
Archetypal principle: Mars-Saturn.

Trachea

Symbolic meaning: (Gas) exchange.
Task/subject: Pipe responsible for supplying air and dividing it between the two lobes (wings) of the lungs.
Archetypal principle: Mercury.

Triple heater

(Meridian and functional circuit [organ] in Traditional Chinese Medicine; see also Meridians)
Symbolic meaning: "Official for Irrigation"; regulates the supply of the body's own fluids; Assignments: Yang, element - fire, complementary to the pericardial sac (pericardium; Yin).
Task/subject: Bodyguard of the "Emperor" (heart), who must be protected.
Archetypal principle: Sun-Saturn.

U

Upper arms

(see also Arms)
Symbolic meaning: Force, strength, power; the personal armies; symbols of power (biceps), home of (striking) power; ability to hold out/bear things.
Task/subject: Holding, lifting, hitting; applying leverage; bringing the world closer, pushing enemies away.
Archetypal principle: Mars.

Upper jaw

(see also Jaw)
Symbolic meaning: Weapons store; static home and base for our upper weapons (teeth); in comparison to the lower jaw (earth element) belongs to the "heavenly" region of the face and the air element; stands for the higher powers of mankind, but also for one's (family) origin; together with the cheekbones, it essentially determines one's facial expression: coupled with high cheekbones, it conveys the somewhat sorrowful-looking facial shape which is common in Slavic countries and corresponds to today's beauty ideal (àcheeks).
Task/subject: Sinking one's teeth into something (first catching hold of something before using the lower jaw to allow the trap to finally spring shut); gritting one's teeth and biting one's way through life.
Archetypal principle: Mars-Saturn.

Ureter

(connection between the kidneys and urinary bladder)
Symbolic meaning: Waste water channels.
Task/subject: Channelling off expended spiritual subjects.
Archetypal principle: Mercury-Moon.

Urethra

Symbolic meaning: Spiritual connection to the outer world; (spiritual) waste water pipe with shut-off valve (sphincter); in men, also the semen duct to the outside; pipeline for waste water and the water of life (seminal fluid).
Task/subject: Discharging, channelling and effective disposal of outlived spiritual matters.
Archetypal principle: Mercury-Moon.

Urinary bladder

Symbolic meaning: Withstanding pressure, deliberately letting go and passing things on; pressure cooker of the body; ability to handle tensions; (old and waste) water reservoir; considered in Traditional Chinese Medicine as the "Storehouse of Bodily Fluids", Assignments: Yang, element - water, complementary to the kidneys (Yin).

Task/subject: Collecting the (spiritual) waste water that has been cleared for excretion and letting it go in large amounts; providing relief for oneself (lower crying); being able to withstand and relieve (psychic) pressure: "pissing off"; pressure equalisation: discharging and relieving oneself; relaxing with confidence, letting the congestion flow (away); being able to hold one's water: "pissing one's pants in fear"; often the storage location of unshed tears, which often result from partnership problems (connection to the kidneys).

Archetypal principle: Pluto-Moon.

V

Vagina

Symbolic meaning: Opening oneself up, giving oneself to another; taking life into the fold; sexual enjoyment; sheath for the male sword; front entrance and exit to the (sexual) underworld; conveyance of life and desire (treasury of desire in eastern teachings of love); the larger and wider, the more the woman can open herself up, the deeper and further she can give herself to another; correlates with the growing commitment and orgasmic ability of women who have given birth to children; mature men prefer this expansiveness and openness to constriction and obstruction, while young, combative men, who still have to prove themselves (their manhood) prefer the tight virginal vagina, which they want to capture and conquer with a certain phallic penetrating force; provides the possibility, together with the male counterpart àthe penis, of overcoming the dichotomy of humankind for a moment: conveying the experiences of unity in the orgasm.

Task/subject: Sheltering and embracing, taking in and letting go; commitment and desire.

Archetypal principle: Moon-Venus.

Vagus

see Parasympathicus

Veins

(see also Blood vessels)

Symbolic meaning: The homecoming routes (Latin venire = 'to come'); the way home for energy: the old, used up life energy rescues itself by heading along these routes back to the fountain of youth (heart-lung system).

Task/subject: Return transport of the depleted, used up blood to the heart.

Archetypal principle: Moon-Mercury.

Vermiform appendix

see Appendix; Large intenstine

Vertebral column

see Spinal column

Visual cortex

(part of the cerebrum)

Symbolic meaning: Creation centre of inner images; magic mirror: makes images out of light stimuli; home-cinema.

Task/subject: Converting light stimuli into images.
Archetypal principle: Sun/Moon-Uranus.

Vocal cords

Symbolic meaning: Classical organ of self-expression; expression of one's own individuality; strings which we cause to resonate and vibrate (in us), and which cause us to resonate and vibrate; conveying the tone (mood) by means of the voice.
Task/subject: Articulation, formation of speech; verbal expression, communication.
Archetypal principle: Mercury-Venus.

Voice

Symbolic meaning: Vocal expression: the tone of the voice shows one's overall tone (mood); communication.
Task/subject: Articulation, formation of speech; expression of information and feelings (the range of one's tones –vocally and mood-wise).
Archetypal principle: Mercury (mediation), Moon (mood), Sun (expression of Self).

Vulva

(external female genitalia)
Symbolic meaning: Protective wall in front of the entrance to the body.
Task/subject: Veiling and protecting the sexual domain.
Archetypal principle: Pluto-Venus.

W

Waist

Symbolic meaning: In principle, second only to the neck as the narrowest point of the body; this bottleneck, respectively the waist size, is decisive for the figure and the feminine or masculine silhouette; in women: the middle magic number in the magical trinity of: bust – waist – hips; men appreciate in women the emphasis of the upper and lower dimensions (hourglass figure), with their clear separation by a slim waist being decisive for the overall impression; in other words, women should have a clear connection to the upper and lower (to the Heaven of the heart and to the Earth and the pelvis), but both of these should definitely not come into contact with each other as a seamless transition; in men a slim waist and a similar-sized pelvis are important in order to be considered as corresponding to the masculine prototype; in this case, a connection to the upper domain (to Heaven) is sufficient – deep-rootedness and a connection to the Earth are less in demand; for this reason, the pelvis should not protrude (Y-shape).
Task/subject: for women: differentiating between the upper and lower planes of life; developing both roots and the heart, but keeping these apart: for men: making room for the heart and developing broad, reliable shoulders, continually tapering downwards towards the waist.
Archetypal principle: Saturn.

Waist (shape)

Symbolic meaning: 1. Narrow: Tight spot (bottleneck) in life; modern ideal of the wasp waist; if reinforced by tight lacing or girdles, this produces the danger of blacking out, since top and bottom are no longer in proper contact (the head of the organism receives too little energy from the base); suppleness;

2. Thick: "life-belt" of fat around the hips allows one to stay above water, although at a problematic level; fear of going under; ideal feminine figure, soft hips; lower bodily centre of gravity.

Task/subject: 1. Separating Heaven and Earth, which should only come into contact with each other at one point;

2. Ensuring that one does not go under, but instead stays afloat; addressing the lower feminine pole on a more sophisticated level; integrating down-to-earth matters into life; nurturing those themes which have a central position in life; bringing together the heart and the pelvis – feeling and desire – and combining these on a broad basis.

Archetypal principle: 1. Saturn; 2. Saturn-Jupiter.

Windpipe

see Trachea

Womb

(Uterus)

Symbolic meaning: Fertility; primordial cave of all beginnings (closeness to Mother Earth with her caves, which provided the first protection for humans, and to the primevally feminine), the fertile primordial swamp, in which life can develop: (the first) nest, sense of security, place of protection for the growing, developing life, the maturing egg cell; organ which expresses the rhythm of the (female) cycle; very strong muscle (female power lies within, and only rarely becomes outwardly visible).

Task/subject: Sheltering and nourishing motherhood and life; opening oneself up and giving life (during birth).

Archetypal principle: Moon.

Womb (external orifice of the)

(Ostium uteri)

Symbolic meaning: Lower mouth.

Task/subject: Demarcation line between the outer and innermost world; gateway to life.

Archetypal principle: Moon-Saturn.

Wrist joint

(see also Joints)

Symbolic meaning: Scope of movement in one's methods for handling things, manipulation capability, flexibility in handling things.

Task/subject: Getting to grips with life and the world.

Archetypal principle: Mercury.

Part 2

Directory of symptoms

Directory of symptoms

B

M

N

A

ABO incompatibility

see Blood group incompatibility

Abdominal inflammation

see Adnexitis

Ablactation dyspepsia

(overly rapid ablactation leading to digestion problems)

Physical level: Digestive tract ("consuming and digesting the world" = Buddhism: Bhoga), stomach (feeling, instinct, enjoyment, centre).

Symptom level: The infant cannot digest, process or accept the (abrupt) separation from its mother's breast; rebellion via the stomach.

Handling: (on the part of the mother): recognising in the cramping of the child's stomach one's own tendency to cramping and conflict; recognising and accepting the cutting back of one's own freedom due to the child; letting go of prescribed opinions and programmes; adapting oneself to the individual situation; reconciling protection (motherliness) and giving birth (letting go).

Resolution: Accompanying the infant carefully to the next stage of independence, which leads both mother and child to greater independence.

Archetypal principle: Moon-Uranus.

Ablatio retinae

see Retinal detachment

Abortion (thoughts of)

Physical level: Womb (fertility, safety and security).

Symptom level: Conscious rejection of the unborn child; fear of the mother role; fear of the challenge (in the physical, mental, spiritual and/or social area); unconsciously letting something in and later not being able to face the challenge; running away from responsibility; inability to respond to life.

Handling: Being on one's guard against judgemental evaluations, and instead seeing through the relativity of these prevailing judgements (in wartime, there are even medals for deliberate killing); creating niches of freedom for oneself; ensuring one's own development possibilities, irrespective of the pregnancy; recognising the development opportunities which pregnancy could bring with it (e.g. growing up, becoming an adult); learning to respond to challenges; reconciliation between conscious and unconscious childhood desires; meditations on one's own role between girl, woman and mother; making oneself aware of Ego issues.

Resolution: From the point of view of esoteric philosophy, life can neither be created nor destroyed, it neither begins nor ends, but simply is; being receptive, ready to accept the great tasks of Fate: commitment and responsibility; becoming truly grown-up: Self-realisation (Self = Ego + Shadow).

Archetypal principle: Moon-Saturn-Pluto.

Abscess

(accumulation of pus due to tissue breakdown; see also Anal abscess, Inflammation, Furuncle)

Physical level: Almost all tissues and areas of the skin (border, contact, tenderness).

Symptom level: Problems with letting out (expressing) issues related to spiritual conflict and allowing them to come to the surface; explosion of repressed conflicts; conflict forcing its way up out of the depths, which crosses the barrier of the skin, wanting to surface into the light of consciousness; border conflict; encapsulated rage, anguish and despair; hot abscess: energetically highly-charged situation, building up towards explosion; cold abscess: (cold) rage, which has been transformed into resignation and disappointment, energetically-empty situation, danger of encapsulation without possibility of discharge (due to lack of energy); sterile abscess: no proof of a pathogen can be found; no conscious (human) opponent, but instead an undefined issue; danger of fistula formation (aggressive energy heading along incorrect and roundabout paths) with discharge into one's own bodily cavities or hollow organs to the point of self-destruction (→blood poisoning).

Handling: Consciously living out aggression: developing fighting skills, boxing, screaming exercises, aggressive dancing, developing an effective conflict culture; experiencing oneself as a volcano; letting out what must be let out at the imagery level; actively breaking through limits: explosion instead of implosion.

Resolution: Courageous conflict resolution by crossing the underlying borders; giving expression to the issue: relief by breaking through the borders of consciousness.

Archetypal principle: Learning how to deal with Mars (energy) and Saturn (border), Neptune.

Absences

(fit-like clouding of one's consciousness; see also Epilepsy)

Physical level: Brain (communication, logistics).

Symptom level: Turning away from this world, fleeing from reality.

Handling: Developing understanding for the fact that the body lives here, but the soul lives here and also beyond; becoming a wanderer between the worlds.

Resolution: Becoming familiar with the other, invisible world and nevertheless living here: being a border crosser.

Archetypal principle: Neptune.

Abuse (pathological)

(see also Addictions)

Symptom level: Confusion of the physical and spiritual level (alcoholics should concern themselves with spiritual subjects instead of with spirits, child abusers with the unresolved childlike aspects within themselves, thus reconciling themselves with their longing for innocence and purity).

Handling: Meditation on the actual (mental-spiritual) objective of the desire; discovering highs and ecstasy within oneself without external aids.

Resolution: Becoming one with the search (for those addicted to drugs or tablets); becoming one with the female aspects in oneself (for rapists); in general: exploring the spiritual (religious) dimension of life in order to get out of the compulsive repetition of excess.

Archetypal principle: Pluto, Neptune.

Acanthosis

(proliferation of the prickle cells of the upper layer of the skin; Acanthosis nigricans = a brown to black hyperpigmentation of the skin; Hyperkeratosis = excessive thickening/keritanisation of the horny layer of the skin)

Physical level: Skin (border, contact, tenderness).

Acathisia

Symptom level: Armouring, particularly at sensitive points (reproduction of the cells of the prickle cell layer of the skin); protection of the most sensitive points through darkening (abnormal pigmentation, particularly on the neck, in the armpits, groin, elbows, anogenital region, lips); camouflaging oneself through ugliness (warty proliferation of the skin, hyperkeratosis, keratosis).

Handling: Owning up to one's fear of getting hurt at the particularly sensitive points; taking conscious defensive and protective measures; hardening oneself with regard to sensitive and weak points.

Resolution: Consciously defending one's own weak points and vulnerable areas.

Archetypal principle: Saturn/Venus-Saturn.

Acathisia

(inability to sit still)

Physical level: Brain (communication, logistics), movement apparatus.

Symptom level: (first clarify and interpret the basic situation): lack of direction, always going round and round in circles, getting off track, e.g. in the case of →Alzheimer's disease.

Handling: Orientation exercises in the mental-spiritual respect; circular dances like the waltz and dances in the round, mandala painting and meditation as conscious rituals; setting off decisively on one's path (with the great objective – unity – in mind).

Resolution: Entrusting oneself consciously to the circle of life (mandala); living openness in all directions; meditations on Heraclitus' aphorism: Panta rhei ('everything flows').

Archetypal principle: Uranus-Jupiter.

Acceleration

see Puberty, premature

Accident

(see also Work accident/Domestic accident, Sport accident/injury, Traffic accident, Trauma)

Physical level: All levels of the body can be affected.

Symptom level: Outbreak of concealed aggression; compulsory lesson in the case of unresolved problems; an ignored conflict breaks into one's life as an apparent misfortune that is provided by Provide/nce (German word for "Fate" = Schicksal from schicken = 'to send' and Latin salus = 'health, well-being') in order to force an awakening; the external threat shows in an obvious way what has been neither recognised, taken for real or taken seriously in the narrower context; calls a form of action or the path a person has taken directly and suddenly into question; decisive break in the life flow; violent interruption of well-worn tracks; being suddenly shaken awake in order to take part in life more attentively again; caricature of one's own problem.

Handling: Reconstructing structure/the sequence of events leading to the accident and transferring it figuratively to one's own situation; understanding the accident event as a kind of break-in on life and helping this suddenly unfolding force to express itself in a more resolved (redeeming) way: instead of the change in routine enforced by the accident, preferring to consciously step out of line, kick over the traces and allow new creative impulses to break into one's life; recognising and accepting what Providence provides in order to save oneself misfortunes.

Resolution: Finding beneficial outlets and creative forms of expression for aggressive Mars-driven energy; voluntarily banking on variety and spontaneous, sudden interruptions in monotonous (life) processes; making the course of one's life more exciting,

more varied and "more dangerous to life": making oneself aware of the fact that life itself is fundamentally dangerous to life, and in every case ultimately ends in the opposite pole - Death; not tempting Fate, but instead opening oneself up voluntarily and at an early stage to its pointers.
Archetypal principle: Uranus.

Achalasia

(constricted entrance to the stomach; see also Vomiting/Nausea)
Physical level: Oesophagus (food pipe, nutrition supply).
Symptom level: Strong aversion to the large chunk that has been swallowed; chronic protest; deeply-rooted fear of any type of absorption; shutting oneself off against what is expected of one; "something makes us sick" or "comes back up again"; great hunger and extreme fear balance each other out; greed and ascesis.
Handling: Becoming honest about one's own attitude of rejection; admitting to oneself that one is not even beginning to properly address the world and life; putting an end to swallowing everything unconsciously; learning to spit out what does not agree with one; learning programme for conscious eating and enjoyment: eating slowly and in small bites.
Resolution: Deliberately choosing to protect oneself against what is detrimental; taking the path of small steps; working from the opposite pole: Bhoga (Buddhism. "consuming and digesting the world").
Archetypal principle: Moon-Saturn.

Achilles tendon tear

(see also Torn ligament)
Physical level: Achilles tendon (spiritual take-off power, steps forward/ progress, moving up), heel (weak point), ligaments/tendons (binding cords that everything hinges on).

Symptom level: Having greatly over-stretched oneself, risked too great a leap; being forced back down to Earth/reality with a hard thud; hubris: having overstepped the mark by setting one's mind on unrealistic ideas; strenuous emotional efforts; abrupt end to ambitious projects; ambition becomes a trip-rope, the (strongest) cord (of the body) tears.
Handling: Taking a break to think; refraining initially from undertaking any further great leaps; getting a firm grasp spiritually on what one is striving for; recognising which connections will only lead to mishaps and should therefore be given up; considering and learning to accept the consequences of physical and spiritual leaps.
Resolution: Having enough time; pausing for thought before activities (gaining an overview); making use of outer calm for inner activity (inner leaps, flashes of inspiration); taking small steps to reach the major goals.
Archetypal principle: Saturn-Mars-Jupiter.

Achromatopsia

see Colour blindness

Achylia

(lack of gastric juices)
Physical level: Stomach (feeling, receptiveness).
Symptom level: Lack of male, Mars-driven power for breaking things down.
Handling: Doing without sourpuss reactions (acidity) in the domestic (Moon) domain; leaving the acerbic (acidic) aspects where they belong.
Resolution: Creating an emotional sphere without using the male powers for breaking things down; accepting and dealing with the world without sourpuss (acidic) reactions.
Archetypal principle: Mars (acid)-Moon (stomach)-Saturn (lack).

Acidosis

(excess acidity)
Physical level: Fluid systems (spiritual subjects).
Symptom level: Too much of the male element (acid gives off H+-ions, while on the opposite pole, bases absorb H+-ions) tips the body's water level (soul) out of balance; excess acidity in the micro- and macrocosm (overtension, muscle rheumatism on the one hand, acid soils, dying forests on the other); a situation which makes one vitriolic (acidic), which eats one up internally and makes one caustically angry; often a disturbed relationship to the feminine element, the maternal aspect in general or one's actual mother; the feminine element, the maternal aspect is often given too little scope in life.
Handling: Using masculine means to get through to the soul; analysis of the archetypally-female body and Mother Nature in order to find ways out of the one-sidedness; being rigorous and strict with oneself, not sparing oneself and not whitewashing life; staring the problems with the opposite female pole straight in the eye.
Resolution: Acknowledging, accepting and realising the masculine pole; using the excess acidity of the entire inner and outer world to help recognise the task of using the resolved (redeeming) characteristics of the masculine pole to balance out the misery that it has led us into with its unresolved tendencies; realising the (masculine) spiritual aspect as the opposite pole to unresolved materialism, which although essentially feminine in nature, has nevertheless been unrestrainedly propagated by the unresolved masculine aspect; ultimate objective working from the opposite pole: harmony between the poles.
Archetypal principle: Mars.

Acne

see Puberty acne, Skin rash

Acoustic neurinoma

(benign growth of the nervus statoacusticus)
Physical level: Brain (communication, logistics), nervus statoacusticus (telephone line).
Symptom level: Growth impulses in the area of balance and hearing instead of on the corresponding figurative levels.
Handling: Practising inner balance and developing the ability to listen inwardly (the disease pattern threatens loss of hearing and balance); meditations on one's own centre, Tai Chi, making pottery on the rotating potter's wheel, mandala painting.
Resolution: Listening (inwardly and outwardly); being in (inner) balance; listening to the commands of the inner voice.
Archetypal principle:
Saturn-Jupiter-Venus.

Acromelagia

(late growth of the extremities of the body due to pituitary gland disease with increased secretion of growth hormone; see also Pituitary adenoma)
Physical level: Enlargement of the hands (grasping, gripping, ability to act, expression), feet (mobility, progress, deep-rootedness), ears (hearing and obeying commands), nose (power, pride, sexuality), chin (strong will, forceful assertion).
Symptom level: Growth on the physical instead of the mental-spiritual level.
Handling: Taking larger steps in the figurative sense; learning to get a grip, learning to listen (inwardly) (meditations on discovering one's inner voice).

Resolution: Stepping out in style in a spiritual sense; having a grip on life; forceful assertiveness; listening and obeying; having a good nose for things (intuition).
Archetypal principle: Jupiter.

Actinomycosis

(radial fungus infection with infiltration of the mucous membranes and formation of small, hard painless inclusions)
Physical level: Particularly the mucous membranes (inner boundary, barrier) of the oral cavity (mouth = absorption, expression, maturity – ability to speak for oneself).
Symptom level: Encapsulations, foreign bodies at the level of maturity.
Handling: Recognising what problems exist with regard to maturity (speaking for oneself), who one is feeding off in this respect (fungi = parasites); greater awareness with regard to foreign elements that one puts in one's mouth.
Resolution: Being mature (committed), i.e. speaking for oneself; following one's own line; finding a healthy Self-border; working from the opposite pole: putting only one's own clean words in one's mouth
Archetypal principle: Pluto.

Adam-Stokes syndrome

(insufficient oxygen supply to the brain)
Physical level: Centre of breathing (exchange, law of polarity) damaged by heart problems, stroke or poisoning; breathing before the final physical end.
Symptom level: Having fallen out of rhythm; battling on in a hopeless situation.
Handling/Resolution: (for helpers: conscious Handling/Resolution on the part of the person affected is

hardly still possible; it is now mostly a matter of the final act of letting go, the conscious departure from the body): playing religious masses or oratorios in the hospital room; reading aloud from the Tibetan/Egyptian Book of the Dead or the Bible.
Archetypal principle: Saturn-Mercury.

Addictions

(see also Abuse (pathological), Alcoholism, Depression, Drug addiction, Binge eating disorder, Messies syndrome, Smoking, Poisoning)
Workaholism: Illusion of being able to achieve everything through performance, to reap all acknowledgement possible and so to become one with everything; taking flight from problems at work.
Archetypal principle: Neptune-Saturn.
Greed: Wanting to possess everything and thus become one with everything; attempt to compensate for one's inner emptiness.
Archetypal principle: Neptune-Venus.
Addiction to success: Wanting to win the love of all people in order to become one with all people; lack of self-esteem.
Archetypal principle: Neptune-Sun.
Addiction to gambling: Wanting to win everything in order to have everything; attempt to become one with everything and be the Number One.
Archetypal principle: Neptune-Sun.
Addiction to collecting: Wanting to have everything complete in order to become complete.
Archetypal principle: Neptune-Venus/Saturn.
Addiction to setting records: Attempt to be the fastest/best and therefore to be the first.
Archetypal principle: Neptune-Mars.

Bulimia/binge eating: Attempt to assimilate everything and to become well-rounded and one with everything. Archetypal principle: Neptune-Venus.
Addiction to information: Wanting to know everything in order to become one with everything; lack of knowledge and above all wisdom. Archetypal principle: Neptune-Mercury.
Addiction to fame and glory: wanting to win the acknowledgement of all people in order to be loved by all people.
Archetypal principle: Neptune-Sun. Sex addiction: wanting to sleep with all people in order to become one with all people (nymphomania, satyriasis); lack of readiness for genuine orgasm and ecstasy or genuine feelings of unity.
Archetypal principle: Neptune-Pluto.

Addison's disease

([partial] disfunction of the adrenal cortex; J. F. Kennedy's disease pattern, whose symptoms he significantly over-compensated for as a womanizer and also with his words "Ask not what your country can do for you - ask what you can do for your country")
Physical level: Adrenal cortex (adrenal gland = centre for stress regulation, water balance and sex life).
Symptom level: Deficiency of the hormones (messenger substances) cortisone and aldosterone and the sex hormones: thirst for the spiritual element (water); having no hunger for life (lack of appetite), and thus becoming less weighty/substantial (weight loss); "shitting oneself" = being afraid (diarrhoea); powerlessness (weakness); excess pigmentation of the skin and mucous membranes: feigning vitality.
Handling: Concerning oneself with spiritual aspects; renunciation instead

of assimilation: giving up power (weight); concentration on the essential; overcoming disappointments; recognising and balancing out material, emotional and spiritual deficiencies; performing devotional exercises; paying attention to the dark sides/shadow issues which give or cost one strength.
Resolution: Integrated female pole; giving oneself completely as a life theme.
Archetypal principle: Moon-Saturn-Mars.

Adenitis

(lymph node inflammation)
Physical level: Everywhere where lymph nodes (police stations) are to be found (neck, groin, etc.).
Symptom level: Conflict, struggle, defensive battles: war at a restricted, local level and at a particular fort, which guards the access to a certain region of the body.
Handling: Confronting and tackling the issues that are forcing their way to the surface in a courageous and open(ly offensive) way instead of waiting until a blockage (node) has formed; defending oneself and learning from confrontations with one's environment.
Resolution: An offensively and courageously lived life.
Archetypal principle: Mars.

Adenocarcinoma

see Lung cancer

Adenoids

(polyps)
Physical level: Pharyngeal tonsils (police stations), mucous membranes (inner boundary, barrier) of the nose (power, pride, sexuality) and sinuses (lightness, airiness).
Symptom level: Allowing the nose to become overgrown, to be chronically

up to one's ears or eyeballs in something and thus sick to the back teeth of it all (impairment of nasal breathing); amazed, permanently perplexed facial expression: "having one's mouth open in amazement", "being gobsmacked"; "dumb-looking", less alert facial expression due to the mouth being continually open for breathing: children do not sniff around and are not curious and nosy, but instead are rather sluggish, lacking in concentration, "hard of understanding" and sometimes also hard of hearing = cut off from the primordial sensory perceptions (smell, taste and hearing), non-sensual existence; not getting enough exchange (air): anyone who does not breathe through the nose also cannot smell, sniff or catch wind of things properly; life is not particularly appetising (no perception of aromas; all food tastes boring); having had enough and being overwhelmed; danger of development being delayed or coming to a complete stillstand; rigidity; permanent conflict; lack of energy due to being stuck in a rut; communication that has been blocked and directed into the wrong channels: necessity to restrict communication; polyps as policemen – "the long arm of the law" who catch one (like octopi) with their tentacles: defence, protection of the organism against intruders.

Handling: homeopathically: becoming aware that one is chronically up to one's ears or eyeballs in something and thus sick to the back teeth of it all; consciously addressing excessive demands and frustrations; recognising conflict in the domain of communication with one's environment; checking one's own communication channels: learning wise restrictions; allopathically: allowing development, developing self-confidence and the will to push on (determination) rather than push away (withdrawal); opening up borders, instead of closing them (oneself) off.

Resolution: Communication and connections with the outside world, which are reduced to the essential; ability to be amazed instead of rigidity; peace and quiet in the middle of life's flow.

Archetypal principle: Mercury-Saturn-Mars (polyps/policemen).

Adenoma

(benign growths originating from the glandular tissue)

Physical level: Various glandular tissues (control, information).

Symptom level: Swelling, tumour; possible hyperfunction of the relevant glandular tissue; often due to a traumatic experience: the trauma energy is absorbed in the corresponding organ or tissue, and compresses itself into a tumour.

Handling: Expanding in the symbolically corresponding domain (e.g. in the case of bronchial adenoma: extending communication).

Resolution: Mental-spiritual growth on the symbolically corresponding level of the relevant outlet gland.

Archetypal principle: Jupiter.

Adhesions

(concrescences, tissue growths)

Physical level: All internal organs in the area of the stomach can be affected (particularly as a consequence of operations).

Symptom level: Things which originally do not belong together grow together and hinder each other painfully.

Handling: Making unusual connections in the mental-spiritual area as well, and if necessary, even accompanied by pain; bringing the various channels of digestion and processing closer together.

Resolution: Unusual, new connections on the figurative level; growing

together of various non-related areas; being one with one's intuition (gut feeling).
Archetypal principle: Mercury-Jupiter.

Adipose tumour

(lipoma)
Physical level: Fatty tissue (overflow, excess reserves), All parts of the subcutaneous fatty tissue can be affected.
Symptom level: Benign proliferation in the area of overflow and excess – the storage capacity; growth of the reserve capacity; expansion overshoots the mark in the isolated area: often arrogance in this subject area; sometimes pressure pains related to one's position: coming under pressure due to developments bursting the banks in the area where the overflow accumulates.
Handling: Allowing material and mental-spiritual reserves to accumulate; observing and processing the excess which is putting one under pressure in a critical way (giving it away, e.g. into the hands of surgeons); allowing reserves to become visible and tangible, showing and using them in life.
Resolution: Accumulating reserves, respectively, excess on extended levels (bank account and one's memory (consciousness) bank).
Archetypal principle: Jupiter.

Adipositas

(see also Obesity, Lipophilia)
Physical level: The whole body can be affected, particularly the stomach (feeling, instinct, enjoyment, centre), buttocks (holding things out, forceful assertion), thighs (steps forward, steadfastness), neck (assimilation, connection, communication), etc.
Symptom level: Outer fullness instead of inner fulfilment; outer protective walls instead of inner security.

Handling: Expanding in the figurative sense, extending one's own scope of influence; carrying weight (importance) instead of being weighty.
Resolution: Fulfilment; taking up and filling the space that is one's due; extension of consciousness.
Archetypal principle: Jupiter.

Adnexitis

(abdominal inflammation, inflammation of the adnexa of the womb; tubes and ovaries; see also Ovaries, inflammation, Ovaries, suppuration, Fallopian tubes, inflammation, Fallopian tubes, suppuration)
Physical level: Female sexual region (fertility, sexuality).
Symptom level: Conflict over the subjects of fertility, reproduction; misunderstanding sex as a performance sport; aggravation of the issue and the affected region.
Handling: Paying attention to cleanliness in the sexual area; recognising frequently-changing sexual intercourse as an expression of a conflict; coming to terms with the area of fertility/sexuality.
Resolution: Fighting with offensive, courageous means for one's own ideas of fertility and having children.
Archetypal principle: Moon-Mars.

Adontia

(congenital lack of teeth)
Physical level: Mouth (absorption, expression, maturity - ability to speak for oneself), upper and lower jaw (weapons store).
Symptom level: Lack of bite and capacity to grit one's teeth ("being a toothless tiger"); vitality deficit: not being able to bite off one's own piece of life; lack of attractiveness: looking old and decrepit; making a completely non-vital impression.
Handling/Resolution: Exercises on learning how to forcefully assert oneself without aggression (model:

Mahatma Gandhi); discovering and making inner beauty a reality.
Archetypal principle: Saturn-Moon.

Adrenal cortex hyperfunction

see Cushing's syndrome

Adrenal cortex insufficiency

see Addison's disease

Adrenal gland medulla tumour

see Pheochromocytoma

Adrenogenital syndrome

(reversal of →testicular feminisation)
Physical level: Genitalia (sexuality, polarity, reproduction).
Symptom level: A woman who lives in a male-looking body; living the life of an exile.
Handling: Getting to know the world of men as a woman in a natural male disguise; reconciliation with the male aspect of the spirit at all levels.
Resolution: Consciously carrying and resolving the aspects of both sexes (anima and animus).
Archetypal principle: Uranus.

ADS (Attention deficiency syndrome)

see Hyperactivity

Aerophagia

(swallowing air)
Physical level: Stomach (feeling, receptiveness), gullet (assimilation, defence), digestive organs ("consuming and digesting the world" = Buddhism: Bhoga).

Symptom level: Feigned willingness to swallow and assimilate something; the air element is swallowed and not intellectually transformed: a misunderstanding causing aggression; "poor sucker": having no say, swallowing everything without objection, having to swallow orders; higher or intellectual expectations: puffing oneself up, puffed up (with importance?); being under pressure to express oneself (burping); not being able to get a word in (children often complain of never having the chance to air their views and having to swallow everything).
Handling: Giving vent to things; swallowing and digesting the air element in the form of thoughts/fantasies/ideas/books, and letting it out again in the form of offensive, innovative ideas; expressing oneself in concrete terms, instead of just producing hot air: recognising where one is puffing oneself up in an exaggerated way; bringing thought and awareness into spiritual areas.
Resolution: Quality-awareness in swallowing and speaking; processing thoughts and feeling and sensing consciously; taking for oneself what one needs in ideal terms.
Archetypal principle: Moon-Mercury.

Affective psychosis

see Manic-depressive disease

Ageing, premature, in children

see Progeria

Age-related symptoms

(see also Senile heart, Senile deafness, Senile hypermetropia, Greying, Chronic diseases, Depression, Insomnia, Sleep problems)

Symptom level, general: Everything recedes away into the distance (senile hypermetropia) – including death, which makes life appear longer; the steps become shorter, also making one's path and life seem longer: the destination recedes into the distance (death is pushed away although it is continually edging closer); sleep becomes shorter, which makes the days appear longer; illusion of having plenty of time, although one has less and less of it; viewed from the opposite pole: impression that time is simply flying past; the return path (in the life mandala) appears much shorter than the outward path; the less intensively life is lived, the faster it flies by.

Symptom level, specifics: Age spots (harmless pigment disorders of the skin): being marked by age; age blemishes (harmless growths with age): unresolved dark sides come to the surface; →hair loss to the point of baldness: losing hair (feathers) in the fray; forgetfulness (short-term memory): losing what is temporally closest from consciousness; calcification (→arteriosclerosis): the power line of vitality becomes restricted and rigid; lines and creases: one's basic spiritual attitude is reflected in one's face, and becomes a mask; wrinkles and crow's feet: reveal the traces left by life; developing features of the opposite sex: masculinisation of women (harsh facial features, →female facial hair) and effeminacy of men (womanly, "softie" facial features); senile insomnia: the dark and still unaddressed aspects of life allow one no rest.

Handling/Resolution: Learning to face up to one's age; accepting and enjoying it; transforming being marked into a form of distinction awarded by life, which has left behind its traces; reconciling oneself to one's own dark character traits; reminder of unsettled bills; losing hair = having to pay (in the same way that losing hair cost Samson dearly); concerning oneself with the guiding golden thread of life and forgetting the trivialities that are close at hand; reducing oneself (one's life) to the essential; learning to face up to the basic features of one's character; bearing the marks of life as distinctions; taking care of the opposite spiritual pole (animus in women, anima in men); addressing open issues on the return path to the centre of the life mandala; spiritual awakening.

Archetypal principle: Saturn.

Aggressiveness

(negative, destructive aspect of aggression; see also Rage, fits of, Amok-running)

Physical level: Brain (communication, logistics).

Symptom level: Pent-up aggressive energy seeks various outlets: via the musculature in the form of restlessness (→hyperactivity), assaults and violent conduct or →accidents; via verbal expression in the form of verbal attacks; on the physical level in the form of infections (→inflammation) and →allergy to the point of → Auto-aggressive/Auto-immune diseases (e.g. →rheumatism, →depression).

Handling/Resolution: Constructive handling of one's own aggressive energy: playing sport, developing a conflict culture, strengthening the immune system.

Archetypal principle: Mars.

Agitation

(see also Nervousness)

Physical level: Vegetative nervous system (news service) of the whole organism from the heart to the skin.

Symptom level: State of emergency in the landscape of the body, uproar in the vegetative nervous system;

being out of balance; readiness (for action), expectant stance.
Handling: Consciously listening to the body and tracking down the tensions, perceiving the unrest in the landscape of the body and taking it seriously.
Resolution: Being open to and ready for everything.
Archetypal principle: Uranus.

Agnosia

(loss of ability to recognise sensual impressions from various sensory areas in the brain)
Physical level: Brain (communication, logistics).
Symptom level: Inability to recognise oneself, e.g. in cases of →Alzheimer's disease, →Cerebral contusion.
Handling/Resolution: Learning to get by and put up with the simplest of perceptions; realising simplicity on the figurative level ("Blessed are the poor [simple] in spirit, for theirs is the kingdom of Heaven").
Archetypal principle: Saturn.

Agoraphobia

(fear of large open spaces; see also Phobia)
Symptom level: Not daring to go out into the big wide world, fear of expansiveness and openness from the mental-spiritual point of view; fear of staking out one's own space.
Handling: Making oneself aware of the last phase of birth: the step from constriction into expansiveness (feeling of being lost in the world); making oneself aware of one's own narrowness (of awareness); accepting one's own smallness; accepting that one is a grain of sand in the cosmos; fulfilling the task of this grain of sand; concentrating on the essential; safeguarding one's own narrow four walls; accepting the emptiness and expansiveness in one's own life.

Resolution: Reconciliation with compulsive confinement, finding security in the narrowest area; owning up to and bearing the fact that one is "all alone in the big wide world"; working from the opposite pole: becoming inwardly expansive, staking out space; finding one's own place, one's own home (in the world); ultimate objective: recognition that the actual real kingdom is not of this world.
Archetypal principle: Saturn-Jupiter.

Agranulocytosis

(lack of white blood corpuscles)
Physical level: Immune system (defence).
Symptom level: Fatal inability to defend oneself against attacks from outside (lack of defensive capability against bacteria because of the lack of white blood corpuscles).
Handling: Exercises in allowing things admission in the figurative sense instead of abandoning all physical resistance.
Resolution: Spiritual willingness for absorption; openness, boundlessness within the boundaries of one's own (path of) fate; balance between setting limits and openness.
Archetypal principle: Saturn-Mars.

Aids

Physical level: Immune system (defence).
Symptom level: Physical openness instead of openness in the mental-spiritual sense, which is not compatible with life in the long term; physical lack of defence and protection with increased defensiveness in the figurative sense; increasing inability to defend oneself immunologically goes along with greater readiness to defend oneself spiritually; sexual →feelings of guilt; suppressed love; threat arising from the driving force of sexual desire; brings the archetypally male pole to despair and compels

regard for the female pole; forces the male principle to its knees and attempts to teach it love; appeal to the sympathy of others; overemphasis of external/material elements to the neglect of internal aspects, feelings and awareness (sex instead of love); prevention of all resistance: teaches at the physical level what unification and love could be on the spiritual level; expression of the suppressed dark goddess (Hekate/Kali) and her terrible anger; symbol of collective dependency and how we are intertwined with each other.

Handling: Battling to gain mental-spiritual openness in order to be able to protect the (vital) borders at the physical level; learning to open oneself spiritually and defend oneself physically: learning to protect the physical level (condoms); learning to bring together content and form (love and sexuality); distancing oneself from physical violence and force (Mars), emphasis on tenderness (Venus), which cannot lead to any (surface) wounds; learning to emphasise the female over the male pole; spiritual opening through candid discussions without reservation; exercises in trust: letting oneself fall; self-control for the purpose of urge control.

Resolution: Truly opening oneself to a person; capacity for binding relationships, "bearing" consequences (in the dual sense of 'taking responsibility' and 'enduring'); surrendering oneself to life as a whole, including its dark sides (also in relationships); unification, becoming one with everything on the mental-spiritual level.

Archetypal principle: Pluto-Neptune (Mars-Venus-Saturn).

Air, swallowing

see Aerophagia

Akinospermia

(immobility of the male sperm; see also Necrospermia, Infertility)

Physical level: Testicles (fertility, creativity).

Symptom level: Infertility due to immobility of the semen; immobility with regard to one's own masculinity; no longer being really able to fulfil the male role; no longer being a real mate (no longer being able to "mate").

Handling: Giving up traditional conceptions of masculinity; reviewing one's own role expectations; recognising and rethinking the lack of fertility; giving up the non-committal "hustle and bustle"; coming more to rest oneself, instead of putting the sperm to rest.

Resolution: Finding one's own life rhythm; being innerly at rest.

Archetypal principle: Mars-Saturn.

Albinism

(general lack of pigment)

Physical level: Skin (border, contact, tenderness) and its adnexa; eyes (insight, perspective, mirrors and windows of the soul).

Symptom level: Complete lack of colour in the border areas (skin): colourless life; complete colourlessness of the symbols related to freedom and power - the antennae (hair); red shimmering window of the soul (eyes): warning; white as the colour of unity on the physical instead of the consciousness level: not being prepared for a life in polarity; remaining stuck in the innocence of the embryonic paradise situation; vitality appears dangerous (avoidance of the sun because of the danger of sunburn).

Handling: Restriction to the essential contrasts in the external impression created; "blowing hot and cold", living a life of contrasts.

Resolution: Doing justice to white - the all-embracing colour of unity - on the consciousness level; inner

brightness; ultimate objective working from the opposite pole: opening oneself up to life with all its colours and shades.
Archetypal principle: **Saturn-Moon.**

Albuminuria

(protein excretion via the urine in the case of kidney problems or over-exertion)
Physical level: **Kidneys (balance, partnership).**
Symptom level: **The building blocks of life are lost through the filter of the kidneys; the kidneys – the organs responsible for balance – let essential things slip through; letting go on the physical instead of the figurative level.**
Handling: **Letting go of important partnership themes; letting go in general, learning to forgive, but also recognising where important things in life are "slipping through the cracks".**
Resolution: **Letting things happen, being able to let go, even in the case of vital matters; the ultimate objective lies in the opposite pole: balance between letting go and retaining.**
Archetypal principle: **Venus.**

Alcoholism

(see also Addictions; Depression; Fatty liver; Liver, cirrhosis; Pancreas, inflammation)
Physical level: **Almost all areas are affected, particularly the liver (life, evaluation, reconnection), stomach (feeling, receptiveness) and nervous system (news service).**
Symptom level: **Attempt to make the hard world appear soft, and to feel soft and round oneself; escape drug: using alcohol to steal away into a more beautiful world full of illusions and dreams, "putting on the beer goggles" to make someone more beautiful; concealing feelings of guilt or pain over failure; expression of insecurity and weakness, lack of courage: drinking in Dutch courage/** liquid courage instead; softening the constrictive feeling of anxieties; "having a skinful" to "fill in" the abyss of inner emptiness and feelings of senselessness; not being able to handle traumas: suppressing the misery of one's own history and/or existence with alcohol; flushing down what would otherwise be too difficult to digest; swallowing everything (down); swallowing whatever comes ("poor sucker", "boozehound"); drunken stupor instead of ecstasy; lack of friends: the bottle becomes the best friend; longing for human closeness and a conflict-free, whole-some, brotherly world by means of conflict avoidance; regression: the babbling, stumbling drunk regresses verbally and motorically to the level of a small child, and once again is dependent on the bottle; sucking on the bottle gives "sucklings" a feeling of security; leads in the long term to →impotence.
Handling: **Making friends with one's own softness and looking for oases of softness (of the female pole) in the hard world; making provision for security in the spiritual and social domains; making one's own life into a well-rounded affair, with the soft sides also receiving recognition; regression exercises in warm water, womb exercises; learning to swallow in the figurative sense, acquiring tolerance for frustration; ecstasy exercises: ecstatic sexuality, engaging in corresponding dances, music, sports such as (wind-) surfing or deep-snow skiing; reconciling oneself with one's own childishness; rituals related to becoming grown up; reconnecting with/retreating to the essential; rituals that involve seeking: Vision Quest; spirituality instead of spirits ("meditating instead of boozing"); attending Alcoholics Anonymous (AA) groups.**
Resolution: **Taking in and taking on whatever comes one's way; searching for sense, unity, being "healthy" in the sense of whole or holy: creating**

a whole-some, ideal world in one's inner reality; re-ligio(n) (from Latin: religāre 'to bind, tie again') as a reconnection to unity, becoming one with everything (true brotherliness); using the opposite pole: coping with the world instead of fleeing from it.
Archetypal principle: Neptune.

Alcohol poisoning

Physical level: Brain (communication, logistics), liver (life, evaluation, reconnection).
Symptom level: End of capability for control, loss of inhibitions, thought disorders, poor judgement, ignoring boundaries: loss of control instead of giving up the restricting inhibitions; giving up critical thinking in favour of feeling and perception; lessening of the power of judgement and the tendency to be judgemental; abandoning one's distance from people.
Handling: Exercises in trust: letting oneself fall; recognising which inner attitudes from deep within separate one from other people; intoxicating experiences, inspiration with regard to one's life goal; getting into the spirit of things (empathising) rather filling oneself with spirits; seeking to achieve closeness and empathy, along with feeling and trust in more redeeming ways.
Resolution: Surrendering oneself to life and one's own task in it; becoming one with the longing for unity, setting out on the spiritual search; feeling a sense of brotherhood on the mental-spiritual level with all sentient beings.
Archetypal principle: Neptune.

Alcohol psychoses

(see also Alcoholism, Alcohol poisoning, Korsakow's Syndrome, Addictions, Delirium)
Physical level: Almost all areas are jointly affected, particularly the brain as the basis of consciousness,
nervous system (connection, communication), liver (evaluation, philosophy of life, religion).
Symptom level: Develops as a rule from a long history of alcohol abuse; the brain then reacts over-sensitively to even the smallest quantities of alcohol (sensitisation to alcohol); the personality façade that is shown outwardly collapses under the toxic effect of alcohol; facets of the personality that have been suppressed deep in the unconscious then find their way into consciousness; loss of inhibitions, thought disorder, poor judgement, loss of control, delusional jealousy, collapse of critical thought and power of judgement, inundation with anxieties from the depths of the shadow world; but also "in vino veritas".
Handling: Reconciling oneself with one's own shadow world (psychotherapy); gentle regression exercises, e.g. in warm water, womb exercises; rituals that involve seeking: Vision Quest; alcohol therapy see also →Alcoholism and →Alcohol poisoning.
Resolution: Accepting what rises up out of the depths of one's own underworld as a task; shadow therapy, which carefully makes the wall between conscious and unconscious spiritual levels more transparent in order to gradually bring shadow aspects to consciousness.
Archetypal principle: Neptune-Pluto..

Alexia

(inability to read)
Symptom level: Largely rejecting this intellectual world.
Handling: Instead of reading letters (in German Buchstaben, originally Buchenstäbchen = 'beech sticks', which illustrated the will of God), learning to understand God's language directly, which is read-ily recognisable in all Creation; devoting

oneself to concrete aspects instead of abstractions.
Resolution: Reading God's Creation like reading a book.
Archetypal principle: Mercury-Saturn.

Alkalosis

(pH-level increase in the blood, opposite pole of →acidosis [excess acidity])
Physical level: Initially in the tissue (stability), later spreading to the blood (life force).
Symptom level: Too many "female" basic (alkaline) elements in the body instead of in the soul.
Handling: Preserving more of the feminine on the figurative level; consciously opening oneself up in a friendly way (instead of reacting in an "acerbic", sourpuss way).
Resolution: Living up to one's own female pole; allowing room for the female in the world; ultimate objective: finding and maintaining balance between the male and female pole (Yin and Yang).
Archetypal principle: Moon-Venus (opposite pole to the "acidity" of Mars).

Allergy

(see also Immune deficiency, Inflammation, Vaccination damage)
Physical level: Skin (border, contact, tenderness): what gets under one's skin against one's will is combatted here; mucous membranes (protective covering, inner border), particularly of the nose (power, pride, sexuality): objectionable matters that those affected turn their noses up at become clear here; lungs (contact, communication, freedom): matters which threaten to stifle one strike here, digestive system ("consuming and digesting the world" = Buddhism: Bhoga): indigestible aspects lead in this case to an uprising.

Symptom level: Raising one's hackles: "being allergic to someone or something"; intolerance, irritability and over-reaction, which attach themselves to certain substances and their symbolism; a part of the world is rejected and combatted in a massive way on the symbolic level using one's own immune defences; allergy as a possible means of saying no; conflict between great aggression and great sensibility; war on the physical plane; over-reaction, escalation, defence, overblown concept of the enemy: going for friends (e.g. food) instead of enemies (e.g. bacteria); strong unconscious aggressiveness, unrecognised and unexpressed aggression: blind projection of aggression, pent-up aggression, suppressed vitality; combatting whatever causes fear, fear of exuberance/vitality: fear of vital breakthroughs (e.g. including those of spring with its (phallically)-pointed buds and sprouts, trees catapulting their seeds and erupting with blossoms and vegetables shooting up out of the ground); power games: enforcing one's will through the avoidance of allergens, tyrannising the surrounding world and thus acting out aggressions; the resulting →feelings of guilt lead to further suppression of aggressions.
Allergens: Symbols for something vital or dirty which is classified as dangerous; frequently symbolically associated with an event in connection with which or a person against whom severe aversion or rage is felt; these can be classified into two overlapping circles:
1. Allergens with erotic-sexual themes (seeds, pollen, animal hair and fruits and everything slimy, soft and mushy),
2. Allergens connected with the themes of dirt, worthlessness and female aspects in the narrower or broader sense. The first small circle is enclosed by the larger second

circle, since its allergens can only have an effect as such if sexuality and eroticism are also unconsciously perceived as dirty and worthless. Both aspects can also often be found mixed together in one allergen. The symbolic reference in such things does not have to be known to the person affected; it is sufficient if it is known to the collective unconscious (e.g. the small child does not know that penicillin is produced from mould fungus).

1st group: erotic-sensual "dirt" Animal hair: Fear of love with an animalistic, sexual connection; every type of fur conveys something ani-malistically-cuddly, soft, warm and thus sensually erotic, and as such, can be combatted allergically: Dog (hair) = eagerness to attack (barking), aggressive masculine forces (the alert watchdog or police dog); snap-pishness (love bites, "loving someone to bits" or "wanting to eat them up"); Horse (hair) = the animalistic/libidinal (young girls often go through a "horse phase" before puberty, in which they practice reconciling themselves with the animalistic/libidinal in a cavalier/knightly and thus chivalrous style); the masculine (the cowboy who masters his world with the strength of his thighs); denying oneself suc-cess, since one cannot stand up for one's masculinity or one's feminine strength; Cat (hair) = pure eroticism (plush pussycat, sex kitten) with a dash of aggression (showing one's claws, wildcat) and freedom (being choosy); acting "cattish", pussyfooting around, stalking ready to pounce, magic, witchcraft.

Blossom pollen, grass seeds ("plant sperm") = fertility, love, sexuality, animalistic instinct (see also Allergy to human sperm below).

Nuts = fertility ("nuts" as a slang word for testicles), love, sexuality, animalis-tic instinct; unsolvable or at least diffi-cult problems ("a hard nut to crack").

Fruits = results of the sexual union of male and female ("the fruit of one's loins"); the attractive, forbidden fruit on the other side of the fence - "stolen fruit tastes sweetest"; Apple = the original symbol of temptation (since the Garden of Eden), aspect of curiosity; desire to tread new paths; Strawberries = the plump, ripe, seductively red fruit; "I am so wild for your strawberry mouth" (François Villon); Peach = attractive, "peachy" skin; erotic, "peachy" bottom; Cherry = slang word for the hymen; "losing one's cherry", i.e. giving up the prize of one's virginity; cherries always hang from the tree in suggestive pairs; Banana = phallic fruit with re-gard to shape, which when mashed up as the basis of muesli or pap for children has something sticky and mushy about it (slimy mucous).

Human sperm = the masculine element judged as unclean and dan-gerous; the woman wants to have no contact with him and to have no issue in common with him (in the form of a child); greatest possible unconscious rejection of the partner.

Insect sting = penetration, sexual act (penetration of the phallic sting, which injects something poisonous that causes one to swell up); emotional stings, stinging taunts; especially bee stings = the busy bee that is self-sac-rificing as part of its very nature; wasp stings = one's own aggressive manner.

Sunrays: 1. Allergy to sun protection agents = sensual aspect of applying cream; the slippery, oiled body as a sex object or symbol of erotic power; 2. Fear of the caressing, erotic and warming contact of the skin by the sun's rays; significance as an allergen nowadays also because of current warnings about the hole in the ozone layer.

2nd group: predominantly dirt, worth-lessness and other "mixed"themes

House dust (excrement of house dust mites) = dirty, unclean, and impure aspects, but also banal elements – the common, the everyday dirt; often as an allergen in people who want to move up in the world or who feel themselves called to higher things, but who lack the courage to draw any consequences from this conviction. Washing agents = dirty, stained, unclean, and impure aspects; the washing agent brings the opposite pole (dirt) to the surface where its sign-ificance is obvious and is combatted accordingly.

(Day)light (as distinct from genuine photo-dermatoses, which are less allergy-based in character than a defensive reaction of the skin to sun and light) = defence and fear of the discovery of secrets: "not wanting to stand in the limelight", "not wanting to shed light on something", "shunning the light of truth", "not wanting to bring anything to light which could expose one", "not showing oneself in one's true light", "where there is shadow, there is also light"; not wanting to shed the light of consciousness on dark and suppressed desires of a sexual nature that are perceived as dirty ("red light district"); fear of kindling the life force ("viriditas" – the divine green power spoken of by Hildegard von Bingen): "getting the green light" and of being prodded into the process of individuation: "let there be light!"; fear of life: "not wanting to see the light of day".

Food and beverages (food as a means for the nourishment of life, vitality) in general = the dirty, impure and dangerous elements in our nourishment; Grains (as cereal pap/sticky dough) = the slippery, slimy, sweet aspects (bread chewed for a long time becomes sweet because of the glucose it contains) are combatted because of their similarity to the slippery sexual intercourse situation; in addition to this, there is conflict over one's humbleness inherited from one's family, which dictates that one should be satisfied with simple things such as bread; Gluten (the "glue" of grains) = the smeary, sticky, binding aspects; Milk = the motherly-female aspects; Protein (proteins such as casein, →milk intolerance) = avoidance of life (protein is one of the basic building blocks of life); Alcohol = the intoxicated-ecstatic high, loss of control; eruption of dark forces, loss of inhibition.

Medications are increasingly coming to be talked about as dangerous, contaminated and harmful (also frequently as allergens); special case: penicillin (the mould fungus Aspergillus penicillinum) = dirt.

Paints, solvents: Since they have increasingly been found to be dangerous and toxic, they are occuring increasingly frequently as allergens (since this is now firmly anchored in the collective unconscious).

Metal: refers exclusively to base metals and their alloys, connection also to (coin) money = rejection of worthless, base aspects; fear of getting one's fingers dirty with money.

Metal alloys as compounds representing the merging/melting together of different elements = sexual parallels, rejection of sexual merging.

Handling: Learning to let out (express) rejection openly; training oneself to say no; learning to fight on different levels in addition to the immune system; aggression exercises (dynamic meditation, confrontation exercises, physical work – energy instead of allergy!) and sensitisation training (learning to distinguish friends from enemies); taking the exercise of aggression away from the body again and thinking and acting more aggressively; daring to live, consciously taking on challenges instead of cultivating avoidance behaviour; acting offensively; becoming more prepared to react, tackling the struggle of life;

learning to enjoy eroticism; desensitisation at the physical level through conscious involvement with the domains that are being avoided and rejected; letting what is being avoided into consciousness and assimilating it, e.g. in the case of a house dust allergy: reconciliation with dirty jokes, consciously washing dirty laundry in order to clean it; psychotherapy in the sense of shadow work.

Resolution: "Love thine enemies"; recognising that antagonistic elements also reside within one; consciously letting in the symbols considered as hostile and accepting them in their entire meaning; recognising that they are in reality friends; living courageously, grasping the red-hot irons (Mars) in life; having the front to face up to life, confronting it (Latin frons, -tis – 'forehead'); overcoming the fear of punishment; taking on challenges gratefully and courageously, and letting them demand one's courage in order to develop from these demands; experiencing courageously-vital eroticism (Venus), allowing oneself to be inflamed by Cupid's arrows (Mars); keeping female and male energy in a state of harmonious tension.

Archetypal principle: Mars-Pluto (suppression of aggression), Mars-Neptune (fleeing from aggression).

Alopecia areata

see Hair loss

Alopecia pityrodes

see Hair loss, Dandruff

ALS

see Amyotrophic lateral sclerosis

Altitude sickness

Physical level: Lungs (contact, communication, freedom), brain (communication, logistics).

Symptom level: With increasing height, the oxygen content of the air falls and consequently also the energy supply to the tissue, resulting in: concentration difficulties, euphoria, weakness, slowing down of movement and thinking capacities to the point of falling asleep and ultimately death; danger when climbing extremely high mountains (beginning above 3,000 m) for those not in proper condition: self-overestimation.

Handling: Making clear to oneself in which areas the air is becoming too thin; recognising the tendency to self-overestimation; aspiring to other pinnacles (peak experiences) e.g. in spiritual and interpersonal areas.

Resolution: Learning self-awareness and humility: the highest mountain peaks are home to the gods, and can only be visited safely with an attitude of humility.

Archetypal principle: Sun-Uranus

Alzheimer's disease

Physical level: Brain (communication, logistics), nerves (news service).

Symptom level: Premature ageing (formerly: presenile dementia); taking flight into old age in order not to have to accept any more responsibility; showing that one is no longer able (to cope) – not remembering anything, not knowing anything, not doing anything; unconscious demonstration of general disability; having lost the connection to one's development path; becoming childish instead of becoming child-like again; giving up responsibility for what is temporally close at hand (short-term memory starts to deteriorate first); losing the way, loss of orientation (no longer being able to find the East, the light): at the end of life, no goal has been achieved, no destination reached; instead, one has lost sight of the path: confusion; letting go of what has sunk down into the shadows; "Twilight of the Gods": the great oblivion; outward unrest (→akathisia) reflects the inner tension: bustling, small steps lead one back to one's starting point (going around in circles); speech disorders (→dysphasia) show that one has nothing more to say, and one's rhythm is no longer in synch; no longer coming into contact with the world; the inability to recognise people and things (→agnosia) shows that true recognition (insight) is no longer possible; in the final stage, not even recognising oneself: opposite pole to self-awareness; becoming incapable of movement (→apraxia) reveals the inability to handle the practical necessities of life; fluctuation between →depression (a summons to concern oneself with death) and euphoria (the realisation of Heaven within oneself); attempt to flee back into childhood, giving up all responsibility to one's environment; possible result of noise and chemical contamination (aluminium contamination from vaccinations, cooking utensils, aluminium film, etc.) and of general over-stimulation (brain as a digestive organ in the spiritual sense is overworked and its capabilities prematurely exhausted).

Handling: Detaching oneself from the past with its ties and binding commitments; setting out on one's path: small steps are better than none at all; becoming calm, allowing the release of tension; returning to the home of the soul; learning to view the world again with child-like amazement (speechlessness); dealing conclusively with death (depression); transforming the caricature of bliss (euphoria) into genuine happiness.

Resolution: Agnosia: transforming knowledge into wisdom, and then renouncing it: "I know that I know nothing"; no longer recognising oneself:

Odysseus, who recognises himself as Nobody; realising the simplicity of a child at the resolved (redeeming) level: "becoming like a child again", living in the here and now; returning to unity.

Archetypal principle: Neptune-Saturn.

Amalgam poisoning

(see also Heavy metal poisoning)

Physical level: Everywhere in the connective tissue (binding commitment, stability), particularly at risk: kidneys, nerves, muscles.

Symptom level: Build-up of deposits in the nervous system (brain, spinal cord, nerves): one's central regulation is brought into question; the overview is gradually lost; in the muscles (→fibromyalgia with typical muscle pains): one's (mental-spiritual) agility has become a problem; in the joints (rheumatic complaints): only being able to articulate oneself with pain; in the kidneys: harmonious relationships with other people are made more difficult by blockages in communication.

Handling: At the dental level, amalgam decontamination with corresponding precautionary measures (cofferdam screening of the tooth that is to be treated from the rest of the oral cavity using a rubber dental dam) and amalgam decontamination at the tissue level; recognising the tendency in one's own life to create new problem areas through the clearing up of old problems; recognising one's own rigidity as a problem (nervous system, muscles and joints all have a relationship with the issue of agility/flexibility).

Resolution: Ensuring clean conditions between the lines and the areas that connect all of these together.

Archetypal principle: Mars-Pluto/Neptune.

Amastia

(congenital absence of the mammary glands)

Physical level: The female breast (nourishment, sensuality).

Symptom level: The attributes of mature femininity are missing, and thus also the ability to nurse and attract a partner in this way.

Handling: Acceptance of the natural Amazonian situation: living out both feminine and masculine subjects and characteristics at the same time.

Resolution: Accepting the androgynous life situation (angels have no breasts).

Archetypal principle: Moon-Uranus.

Amenorrhea

see Menstruation, absent

Amincolpitis

(see also Sexual diseases)

Physical level: Vagina (commitment, desire).

Symptom level: Fishy smell in the genital area caused by sexually-transmitted gardnerella bacteria; continual weeping discharge; the lower area of one's own sexuality stinks, both to oneself and the partner; unconscious rejection of sexuality: (unintentionally) making oneself unattractive.

Handling: Addressing the objectionable problem that one is turning one's nose up at; protecting oneself against questionable intruders, turning away uninvited guests, protecting the genital area.

Resolution: Making a considered choice in order to really be able to open oneself up inwardly.

Archetypal principle: Pluto-Venus.

Amnesia

(memory loss)

Physical level: Brain (communication, logistics).

Symptom level: No longer wanting to remember anything, no longer wanting to have a clear picture of things; forgetting one's prior life or individual events, deleting them from one's memory and thus from one's life; no longer wanting to have anything to do with them, and therefore taking flight into forgetfulness.

Handling: Exercises in letting go, learning to trust: consciously and ritually diving head-first into the water; falling backwards into someone else's waiting arms; letting oneself fall blindly into waiting arms amongst a circle of friends; allowing oneself to be helped; discovering the part of life where a new beginning is due.

Resolution: Release from the past; letting go of the old, arriving in the here and now; true identity.

Archetypal principle: Neptune.

Amniotic sac, infection

(amnionitis, in cases where the waters break prematurely or as the result of a very long delivery time or the main complication in the examination of the amniotic fluid [amniocentesis])

Physical level: Womb (fertility, safety and security).

Symptom level: Life-threatening conflict, which can originate both from the mother or from the child; aggression of the child against the nest (foetal membrane), in which it feels itself trapped; rage against the eggshell, which hinders its attempts at freedom; the mother holds the child back for too long; aggression of the mother against the child, which is driven out of the protective, nourishing womb.

Handling: Becoming aware of and confronting the conflict over pregnancy.

Resolution: Facing up to the situation, and in this final conflict, consciously crossing over to the side of

the child; fighting side by side for its life.
Archetypal principle: Moon/Saturn-Mars/Uranus.

Amoebic dysentery

see Dysentery

Amok, running

(see also Aggressiveness)
Symptom level: Suddenly and recklessly directing long-suppressed aggression (Malayan amok = rage) outwardly, usually against innocent bystanders: rupture of the dam of aggression; bursting of the dam of emotions; explosion, after the pressure release valve has been blocked for a long time; a shadow aspect issue blazes a path to the surface with sudden aggressive momentum; in the traditional Malay-Indonesian culture, a person running amok was regarded as the temporarily-insane victim of "dark inner forces" and went unpunished.
Handling: Expressing one's opinion, and learning to bear the resulting consequences; learning to give vent to aggression in good time; exercises in letting out aggression, such as dynamic meditation, martial arts, sport and movement as safety-release valves for aggressiveness.
Resolution: Self-control (presupposes recognition of one's own aggression) instead of suppression; integrating aggression into life as a healthy aspect of vitality; ultimate objective based on inclusion of the opposite pole: reconciliation of war (Mars) and peace (Venus); finding harmony in the centre between the extremes (the poles): making friends with Harmonia, the Goddess of Harmony, who is a daughter of Venus and Mars.
Archetypal principle: Mars-Pluto-Uranus (sudden eruption of suppressed aggression).

Amputation

(see also Accident, Gangrene, Diabetes mellitus)
Physical level: All limbs and organs can be affected.
Symptom level: Unconscious sacrifice of a part of the body, feelings of guilt with regard to transgressions or "evil" deeds (in countries with Medieval legal standards still a punishment for crimes today; thieves have their hand chopped off).
Handling: Voluntarily atoning for corresponding misdeeds; making sacrifices spontaneously and of one's own accord.
Resolution: Sacrificing oneself in the figurative sense instead of sacrificing parts of the body.
Archetypal principle: Pluto.

Amyotrophic lateral sclerosis (ALS)

Physical level: Motor nervous system (news service), first upper and second lower motor neurons.
Symptom level: Degeneration of the nerves from the brain via the spinal cord to the peripheral nerves with resultant multiple spastic paralysis, including the respiratory musculature (frequently resulting in →lung inflammations because of problems with swallowing); giving up one's connection to the executive organs; as a result, one's spirit and soul are less and less able to pervade the body; men are affected more frequently than women, including a conspicuously high number of competitive sportsmen, particularly footballers.
Handling: Voluntarily assigning the body to the second league; placing the soul and spirit in the central point of focus, taking them more seriously and rejoicing in them; the astrophysicist Stephen Hawking has been living with this disease pattern for over 40 years; he constitutes an exception in

this respect, but shows in any case the potential that exists.

Resolution: Conscious spiritualisation of one's own life; placing the focus on spiritual development: voluntary relinquishment of the demands on one's body; overcoming the physical aspects: platonic love; becoming one with the universe in a spiritual sense: liberation.

Archetypal principle: Saturn-Pluto.

Anaemia

(see also Iron deficiency, anaemia)

Physical level: Blood (life force), especially erythrocytes (energy carriers of the life flow).

Symptom level: Too few blood corpuscles or not enough pigment: too little colour and intensity in life; lack of vitality, lack of (life) energy, →fatigue, feeling of weakness; no joy in life, lack of courage to face life; refusal to take up one's own due share of life energy and put it into action; little interest in life; illness as an alibi for one's own passiveness; (spiritual) inability to open oneself up to the life energy, psychological lethargy; the pale, colourless appearance stands for a colourless life; pale with fear or exhaustion: the continual monthly recurring blood sacrifice of the period cannot be compensated for; haemoglobinemia (breakdown of the blood pigment): the colour seeps out of one's life.

Handling: consciously going about life in a calm way; sinking into one's calming centre; learning genuine modesty; consciously turning away from the hecticness of outer life in the sense of religious rituals in silence: finding strength in and from weakness.

Resolution: Finding the calming pole in one's own centre; being satisfied with the essential aspects; opening oneself up to one's inner life.

Archetypal principle: Mars-Saturn-Moon.

Anaesthesia

see Insensitivity to pain

Anal abscess

(see also Abscess)

Physical level: Skin (border, contact, tenderness), anus (entrance and exit of the underworld).

Symptom level: A dark conflict connected with the underworld breaks through the border in the sensitive domain of excretion – the letting go of shadow aspects; explosive fuel for conflicts and pressure from the underworld seek an outlet and "bust one's ass".

Handling: Letting out the matter(s) of conflict); confronting oneself with the dark aspects, even in difficult domains and allowing these to come to light; meeting elimination of spiritual elements with attentiveness and openness.

Resolution: Actively and courageously bringing dark anal subjects to light.

Archetypal principle: Mars-Pluto.

Anal eczema

(see also Eczema, Skin rash)

Physical level: Skin (border, contact, tenderness), anus (entrance and exit of the underworld).

Symptom level: Something dark breaks through the border in a sensitive domain; something that has been held back and repressed until this point attacks the border of suppression in order to force its way into view (into consciousness): fearfully warding off an anal and/or dark (unconscious or concealed) conflict that is trying to force its way out; damage to one's (structural) integrity in the anal domain from the inside out; the appearance of the clean, honest skin is disfigured by the impure; unsightly superficial situation: unclean conditions in one's own backyard;

smearing (oozing out) spiritual energy (secretion) in the area of the exit from the underworld: always having a slightly damp rear exit; suppressed fear, the pressure seeks an outlet: "having shit for brains".

Handling: Letting internal aspects come out into the open, allowing matters from the bottom to rise to the surface; voluntarily opening up the inner borders to previously-repressed anal subjects; allowing oneself to be pushed from repression to openness; allowing the supposedly unclean across the border of consciousness - confronting and accepting it; bracing oneself for wounds from within, e.g. from realisations rising to the surface; becoming vulnerable in the sense of sensitive; clarifying what one wants to get rid of by the back way without allowing it to come to light; pragmatic therapy: treatment with one's own urine (the waste region with the waste water); directing one's attention to the anal area and taking care of it.

Resolution: Standing up for oneself, including one's dark sides (ensuring a clean rear exit through openness on the mental-spiritual level for one's dark, and seemingly-unclean aspects); allowing dark anal aspects to flourish and illuminating them with the light of consciousness.

Archetypal principle: Pluto.

Anal fissures

Physical level: Anus (entrance and exit of the underworld), skin (border, contact, tenderness).

Symptom level: Tears and cracks in the mucous membrane of the anus (first clarify and interpret the basic situation, frequently →Constipation): trying or pushing (oneself) too hard; having to dispose of tough nuts that are too difficult to crack, and thereby injuring oneself and tearing oneself apart; being "split" with regard to anal-related themes of letting-go;

worn and torn rear exit: unclean conditions in one's own backyard; bleeding from the rear (area): losing life force (making a blood sacrifice); wanting to solve many things via the back way; often people with →helper syndrome, who bend over backwards for others and even "bust their ass", usually without receiving the necessary recognition, and without admitting their true motivation to themselves.

Handling: Exploring the question of whom or what one is "busting one's ass" for; preferably disposing of tough nuts from the shadow kingdom in the figurative sense; clarifying what one is paying so dearly for by dealing with things the back way; expressly putting oneself out for other people/things.

Resolution: Clean, healthy rear exit through openness on the mental-spiritual level for the dark, seemingly-unclean subjects.

Archetypal principle: Pluto.

Anal fistula

(see also Crohn's disease)

Physical level: Anus (exit of the underworld).

Symptom level: Misdirected attempt to find a new exit from the shadow world; looking for roundabout ways, hidden paths, ways out of dark themes; searching for ways out which bring nothing but disadvantages; presumptuous attempt to rework Creation (of the body); danger of spreading dark vexing matters (intestinal bacteria).

Handling: Looking for new possibilities to let shadow subjects come to light; adopting unconventional approaches in order to devote oneself to one's own underworld; dealing with conflicts over letting go in a new and unusual way.

Resolution: Finding one's own unusual ways of disposing of outlived themes; breaking through old

borders; using unconventional ways of letting go; becoming more creative with shadow work.
Archetypal principle: Pluto-Uranus-Mercury.

Anal itching

see Anal pruritus

Anal pains

Physical level: Anus (exit of the underworld).
Symptom level: Cry for help from the anal region; painful nuisance, irritation ("a pain in the ass"); the exit of the shadow kingdom needs attention and care; repressed feelings of guilt and unconscious tendencies towards self-punishment (the backside is painful as if one had received several smacks on the bare bottom; one takes on the responsibility of giving oneself a sore behind).
Handling: Turning one's attention to underworld and shadow issues with courage and energy; relentlessly addressing one's old toxic residues.
Resolution: Bringing light (energy) into the dark.
Archetypal principle: Mars-Pluto.

Anal prolapse

(prolapse of the anal mucous membranes and the last section of the rectum)
Physical level: Anus (entrance and exit of the underworld).
Symptom level: Rather than being so "fed up" that it makes you sick, a piece of the intestine hangs out of the anus so that things come out via the backdoor instead (in vulgar terms: "things give one the shits"; the shadow kingdom forces itself into the light of consciousness via the backdoor; the exit of the shadow kingdom becomes turned inside out, and the sphincter muscle fails: the gates of hell can no longer be controlled.

Handling: Voluntarily approaching the shadow kingdom; allowing one's own dark sides to come to light and owning up to them: recognising which ignored spiritual subjects are thrusting themselves forward via the backdoor ("letting something hang out" = showing it); realising what pressure the shadow kingdom has come under; learning to confront and let out (express) shadows (psychotherapy).
Resolution: Reconciliation with one's own shadow kingdom; integration of the shadow into one's "Ego "= self-realisation: "Ego" + shadow = Self (according to C. G. Jung).
Archetypal principle: Pluto.

Anal pruritus

(anal itching)
Physical level: Anus (exit of the underworld).
Symptom level: State of irritation at the exit; something is itching in the domain related to letting go; stimulus to get rid of something that is old and outlived, "busting one's ass", leaving something behind oneself; wanting to rip open the entrance to the underworld; bristling with excitement with regard to the shadow kingdom.
Handling: Learning to "shit" all over the past with relish.
Resolution: Joyfully letting go of the old and enthusiastically opening oneself to the underworld and the Plutonic domain.
Archetypal principle: Pluto-Mars.

Anal rhagades

see Anal fissures

Analgesia

see Insensitivity to pain

Anankasm

see Neurosis

Anaphylaxia

see Allergy, Collapse

Aneurysm

(dilation of the walls of the arteries or heart)

Physical level: Artery walls (arteries = energy pathways).

Symptom level: frequently based on wall damage (infarction) or blockages of the heart vessels; areas of the wall that have died off (→necroses following infarction) remain potential weak points, whose rupture leads to leakage of blood into the pericardial sac so that the heart is throttled from the outside (cardiac tamponade): distension in the central area based on weakness; thinning and dilation of the wall leads to weak points; ball-Moon-like dilations of the arteries due to changes in the wall structure can lead to rupture: instant death if the heart (heart or aorta wall) breaks.

Handling: Extending and expanding the pathways of one's own life energy in the figurative sense; directing the life energy along new channels; letting one's own life force flow outwards; becoming aware of the weak points in one's own energy system; allowing the basically continual threat to life into one's consciousness; making oneself aware of pressing and oppressing heart issues.

Resolution: Allowing the heart to expand and grow beyond its limits in the figurative sense; giving way to the pressure of the heart in good time.

Archetypal principle: Saturn-Neptune.

Angina pectoris

(cardiovascular restriction/coronary sclerosis)

Physical level: Heart (seat of the soul, love, feelings, energy centre), blood vessels (transport routes of the life force).

Symptom level: Preliminary stage of →cardiac infarction: giving the heart too little nourishment (energy, oxygen), strangling it due to cramping or as the result of the "cementing in" of the energy supply lines; a closed heart leads to a closed mind; narrowness = fear: angina; hardened, petrified heart, "heart of stone"; feeling of destruction; oppressive situation; call for help by the left/female side; spasm and struggle over matters of the heart; the attempt to earn oneself love or even to buy it ends in disappointment; the heart as a skeleton closet filled with hate, rage and tears.

Handling: Granting oneself rest; attuning one's life to one's heart; paying attention to the voice of the heart: listening to the heart and obeying its voice; owning up to feelings of anxiety and hate, getting to know one's own narrowness in central points, and accepting this as a fact; crying in a heart-melting way; not using the heart as a skeleton closet (anymore); concentrating on one's own centre and the (essential), the essence of life; obeying the gentler stirrings of the heart, recognising the bid for power in the often present →helper syndrome, helping oneself in matters of the heart; practical: mandala meditations and exercises, Tai Chi for concentration on one's own centre.

Resolution: Concentration on the heart, bringing it into the central focal point of life; circling around the centre, dancing the dance around one's centre; ultimate objective working from the opposite pole: creating room for the heart again; opening oneself up and becoming expansive towards other people and their needs: once the heart can nourish itself again, "Love thy neighbour as thyself"; opening to hearty and heartfelt stirrings; sacrificing "Ego"-forces and desires for power, developing self-esteem and self-love.

Archetypal principle: Sun-Saturn.

Angina tonsillaris

see Tonsillitis

Angioma

see Strawberry marks

Angiospasm

see Vascular cramps

Ankle fracture

Physical level: Ankle, ankle joint (take-off point).
Symptom level: Through taking a false step or twisting one's foot awkwardly, the outer part of the ankle in particular breaks off or splinters: having sprung a crack in the (joint) socket; having sprung a crack in the ankle joint signifies a hard landing and hinders further leaps: keeps one bound to the ground/Mother Earth; those affected are no longer on the go, but instead have pretty much already arrived; smooth, harmonious steps forward (progress) are called into question for the time being.
Handling: Watching where one is treading (one's footholds); allowing oneself to arrive at one's allocated place; committing oneself more fully once there; putting down roots, learning to stay put.
Resolution: Giving things a rest; taking time for reflection, which has the effect that nothing can proceed further externally, but quite a bit internally.
Archetypal principle:
Uranus-Saturn.

Ankle joint inflammation

see Rheumatism

Ankylosis

(stiffening, rigidity of the joints)
Physical level: Joints (mobility, articulation).
Symptom level: Stiffening of the joints due to capsular shrinkage, cartilage atrophy, inflammations; loss of mobility and articulation capability in this area; restriction of overall mobility; lack of flexibility, and instead rigidity in the relevant domain associated with the particular joint; pig-headedness, obstinacy, resistance.
Handling: Becoming sterner and stricter in articulation; adjusting one's statements on particular areas (subject depending on the joint); recognising and acknowledging one's own rigidity, putting up resistance on the spiritual level.
Resolution: Replacement of the physical articulation level by the verbally-expressed mental-spiritual level; restriction and orientation of movements to the essential; recognising and acknowledging important points of resistance, resisting movements and developments which are at cross-purposes to one's own life.
Archetypal principle:
Saturn-Mercury.

Anorexia

(Anorexia nervosa; see also Bulimia, Addictions)
Physical level: The whole body, particularly in its feminine forms; stomach (feeling, receptiveness); almost exclusively affects young girls, and only very rarely, effeminate young boys.
Symptom level: Rejection of the transition from girl to woman; conflict between spirit and matter, purity and drive, greed and ascesis, hunger and relinquishment, egocentricity and devotion; fear of orgiastic experiences (of unity), but at the same time longing for unity; unfulfilled greed struggles accompanied by the longing

for ascesis; fear of lively vitality and simultaneous burning hunger for what is lively and vital; the objective: purity and spiritualisation, chastity and asexuality, dematerialisation; unconscious or semi-conscious desire to simply disappear; ascesis ideal: not granting oneself anything enjoyable (love, food); saying 'no' to physicality: wanting to make oneself scarce; taking flight from polarity, which is perceived as impure with its oppressive feminine aspects; fear of sexual love; resistance to sexuality, femininity, motherhood; loathing of feminine aspects and all forms of receptiveness and taking things on board; longing for loving attention; exercise of power; unconscious rebellion against the prevailing feminine ideal; not being satisfied with one's given body, not making peace with it.

Handling: Accepting oneself as a woman: puberty rituals; reconciliation exercises with polarity ("Be hot or cold, the lukewarm I will spit out of My mouth"): committed taking and receiving, committed giving and giving away freely; being honest towards oneself and one's shadow; leaving the ivory tower of disembodied purity; acknowledgement of the feminine, maternal principle; getting to know and appreciate Venus subjects: learning to enjoy fulfilling sensuality; resolved (redeeming) cleansing exercises of giving of oneself, such as fasting, sweating, excretion (vomiting as a method of older-style naturopathy); practice/spiritual exercises in strictness and consistency towards oneself: spending time in a cloister on a trial basis in order to experience the ascesis ideal; transforming the attempt to flee from polarity into the attempt to overcome it in the sense of following one's development path in the direction of unity; striving consistently for experiences of unity and peak experiences; exercises in realising the centre between the poles: Tai Chi, making pottery on the potter's wheel, mandala painting and meditation; psychotherapy in order to reconcile oneself with one's own rounded forms and creative fertility.

Resolution: Reconciliation with being a woman: becoming a woman by discovering the force of the feminine in oneself and finding a new perspective within oneself (e.g. by receiving the seed to conceive a child, to whom one gives life); (ritually) coming to terms with the transition from puberty; leaving childhood and one's youth behind; experiencing (making) love with its enjoyable, simultaneously spiritual and physical taking and giving; appreciating ecstasy (e.g. sexual) as a foretaste of unity; reconciliation with unity as the all-embracing sum of all manifestations, which also includes the shadow realm.

Archetypal principle: Moon-Saturn/Uranus/Neptune.

Anorgasmia

see Orgasm problems

Anovulatory cycle

see Ovulation, absent

Antibody deficiency syndrome

(see also Agranulocytosis and Aids, which ultimately is also an antibody deficiency syndrome)

Physical level: Immune system (defence).

Symptom level: Defencelessness against external and internal attacks (not only foreign pathogens coming from the outside, but also the body's own germs, for example, those coming from the intestines can also become threatening).

Handling: Disarmament on the consciousness front: i.e. opening the

spiritual borders instead of foregoing all defence on the physical front.
Resolution: Recognising the boundlessness of life and beginning to live; everything is connected to everything else, and disconnections only take place in one's consciousness.
Archetypal principle: Mars-Saturn/Neptune.

Anuria

(urine excretion disorder)
Physical level: Kidneys (balance, partnership).
Symptom level: The spiritual waste water (urine) – the outlived spiritual contents – can no longer be let go of; the lack of urine production results in autointoxication – self-poisoning (uraemia, →kidney insufficiency).
Handling: Continuing to take old spiritual matters seriously and making their essence one's own; making clear to oneself that one can no longer let go on the spiritual level.
Resolution: Reconciling oneself with the spiritual poison which over time circulates in one's life; becoming one with everything on the figurative level: transforming the (spiritual) poison into an exilir for healing (making whole).
Archetypal principle: Moon/Venus-Saturn/Pluto.

Anus (artificial)

see Anus praeter (naturalis) below

Anus praeter (naturalis)

(artificial anus; see also Rectal cancer)
Physical level: Rectum (underworld), anus (entrance and exit of the underworld).
Symptom level: Problem with letting go; the point of release is relocated forwards from the rear to the centre; exclusion of the underworld from life; secret desire for circumvention or

overcoming of the unconscious; the excreted becomes visible.
Handling: Recognising where one tends to let out unpleasant things at an inappropriate place in the figurative sense; shadow therapy: looking at things in one's (own) life which one does not want to allow into the light of day under any circumstances; occupation with the old, outlived (excrement) on the consciousness level; consciously processing and disposing of the excretions from the shadow kingdom (bringing them forward to the light side).
Resolution: Integration of one's shadow and reconciliation with the "Ego" for the purposes of self-realisation ("Ego" + shadow = Self).
Archetypal principle: Pluto-Uranus.

Anxiety

(see also Phobia; Flying, fear of; Nightmares/Anxiety dreams; Depression; Neurosis; Panic)
Physical level: Noticeable above all around the neck (assimilation, connection, communication) and in the breathing pattern (exchange, law of polarity).
Symptom level: Narrowness, restriction (Latin: angustus = 'narrow') as if tightly bound (choking), hindered in the free flow of breath; desire to escape; often unaddressed birth trauma (birth = primordial or first restriction in life); feeling of being stifled by the restrictiveness, of being held captive, of being caught in a trap, of remaining stuck (birth), being boxed in and restricted; one's own needs in life are seemingly being stifled.
Handling: Accepting and letting in the fear until it loses its capacity to terrorize, can be identified and thus transforms itself into expansiveness; (voluntarily) giving one's fear space; confrontation of the restriction: connected breathing (similar to rebirthing) [Leonard Orr]; having the front to

face up to the fear; experiencing one's birth again and consciously integrating it (reincarnation therapy); finding stability (support): regaining the security and stability of the womb: acquiring basic trust (through peak experiences, respectively experiences of unity); voluntary "restriction" = concentration (in various respects); consciously holding oneself (which can then be transformed into letting go): holding therapy.

Resolution: Concentration on the essential, the present moment; living in the present moment, because fear lives from the past or future; ultimate objective lies in the opposite pole: becoming expansive, open and free despite the restrictivemess; expansiveness.

Archetypal principle: **Saturn, Pluto.**

Anxiety dreams

see Nightmares

Anxiety neurosis

see Anxiety and Neurosis

Aortic insufficiency

(see also Heart valve insufficiency).
Physical level: Heart (seat of the soul, love, feelings, energy centre).
Symptom level: Over-exertion of the heart (left ventricular hypertrophy) with chamber enlargement and huge blood pressure amplitude due to the deficient valve function of the heart ventricle: over-exertion (left ventricular insufficiency); marching on the spot, running a marathon while standing still (myth of Sisyphus); notorious 'yes'-saying, spiritual condition similar to →angina pectoris and →cardiac infarction, with dangerous long-term effects; after every act of giving, inappropriately taking back straight away; complete openness to the blood flow; fear of one's own impulsive life force; directional and orientation problems

in matters of one's central life energy; allowing the life energy to seep away again immediately at the point of its strongest impulse.

Handling: Learning to give oneself more time; recognising regressive tendencies; openness at the figurative level of the heart instead of at the physical level; learning to give without taking.

Resolution: Harmony between giving and taking; complete openness at the level of the heart; balance between saying 'yes' and 'no' (in order to be truly open, one must also be capable of saying 'no'); working from the opposite pole: giving one's life energy the necessary support once it has been set in motion so that it continually moves forward.

Archetypal principle: **Sun-Neptune.**

Aortic isthmus stenosis

(congenital heart defect)
Physical level: Heart (seat of the soul, love, feelings, energy centre).
Symptom level: Constriction of the aorta behind the outflow area of the vessels for the upper half of the body: drastic preference for the upper, male half of the body to the detriment of the lower, female half; greatly restricted life (to the upper area); hardly any openness (life energy) for the lower, female part of life, such as sexuality and procreation of offspring, but also neglect of progress (difficulties with walking).

Handling: Becoming aware of the rejection of one's own female aspect; recognising and acknowledging one's own one-sidedness; giving oneself entirely to the upper, male pole, with the objective of exploiting one's possibilities to the full; putting aside the energetically under-supplied issues of fertility, eroticism and progress, until the resolution of the upper tasks has progressed further; only then focusing on the lower themes by drawing from the strength of the upper pole.

Resolution: Exploiting and resolving (redeeming) the possibilities of the upper, male levels; taking mental-spiritual subjects more seriously than physical subjects; ultimate aim through inclusion of the opposite pole: to gain the lower level of the body (female pole) in both the symbolic respect as well as at the physical level through cardiac surgery intervention (aortoplasty).

Archetypal principle: Saturn-Sun.

Aortic stenosis

(congenital or acquired restriction of the aorta)

Physical level: Heart (seat of the soul, love, feelings, energy centre), aorta (main [traffic] route of the life flow).

Symptom level: Constriction directly at the outflow area of the aorta, with the result that the complete organism is under-supplied (compare →aortic isthmus stenosis, which only affects the lower body); the heart works against great resistance, while the outflow valve remains closed: enormous pressure in the heart, low (blood) pressure in the body; effects on the heart: left ventricular hypertrophy as the trigger for →angina pectoris to the point of cardiac infarction; effects on the body: low blood pressure, dizziness, blackouts when under stress; general effects: the body and heart receive too little (nourishment); no (blood) pressure in life; the emotional plane of the heart and the flow of life energy threaten to dry up; limited life.

Handling: Becoming aware of one's one-sidedness; drastically reducing one's own needs and learning to be satisfied with less.

Resolution: Preference for mental-spiritual life themes rather than physical issues; ultimate objective

working from the opposite pole: to also gain the lower physical level (female pole) through cardiac surgery intervention (aortoplasty); keeping the life flow in motion.

Archetypal principle: Saturn-Sun.

Apathy

(see also Depression)

Symptom level: Lack of willingness to contribute to the struggle over and for one's life: sleeping one's life away; refusal to take part in life and its sufferings (Greek. a-pathos = non-suffering); turning away from life, feelings of senselessness; trying to please everybody, but without any inner participation; complete lack of passion, motivation and involvement; indifference.

Handling: Conscious return to oneself; consciously cutting oneself off from overpowering feelings; exercises in simplicity and attentiveness, relinquishment: e.g. Zen; withdrawal into solitude: finding strength in and from rest and calm; instead of avoiding suffering, overcoming attachment: wise restriction to the essential (Buddha: "All suffering comes from attachment").

Resolution: Recognising everything as "in-different" (= not different, i.e. equally valid) in the Buddhist sense (Uppekha); ascesis as an art of life, self-sufficiency, being alone in the sense of al(l in)one.

Archetypal principle: Saturn.

Aphasia

(speech disorder, e.g. after cerebral contusion, stroke, spiritual trauma)

Physical level: Brain (communication, logistics).

Symptom level: The speech centre is blocked, with the result that all other senses and (previously- neglected?) channels of communication are addressed instead: the language of the emotions and feelings gets a chance; possible correction of intellectual top-heaviness.

Handling: Recognising what has rendered one speechless; hearing and listening carefully instead of speaking; feeling, sensing, communication without words: learning to convey those things which cannot be conveyed verbally; developing new means of expression for oneself; input instead of output.

Resolution: (Appreciating) silence, listening inwardly ("silence is golden"); listening with the heart; contemplative life.

Archetypal principle: Mercury-Saturn.

Aphonia

see Hoarseness

Aphtosa

(small inflamed ulcers [viruses], see also Stomatitis aphtosa)

Physical level: Mouth (absorption, expression, maturity – being able to speak for oneself), tongue (expression, speech, weapon), palate (taste).

Symptom level: Harmless, but very painful conflicts in the area of taste; oral enjoyment becomes a painful procedure; rotten compromises with regard to the purity and wholesomeness of meals; frequently in children: too much indigestible muck in the mouth, respectively too much of what is unconsciously perceived as unclean and impure, and in any case, detrimental; indication of a lack of attentiveness and hygiene in the figurative sense; after periods of fasting, they betray a lack of awareness and consciousness which one had actually resolved to put into effect.

Handling: Offensive, courageous confrontation with issues of taste and choice of food (e.g. after fasting); posing the question: "What is good for me?"; giving way to the symptoms, more or less forcing them (in the case

of mouth rot [stomatitis aphtosa]) to fast: finding enjoyment on other (sensual) levels.

Resolution: Being able to fend off what is not good for one; uncompromising attitude in matters of quality, quantity and consciousness.

Archetypal principle: Mars-Moon.

Aplasia

(congenital absence of organs or parts of the body, e.g. following damage caused by the former sedative medication – Thalidomide/Contergan)

Physical level: The whole organism can be affected.

Symptom level: Absence of the subject represented by the organ.

Handling: Practice in getting by without the corresponding subject, and thereby recognising and acknowledging its importance; compensation in consciousness.

Resolution: Resolving the subject (that is absent in the body) on the mental-spiritual level.

Archetypal principle: Differs according to the missing organ.

Apnoea

(respiratory arrest; see also Sleep apnoea)

Physical level: Lungs (contact, communication, freedom), respiratory centre in the brain (communication, logistics).

Symptom level: Detachment from the polar world of inhaling and exhaling; being cut off from polarity; coming close to a transcendental experience of unity; departure from polarity (in moments of transcendental experience, breathing stops as a sign of contact with unity).

Handling: (on the part of the carer, as usually this is no longer consciously possible on the part of the person affected): resuscitation in the sense of a return to polarity by

125

means of artificial respiration and heart massage from the outside or, depending on the situation, palliative, end-of-life care; breathing exercises: practising taking while also letting giving happen; exercises in connected breathing; practising exchange on the mental-spiritual level; spiritual exercises directed towards polarity.
Resolution: Learning to get by with less exchange and communication, restriction to the essential in energetic terms, becoming more sparing with one's own energy.
Archetypal principle: Saturn-Mercury.

Apoplexy

see Stroke

Appendicitis

Physical level: Vermiform continuation of the appendix in the large intestine (the cul-de-sac of cul-de-sacs in the unconscious, in the kingdom of the dead), police station and weapons forge (defensive organ) of the underworld.
Symptom level: War, conflict in the underworld (in the cul-de-sac of cul-de-sacs); feeling of being stuck in a dead-end; often first severe shadow confrontation of the child: conflict in the border area between "innocent childhood" and the "dangerous adult world"; confrontation with the expectations and role patterns of one's own family tradition, which appear largely or completely indigestible; inability to digest the hard core of things; intrusion of the shadow kingdom into one's day-to-day world: suppressed dark aggressions burst forth.
Handling: Recognising the dead ends that one does not want to give up the fight in; offensively confronting one's shadow (the "bogeyman"); courageously bringing what has been repressed and suppressed back into the light of awareness; enabling the

child to find ways into the "dangerous adult world" (puberty rituals).
Resolution: Acknowledgement of one's dark inner partner, of the opposite pole; reconciliation with the dark sister, the dark brother.
Archetypal principle: Pluto-Mars.

Appetite, excessive

see Binge eating disorder

Appetite, lack of

(inappetency; e.g. in the case of liver diseases, depression)
Physical level: Consciousness, brain (communication, logistics), stomach (feeling, receptiveness).
Symptom level: No desire for life and absorption; refusal to take any further active part in normal life, to get involved with it and to embrace it; turning away from the energy supply; starving oneself in energetic terms; secondary refusal to digest life; having no hunger for life, playing dead; no longer feeling any desire to take part in exchange, to let new things close to and into oneself; often also feelings of guilt; self-denial.
Handling: Recognising what is no longer to one's taste in the figurative sense; consciously and voluntarily doing without; conscious fasting; reduction to the essential and most necessary; distancing oneself, being completely on one's own, reflecting on oneself and one's own inner strength, finding and being with oneself; discovering the new in oneself; ascesis exercises as an art of living; practicing Bhoga (Buddhism: "consuming and digesting the world").
Resolution: Contentment, conscious fasting; withdrawing into seclusion (cloister), hermit existence; absorbing Pranic light nourishment (Note: not to be understood as a recommendation!).
Archetypal principle: Saturn.

Apraxia

(inability to perform coordinated movements although not paralysed)
Physical level: Brain (communication, logistics).
Symptom level: No longer being able to deal with the world, e.g. in the case of →Alzheimer's disease, → cerebral contusion (wanting to get a grip on something, without being able to grasp it).
Handling: Acknowledging one's own inabilities; turning away from a practical life in order to achieve higher understanding, preferring inner worlds; learning to move in other worlds.
Resolution: Preparations for the change from outer to inner life.
Archetypal principle: Saturn-Neptune.

Arachnophobia (fear of spiders)

see Phobia

Arm dislocation

Physical level: Shoulder joint (movement and stability).
Symptom level: Disregarding sensible (physical) limits; being beside oneself and losing one's composure; overestimating oneself, overbearingness; being on the wrong track; failing to get a grip, over-extending oneself, dealing with too much; overstretching things: overdoing the theme of mobility, overestimating or over-straining one's own capabilities.
Handling: Daring to go beyond one's own (spiritual) limits; risking the grand scoop, the golden touch (the golden gateway); seizing the right moment; physical therapy: putting things back into alignment; in the figurative sense: putting things back into alignment in good time and getting to know and respect one's own scope for movement.

Resolution: Courageous (spiritual) flexibility; realising the great chance (plan) in life; growing beyond oneself; ultimate objective working from the opposite pole: bringing something that has been dragged too far off track back onto the right path.
Archetypal principle: Uranus-Mars.

Arm fracture

Physical level: Arms (force, strength, power).
Symptom level: The message depends on which arm is broken and how the accident occurred: broken relationship with the world; no longer having a proper grasp of life, and therefore also not coming to grips with it; inability to act; being up in arms.
Handling: Breaking out of the rut of one's life pattern: daring to really live and regarding life as a challenge, bringing variety into one's life; creativity on the spiritual instead of the physical level instead of forcing the body to create joints where none exist, calmly carrying flexibility over into areas on the figurative level where previously it was not usual.
Resolution: Flexibility; articulation capability.
Archetypal principle: Uranus-Mars, Mercury.

Armoured heart

see Pericarditis

Arrhythmia

see Heart rhythm disorders

Arterial calcification

see Arteriosclerosis

Arterial dilation

see Aneurysm

Arterial inflammation

(arteritis)
Physical level: Vessels (conduction pathways), arteries (energy supply routes).
Symptom level: Unconscious chronic conflicts over energy distribution: "street battles".
Handling: Concerning oneself with the distribution of energy.
Resolution: Courageous, offensive battles over the use of one's own energy; perceiving new possibilities of energy usage.
Archetypal principle: Mercury-Mars.

Arterial wall inflammation

see Panarteritis

Arteriosclerosis

(arterial calcification; see also Angina pectoris, Claudicatio intermittens, Cerebral circulation disorders)
Physical level: Arteries (energy pathways), blood vessels (transport routes of the life force).
Symptom level: Most frequent cause of heart and brain infarction: partial or general "cementing in" of the life flow; hardening in the domain of the life flow; calcified vessels correspond to constricted, walled-in energy pathways: typical of people who subordinate their life to external constraints (family, company, possessions) and allow themselves and their life to run along fixed paths which do not correspond to their interests and talents; doing everything for security (of the path in life), and having too little left over for one's own individual development possibilities; reduction of flexibility and elasticity with advancing age; increasing internal pressure; spiritual constriction; a female pole that has come up too short; tense, inflexible and ultimately hardened situation in the domain of the communications channels of the life energy.
Handling: Concentration on the essential in energetic terms; strict to highly stringent apportionment of one's own energy; putting a stop to energy wastage; recognising struggles that are acting as a substitute and firmly bringing them to an end: addressing the decisive level; concentrating on central matters/the essential; genuine efficiency instead of frittering away energy or trying to act important; comparable example from the macrocosm: the cementing-in of river beds only brings short-term and short-sighted advantages, in the long term, it does harm.
Resolution: Realisation of energy-saving solutions; elevating "the highest first" to a principle (e.g. solving authority conflicts at the highest level).
Archetypal principle: Saturn.

Arteritis

see Arterial inflammation

Arthritis

see Rheumatism

Arthrosis

Physical level: Almost all joints (mobility, articulation), particularly the hip, knee, ankle and finger joints.
Symptom level: (general): function-impeding changes in the joint; wear and tear, worn-out joint; restricted movement and articulation capability, rigid posture; uncramped interaction (between the bones) is no longer possible, the oil in the gearbox has long since been used up (seized piston situation); a worn joint reflects the need for greater closeness in interacting, in other words, for the closest possible connection (the bones eat into each other, the distance of the joint gap is gone).

128

1. Hip joint (stepping forward)

Symptom level: Excessive demands on structural equilibrium and dynamics in the past; deterioration of one's articulation capability on the affected level of stepping forward; progress, and in fact, every individual step forward is painful; the process of getting ahead in life is called into question; great steps/leaps are no longer possible with ease.

Handling: Acknowledgement of one's own rigidity, of the pains brought about by any progress; consciously sensing the effort required for every step forward.

Resolution: Giving things a rest outwardly and instead taking great steps inwardly; setting out on inner journeys.

Archetypal principle: Jupiter-Saturn.

2. Knee joint (humility)

Symptom level: Deterioration of one's articulation capability on the affected level of kneeling; gestures of humility – such as going down on one's knees – are painful, (occupational illness [pattern] of tile-layers, who outwardly crawl around all their life on their knees, thus paving the way for others); getting ahead in life is often only possible with pain; the symptoms draw attention to the upcoming subject of humility or the axis: humility – humiliation.

Handling: Owning up to one's own rigidity and the pains brought about by every act of kneeling and striding forward; consciously sensing the effort of will which every act of kneeling down would cost; conscious practice of humility on the mental-spiritual level; relieving the physical levels of the burden and instead being prepared to lower oneself far enough on inner levels to take one's own situation seriously.

Resolution: Inner humility.

Archetypal principle: Saturn.

3. Ankle joint (take-off point)

Symptom level: Deterioration of one's articulation capability at the level of leaping; difficulties in finding the right chance to make the leap; no longer being on the go; not being able to take any great leaps anymore, every leap causes pain; end of the spring in one's step; getting ahead in life is often only possible with pain; painful ankle joints draw attention to the upcoming subject of making the leap.

Handling: Admitting to oneself that one has (crash) landed back on Earth and can no longer move up in the world without pain; consciously lowering oneself; practice in landing; parting with high-flying dreams.

Resolution: Making the leap inwardly instead of outwardly; inner elasticity and dynamism, being lively and full of beans inwardly.

Archetypal principle: Uranus.

4. Wrist and finger joint (grasping, ability to act)

Symptom level: Deterioration of one's articulation capability at the level of grabbing, gripping and grasping; problems coming to grips with life; manipulating things causes pain; the ability to act is painfully restricted; painful wrist and finger joints draw attention to the issue of letting go, which the symptom forces one to do.

Handling: Admitting to oneself that one can no longer grab hold of things, and should let go; exercises in letting go; conscious departure from all manipulations.

Resolution: Letting go of the outer life in favour of one's inner life; coming to grips with one's inner life; inner composure.

Archetypal principle: Mercury.

Articular effusion

Physical level: Joints (mobility, articulation).

Symptom level: 1. Water from the surrounding tissues floods the joint and drowns it; weeping into the joint, and swamping it with water; 2. Accumulation of blood; 3. Swelling, pain, overheating.

Handling: 1. Addressing the subject of the affected joint with spiritual means; learning to understand the tears that have been shed over the corresponding subject; 2. Accumulating life force for the expression of the individual dynamism reflected by this joint and using it for new and lively mobility; 3. Granting the conflict importance; recognising the red hot iron which lies embedded here; taking the call for help of the affected region seriously; making something out of it and learning from it; investing energy in the resolution of the conflict.

Resolution: 1. Resolving the corresponding subject with spiritual energy (e.g. in the case of knee joint effusion, promoting the articulation of humility with spiritual energy); 2. Finding joy for life via the subject related to the affected joint; 3. Placing the subject at the centre of one's attention with courage and commitment and resolving it in the sense of growing from it, healing in the sense of becoming more whole; allopathically: coming to rest, pressure relief via joint puncture; cooling applications.

Archetypal principle: Mercury-Moon-Mars.

Ascites formation

([cavity] hydropsy, tendency to oedema; with cardiovascular, lung, kidney, liver or cancer diseases)

Physical level: Abdominal cavity (safety and security) and related parts of the body.

Symptom level: Water = spiritual blockage; the spiritual element becomes separated from the blood flow (life force) and drains away: having a heavy spiritual load to bear; dragging around spiritual aspects; backing-up of the life energy in front of the centre

of feeling (heart) and centre of meaningfulness (liver): the spiritual leaves the flow of vitality and no longer takes part in the cycle of life, but instead hinders it: in the case of pericard hydropsy, by hindering central functions; in the case of classical ascites, by hindering the digestive work in the abdominal cavity, and in the case of hydrothorax, by hindering respiration.

Handling: Paying attention to the spiritual element, taking it seriously and allowing it to become fertile; allowing oneself time for impulses of the soul.

Resolution: Making room for spiritual subjects; allowing (gut) feelings to make themselves felt; working from the opposite pole: keeping spiritual forces in flow.

Archetypal principle: Moon.

Asphyxiation attacks

(see also Croup)

Physical level: Air passages (communication, contact).

Symptom level: Demonstrative attempt to break off contact with the world; indication that the air for breathing is not adequate in the corresponding situation; being strangled, feeling oneself stifled, not having enough life energy and room; not being able to live as one would like.

Handling: Consciously reducing contacts, withdrawing oneself, voluntarily restricting one's living space, not consuming so much energy, wisely cutting back.

Resolution: Recognising loneliness and seclusion as an opportunity, being there completely for oneself and with oneself alone.

Archetypal principle: Pluto-Mercury.

Aspiration pneumonia

(see also Lung inflammation)

Physical level: Lungs (contact, communication, freedom).

Symptom level: Something has gone down the wrong way; food (material nourishment) incorrectly goes down the (wind)pipe designed for Pranic (immaterial nourishment) and ends up in the lungs.

Handling: Dealing with conflict over problematic choices between immaterial (mental-spiritual) and material nourishment in consciousness.

Resolution: Courageous spiritual confrontation with one's own nourishment choices (both immaterial and material); finding the right channels for digesting things in consciousness.

Archetypal principle: Mercury-Mars.

Astigmatism

(abnormal curvature of the cornea)

Physical level: Eyes (insight, perspective, mirrors and windows of the soul).

Symptom level: Skewed view (of things), seeing certain areas of one's own life in a distorted and skewed light, warped views, warped vision: the eyeball is not a well-rounded affair (the light rays cannot be bundled together at a single point, with the result that no sharp focal point can be achieved [Greek stigma = point]); distorted view of the world, frequent discrepancy between the traditional world view and one's own ambitions; inability to look oneself in the eye as one truly is.

Handling: Following unconventional, warped points of view; consciously perceiving the world in an idiosyncratic way; developing a broad point of view, disregarding concentration that is too close; allowing different views of the world to be valid; developing a more whimsical, original and individual view of the world; allopathically: ensuring perspective in the areas of warped vision.

Resolution: Creative view of the world; accepting one's own individual world view and making it binding not for others, but instead for oneself

Archetypal principle: Sun/Moon-Uranus.

Ataxia

(disorder affecting smooth motor co-ordination)

Physical level: Brain (communication, logistics), motoric system (mobility, progress).

Symptom level: Jerky, staccato movement pattern: interruptions in the flow of movements and actions.

Handling: Allowing erratic impulses that sometimes overshoot the mark; learning to pause and accept interruptions.

Resolution: (working from the opposite pole): finding and walking along the golden middleground; being in flow: discovering the deep inner flow of existence and going along with it.

Archetypal principle: Uranus.

Athetosis

see St. Vitus's dance

Athlete's foot

(see also Dermatomycoses)

Physical level: Skin (border, contact, tenderness), feet (steadfastness, deep-rootedness), toenails (lower claws, aggression).

Symptom level: The contact to Mother Earth/woman/world is not clean; a forgotten conflict over one's own steadfastness wants to return to consciousness and be dealt with; being too weak to defend one's own skin (weak defensive situation); one's own border fortifications (skin) and weapons store (claws) are occupied by foreign invasion troops, which then become parasites; above all, it is non-living tissue, which falls victim to fungal invasions (fungi are saprophytes, which live on dead organic matter).

Handling: Reducing defensiveness with regard to one's own standpoints; becoming more willing to compromise and co-operate, fostering the involvement with foreign impulses; letting in foreign elements; making room for foreign elements and making them one's own instead of letting oneself to be taken over by what is foreign; opening up those areas which are no longer used and consequently no longer needed, i.e. lifeless areas, which have died off, to foreign life impulses; wrestling with unclean, unclear standpoints, reconsidering them aggressively, and if necessary, revising them; taking in vital (living) nourishment, which yields nothing to the fungus; consciously making the daily choice: either nourish the fungus with dead nourishment that has no nutritional value, or oneself with vital (living) nourishment; clarifying the question of one's own parasitism: "Where am I sponging off others?"
Resolution: Integration of foreign impulses and life forms: "Live and let live"; creating one's own living terrain (in consciousness)
Archetypal principle:Neptune/ Saturn-Pluto.

Athlete's heart

see Cardiac enlargement

Atonia

(pronounced slackening of the muscles)
Physical level: Musculature (motor, strength). Symptom level: Surrender of dynamic movement powers; loss of the ability to build up tension.
Handling: Exercises to relieve tension for the spirit and soul.
Resolution: Surrendering oneself to weakness: yielding freely (devotion); mental-spiritual serenity (Buddhist: Uppekha = equanimity); working from the opposite pole: the archer's bow loses its strength if it is first over-stretched and then let go completely: finding (one's own) happy medium between slackness and over-tension.
Archetypal principle: Mars-Neptune.

Atresia

(absence of natural bodily orifices)
Physical level: Body surface.
Symptom level: Absence of outlets for the particular subject associated with the relevant part of the body.
Handling: Surgical therapy in order to apply strong pressure to open the area (by force); consciously opening it later in the mental-spiritual respect.
Resolution: Paying attention to the corresponding subject and giving it access to consciousness.
Archetypal principle: Saturn-Pluto (otherwise according to the relevant orifice).

Atrophy

(regression of organs or tissue; see also Muscular atrophy)
Physical level: Possible in many areas, both externally and internally.
Symptom level: Regression of certain structures in an otherwise vibrant body.
Handling: Giving up, letting go of the subjects symbolised by the atrophying regions or organs.
Resolution: Withdrawing one's life energy from certain subjects and separating oneself from them.
Archetypal principle: Neptune.

Attention deficiency syndrome (ADS)

see Hyperactivity

Auditory canal eczema

(see also Eczema, Skin rash)
Physical level: Outer auditory canal (sound collector, ear trumpet).

Symptom level: Itching rash at the entrance area to the hearing organ: one is itching to hear something; something dark, unpleasant, but also stimulating breaks through the barrier in order to be heard; aggressive outpourings (rash outbreak) in the domain of listening to (obeying) commands.

Handling: Instead of continually boring deeply into one's ears with scratching, boring deeply into the depths of the unconscious; devoting oneself to listening carefully inwardly: What dark subjects want to break out? What is so urgently making one itch?; looking after the auditory canal and one's hearing (for example, regularly dabbing the former with one's own urine).

Resolution: Openness for messages from the depths (generally classified as unpleasant).

Archetypal principle: Saturn/Venus-Mars.

Auditory canal inflammation

(otitis externa)

Physical level: Outer auditory canal (sound collector, ear trumpet).

Symptom level: Conflict over the filtering of what has been let in (sensory overload); inflammation of the outer auditory canal due to minor injuries, possibly on the basis of insufficient earwax (badly-oiled hearing organ): conflict over what has been heard, and over listening carefully and heeding (obeying); rage over what has been heard or the unheard of, which then ignites a heated conflict; this even temporarily prevents hearing so that one can listen better inwardly and heed (obey) the inner voice: "Did what was heard also hit a chord? Did it accord well to listen to it at all, or was that already unheard of in itself? Was something unheard of heard? aggressive confrontation in

the domain of heeding (obeying) with regard to the inner voice.

Handling: Exploring the depths of the unconscious instead of continually poking around in one's ears in order to provide relief from the swelling of the inflammation; carefully listening inwardly to the unheard of and discordant elements which were overheard; looking after the auditory canal and one's hearing (e.g. regularly dabbing the former with one's own urine [spiritual water] during the inflammation).

Resolution: With courage and combat strength, learning obedience with regard to one's own inner voice; owning up to one's conflicts over taboo areas (unheard of and discordant elements) and bringing light into the darkness.

Archetypal principle: Saturn-Mars.

Autism

Symptom level: Closing oneself off completely from the outer world (see the films Rain Man and House of Cards); in many patients, outbreaks of aggression; living in one's own inner world; inner asylum: outer asylum as the response of a helpless society; taking flight from the social environment, from the need to come to compromises with others; instead of living in a uni-verse, patients live in a multi-verse: the skills for dealing with generalities are not in their blood, but as a counterbalance, they appreciate concrete details all the more; sometimes they have access to Pythagorean worlds of mathematics and numbers; recognition that everything in the universe is number and sound: unbelievable (for normal people), wonderful abilities in playing with numbers; in the grand scale of things, they are failures, but at the same time, are geniuses in small niches of reality; (Selective Mutism): in effect, a paraphrase for autism, that is, relating only to individual persons;

falling silent due to psychological problems, temporary refusal to speak by children.

Handling: (for jointly-affected parents): trying to tap into unusual contact and communications channels (e.g. via computer) since patients are barely accessible and not capable of normal contact; letting oneself get involved in another, extraordinary world; attempting to stimulate offensive self-expression, bringing out vitality in a more resolved (redeeming) way.

Resolution: Inner reflection in the sense of being al(l)-one.

Archetypal principle: Saturn/ Uranus-Mercury.

Auto-aggressive/ Auto-immune diseases

(see also Lupus erythematodes, Allergy, Colitis ulcerosa, Rheumatism, Fibromyalgia, Cancer, Pain, Aggressiveness)

Physical level: Immune system (defence); all areas of the body can be affected, e.g. joints (forms of rheumatoid arthritis); large intestine (Colitis ulcerosa); thyroid gland; liver; skin (Lupus erythematodes); vessels (vasculitis); blood (haemolytic anaemias).

Symptom level: One's own structures are violently attacked from the inside out; the body's immune defence powers are aimed against one's own structures, instead of outwards against external enemies: becoming one's own worst enemy; eating oneself up with the unexpressed aggression that is forcing its way to the surface; expression of the strongest form of suppression.

Handling: Voluntarily calling one's own structures into question; allowing oneself to be stirred up more and more intensely in the figurative sense: directing the battle to a higher level;

dealing with oneself in a forceful way – and thereby taking the load off the immune defence system; self-control instead of suppression; exercises which get under one's skin; scratching at the (superficial) gloss and calling existing entrenched life patterns into question; discovering fasting as a possible means of returning to the essential.

Resolution: Courageous questioning of one's own attitudes/life patterns and their offensive restructuring.

Archetypal principle: Pluto-Mars.

Auto-intoxication

see Self-poisoning

AV block

(see also Heart rhythm disorders)

Physical level: Stimulus-conducting tissue in the heart: transition from the sinus node to the AV node (heart = seat of the soul, love, feeling, energy centre; muscle = strength).

Symptom level: The signals from the first rhythm centre in the atrium to the second at the base of the chamber are completely or partly blocked: the messages of the heart cannot, or at least not completely, be transmitted from the upper to the lower heart level; first-, second- or third-degree blockage, depending on how many impulses are being swallowed up; information blockage in the centre of one's (emotional) life; the right way is barred; being slow on the uptake as far as the transmission line for matters of the heart is concerned.

Handling: Consciously leaving out many stimuli; not following every impulse (of the heart); not having too many irons in the fire; now and again consciously allowing opportunities to pass one by; only following every second or third impulse; becoming aware of the central blockage (in matters of the heart).

Resolution: Being calmer in matters of the heart; allowing oneself time, not forcing anything, learning to pass up offers; slowing down and calming the rhythm of life.

Archetypal principle: Uranus-Sun.

Avian influenza

(former designation: bird flu; see also Influenza, Psittacosis)

Physical level: Head (capital of the body), nose (power, pride, sexuality), neck (assimilation, connection, communication), lungs (contact, communication, freedom), musculature (motor, strength).

Symptom level: Extremely rare disease pattern which results from mutation of a virus specific to animals, or more exactly birds; a mutation of this type has arisen (definitely) at least once in the last 100 years with terrible ramifications, and possibly also a second time; this does not mean, however, that it will happen again soon; the hysteria triggered by the fear of avian influenza serves above all to induce the vaccination-weary population to once again get themselves vaccinated (an influenza vaccination would not, however, offer any protection against avian influenza, and as yet, no vaccine against avian influenza actually exists); the real danger to date still lies in the weakening of the immune defence system on the basis of the fear-mongering (→vaccination damage), and in this respect, birds - as symbols of the soul - are particularly suitable for triggering collective spiritual fear; in actual fact, our freedom is indeed endangered; people had become too free and independent in their decisions (e.g. against vaccinations) and are made compliant again by such methods.

Handling: Setting limits, keeping one's inner space free; voluntary withdrawal from external activities, actively keeping external demands at arm's length; offensively shutting oneself off from the inflow of further influence, clearing up unclear situations; opening oneself up for spiritual truths.

Resolution: Being in flow; clearing up deadlocked problems; taking into account the characteristic qualities of the prevailing time period (autumn and spring as seasons of change enforce calm and attentiveness for new developments).

Archetypal principle: Uranus-Pluto.

Avolition

see Depression

B

Back pains

(see also Posture defects)

Physical level: Back (strenuous effort, uprightness), spinal column (dynamics and hold, uprightness).

Symptom level: One's inner and outer stance do not correspond with one other; rising up in protest, since the inner stance/shadow realm cannot be lived out; compensatory measures to counterbalance one's honest but unpopular stances cause pain in the long term due to the fact that upholding these measures is a continual strain that costs of great deal of energy expenditure: lack of uprightness ("crooked as a dog's hind leg"); bending over backwards; no longer being able to be straight with oneself; having problems in standing up for oneself; being bowed down by grief: unprocessed grief has an oppressive impact on one's stance; being placed under pressure by existential burdens (intervertebral disc problems); the feminine pole (the soft intervertebral disc) in the life axis of the spinal column is trapped and squashed flat between two hard (masculine) vertebral bodies; pains in the cervical and thoracic vertebra area: cries for help with regard to emotional support; pains in the lumbar vertebra area: cries for help with regard to existential (material) support; unconscious conflict over the existentially-decisive next steps; tension in the back: free self-expression is held back; one's own strength finds no backing.

Handling: Uncovering and owning up to one's unconscious deficits in relation to uprightness (including towards oneself); finally forcing oneself to wrestle with the original, honest but incorrect posture, and starting from this basis, working on genuine uprightness; re-examining strains which weigh heavy on one's back for their coherency; relieving the back of burdens which have become superfluous, and at least making oneself aware of other burdens which have been taken on unconsciously; transforming tensions into conscious potential and actions; Tai-Chi exercises for developing a culture of movement.

Resolution: Standing up for oneself and one's conscious inner stance.

Archetypal principle: Saturn-Mars.

Balance disorders

(see also Menière's disease, Kinetoses, Rotary vertigo, Pregnancy complaints)

Physical level: Balance organ in the inner ear (balance sensor).

Symptom level: Different contradictory items of information come together in the central control headquarters; e.g. in the case of seasickness and the corresponding giddiness: the eyes report that everything is at rest, but the balance organ reports rolling movements; feeling oneself to be on unsteady ground; not being fully aware of one's own situation; deceiving oneself with regard to one's own adaptability; not feeling oneself in one's own element; movements that are too rapid for one's own consciousness; not being able to trust one's eyes; being out of balance, torn this way and that, wavering between two decisions; "feign"ting (giddiness/[self]-deception) is the precursor to a fall and the Fall is the original trauma (sin) of mankind (i.e. the Fall from Grace); the desire for giddiness/(self-) deception and to feel giddy/deceive (oneself): after the Fall from Grace, the first people started to be "wrapped" in clothing (fig leaves) and "rapt" in each other (sexually): waltzes and the amusement rides at funfairs stand for the enticing giddiness/(self-) deception; "feign"ting: deceiving oneself; also an expression of escapist tendencies (caught in the wrong bed, one sits up briefly in alarm, before falling back again in a "feign"t); taking flight from a situation which is developing too quickly (standing up too quickly with low blood pressure and the corresponding pattern).

Handling: Bringing the conflicting information into accord, e.g. in the case of seasickness: going out on the deck of the ship and consciously perceiving the movement of the water or closing one's eyes to exclude them as a source of error; trusting the unsteady ground and rolling with the punches; consciously trusting oneself to the foreign element, giving in to it; adjusting speed and shifting things down a gear to correspond to one's own processing speed; allowing one's (apparent) balance to be thrown off, trusting oneself to the true circumstances; finding a new balance and making decisions on a new, more realistic level; developing an inner point of view (and stance) on the situation.

Resolution: Surrendering oneself to the situation.

Archetypal principle: Venus-Neptune.

Balanitis

(inflammation of the glans with discharge of an [often stinking] secretion)

Physical level: Glans (spearpoint of masculinity), inner foreskin (curtain in front of the tip of the weapon).

Symptom level: "Fire in the hole", burning member: danger in the foremost superficial area of masculinity; conflict over the spearhead of masculinity; painful irritation at the spearhead: the member is irritated or over-irritated, "the lance-tip has a burning desire to be cooled"; the member is over-worked (has become too hot?); self-punishment for overly intensive or misdirected use (masturbation?); self-punishment for uncleanliness (on the physical or figurative level); the man finds that something stinks with regard to the spearhead of his masculinity; it has gone bad: is unclean, stinking, reddened and out of shape; terrible, unpleasant experience in the sexual area which stinks to high heaven for him.

Handling: Becoming aware of the dangers in the area of superficially phallic masculinity; offensively and courageously having out the conflicts over the spearpoint of masculinity; ensuring relief: putting one's masculinity into practice more or less consciously instead of overheating the member; coming to grips with the subject of masculinity and conquering it in the heat of battle; consciously placing judgement/punishment in higher hands; reconciling oneself with desire; looking after one's own weapons (taking greater care in the hygienic or psycho-hygienic respect); trusting oneself to get involved in the battle of the sexes with provocative women.

Resolution: Exercising courageous care of the weapon in all respects: not allowing the weapon become run down; responsible and skillful use

of the weapon with desire and love; demonstrating masculinity in a playful, yet combative way.

Archetypal principle: Mars-Mars.

Baldness

see Hair loss

Bartholinitis

(inflammation of the Bartholin's glands)

Physical level: Labia (entrance gates to the sexual underworld), vulva (protective wall).

Symptom level: Due to an →abscess or a →cyst, the vaginal vestibule e is no longer sufficiently moistened and lubricated by the gland; swelling caused by the inflammation also hinders sexual intercourse; not being ready for sexual intercourse; blocking the entrance to the temple of desire; resistance, nothing goes smoothly any more; her partner and his unwelcome desires rub her the wrong way; reluctance, boiling rage instead of hot eroticism.

Handling: Trusting oneself to say 'no', and shutting the gates to the sexual underworld with vehemance rather than with pain; articulating one's own sexual needs courageously and openly, pursuing one's own desires and ideas.

Resolution: Sexual self-determination; accepting responsibility for one's own sexuality; fighting the battle of the sexes at the level of erotic desire and lust.

Archetypal principle: Venus-Mars.

Basalioma

(carcinoma without the tendency to metastasise, but with the tendency to return after operative removal; see also Cancer, Skin cancer)

Physical level: Occurs only in the area of the head (head = capital city of the body), particularly on the face (visiting card, individuality, perception, façade).

Symptom level: Too much sunlight (UV light) leads to thickening of the horny skin (→keratosis) and later (frequently) to basal cell carcinoma: this eats away/disfigures the face; has all the tendencies of cancer (processes), only less malignant since there is no dissemination into the rest of the body; it restricts itself to disfigurement of the face: being eaten up by unexpressed emotions, sentiments and feelings; ulcerous changes in one's facial expression to the point of forming a horror mask.

Handling: Bringing more inner light instead of outer light into the game (of life); addressing one's own individuality (→cancer); attacking one's own (false) mask in order to find and accept the real shadow expression beneath it; expressing emotions and feelings, and above all, also their dark forms on one's face ("it's written all over your face": basal cell carcinoma patients initially have nothing written on their face, until everything suddenly comes all at once).

Resolution: Having the sun in one's heart; coming to terms with one's shadow all the way down into the depths of the soul; courageous, offensive self-expression.

Archetypal principle: Pluto-Venus.

Basedow's disease

(see also Thyroid gland hyperfunction, Goitre)

Physical level: Thyroid gland (development, maturity), neck (assimilation, connection, communication).

Symptom level: Protruding eyeball (exophthalmus): the whole iris becomes visible, giving the eyes a greedy expression as if they would like to leap out of the sockets; eyes wide open in fear, as if they had glimpsed primordial dread; goitre (thick neck) reveals the subject:

never being able to get one's fill of something; racing pulse and corresponding heart palpitations: agitation, fear, desire to flee; unrest and excitability: demand for activity; weight loss: eating one's heart out for something; trembling: general fear of life; the frequently accompanying hair loss shows the sacrifice of freedom, strength and radiant aura.

Handling: Learning to look closely at things, to step up to them; learning to take for oneself what one needs; converting activity into (inner) movement; firing oneself up for hot subjects; plunging into life, living (experiencing) more intensely; becoming absorbed in one's task and becoming committed; transforming fear of life into concentrated handling of the relevant subjects; identifying the subject that is worrying one; confronting inner dread; making sacrifices for the task which is stirring one's heart and keeping it on the go.

Resolution: Daring to address the subject which is making one's heart pound in one's throat and one's eyes burst their sockets.

Archetypal principle: Mercury- Mars.

Bechterew's disease

(Morbus Bechterew)

Physical level: Spinal column (dynamics and hold, uprightness).

Symptom level: One's own world axis ossifies into a bamboo pole: unconscious surrender of the female pole (intervertebral discs) and thus of mobility and flexibility; fossilisation of one's own centre and axis; embodied Ego claim; embodied inflexibility, rigidity; one's degree of rigidity and inflexibility is shoved right under one's nose; being forced back down to Earth by the head.

Handling: Showing more consistency and backbone towards oneself; becoming aware that the female pole is coming up short and to what degree this is causing a rigid, unbending state; developing masculinity in a stable form which can be relied on; achieving genuine spiritual straight-forwardness instead of physical straightforwardness; consistency and firmness with regard to one's own life axis: e.g. seeking out a fixed place where one can embed one's "totem pole" and that one can come home to inwardly; seeking a fixed centre and support in life: bringing genuine stability into one's inner life; display-ing inner firmness and uprightness towards oneself and others; providing backing for oneself: proudly standing behind one's own Ego claims; re-maining concentrated on the next few steps; noting what is happening right at one's feet; practising not allowing oneself to be drawn out of one's centre; consciously aligning oneself with Mother Earth, voluntarily turning towards her and the feminine aspect in general.

Resolution: Remaining straightfor-ward and in alignment with oneself; cultivating the utmost modesty and self-restraint; adopting clear posi-tions and standpoints; bringing the twisting and dynamic aspect of the verterbral column (Latin vert(ere) = 'to turn') back into play as soon as inner stability is ensured and one has straightened oneself out inwardly while nevertheless turning one's gaze in humility to (Mother) Earth.

Archetypal principle: Saturn-Saturn.

Bedsores

see Decubitus

Bed-wetting

Physical level: Urinary bladder (with-standing and relieving pressure).
Symptom level: Letting off pressure at night when conscious control is lessened; the overwhelmed day-to-day control mechanism of the head

fails at night: total release; giving back the pressure received through-out the day; exercise of power; crying down below; often problems with the mother.

Handling: (On the part of the par-ent/guardian): becoming aware of the day-to-day pressure on the child: sensing the fear behind the pressure; motivating the child to accept demands and pressure as a challenge; creating room for relax-ation throughout the day; reacting to excess pressure with games, en-abling pleasurable letting go; creating outlets for natural crying (encouraging tears of joy and of sadness instead of disparaging them); giving the child opportunities to let him/herself go, regress completely.

Resolution: (for the child): being able to defend him/herself face-to-face throughout the day; being able to handle (one's own) emotions.

Archetypal principle: Moon-Pluto.

Belching, acidic

Physical level: Stomach (feeling, re-ceptiveness), oesophagus (food pipe, nutrition supply).

Symptom level: Expression of concealed resistance to what has been swallowed; feelings that have been swallowed, but are indigestible force their way to the surface; sour-ness (acid) rises up and wants to be expressed; concealed aggression: "giving vent to things", "letting off pressure"; resentment: "something leaves a sour taste in one's mouth" – above all, the inability to articulate oneself appropriately; being "fed up to the back teeth" with a situation.

Handling: Practising means of expressing oneself that come from one's own depths and make use of one's own physicality: allowing oneself feelings of reluctance and sourness; expressing aggression, letting suppressed aspects come to the surface; learning to give vent to things; freeing oneself from what is weighing down on one, being aware of one's resentment.

Resolution: Giving free rein to one's gut feelings, speaking and acting on the basis of gut feelings.

Archetypal principle: Moon-Mars.

Biermer's disease

see Pernicious anaemia

Bile duct carcinoma

see Gall bladder cancer

Biliary colic

(see also Colic, Gall stones)

Physical level: Gall bladder (aggression, poison and bile).

Symptom level: Pains similar to the contractions associated with labour, which drive the stone (of contention – consisting of petrified aggressions such as anger and rage) forwards and outwards and launch a field offensive against the obstacle in ever-recurring waves of attack; being rattled in the truest sense of the word; those who have swallowed down bile and poison for too long instead of spitting it out must reconcile themselves with such precipitations of balled up, toxic rage; overcoming a difficult birth with severe contractions: managing a new beginning; bringing the balled up and solidified toxic aggression into the world after all; emphatically breaking up what has become stuck (repressed); freeing up of the energy backlog caused by the blockage.

Handling: Using rhythmic force to free oneself from stones which one has placed in one's own way; overcoming one's own inertia (symbol: stone); using steadfast perseverance to get rid of what has become stuck (repressed); however, not making a continuous effort, but instead bringing

about the (re)solution with efforts that occur in a rhythmic ebb and flow; letting out one's own toxic aspects: preferring to spit poison and bile rather than giving birth to gall stones; open (to view) demonstration of one's own aggressive energy; bringing one's own aggressive energy back into flow in an open(ly offensive) way; courageously undertaking the first steps; letting go (in a painful way) of what is standing in the way of a relaxed life; overcoming hindrances instead of sidestepping them: the alternatives (also after an operation): either light food or living offensively.

Resolution: Making oneself aware in what respect this gall stone is a "stone" of contention (poison? [bile] acid? biliousness?) and in future, bringing this subject out into the open in a more conscious and conciliatory way; letting go of and overcoming hindrances which stand in one's way.

Archetypal principle: Pluto-Mars.

Bilirubinuria

(transgression of bile fluid into the blood in →liver diseases and excretion of bile pigment with the urine)

Physical level: Liver (life, evaluation, reconnection).

Symptom level: Resentment and unexpressed aggression get mixed up (meddle) with the life flow and discolour it right down to the spiritual waste water.

Handling: Letting one's own aggression live; letting out one's resentment at a suitable point.

Resolution: Also allowing aggressive forces to participate in one's life as part of one's own vitality.

Archetypal principle: Mars-Pluto/ Jupiter.

Binge eating disorder

(see also Obesity, Appetite, lack of [as the opposite pole])
Physical level: Consciousness, brain (communication, logistics), stomach (feeling, receptiveness).
Symptom level: Not getting enough, having a hole in one's stomach, feeling empty; hunger for love and love of life; food as a substitute for life and love; unbounded appetite to devour life; excessive desire to take part in life, to let oneself get involved in it and to pack in as much as possible; filling oneself up, fullness instead of fulfilment.
Handling: Allowing oneself to live indulgently with all the joy (of life), letting oneself get involved with it; taking one's own slice of life; claiming and collecting what is due to one.
Resolution: Finding fulfilment, becoming one with all; integration.
Archetypal principle: Jupiter.

Bipolar disorder

see Manic-depressive disease

Birth complications (general)

(see also Premature birth, Caesarean section, Placental insufficiency, Placenta praevia, Placental separation, Stillbirth)
Physical level: Womb (fertility, safety and security).
Symptom level: The intial birth pattern is characteristic of all later handling of new beginnings and breakthroughs and for many later anxiety symptoms: "Everything lies in the beginning" as a basic insight of esoteric philosophy.
Handling: (in later life): making oneself aware of the patterns imprinted by birth and realising its basic themes on the most resolved (redeeming)

levels possible; e.g. in the case of a Caesarean section child: instead of always waiting for outside assistance, accepting this where it is available, but otherwise learning to first and foremost resort to the helping hand at the end of one's own forearm; instead of thinking "The others should see to it that something becomes of me", preferring to think "The others should see what is going to become of me!"; clarifying and accepting the birth(pattern) in therapeutic processes, and if necessary, coming to terms with one's own birth trauma.
Resolution: Reconciliation with the Mars-driven, aggressive forces inherent in all beginnings.
Archetypal principle: Mars-Moon.

Birth complications: breech presentation

Physical level: Womb (fertility, safety and security).
Symptom level: (in the case of the child): opposition, non-compliance, protest: "You can just (kiss my ass)"; greeting the world with different cheeks; meconium (child's first fecal discharge) is let out in greeting: "shitty" transition into the world of air; frequently children who are not the sex openly or secretly wished for by the parents; avoidance of the Mars principle and a courageous, headlong leap into the polar world; early, anxious turning away from life; later strategy of keeping one's head held high at all costs; pig-headedness.
Handling: (On the part of the later adult): learning commitment.
Resolution: Reconciliation with the Mars principle.
Archetypal principle: Moon/ Mars-Saturn-Uranus.

Birth complications: carrying over term

Physical level: Womb (fertility, safety and security).

Symptom level: 1. (On the part of the mother): refusal to give up the child; not wanting to let go (of the child); lacking the strength to cast out the child; 2. (On the part of the child): shying away from the courageous, headlong leap into life; lack of (basic) trust; not wanting to separate oneself from the cosy nest (snugness).

Handling: 1. (On the part of the mother): avoiding overprotection of the child; all compensation measures harbour the danger of pushing things too far (e.g. overfeeding to the point of stuffing the child full; becoming aware that being a mother means not only sheltering and protecting, but also giving birth and giving up; 2. (On the part of the later adult) recognising the danger in good time of sitting still for too long everywhere, of overstretching things, and staying too long; bracing oneself for a certain hostility towards development in order to be able to meet it.

Resolution: 1. Giving the child its own (living) space; 2. Plucking up courage; tackling necessary things in good time.

Archetypal principle: Moon/ Mars-Jupiter-Pluto.

Birth complications: cervical rupture

Physical level: Cervix (gate to the primordial cave of all beginnings).

Symptom level: 1. The mother does not open the gateway for the child into the polar world of her own (free) will; not wanting to give it up; 2. The child forces its way into freedom with brute force: "ramming its head against the wall".

Handling: 1. (On the part of the mother): releasing the child into independence, delivering it; opening and broadening oneself to new ways of life; 2. (On the part of the later adult): grabbing one's right to life at almost any price; forcing one's will (head) through without consideration for others and going one's own way in the sense of individuation.

Resolution: (for both): allowing oneself to be torn apart in order to enable new life; self-sacrifice, giving of oneself to the extreme.

Archetypal principle: Moon-Mars/ Uranus.

Birth complications: perineal tear

Physical level: Vagina (commitment).

Symptom level: In the case of an unsuitable (lying) position of the mother during the birth, the head of the child presses on the perineum instead of on the opening and tears it; overstretching oneself, "busting one's ass"; being forced to a level of openness which simply does not fit.

Handling: (On the part of the obstetrician): not laying the mother flat on her back (episiotomy in order to prevent later descent is also now refuted by traditionally-accepted medicine; accepting small perineal tears, since these heal just as well as stitches); during the preparation for the birth, already warmly recommending better positions to the woman, e.g. one in which she remains standing or crouching on her own two feet, and in which, given this independent standing, she also preserves responsibility.

Resolution: (On the part of the mother): giving the child the gift of life from a position of strength, such as crouching.

Archetypal principle: Mars-Moon.

142

Birth complications: premature amniotic sac rupture

Physical level: Womb (fertility, safety and security).

Symptom level: (On the part of the mother): showing the child the door (into the open air) too early (→premature birth); leaving it high and dry in relation to the water of life; no longer wanting to make the maternal cave available (→amniotic sac infection).

Handling: (For both the mother and the later adult): watching out for rash, ill-considered decisions.

Resolution: Mastering the art of choosing the right moment.

Archetypal principle: Moon/ Mars-Uranus.

Birth complications: premature contractions

Physical level: Womb (fertility, safety and security), birth canal (the slide into life).

Symptom level: The child is on its way (in life) too early; 1. (On the part of the mother): attempt to be rid of the child prematurely, throwing it out and showing it the door (into the open air), unconscious attempt at expulsion; 2. (On the part of the child): pressing ahead prematurely, taking flight, restlessness.

Handling: 1. (On the part of the mother): in raising the child: allowing it its own time and giving it its own space; taking the child to heart; exercising patience; gratefully accepting the premature delivery from required care; submitting to rest and relaxation; 2. (On the part of the later adult): looking ahead (being cautious) and looking out for others (being considerate); learning to recognise the dangers of impatience: reworking is usually more strenuous than having the necessary staying power; learning to handle one's own pace; transforming hectic activity and restlessness into energetic action.

Resolution: (for both): bringing things to a close; sticking with things right to the end.

Archetypal principle: Moon/ Mars-Uranus.

Birth complications: shoulder dystocia

Physical level: The head (main part) of the child is already born, however, the shoulder (load-bearing capacity, stance) remains stuck at an angle in the mother's pelvis (basis of life).

Symptom level: More frequently in overweight mothers, diabetes sufferers or following excessive weight gain during pregnancy, and in general in the case of overterm, respectively children with a birth weight of over 4500g; general: disproportion, exaggeration, indecisiveness, stretching things to the limit; making it unnecessarily difficult to bear for oneself and others; 1. (On the part of the mother): not giving up the child, having fed and carried it too well and for too long, and thereby endangering its being born and its independent standing; 2. (On the part of the child): not letting the last step into life simply take its course; being in the wrong (position) and getting stuck, being oblique and obstructive, spreading oneself out, puffing oneself up and risking one's later ability to act (danger of plexus paralysis).

Handling: 1. Nourishing and providing for the child for a long time in the figurative sense; releasing it into an independent standing in life only step-by-step, while continuing to care for its well-being; 2. (On the part of the later adult): meeting even unusual situations/positions with great firmness; consciously recognising and resolving skewed positions, taking oneself seriously and consciously taking up space.

Resolution: 1. Giving everything to one's own child; 2. Living out life-enhancing determination; progressing step-by-step into an independent stance and self-responsibility; learning to stand on one's own two feet in stages.

Archetypal principle: Moon/Mars-Saturn.

Birth complications: tearing of the pubic bone joint

(symphysis rupture)

Physical level: Pelvis (basis of life, resonance base), pubic bone (base of the mound of Venus, protection of the sexual region).

Symptom level: Rupture of the pelvic bowl, which has already been loosened by the high oestrogen level prior to the birth, as a result the child surging forward; 1. The mother is not up to the onslaught; it penetrates to her very substance and the bones; taking self-abandonment too far; 2. (In the case of the child): becoming too big for its boot(ie)s in an "egoistic" way; forcing one's will (head) through without consideration for others; make-or-break struggle since the big-headed, thick-skulled child experiences too little backing from the mother.

Handling: 1. (On the part of the mother): doing all one can for the child in the figurative sense and tearing oneself apart for its life interests; opening oneself even more and creating room beyond all limits, adapting oneself and even giving way to being overstretched; 2. (On the part of the later adult): harming one's own mother, one's own origin; destroying the nest.

Resolution: Putting oneself out to the extreme, going to the absolute limit;

tearing oneself apart for life (or letting it happen).

Archetypal principle: Saturn-Uranus

Birth complications: transverse presentation

Physical level: Womb (fertility, safety and security).

Symptom level: (in the case of the child): no longer wanting to co-operate; perfect non-compliance, destructive contrary stance: "I will be deliberately obstructive, the others should take care of what is to become of me" (→Caesarean section); early defiance phase ("going against the grain"); being at cross purposes with one's own development path; not learning to push one's way through restrictiveness and fear; coming into the world without being born; waiting to be freed instead of freeing oneself (Princess attitude): waiting for deliverance instead of striving to achieve it oneself.

Handling: (in the case of the later adult): scaling back attitudes of expectation; catching up on restrictive experiences as an initiation into the world of polarity with its fear.

Resolution: Being in agreement with one's own path (including Caesarean section).

Archetypal principle: Moon/Mars-Saturn.

Birth complications: umbilical cord prolapse

Physical level: Neck (assimilation, connection, communication), womb (fertility, safety and security).

Symptom level: 1. (In the case of the mother): tendency, also later, to smother the child (e.g. with "love"), to overwhelm (crush) it; love which takes one's breath away; being mixed-up, inner chaos; 2. (In the case of the child): auto-aggression, manoeuvring oneself into a trap; attempt to strangle oneself: "I would rather kill myself, than let go and entrust myself to the general flow"; fear of what is to come, being rash and aggravated or resentful; often in combination with transverse presentation in order to be freed by means of →Caesarean section; the child just hangs loose, also in the figurative sense; it musters no strength to free itself; the battle for life is rejected, threatening with one's own strangulation.

Handling: 1. (On the part of the mother): keeping the danger of overprotection in mind; controlling one's great desire for dominance; 2. (On the part of the later adult): becoming aware of one's own Plutonic (all-engulfing and all-entangling) powers; learning to see through destructive forces and recognising →suicide as an escape.

Resolution: (for both): recognising the "death and rebirth" principle as one of the primordial subjects of being human; being able to handle metamorphosis processes; unfolding (developing) oneself instead of getting entangled.

Archetypal principle: Moon/Mars-Pluto.

Birth complications: vaginal tear

(colporrhexis; can include perineal tear)

Physical level: Vagina (commitment, receptiveness).

Symptom level: The final gateway, after the womb has already released the head of the child, is too narrow; imbalanced relationship between mother and child; 1. The mother has either overnourished the child for too long and over-estimated her own capacity to broadly open herself and make room for another, or the father has been too overbearing in relation to her, which similarly results in an over-estimation; can later lead to the point of total self-sacrifice for the child, tearing oneself apart in the truest sense of the word for the common child; 2. (On the part of the child): taking up too much room, charging forward too inconsiderately, over-stretching one's mother.

Handling: 1. Giving oneself fully and opening oneself up to the birth process, freely choosing the individually-fitting stance to the birth; 2. Forging one's path into life with all one's strength; going one's own way uncompromisingly.

Resolution: 1. Sacrificing oneself for the next generation, clearing the way; 2. Remaining true to one's own path, courageously fighting to clear the path.

Archetypal principle: Moon/Mars-Uranus.

Birthmark

(naevus; see also Liver spot)

Physical level: Skin (border, contact, tenderness).

Symptom level: Having been given a sign (mark of distinction) at birth from one's mother (one's forebears) to take along with one: legacies, reminders of one's origin and tasks that have been brought along (from other times); often vestiges of experiences (wounds, scars) in previous existences, which still leave traces behind and indicate an issue worthy of note; the mark of Cain: being marked (with distinction), branded; vascular tumours/port-wine stains (Latin: nevus flammeus = 'flaming, fire-coloured birthmark'): a wary child that has been burnt before (see the port-wine stain of M. Gorbachev, which certainly marked him in earlier times and still marks him with distinction today).

Handling: proving oneself to be worthy of the mark; living up to the distinction.
Resolution: Accepting and resolving inherited tasks.
Archetypal principle: Saturn/ Venus-Mercury/Pluto.

Bite injury

(see also Accident)
Physical level: All areas of the body surface can be affected.
Symptom level: Openness to attacks and assaults.
Handling: Opening oneself up to energy impulses from outside (Aikido, martial arts); allowing oneself to be stimulated by outside energies (encouraging attacks, e.g. in discussions); becoming inwardly expansive, outwardly strong, e.g. confronting the dog while being inwardly open but outwardly courageous (often prevents the dog biting); inner processing of the animal that has manifested itself in the outer world: the aggressiveness of the dog; the seductive dangerousness of the snake, etc.; confronting one's own snappishness.
Resolution: Openness to dangers: alertness and readiness instead of avoidance behaviour (confronting dogs offensively, looking them straight in the eye); confronting aggressions; facing up to challenges.
Archetypal principle: Mars..

Bladder diverticule

(sack-like bulging of the urinary bladder)
Physical level: Urinary bladder (withstanding and relieving pressure).
Symptom level: Extra storage tank which contains, and over time, retains the waste products of the (spiritual) waste; this frequently leads to (inflammatory) conflicts over these residues (of urine).
Handling: Becoming aware of one's hidden spiritual pockets and secret compartments, and critically sifting through their contents; risking confrontations with this long held back spiritual waste.
Resolution: Opening up new areas in the spiritual respect; courageous cleaning up in the catchment basin of one's spiritual waters.
Archetypal principle: Pluto-Moon.

Bladder fistula

see Urinary bladder fistula

Bladder, inflamed / irritated

see Urinary bladder inflammation

Bladder stones

see Urinary bladder stones

Bladder weakness

see Incontinence

Bleeding after menopause

Physical level: Genitalia (sexuality, polarity, reproduction), blood (life force).
Symptom level: Persistent bleeding after menopause because there is still too much oestrogen and too little progesterone in circulation; the build-up of the uterine lining which is now being shed shows that growth impulses have become pressing: not yet being done with the issue of having children and the central female phase; not being able to detach oneself from youthful womanhood; denying oneself the natural ageing process; often in combination with →myomas.
Handling: Letting go of the mother aspect; growing into the new role in life.
Resolution: Cultivating fertility on the spiritual level, sacrificing life energy

for others; becoming a "grand" mother in a wider sense (e.g. committing oneself to social causes).
Archetypal principle: Moon-Mars/ Pluto.

Bleeding after sexual intercourse

(see also Dyspareunia)
Physical level: Vagina (commitment, desire).
Symptom level: Usually occurs together with a hormone imbalance (lack of the "female" oestrogen), more rarely as a result of injury; putting up resistance to the challenging mascu-linity, being unwilling and unable to open (oneself) up; self-punishment for unacknowledged desire, unconscious desire for everlasting virginity and purity.
Handling: Entering into womanhood with all its consequences; giving one's own life force to womanhood instead of making a blood sacrifice every time; questioning the female archetype of the Mother Mary.
Resolution: Reconciliation with the world of contrasts, one's own female role and the sacrifices which it natu-rally demands.
Archetypal principle: Pluto/ Venus-Mars.

Bleeding blockage

(haematocolpos)
Physical level: Vagina (commitment, desire), vulva (protective wall).
Symptom level: The menstrual blood collects in front of the hymen, which is stuck together and impermeable, thus preventing the outflow of blood, danger of →inflammation; conflict over the breakthrough of female en-ergy; the acknowledgement of one's own womanhood is circumvented; female sexuality is overlaid with ta-boos; fear of masculine penetration;

unconscious desire to remain a child (to stop the menstrual flow).
Handling: External, operative sup-port (defloration) in order to enable the release of the menstrual blood; becoming aware of feelings of guilt, anxieties and shock experiences surrounding the subjects of femininity, womanhood and sexuality.
Resolution: Enjoying feminine vitality and joy for life; fulfilling sexuality.
Archetypal principle: Moon/ Venus-Saturn.

Bleeding tendency

(haemorrhagic diathesis)
Physical level: Blood (life force).
Symptom level: Loss of vitality, fatigue, weariness, loss of the joy for life.
Handling: Making sacrifices; exer-cises in letting go, letting things hap-pen, deep relaxation; exercises which harmonise the life flow, such as Tai Chi, Qi Gong.
Resolution: Consciously giving away one's own life force; letting go of the demands of the Ego.
Archetypal principle: Mars-Neptune.

Blepharitis

see Lid inflammation

Blindness

(vision below 10%; see also Colour blindness)
Physical level: Eyes (insight, per-spective, mirrors and windows of the soul).
Symptom level: Not wanting to see, blindness of the consciousness; com-pulsion to look inwards: only the inner images remain (residually) when the outer images are taken away.
Handling: Introspection: journeys inwards instead of outwards; learning to see in inner worlds: learning to open up the outer world by mastering inner vision.

Resolution: (see also the life story of Helen Keller): true vision, higher insight: great visionaries, who saw the reality behind the external forms, were often blind (e.g. Teiresias in the Oedipus myth); Resolution of one's inner tasks, conquest of the inner world; glimpsing the inner light; learning to look inwards with the eyes of love.
Archetypal principle: Sun/Moon-Neptune.

Blisters

see Burns

Blisters, suppurating

see Impetigo

Blood (in the stools)

Physical level: Digestive tract ("consuming and digesting the world" = Buddhism: Bhoga).
Symptom level: Lifeblood has gone astray into the waste disposal system/in the underworld (as always, first clarify the traditionally-accepted medical cause, then identify and interpret the underlying problem): life energy is being lost via the waste disposal system; the red vitality (symbol) is transformed into the black death (symbol); blood sacrifice.
Handling: Directing the life flow into the shadow kingdom: performing lively shadow work; devoting life energy to wayward projects; concerning oneself with "death and rebirth" (eternal change).
Resolution: Reconciliation with Pluto-Hades (shadow therapy) – the god of the kingdom of the dead, who is also the god of wealth: creative potential often lies concealed in the shadow kingdom; reconciliation with death as the objective of life.
Archetypal principle: Pluto-Mars.

Blood (in the urine)

see Haematuria

Blood (thickening of)

(see also Blood coagulation, Thrombosis, Embolism)
Physical level: Blood (life force), especially erythrocytes (energy carriers of the life flow), blood vessels (transport routes of the life force).
Symptom level: The blood flow becomes slower and more lethargic and tends towards stagnation, the life energy becomes bogged down; this bogged-down energy transport threatens the dependent parts of the body with starvation (example: heart or lung infarction) or the formation of thromboses (blood clots), which are then carried off into the smallest peripheral vessels, where they lead to blockage and supply problems (→lung embolism); life is no longer in flow, stagnation in central questions.
Handling: Homeopathically: going about life more calmly, letting the life energy flow more deliberately and carefully, ensuring more substance in life, intensifying the concentration of energy; allopathically: intensifying the life flow, living more fluidly, ensuring swifter process flows, giving the soul a greater share in the life flow.
Resolution: Homeopathically: concentrating on the essential with respect to the life energy; letting the flow of life become more substantial; Allopathically: getting more fully into the flow in the figurative sense, integrating more of the spiritual element (water) into the flow of life.
Archetypal principle: Mars-Saturn.

Blood (vomiting)

(haematemesis; in cases of bleeding →stomach ulcer or →oesophageal varices)

Physical level: Stomach (feeling, receptiveness), oesophagus (food pipe, nutrition supply).

Symptom level: (Interpret the basic symptom as the first priority): spitting out lifeblood (energy): inner wounds burst open; losing vitality; paying for something with one's own blood ("being bled dry").

Handling: Developing a willingness to make sacrifices; learning to pay bills that are still outstanding.

Resolution: Sacrificing one's life energy in order to resolve a problem.

Archetypal principle: Mars-Neptune/Uranus.

Blood clot

(see also Blood, thickening of, Thrombosis, Embolism)

Physical level: Blood (life force), blood vessels (transport routes of the life force).

Symptom level: The flow of life has become sluggish; solidification of what has been set loose, congealment of the flowing; obstruction/blockage of one's life (flow).

Handling: Taking more time for oneself; slowing down the tempo of life, not rushing into anything; consolidating, getting something out the flow of life, and making something of it; crystallising out the essence; blocking out or cutting back on certain areas of life (affected by the embolism).

Resolution: Using the flowing life energy for concrete projects.

Archetypal principle: Mars/Mercury-Saturn

Blood count (haemogram), disturbed

Physical level: Blood (life force).

Symptom level: Count of the 1. Erythrocytes (red blood corpuscles) too low: →anaemia; too high (polyglobulia): over-abundant energy

supply, danger of vessel blockages (vitality blockages); doping problem in modern endurance sport; 2. Leukocytes (white blood corpuscles) too low: general →immune deficiency; too high (leucocytosis): non-specific defences running at high speed; admittedly, the enemies are not yet known, but there is a general readiness for battle on a broad front; 3. Lymphocytes too low: immune deficiency to the point of a total collapse of immunity (e.g. if T-lymphocytes are too low as with →Aids); elevated: indication of infection (→inflammation) or unconscious defensive battle; 4. Thrombocytes reduced (→thrombocytopenia): tendency to bleed even to the point of being in danger of bleeding to death from minor injuries; one's vitality slips away.

Handling: 1. Making the energy supply the central focal point of life; 2. Putting the general defensive situation in order; reconsidering one's general defensive potential; 3. Revising the defensive situation with regard to special themes; 4. Letting the current of life flow more easily in the figurative sense; allopathically: taking care to preserve one's own vitality, sparing the life force, safeguarding life energy.

Resolution: 1. Bringing vitality into harmony with one's needs in life; 2. Bringing general readiness for battle into harmony with one's life situation; 3. Bringing special defensive capabilities into harmony with the threatening situation; 4. Remaining in the flow (of life).

Archetypal principle: 1. Sun-Mars; 2. and 3. Mars; 4. Mars-Saturn.

Blood group incompatibility

(AB0 incompatibility)

Physical level: Blood (life force), immune system (defence).

Blood poisoning

Symptom level: High-risk pregnancy, incompatibility between the mother's and child's vitality; resistance from the mother against the child, non-acceptance of the child as one's own (flesh and blood).

Handling: Mental-spiritual confrontation with the child; meditation on the mother role.

Resolution: Accepting the child as an independent being (see Khalil Gibran "On children" in: The Prophet); reconciliation with the child's vitality, giving one's own a lower priority.

Archetypal principle: Moon-Uranus.

Blood poisoning

(sepsis)

Physical level: Blood (life force) and lymph channel (immune) system of the whole body.

Symptom level: Stirring elements (pathogens - from Greek. pathos "suffering, feeling, emotion") flood one's complete existence (the whole body) and poison the life flow; above all in people who have taken too much of a back seat and given their own interests in life too low a priority; general mobilisation (fever) against the foreign intruders: the battle (antibodies versus pathogens) shakes one to the core (attacks of the shivers), the pulse and heart race, the metabolism moves into high gear; in the worst case, gradual giving up (drowsiness) followed by the withdrawal of one's own troops (blacking out and thus powerlessness), capitulation (cardio-vascular failure) and total surrender (death).

Handling: Allowing oneself to be touched by stirring subjects existentially, instead of throwing the doors wide open to stirring elements in the form of pathogens; opening oneself up to unfamiliar subjects, ideas and impulses; becoming open to what is unaccustomed, the foreign; approaching the confrontation with these external impulses wholeheartedly and thereby risking one's neck with regard to old ideas and attitudes; consciously taking on the risk that old points of view might go under in the event of critical confrontations; giving in to the foreign, the new, giving up one's own force of habit, and allowing oneself to be taken over by the new ideas; transforming oneself; on the Physical level: coming to the aid of the system with foreign troops (mercenaries = antibiotics).

Resolution: Existential stirring up and transformation; risking and decisively fighting spiritual battles; giving in completely, going all the way.

Archetypal principle: Mars-Pluto/Neptune.

Blood sugar level, low

see Hypoglycemia

Blushing

Physical level: Face (visiting card, individuality, perception, façade).

Symptom level: Signal; indication of an overlooked subject charged with fear and embarrassment: "turning bright red"; the flaming cheeks become one's own personal red beacon in order to blazon the truth and make one honest against one's will; suppressed narcissistic desire for attention; wanting to stand in the centre of attention (delusions of grandeur: "I am the best").

Handling: Becoming aware of one's shamefacedness and learning to stand behind it; consciously risking entering one's own personal red-light district and having the corresponding experiences; recognising that the reddening of the cheeks, neck and chest in the relevant situations is neither worrying nor embarrassing, but natural; living out the overlooked subject more and more, and thereby

integrating it into consciousness so that it thrusts itself less and less into the foreground at every "inappropriate" opportunity; working on self-awareness (pre-requisite: basic trust, which develops in early pregnancy).
Resolution: honestly standing behind oneself (and one's own [secret] desire for attention and recognition); satisfying sexuality, which above all drives the blood down into the lower areas of the body and only incidentally slightly reddens the cheeks.
Archetypal principle: Venus/Mars-Neptune/Sun.

Body hair, excessive

see Hypertrichosis

Boeck's disease

see Sarcoidosis

Bone cancer

(see also Cancer)
Physical level: Bones (stability, strength).
Symptom level: Aggressive destruction of the stabilising and supporting structures, accompanied by the danger of causing them to break; degeneration in the structural domain: wildly and ruthlessly rampant growth; having strayed so far off track from one's inherent development path with regard to continuity, form and structure that the body has to help the (forgotten/repressed) issues to express themselves; cracks in one's self-esteem (which are frequently the trigger) show themselves later in the breakdown of one's physical structure (interpret the relevant skeletal region: spinal column = life axis, etc.); the mental-spiritual growth in this area has been blocked for so long that it now forges a path in the body and strikes out in an aggressive and uncontrolled way; the cancer realises

physically in the structural area that (turnaround) which would be spiritually necessary in the corresponding area of consciousness.
Handling: Radically questioning the old structures and stabilising elements of one's own life that have been passed down to one, and if necessary, destroying them, even if this involves the danger of having to break completely with much of the old; opening oneself up in the area of structure and form to one's own outlandish ideas and bold fantasies and courageously allowing them to flourish and expand without control; thinking back to early dreams of one's own forms of expression; bringing these (back) to life and putting them into practice with wild decisiveness; in the certainty of having nothing more to lose, mustering courage for self-realisation/one's own path; taking the growth impulse away from the body and directing it to more resolved (redeeming) levels; considering all the measures mentioned under →cancer: since cancer affects the complete organism, it must also be met across-the-board.
Resolution: Breaking with old structures that are actually foreign to one's own being, making a break in the general continuity; struggling aggressively and in an open(ly offensively) way for one's own (life) forms and structures; providing expression for oneself in the structural domain (i.e. in the world of forms) instead of allowing the body to speak up for itself; recognising the necessity to switch from the physical and thus (life-) threatening level to the challenging, but life-saving mental-spiritual level, and relying in this realm on expansive growth in the affected Archetypal domain; discovering love that transcends all boundaries; setting oneself above external rule and standards laid down by oneself or others, and living and expressing oneself solely

in accordance with the obligations of one's own highest law.
Archetypal principle: Saturn-Pluto.

Bone caries

(see Bone marrow inflammation)

Bone fracture

(see also Arm fracture, Leg fracture, Greenstick fracture, Accident, Work accident/Domestic accident, Sport accident, Traffic accident)
Physical level: Bones (stability, strength).
Symptom level: A break(down) of the deepest inner structure, crash-landing; enforced rest, a break in continuity; overlooking/missing the end of a development; breakup of the old; sudden break in a path which was marked by too much activity and movement; over-stretching and pushing things too far; breaking up of rigidity: new flexibility is enforced violently (in practical terms, it is a new joint which forms); unwillingness to bend; attempt to break ranks.
Handling: Resolutely questioning what has provided stability up to this point and digging down to the deepest depths of what is familiar; making a break in the uniform progression of one's life path; consciously adjusting oneself to the end of every development; developing the willingness to break off from and get over old forms, breaking up entrenched patterns; creating new space for movement; extending the radius of one's own mobility even if drastic measures are required; preferring to break with old thought patterns and habits rather than letting oneself be broken by Fate; voluntarily giving things a rest; ensuring that the energies one is using remain controllable; learning to bend voluntarily and in good time and adapting oneself to necessary turnarounds; undertaking changes in direction (re-orientation): helping

new elements to break through; rebelling against overly rigid norms that have been set in stone and breaking through them.
Resolution: Venturing to truly live life and regarding it as a challenge; bringing variety into one's firmly-established track in life; consciously and voluntarily gaining hold of more room to move in life; ensuring expansion of one's own binding connections.
Archetypal principle: Saturn-Uranus.

Bone marrow inflammation

(bone caries, osteomyelitis)
Physical level: Bones (stability, strength).
Symptom level: Inflammation of the bone marrow: conflict which goes right down to the bone; allowing one's stability and structure to be eaten away; aggressive, all-consuming conflicts over norms and laws; war extending to the very depths of one's own weapons production centre (immune defence system in the bone marrow).
Handling: Pursuing conflicts offensively and courageously down to the very depths; allowing one's accustomed stability and familiar structures to disintegrate in favour of new ones; risking an open(ly offensive) struggle with norms and laws; encouraging conflicts over one's own structures; questioning one's own staying powers (ability to hold out); recognising that the structures which give us stability are actually soft at their innermost core.
Resolution: Bringing everything about oneself into question right down to one's deepest depths; courage for confrontation that goes down to the bone.
Archetypal principle: Saturn-Mars.

152

Borreliosis

(bacterial infection transmitted by tick bite; see also Bite injury)

Physical level: Initially all parts of the skin (boundary, contact, tenderness) can be affected, then after a dormant phase, the infection spreads to organs and nerves.

Symptom level: Bites from sneaky, small and dangerously poisonous vampires; war on the surface, which later spreads to various subject areas and also attacks the information system (nervous system); being touched to the quick/hitting the raw nerve (of life).

Handling: Concerning oneself with the Plutonic principle (allowing oneself to be "stung by the tarantula" from time to time; addressing one's own deviousness and poisonousness; examining who is hanging onto one like a tick, or who one is clinging onto tightly oneself, and courageously detaching oneself; tracing superficial conflicts to their depths; confrontation also with subjects which get on (and hit) one's nerves; making small voluntary sacrifices to competitors for the life energy in good time in the form of donations in order to not make oneself their involuntary victim, and as a side effect, then fall victim to more serious conflicts (e.g. in the sense of Buddhist offerings to helpful and dangerous spirits); allopathically: practising setting limits in good time.

Resolution: Reconciliation with the "death and rebirth" aspect of the Plutonic principle, which relentlessly goes all the way; voluntarily sparing oneself nothing based on the recognition that one is spared nothing anyway, and therefore being ready for anything.

Archetypal principle: Mars-Pluto/ Neptune.

Botulism

(poisoning from meat, sausage or fish products, mainly due to spoilt canned foods in which there has been a build-up of the dangerous nerve toxin caused by botulism bacteria; the disease must be treated with a specific serum)

Physical level: Paralyses in the area of the nervous system (news service).

Symptom level: No longer being able to see through (understand) things (vision disorders); no longer being able to swallow (absorb) things (swallowing disorders); learning instead to give away things (pumping out the stomach as the initial measure); no longer being able to take part in communication (respiratory disorders) to the point of a total polarity boycott (respiratory paralysis as a total communication blockade); general blockage of all signal communications (paralyses due to nerve toxin; nowadays made use of in Botox therapy: injection of ptomaine (cadaveric poison) in order to remove wrinkles and even into the armpits in order to paralyse the secretion of sweat – from a naturopathic point of view, a life-threatening measure which leads to self-poisoning).

Handling: (considerations after overcoming the disease): becoming aware of what one is being poisoned by, what one cannot process; cultivating insight instead of external overview; ceasing to let everything in, to swallow everything; performing voluntary rituals of giving away; granting phases of rest to the nerves.

Resolution: Becoming empty (in the sense of the great emptiness, of Nirvana); overcoming polarity in tendential form (breathing stops during experiences of unity).

Archetypal principle: Mercury-Neptune.

Bow legs

see Part 1, Leg shape

Brachialgia

Physical level: Arms (force, strength, power).
Symptom level: Pains in the arm area due to pinching of the corresponding nerves (Plexus brachialis), often on the basis of neck and spinal column problems: things are not in the right place on the life axis, being "out of alignment" in the upper area, with the result that one becomes incapable of action; no longer being able to raise a finger, being stumped (at the end of one's tether).
Handling: Leaving one's arms at rest and concerning oneself with the main problems in one's own world axis; sorting out what has inwardly ended up "out of alignment".
Resolution: Laying down one's arms (surrendering) and looking at what needs to be put right (at higher levels, where the actual problem lies).
Archetypal principle: Mercury-Mars-Saturn.

Bradycardia

(slowing down of the heart rate to below 55 beats/minute)
Physical level: Heart (seat of the soul, love, feelings, energy centre), sinus node (chief rhythm producer).
Symptom level: Completely normal in endurance athletes and a sign of excellent cardiovascular functioning; pathological bradycardia, e.g. with complete failure of the sinus node and take-over of the peak of the hierarchy by the low-frequency AV nodes.
Handling: Calming oneself in the deepest sense: slowing down the pace of life; dealing with the essential things slowly and step-by-step; going about matters of the heart more calmly; taking things easier (smaller steps), reducing the tempo of life.

Resolution: Living slowly and with awareness.
Archetypal principle: Sun-Saturn.

Brain abscess

(see also Abscess)
Physical level: Brain (communication, logistics).
Symptom level: Entrance via the ears (hearing and obeying commands), nose (getting wind of things), due to trauma (→accident) or metastatically (dissemination; e.g. in →childbed fever); central life-threatening conflict, which cannot penetrate into consciousness; →headaches and dizziness due to self-deception -"feign"(t)ing spells (→balance disorders): something is out of order in the central control area, one is deluding and deceiving oneself; stiffness of the neck: hard-headedness (stubbornness) becomes apparent; feeling of weakness: decline of the life forces becomes noticeable; greatly increased blood sedimentation: the cohesion of the lifeblood declines, the blood corpuscles separate themselves rapidly from the serum, degeneration of the life energy; slowing of the pulse: the cycle of life (circulation) becomes weaker and develops towards fever, weakening in the defensive struggle essential for life.
Handling: Making oneself aware of the origin and the roots of the central conflict: courageously waging the decisive struggle for life; transforming hard-headedness and obstinacy into determination and consistency; applying (sacrificing) one's own life energy for the central problematic issue.
Resolution: Facing up to the decisive battle courageously and in an open(ly offensive) way, defending oneself and fighting back.
Archetypal principle: Mercury-Mars.

Brain concussion

(commotio; see also Cerebral contusion, Accident, Work accident/ Domestic accident, Sport accident, Traffic accident)

Physical level: Brain (communication, logistics), head (capital of the body).

Symptom level: Shake-up of one's system of thought; of one's habitual patterns of thinking prior to that point (somebody who normally cannot be shaken by anything else can still be shaken [reached] in this way); retraction of the dominance of the head; warning shot across the bows, "blow to the brain", "getting one's block knocked off", "it knocks one for six"; having gone at least one step too far; violent correction of a wrong path that has been taken; the attempt to ram one's head through the wall has failed painfully; having deceived oneself; brief surrendering of responsibility and being without power over oneself and the world; stealing away from responsibility; not knowing what is going on in one's own life and how decisive things are taking place; attempt to put oneself out of action; switching the brain off in order to no longer have to own up to a situation (retrograde amnesia = not remembering the circumstances of the accident); possibly a way out of an unconsciously unbearable situation by fleeing to another level.

Handling: Amending one's previous habitual thought patterns which have led to the point of catastrophe; allowing the head (and oneself in general) extensive rest periods; paying attention to warnings, proceeding more carefully; thoroughly reviewing the path taken; taking pause for thought in good time, getting down off one's high horse; learning to overlook certain things: learning to forgive and forget; voluntarily giving up responsibility and power from time to time

in order to rest; instead of throwing up physically, throwing oneself up to a spiritual level; front-ing up to confront-ations in the figurative sense.

Resolution: Recognising the turning point in the catastrophe (Greek he katastrophe = 'catastrophe and turning point') and taking it as a starting point for turning around and turning inwards; allowing oneself to be shaken and then rethinking things.

Archetypal principle: Uranus-Mercury.

Brain tumour

(see also Cancer)

Physical level: Brain (communication, logistics).

Symptom level: Wild and relentlessly proliferating growth in one's own central control headquarters: process that demands space; having strayed so far off track from one's inherent development path with regard to governance that the body - acting on its own intiative - helps the issue to express itself; the mental-spiritual growth in this area has been blocked for so long that it now forges a path in the body in an aggressive, random and ruthless way; the cancer realises physically in the area of the (switching) control centre that (turnaround) which would be spiritually necessary in the corresponding area of consciousness; →headaches as an indication of a way of thinking contrary to one's own nature.

Handling: Making oneself aware of where one is simply "spinning a tale"; recognising illusionary spiritual growth and making it a reality; opening oneself up in the area of government to one's own wild ideas and bold fantasies, courageously and daringly allowing them to grow and flourish; meeting the need for expansion in good time on figurative levels; thinking back to early dreams of one's own life and being wildly decisive in bringing them (back) to life and putting them into practice; mustering courage from "having nothing more to lose"; considering all the measures mentioned under →cancer; since cancer affects the complete organism, it must also be met across-the-board.

Resolution: Discovering love that transcends all boundaries, setting oneself above external rule and standards laid down by oneself or others, and pushing the buttons and calling all the shots in accordance with the obligations of one's own highest law; recognising the necessity to switch from the physical and thus (life-) threatening level to the challenging, but life-saving mental-spiritual level, and relying in this realm on expansive growth.

Archetypal principle: Moon/ Mercury-Pluto.

Breast cancer

(mammary carcinoma; see also Cancer)

Physical level: The female breast (motherliness, nourishment, safety and security, sensuality, desire).

Symptom level: Fear of living as oneself; being torn between the old and new female role (conflicts with regard to emancipation and tradition); not knowing one's own spiritual identity, living in a world of alien feelings; neglect of one's individual feminine path; alienation from one's own femininity (world of feeling, motherliness, etc.); unresolved (entangled) mother relationship, disappointed motherly love; "degenerated" association with the affected region (e.g. not being able to do justice to the mother theme); unlived/unexpressed offensive strength strikes out; aggression forges a path in the body; deep, unprocessed anguish has led to resignation; unconscious retreat; being hurt and angry to the core, without

reacting malignantly on the outside (inner defiance, desire for revenge), but instead, being full of reproaches and allocations of blame; refusal to strike out, to put the pressure on, to become forceful (intrusive), to make accusations; proud of not being egotistical; the soft, feminine way of handling life has become a hindrance (Amazonians).

Left breast: the archetypally soft, feminine aspect comes to the fore (the breast as a nourishing organ, Archetypal principle: Moon; mother(hood) problems, nesting and security issues (anima subject);

2. Right breast: the offensive feminine aspect comes to the fore (the breast as the female "weapon", the breast tip as the invasive element, Archetypal principle: Venus); partner and/or father conflict (animus subject).

Handling: Finding the way back to one's feminine rhythm; learning to live out one's own femininity at whatever cost; standing behind one's own femininity; concentrating on what is one's own and individual to oneself, and asserting it or opening up and losing oneself entirely and willingly in the traditional feminine role; dealing offensively with issues related to the breast (mamma): cultivating and nourishing motherliness, nourishing oneself; using the breast offensively: conquering one's own part of (feminine) life; finding one's own strength and applying it courageously; outwardly manifesting rage and emotions; making a clean breast of things, shouting out one's heartache; getting back to the essential; conscious return to one's own desires; if need be, perhaps even conscious relinquishment of one aspect of femininity; considering all the measures mentioned under →cancer: since cancer affects the complete organism, it must also be met across-the-board (this includes psychotherapy in the sense of therapy involving disease pattern interpretation, as well as clarification by traditionally-accepted medicine and – where indicated – also operation).

Resolution: Finding one's identity; getting back to one's vital essence and integrity with regard to one's own original expectations of life; reconnecting with /retreating to one's actual life theme: living one's own dream; resolving (setting free) one's own womanhood with penetrative strength in order to then bring tenderheartedness and motherly understanding into one's life; selfless devotion only after one's identity has been found and is being lived out; recognising the need to switch from the physical and therefore (life-) threatening level to the challenging, but life-saving mental-spiritual level, and relying instead on expansive growth in this realm; discovering all-pervading, unconditional (undying) love (e.g. motherly love) that transcends all boundaries; taking one's own feminine path to self-responsibility.

Archetypal principle: Moon-Pluto/Neptune.

Breast cysts

(Mastopathia fibrosa cystica; see also Mastopathy, Hormone disorders, female, Cysts, Breast nodes, benign)

Physical level: The female breast (motherliness, nourishment, safety and security, sensuality, desire).

Symptom level: Occurs in three-quarters of the women in industrialised countries; expression of a confused hormone system; often in combination with →premenstrual syndrome and simultaneously with →ovarian cysts; usually disappears with the onset of menopause; not being in balance; often affects women who identify themselves with the young girl role and who do not manage the transition to the motherly role very well; encapsulated tears on

the basis of spiritual injuries in the domain of pregnancy and nursing as well as on the basis of shock experiences and disappointments; hardening of feelings; feelings of guilt because the giving of motherly femininity, of spiritual nourishment does not function properly; not receiving enough loving attention; conflict in the area of nourishing and being nourished.

Handling: Consciously keeping feelings and valuable experiences to and for oneself and burying them in one's bosom; being worthy of looking after oneself properly; discharging emotional and spiritual tensions, releasing (resolving) tensions in the domestic area.

Resolution: Living in harmony with the female cycle of rest and activity; paying attention to life's rhythms; ensuring gentle tenderness and feelings of security and enjoying these.

Archetypal principle: Moon, Saturn.

Breast milk intolerance

see Milk, intolerance

Breast milk production, deficient

(hypogalactia; see also Nursing problems)

Physical level: The female mammary glands (motherliness, nourishment).

Symptom level: The child receives too little, because the mother has too little to give (deficiency situation) or gives too little (stinginess with spiritual nourishment): the mamma (Latin for 'breast') has nothing to give; economy of feelings, holding back spiritual elements, without having any advantage from them oneself; not being able to live up to the mother role; doubts about one's own maternal capabilities are almost always the result and sometimes also the cause.

Handling: Concentrating on the child; learning to take what is necessary for oneself (physical and spiritual nourishment) and to pass it on accordingly; consciously growing into the mother role; not giving up (so quickly - both the mother and the child) (even adoptive mothers can nurse under the right circumstances); learning to share one's own life energy: developing willingness to make sacrifices.

Resolution: Consciously sensing and fostering the chain of life; giving oneself to the new task as a mother and life source for the newborn.

Archetypal principle: Moon-Saturn.

Breast milk production, excessive

(hypergalactia)

Physical level: The female mammary glands (motherliness, nourishment).

Symptom level: Overshooting the mark in breast milk production: overblown desire to nourish (as an over-compensation for spiritual nourishment that is lacking?); piling food upon the child instead of loving attention (overprotection on the nourishment level).

Handling: Offering sufficient spiritual nourishment; consciously turning one's loving attention to the child; making oneself aware of one's own overreaching need to feed and measuring it up against one's own life history: "Was I overfed myself, or has there been too much that I've done without?"; avoiding (physical and spiritual) overfeeding.

Resolution: Nourishing the soul, the spirit and the body and paying close attention to the order of this sequence.

Archetypal principle: Moon-Jupiter.

Breast nodes, benign

(usually fibroadenoma; see also Mastopathy)

Physical level: The female breast (motherliness, nourishment, safety and security, sensuality, desire).

Symptom level: Something which is causing anxiety becomes knotted in the breast; such knots (nodes) stand for a problem which could not be broken down (resolved) on the spiritual level, and which therefore makes itself noticeable in this way, i.e. by threatening with the fear of cancer and therefore also death.

Handling: Accompanied by the corresponding fear, actively and consciously addressing the problem of cancer and dying; reliably and self-responsibly having the node diagnosed (using traditionally-accepted medicine) and doing this immediately (not after one's own observation period).

Resolution: Identifying, clearing, addressing and breaking down (resolving) the knots (in one's own consciousness); in the event of a "benign" diagnosis, using and enjoying the "gift of life" accordingly and developing ones female strengths.

Archetypal principle: Moon/ Venus-Jupiter/Saturn.

Bronchial asthma

(see also Allergy)

Physical level: Lungs (contact, communication, freedom), immune system (defence).

Symptom level: 1. Biting off more than one can chew; attempt to take too much and not give (enough); disturbance of the polarity of giving and taking: threat of being smothered by the (excessive) amount taken in; wanting to keep everything and thus poisoning oneself, cutting oneself off from abundant fullness: "never being able to get one's fill"; longing for love, but without being able to give love; great need to be cared for and mothered. 2. Aversion to contact; fear of the step into freedom and independence; autonomy is experienced as a loss of care and therefore as a threat (to life); inwardly: shortness of breath, anxiety, constriction; outwardly: inflated claim to dominance and power (barrel chest, →lung emphysema); resistance to lively vitality, wanting to shut oneself off/isolate oneself from lively vitality; escape into ideals and formalisms. 3. Puffing oneself up, one would like to "give vent to something"; aggression remains stuck in the lungs: "coughing up" what one really thinks, "gasping with rage". 4. Exercise of power and self-sacrifice by "putting the squeeze" on others with life-threatening attacks; imbalance between power and powerlessness (blacking out): "being speechless or lost for words"; " it akes one's breath away" when confronted with the dominance of others; longing for clean air and majestic mountain tops; wanting to stand above things and other people: "Me alone and after me, the deluge"; shedding tears inwardly. 5. Resistance to the dark areas of life, usually top-heavy (cerebral); relocation of sexuality into the chest (mucous production at a problematic level). 6. Aggression: expectoration (from Latin ex- "out" + pectus (gen. pectoris) "breast.", i.e. making a clean breast of something), spitting something in someone else's face, namely, one's life and its complete softness so to speak. 7. Not being able to breathe freely: not being able to live in one's own way; other people (the mother?) do not allow enough room for one to unfold (develop); autonomy is sacrificed.

Problem areas summarised in keywords: 1. Giving and taking, 2. Wanting to shut oneself off, 3. Aggression, 4. Claim to dominance

and smallness, 5. Sexuality, love and dirt, 6. Aggression, 7. Freedom and space.

Handling: 1. Breathing therapy: experiencing and accepting the balancing of the tensions between giving and taking using connected breathing; 2. Blunt openness and honesty; 3. Living out healthy aggression; articulating aggression in words: "giving vent to something"; living in an offensive manner; 4. Realising and accepting smallness in one's consciousness; learning to forcefully assert oneself without using the symptoms to exercise power; 5. Learning to give and accept love; elevating sexuality into one's consciousness instead of the chest; letting in what has been avoided, re-accepting one's own "dirt and filth", coming to terms with it and integrating it (example: own urine therapy); 6. Living out healthy aggression; 7. Giving oneself space and freedom for self-realisation and also giving this to others.

Resolution: Expansion in one's consciousness; taking up space in the figurative sense; elevating oneself above polarity, but being able to see both sides of the coin; acknowledging the "death and re-birth" principle in inhaling and exhaling; consciously making high-flying dreams real; being al(l)-one for oneself in the sense of self-sufficiency and autonomy.

Archetypal principle: Mercury(-Uranus).

Bronchial carcinoma

see Lung cancer, Smoking

Bronchiectases

Physical level: Bronchia (connecting channels between the inner and outer world), lungs (contact, communication, freedom).

Symptom level: Rarely reversible dilation of the branches of the bronchia to the point of forming large cavities in the lungs, which then hinder the exchange of gas because they take up so much room; 25% congenital, 75% acquired (through infectious diseases in childhood →pulmonary consumption,→ lung abscess, →mucoviscidosis; expectoration (sputum by the mouthful); early conflicts leave behind traces and continue to take up room because they have not been definitively resolved.

Handling: Expanding oneself in mediative, communicative areas and taking up room; opening one's mouth and letting out what has to come out; expressing aggression on appropriate levels instead of spitting it out in the morning (sputum); recognising spitting as an expression of aggression ("spitting at someone's feet/in someone's face").

Resolution: ensuring room for oneself for exchanging (ideas); becoming mature in terms of being able to speak for oneself and opening one's mouth; expressing oneself verbally.

Archetypal principle: Mercury-Jupiter/Mars.

Bronchitis

Physical level: Bronchia (connecting channels between the inner and outer world).

Symptom level: Conflict over the contact channels; suppressed conflicts (that should be carried out verbally) become stuck; critical thoughts are held back; one coughs, instead of "coughing up" what one really thinks of others; blockage of the communications channels with spiritual subjects (mucous); compensation for smarmy hypocrisy (slick, glib commitment; slippery, elusive confrontation); in the case of spastic bronchitis: cramped aggressions due to having been long suppressed; the respiratory passages are constricted by this constant effort; restricting oneself in order to be able to take a

small gasp of air; in small children often the taking on of the chronic conflicts of the parents, who have not been able to solve these themselves, and thus leave them to the children (particularly apparent in parents who smoke, who have already exposed the children to this burden while in the womb and [through their smoking] continue to do so).

Handling: Seeking offensive confrontation and fighting it out on the verbal level; trusting oneself to cough up what one really thinks of others; letting spiritual tasks move one to pause inwardly; making the effort to oil the connecting channels well so that communication can flow smoothly.

Resolution: Willingness to face conflict: taking on challenges courageously; allowing oneself to be stimulated by new and foreign subjects and exchanging views in a smooth, well-oiled way.

Archetypal principle: Mercury-Mars.

Bruises

(Haematoma, see also Connective tissue weakness)

Physical level: Skin (border, contact, tenderness), connective tissue (connection, stability, binding commitment), blood vessels (transport routes of the life force).

Symptom level: Easily piqued (offended): quick to be impressed, hurt (insulted) and to bear grudges (black marks); offensive thoughts become visible in the body; great impressionability (on the physical instead of on the consciousness level); having a long memory for all offences (shocks) and everything offensive (shocking); victim of aggression; injury of the vitality flow; defect in one of the channels of the life energy; overlooking the proddings of Fate: small pushes and shoves on the physical level (harmless and healthy in the sense of treatment with one's own blood).

Handling: Consciously allowing oneself to be impressed, stimulated and prodded; applying one's own sensibility on more resolved (redeeming) levels, training one's memory in order to take better note of such stimuli; taking into account the opposite pole: going voluntarily instead of letting oneself be pushed; taking on the initiative oneself instead of always waiting for external prodding; opening oneself up to foreign prompts; letting in external impulses and allowing their effects; courageous exercises in taking things on (accepting) and being able to take them (bearing): Tai Chi, Aikido, martial arts; using external impulses in order to pause for a moment and come to one's senses; making oneself aware of the tendency to react blackly to binding commitment and fixed relationships.

Resolution: Momentary pausing in the life flow; sensibility, developing sensitivity and receptiveness, impressionability on the spiritual level.

Archetypal principle: Mars-Moon.

Bruising

(see also Accident, Work accident/ Domestic accident, Sport accident, Traffic accident)

Physical level: Skin (border, contact, tenderness).

Symptom level: Caught between different stools; stuck between a rock and a hard place; wedged in without noticing it (vice).

Handling: Becoming aware of the conflicting forces in one's own life; learning to withstand spiritual tensions.

Resolution: After having learnt to hold out pressure and put up resistance to it, also integrating the opposite pole: showing one's true colours in the figurative sense and making decisions.

Archetypal principle: Mars-Saturn.

Bruxism

see Teeth, grinding overnight

BSE (Bovine Spongiform Encephalitis)

see Creutzfeldt-Jakob disease

Buffalo hump

(see also Fatty hump, Fatty neck, Hunchback)

Bulimia

(see also Anorexia, Binge eating disorder)

Physical level: The whole body, particularly those aspects related to the feminine form; stomach (feeling, receptiveness).

Symptom level: Rejection of the transition from girl to woman (and in extremely rare cases, also from boy to man); not accepting one's own (almost always) female body, and instead struggling against it: the body makes one want "to be sick"; taking flight out of the state of polarity that is perceived as unclean with its feminine, respectively its sexual elements, which are bearing down upon one in a threatening way: devaluation of feminine fullness and roundness and one's own sexuality; futile search for inner fulfilment through the frenzied filling of the stomach; attempt to fill up the inner emptiness with a feeding frenzy; frantic taking and frantic giving; not granting oneself anything enjoyable (love, food); vomiting as a form of punishment and cleansing at the same time; violently parting with what was illegally assimilated so to speak; fear of orgiastic experiences (of unity) while at the same time longing for unity (insatiable greed struggling with the longing for ascesis): rapid switch between ascesis (vomiting in the sense of cleansing, purging) and orgiastic fullness (feeding frenzies, binges); conflict between the material and the spiritual world: problems with polarity in the search for the happy medium (eating = orgiastic element, vomiting = self-chastisement, cleansing); assimilation is restricted to the material; a broadening of consciousness is lacking; the hunger for life is appeased by eating instead of by experiences: "swallowing everything and keeping it bottled up"; "putting on weight due to comfort eating"; looking for confirmation, reward and love on the wrong level, instead of opening oneself up to love. Handling: In phases of anorexia: conquering spiritual worlds; in binge phases: letting in the physical world; accepting oneself as a sexual being (puberty rituals); developing readiness to involve oneself with polarity and give up one's innocent, pure childhood (becoming like a child, not remaining like one!); making oneself aware of the longing for purity and virginity; indulging oneself: consciously taking in impressions, experiences, sensations; active taking and receiving, learning to give in general and to give away freely; getting to know and to appreciate Venus-related themes: learning to enjoy fulfilling sensuality; practising more redeeming cleansing exercises for parting with things, such as fasting, sweating, excretion (vomiting is a method of older-style naturopathy, as enemas still are today); spiritual exercises in strictness and consistency towards oneself instead of child-like softness; transforming the desire to flee from polarity into the attempt to overcome it in the sense of the development path towards unity: overcoming the world (mythologically: the dragon) rather than avoiding it; frequently a station on the way from anorexia to recovery: in this case, also recognising and acknowledging it as such; taking

up the struggle with the demands of femininity, respectively with the sexual role: reconciliation with one's own determination (as a woman); extending one's domain of experience on spiritual and intellectual levels: using one's partner as a sweet temptation to nibble on, devouring books as a transition to normal enjoyment; recognising the hunger for life in the feeding frenzies and transferring this to mental-spiritual levels; taking in all impressions which come one's way, and processing what agrees with one; striving consistently for peak experiences/experiences of unity; exercises for reconciling oneself with polarity ("So, because you are lukewarm, and neither hot nor cold, I will spit you out of my mouth" Revelation 3:16); recognising the underlying system in the rapid swinging of the pendulum and identifying the centre as the goal: seeing through the rejection of life (vomiting) and the excessive hunger (for life) as being one-sided; exercises for realising the centre between the poles: Tai Chi, making pottery on the rotating potter's wheel, mandala painting and meditation as rituals, riding; opening one's "Ego"-borders, allowing other people to get closer and come in.
Resolution: Becoming an adult (woman) (e.g. by receiving (conceiving) a child, to which she then gives the gift of life); (ritually) mastering the transition of puberty; leaving childhood and youth behind; reconciliation with earthly things; living out love with its joyous, simultaneously spiritual and physical giving and taking: merging with one's loved ones or one's special loved one; finding them good enough to eat and enjoying it all; knowing how to appreciate ecstasy (e.g. sexual) as an appetizer for the unity to come; practising consuming the world (Buddhism: Bhoga), instead of eating up the world of the refrigerator; reconciliation with unity as the

all-embracing sum of all manifestations, which also includes the realm of shadows.
Archetypal principle: Moon-Pluto/ Uranus.

Burns

(see also Accident, Work accident/ Domestic accident, Traffic accident)
Physical level: Skin (border, contact, tenderness).
Symptom level: Fire = masculine element and expression of masculine energy; inwardly unlived fire energy overcomes one and threatens from outside; the body extinguishes the scene of the fire by transporting water (spiritual element) to the area (this extinguishing water collects in blisters): those who do not dare to grasp the red-hot irons and address the burning subjects of life frequently encounter them externally; playing with fire and getting too close to it; playing with danger, incorrect assessment of dangers: "a burnt child dreads the fire"; deceiving oneself: "getting burnt"; anger ("boiling with rage") frequently leads to burns: the unrealised spiritual subject is encountered externally; conflict-laden confrontations with love/sexuality: "catching fire", "bursting into flame", "getting one's fingers burnt" when one comes into contact with a guy who is too "hot" or a corresponding woman; border infringement, calling the Ego into question.
Handling: Burning down the borders; all fired up to set initiative alight; "not letting any chances go up in flames"; playing with (the) fire (of inspiration); letting oneself be inflamed, being on fire for one's "flame"; opening the Ego borders; burning with desire for other people: following in Eros' footsteps, who shoots or thrusts his flaming darts into people's hearts; seeing through deceptions: e.g. recognising that hot, burning issues cannot be resolved by burn blisters; counteracting

the masculine element that is threatening from the outside with spiritual energy on the inside.
Resolution: Rejoicing in the glow of love; letting one's heart burn; discovering and making one's own inner fire a reality: bringing fire into one's soul.
Archetypal principle: Venus/ Saturn-Mars.

Burnout syndrome

(chronic burnout; see also Depression, Sleep problems)
Physical level: The whole organism can be affected.
Symptom level: Burning oneself up and consuming one's energy at the "wrong" point; chronic →fatigue, which is only minimally improved by sleep; feeling beat (exhausted); the energy reserves have been exhausted down to the deepest level ("empty batteries"); feeling of not being able to perform well enough, never managing to catch up and no longer being able to live up to the demands of life; auto-aggressive exploitation; desire to flee from a demand that can no longer be met (in one's profession, family, partnership); preliminary stage of depression.
Handling: Ensuring inner calm; consciously withdrawing oneself from the daily confrontations in the battle of life; distancing oneself; identifying and stopping energy leaks (e.g. unresolved life crises, rotten compromises) if necessary with the aid of psychotherapy; exhausting oneself spiritually until emptiness is restored; burning at the "right" point: developing genuine enthusiasm and motivation (a burning heart), e.g. finding work which one truly enjoys.
Resolution: Drawing on one's own primordial sources of strength; realising emptiness on the ultimate level in the sense of the Buddhist Nirvana: meditation.
Archetypal principle: Neptune.

Bursitis

(Latin: bursae "small sacs)
Physical level: Usually in the knee area (humility).
Symptom level: What was intended as protection and for cushioning comes under pressure itself; the consequence is often large outpourings of liquid (effusions) as an attempt at padding (water cushion); usually resulting from stress overload, e.g. through long periods of crawling around on one's knees at the feet of other people, such as when cleaning their floor or laying their tiles: suppleness and smoothness are hindered in the area of humility; conflict over suppressed rage about one's own subservience, which is not accepted on the spiritual level; having served others and undertaken a great deal in order to please them, perhaps also in a slick and smooth way, and adopting behaviour which one can no longer face up to (sycophantic crawling); great desire for acknowledgement and being actively involved; growing need for more protective padding and better cushioning.
Handling: Clarifying where one is demanding too much of oneself, where one is being too relentless (on oneself) or too strongly rubbing (others) the wrong way; submitting to the necessary subservient stance or rising above it (changing career); transforming the subservience enforced by circumstances into humility; recognising what one must force oneself to do (too little influence of the soul on one's own stance, and too much willpower); serving oneself and thereby providing acknowledgement for one's own way of being .
Resolution: Acknowledging the period of rest and stillness which the body is enforcing for itself, and in the long term, granting this to the body voluntarily; allowing humiliation to grow into genuine humility.

Archetypal principle: Saturn/Moon-Mars.

Buzzing in the ears

See Ear noises

C

Cachexia

(loss of strength, consumption)
Physical level: Affects the complete organism.
Symptom level: Surrender of the body: emaciation, physical collapse in disease patterns ultimately aiming at death; the systems gradually cease to function: slow dying; the body gives up, frequently instead of a conscious spiritual letting go.
Handling: Preparing oneself for leaving the crumbling dwelling place of the body: allowing the soul to come to the fore; concerning oneself with the soul instead of investing further in the physical dwelling place which is soon be left; the given task is now to give up: to give up the body as consciously as possible in order to be prepared for the journey of the soul, the free flight of the bird of the soul; arranging for spiritual provisions for the journey: oratorio music, reading the Books of the Dead, dying rituals.
Resolution: Consciously consigning oneself: "Thy will be done."
Archetypal principle: Saturn (as the Grim Reaper for the body and guardian of the threshold for the soul).

Caesarean section

(see also Birth complications, general)
Physical level: Womb (fertility, safety and security), abdominal wall (protection).

Symptom level: 1. (On the part of the child): desire to hang around in Paradise – the land of milk and honey – of the womb; missing the moment to make the break; giving oneself weight and weightiness (importance); life pattern: "The others should see to it that something becomes of me"; 2. (On the part of the mother): Refusal to give up the child, not wanting to separate herself; not having experienced (enjoyed) the pregnancy consciously enough; giving oneself too much weightiness (importance); fear of being too narrow and restrictive, of becoming unattractive; lack of conscious initiation into motherhood; fear of pain in the case of a consciously-chosen Caesarean section; general rejection of the enormity of the task: call for help to the helpers: "I can't do it, don't want to do it and can't manage it!"

Handling: 1. (On the part of the child/later adult): learning to deal with limits and to overstep them where necessary; learning to take on responsibility for oneself, but also allowing oneself to be helped; learning to rely on one's own strength in order to overcome tight squeezes; getting the right take-off; critically addressing one's own life pattern: understanding in good time that others are only willing to see to it that something will become of one right at the very beginning; 2. (On the part of the mother): learning to take conscious leave and to take a step back in the course of becoming (being) a mother; learning to accept the beauty of motherhood, of taking on maturity; processing one's own birth trauma with regard to the primordial fear of restrictiveness; consciously allowing oneself to get involved in the initiation into motherhood (rituals).

Resolution: Finding the happy medium between sitting things out and impatiently pressing ahead; dealing consciously with the pattern of just sitting tight and simply waiting: ensuring for oneself that something becomes of one.

Archetypal principle: Mars-Moon.

Calcification

see Arteriosclerosis

Calculi

see Stony concretions

Calf muscle cramps

Physical level: Lower leg (take-off power, elasticity), calves (emotions). Symptom level: Lack of mineral salts: the salt is missing from the soup of life; pent-up emotional tension; being overstretched, tensely cramped; no longer being able to make any great leaps; breaking down, not being able to take it anymore; signs of unacknowledged inner resignation and surrender: no longer being able to achieve the take-off; not managing the leap into life; frequent symptom in pregnancy, which does not allow any more great leaps.

Handling: Exerting oneself strenuously and pulling oneself together; truly living out these stances instead of playing them out on the stage of the body; bracing oneself against threatening aspects; confronting fears; in the case of night-time calf muscle cramps: tackling unconscious fears.

Resolution: Conscious tension and strenuous effort in order to realise the greater goal.

Archetypal principle: Uranus.

Calluses

Physical level: Stress points of the skin (boundary, contact, tenderness). Symptom level: Benign callus proliferations, formation of armour at points of relative overloading: attempt

of the organism to protect itself against wear and tear injuries.
Handling/Resolution: Providing oneself with better protection against overloading in the figurative sense.
Archetypal principle: Saturn.

Cancer

(see also Auto-aggressive /Auto-im- mune diseases, Aggressiveness)
Physical level: Can affect almost all regions and organs of the body.
Symptom level: Neoplasma: some- thing new grows, takes on shape and form; growth on the wrong level; deep anguish, unprocessed wound(s), feelings of guilt which have become unbearable (also towards oneself and the life that has been missed out on), and particularly frequently, shock experiences block one's own immune defence powers and become a trigger: cancer begins immunolog- ically after a collapse of the immune defences (if the immune defences are intact, developing cancer cells are wiped out by the immune defence system - a process which probably happens often); an unacknowledged self-destructive life problem lays the foundation: dragging oneself along slowly in crab-like fashion (Latin: cancer = 'crab') (not progressing further along one's path); degener- ation: striking out and not being true to one's type, deviating from one's (inherent) path; straying so far off track from one's line of development in the subject area concerned) that the body has to help the (forgotten/ repressed) issue to express itself to ensure that it is not completely lacking; the cancer realises physically that (turnaround) which would be spir- itually necessary in the corresponding area of consciousness; degeneration of the cells as a desperate struggle for survival of a cell that has been aggravated to death (e.g. by poisons), comparable to the desperate swelling

of the shoots of trees threatened by forest dieback; cancer as an initia- tion: an incisive event, the decisive caesura (Latin: 'cut') in life; error in the concept of realising freedom and immortality; suppression of the possibilities for boundary experiences at the edge of one's limits and of life impulses; clinging to the norm; per- fect social adaptation (normopathy); aggression and egoism in the cancer process: aggressively-suppressed policy of elbowing one's way through, might is right, infiltration, invasion, extortion, exploitation of slave(-cell) s; cancer takes over the task of the soul: self-realisation/ego-trip; break- ing the rules of normal co-existence; top-heavy, wanting to ram one's head through the wall (growth problem); total up-ending of the honourable ide- als held by subordinates in favour of the total ego principle; unlived desire to ruthlessly push through one's own interests; dark side of the feminine (Hekate/Kali): the shadow side of love as a form of revenge by the long-tor- mented feminine principle; instead of communication with one's envi- ronment, total egoism, omnipotence, claims to immortality; the search for immortality and omnipotence (of the soul) lives itself out in the cancer cells instead of in consciousness; love (as the principle transcending all bound- aries) expressed on the wrong level; regression process: re-connection to the origin, the source of re-ligio(n) (from Latin religāre 'to bind, tie again') has sunk into the regressive tenden- cies of physical cancer cells; growth and progress as the perverted goal in our time and society; recognising metastases as similar to the affiliated (Latin filiae = 'dark, doom-bringing daughters') branches and subsidiary companies that we are criss-crossing the body of the Earth with; collective pattern of ruthless expansion and realisation of one's own interests; re- flection of the exploitation of the Earth by humankind; polarisation of the Ego versus a sense of community: lack of consciousness for greater, embracing unity.

Handling: Taking stock: "Has the path up till now corresponded to one's own (inherent) one?"; opening oneself up in the subject area concerned to one's own outlandish ideas and bold fantasies; courageously, and by all means, even daringly allowing them to grow and expand; relieving the body of the struggle for survival on the mental-spiritual level; letting new elements (neoplasma) grow; thinking back to early dreams and one's own goals and wishes in life, bringing them (back) to life and putting them into practice with wild decisiveness; taking the growth impulse away from the body and directing it to more resolved (redeeming) levels; in the certainty of having nothing more to lose, mustering courage for one's own self-realisation/one's own path; rising up against (restrictive, rigid, iron-clad) rules; shattering norms which hinder self-realisation; instead of slotting into small-scale systems of order (normopathy), finding one's place in the great order of things (re-ligio[n]); kicking over the traces, stepping away from the (established) line in order to really get to know the Ego; decisive and forceful self-assertion; bringing one's own self-rigidity and isolation into question: expansion of consciousness; acknowledging the boundlessness and immortality of the soul; reconnection in the sense of re-ligio[n] ("Where do I come from? Where am I going? Who am I?"); growing beyond the Ego; returning to (one's own) primordial beginnings; reconnection to the primordial basis of being; learning to say 'no', to stand up for oneself; even living with one's own mistakes is better than taking on foreign virtues; taking up the struggle for survival in an open(ly offensive) and aggressive way on the level of inner imagery; reincarnation therapy, Simonton therapy, breathing therapy.

Resolution: Providing expression for oneself, instead of allowing the body to speak up for itself; recognising the necessity to switch from the physical and thus (life-) threatening level to the challenging, but life-saving mental-spiritual level, and relying in this realm on expansive growth; discovering love that transcends all boundaries; setting oneself above external rule and standards laid down by oneself or others and living and realising oneself solely in accordance with the obligations of one's own highest law; boundary experiences at the edge of one's limits in the sense of peak experiences; striving for immortality in spirituality instead of in the physical body (giving pride of place to the immortal soul); studying the battle with the Hydra in the Herakles myth: when Herakles is bitten by Cancer (the crab), he does not retreat into unresolved regression; instead, he takes on the challenge, faces up to the struggle, crushes the crab and goes on to destroy the monster.

Archetypal principle: Pluto-Jupiter (cancer), and in connection with all the possible regions and organs, the various related Archetypal principles.

Cancer, fear of

(carcinophobia; see also Anxiety, Cancer, Hypochondria)

Symptom level: Pressing and restricting thoughts (often after cancer illnesses in the family), fear of life = fear of death; fear of living and suffering; great expectations about one's own life on an unresolved level; unconscious desire to fail in life.

Handling: Exploring one's own cancer pattern (social adaptation pattern, normopathy structures), and in consequence, going one's own way; making one's expectations on one's

own path (in life) a reality; recognising that all life is suffering (Buddha).
Resolution: Reconciliation with one's own mortality; recognition that living and dying belong together like light and shadow (Tibetan/Egyptian Book of the Dead); living in accordance with one's own structure and purpose.
Archetypal principle: Pluto/Saturn.

Candidamycosis

(thrush; see also Dermatomycoses)
Physical level: Primarily the outer skin (border, contact, tenderness), inner mucous membranes (inner border, barrier), but also in the case of weakened immunity (e.g. →AIDS) or long-term antibiotic therapy (organ mycoses).
Symptom level: Despite the protective shield provided by an acid coating and resistance by defensive cells, one's own borders are occupied by brazen and freely-spreading foreign troops (fungal growths [myceles] branching out in all directions): being too weak to defend one's own skin and to digest impressions in a lively enough form (intestinal fungus); all non-living material is endangered by the fungal infestation (fungi are saprophytes, which live on dead organic matter); the violent conflict only begins later and then deep within the body's terrain; agonizing and ghastly treatment of oneself.
Handling: Owning up to how much dead matter one is dragging around with oneself; opening up one's own borders in the mental-spiritual respect instead of defending them; making room for new and foreign elements, and making them one's own; opening up one's own lifeless areas that have died off to new and different life impulses; allowing these foreign life impulses to firstly get as close as possible and then getting to know them based on one's own experiences before the critical and violent conflict with them begins; concrete exercises: allowing others to have a piece of one, e.g. taking on (accepting) and taking in (welcoming) foreigners, getting involved with them and confronting them critically in an open(ly offensive) way in those areas in which they want to overextend their way of life into one's own terrain; taking in vital (living) nourishment, which the body can convert into living structures, but which the fungi cannot make use of.
Resolution: Acceptance and integration of other impulses and life forms; creating one's own living terrain (in consciousness).
Archetypal principle: Pluto.

Carbuncle

see Furuncle

Carcinoma in situ

(superficial cancer of the external orifice of the womb; see also Cancer of the mouth of the uterus, Sexual diseases, Cancer)
Physical level: External orifice of the uterus (lower mouth), mucous membranes (inner boundary, barrier), womb (fertility, safety and security).
Symptom level: Border combat and battle of the sexes, which reflects inner spiritual struggles; inability to protect oneself adequately against sexual attacks and assaults.
Handling: Dealing with conflicts over issues of sexual self-determination in an offensive way; recognising one's own wounds and chronic over-irritation in this area; learning to protect oneself against assaults and attacks on one's own femininity by foreign interests; considering all the measures mentioned under →cancer: since cancer affects the complete organism, it must also be met across-the-board.
Resolution: Safeguarding one's own interests in the case of conflicts

in the intimate area; recognising the necessity to switch from the physical and thereby (life-)threatening level to the challenging, but life-saving mental-spiritual level and relying in this realm on expansive (spiritual) growth; discovering love that transcends all boundaries, setting oneself above external rule and standards laid down by oneself and others, and living and developing oneself solely in accordance with the obligations of one's own highest law.
Archetypal principle: Moon-Pluto.

Carcinophobia

see Cancer, fear of

Cardiac asthma

Physical level: Heart (seat of the soul, love, feelings, energy centre), lungs (contact, communication, freedom).
Symptom level: Asthma and constriction in the lungs due to deficient heart performance (the left chamber of the heart cannot pump blood into the body's circulatory system, with the result that it builds up in the lungs): threatening to be stifled by one's own life energy, which can no longer be brought into circulation; being too full of unlived energy; the basic problem of the heart is brought into focus.
Handling: Less is more: taking it easy with regard to the outer world (the great cycle of life or the body's circulation), and devoting oneself instead to the inner energy blockage; concentrating on the heart and heart-related subjects, making an effort in this respect and getting down to the essential.
Resolution: (Allopathic approach) bringing one's outer and inner worlds into harmonious interplay.
Archetypal principle: Sun/Mercury-Saturn.

Cardiac enlargement

(Cardiac hypertrophy, athlete's heart)
Physical level: Heart (seat of the soul, love, feelings, energy centre).
Symptom level: 1. Concentric cardiac hypertrophy (relatively harmless and to a minor degree even healthy cardiac enlargement frequently caused by doing a lot of sport) and 2. Eccentric cardiac hypertrophy (the left or right side of the heart is enlarged in a lopsided way, which relates back to vascular or valve problems and can be life-threatening); (over-)stressing of the physical heart; expanding beyond one's (physical) limits.
Handling: demanding more of one's heart in a spiritual respect in order to grow from these demands; allowing it to grow beyond itself in the figurative sense; expanding the heart and opening it up to life and its demands; giving more weight to the heart and its subjects; in the case of eccentric hypertrophy, first doing justice to the basic problem: e.g. clearing up →high blood pressure or following up the matter of valve defects (→heart valve insufficiency) and its significance
Resolution: Big-heartedness and conquering one's own limits.
Archetypal principle: Sun-Jupiter.

Cardiac hypertrophy

see Cardiac enlargement

Cardiac infarction

(see also High blood pressure, Circulatory disorders, Vascular blockage)
Physical level: Heart (seat of the soul, love, feelings, energy centre), blood (life force).
Symptom level: Undersupply of the heart with life energy (blood): the heart is starved, either completely or partly; not being able to take (on) love, not opening oneself up to it; death cries/throes of an already

strangulated part of the heart (cardiovascular restriction, →angina pectoris); closed-heartedness, hardening (coagulation), petrification as a pre-condition ("heart of stone"); blockage/stiffening in the flow of one's (heart) feelings; due to overvaluation of one's Ego powers and dominance, being cutting off from the flow of the living; the individual striving for dominance/ performance, fear of criticism and failure; build-up of aggression (restrained aggression) and eventual discharge of the backlog of aggressive energy (e.g. in the rupture of the heart wall); low feeling of self-esteem, which aims at improvement through good functioning and the striving for recognition and love, but only succeeds to a certain extent: in the case of an infarction, the worst case scenario occurs = collapse of the feeling of self-esteem; inhibition with regard to formulating one's own spiritual needs; lack of a higher goal; social isolation, loneliness: "lonely heart", "broken heart"; infarction as the closing in of one's feelings; dissatisfaction; basic undertone (mood) of irritation; chronically-expectant attitude, tense politeness, rigidity; fear of being hurt; inability to achieve any deeper release of tension; centre of the body as a city of the dead (necropolis); a scarred heart: something vital to life and highly vital (full of life) is replaced, as an emergency measure, with relatively lifeless material; taking leave from an area of the heart, in which nothing more will remain than an inferior substitute.

Handling: Becoming aware of the undersupply (strangulation) of one's heart (muscle) with (life) energy, time and caring attention; answering the heart's cries for help that are being sent in the cries of pain from tissue that is hungering for loving attention (nourishment); admitting to oneself that the Ego with its demands has conquered first place in life over and above matters of the heart; being consistent and hard with oneself (the Ego and its demands); finding one's own standpoints; becoming aware of the alternative – the Archetypal axis of flowing and holding back; facing up to the battle over one's own centre: resigning (shutting up) or getting into the flow; bringing life into flow; not turning one's heart into a skeleton closet (full of hate, rage, revenge, sorrow, pain); achieving inner peace before the ultimate peace of the grave; allowing oneself weakness and vulnerability; cutting oneself off from (everything) on the outside in favour of the inner centre; recognising the basic fear of losing one's self, but making clear to oneself that one "merely" has to lose one's Ego in order to arrive at the centre.

Resolution: Consciously making the heart a living (or dying) city; recognising it as the centre of the life flow and opening oneself up to its needs; showing humility and concentrating on and restricting oneself to the essential; finding the way to self-acceptance and love.

Archetypal principle: Sun-Saturn.

Cardiac insufficiency

see Senile heart, Heart failure

Cardiomyopathy

(see also Myocarditis, Heart failure)

Physical level: Heart (seat of the soul, love, feelings, energy centre).

Symptom level: Various forms, usually slack extension of the heart muscle with thinning of the musculature.

Handling/Resolution: Expanding the heart in the figurative sense so that it can remain physically in (its accustomed) form.

Archetypal principle: Sun-Jupiter-Saturn.

Cardiostenosis

see Achalasia

Cardiovascular problems

(circulatory regulation disorders, usually on the basis of low blood pressure; see also High blood pressure, Low blood pressure)

Physical level: Heart (seat of the soul, love, feelings, energy centre), blood circulation (circuit of the life energy, supply and disposal).

Symptom level: Not being flexible enough to come to terms with changing positions/situations in life; changes (in position/situation) lead to adaptation problems; supply bottlenecks, which can only be overcome following a period of adjustment; contact and enjoyment disorder.

Handling: Taking more time to adjust oneself to the changing ups and downs of life; accepting these rather than avoiding them; making oneself aware of one's resistance to all changes (in position/situation) and seeing through one's "hopefully nothing will happen" philosophy of life; recognising undersupply as a life principle of a conservative stance to life which stabilises and sometimes even glorifies the relevant status quo; striving for an even, steady life flow; spiritual exercises: fasting, meditation, autogenic training, Tai Chi, mandala painting.

Resolution: Adjusting and giving in to the prevailing life flow.

Archetypal principle: Sun-Moon.

Cardiovascular restriction

see Angina pectoris

Carditis

see Endocarditis, Myocarditis, Pericarditis

Caries

Physical level: Teeth (aggression, vitality).

Symptom level: Decaying life force, letting one's own teeth be eaten away, battered weapons; suppression of aggression, the ability to put up a fight, to get one's teeth into things; avoidance or inability "to bare one's teeth", inhibited bite; lack of forceful assertiveness ("gritting one's teeth and biting one's way through life"); real bite is lacking; rotten compromises; loss of vitality, energy and potency; problems with aggressive expression (sinking one's teeth into things) and hashing out the essential (grinding things out); loss of feeling of self-esteem with the loss of the health of the teeth; feeling oneself worthless and unworthy ("never look a gifthorse in the mouth"); gnawing over problems or finding them difficult to chew; preference for bland, soft food which represents no challenge for the teeth and the Mars force, but instead causes them to degenerate.

Handling: Learning to fight for one's own weapons; practising caring for one's own weapons and putting this into practice: cleaning the teeth and living (out) aggressions (one's vital powers), "probing someone deeply to get to the roots of something"; equipped with the knowledge of the symbolism of the teeth, learning to appreciate their value correctly and doing something for them so that they can also do something for one in return; ensuring healthy teeth and vitality in the course of one's life in order to thereby build up a feeling of self-esteem; conquering a "sweet" partner instead of nibbling other sweet temptations; learning to actively soften the hard things in life, breaking up the rigidity; granting oneself a proper diet which makes a worthy opponent for the teeth.

Resolution: Recognising that being on a war footing with Mars is dangerous, because here he is in his element: preferring instead to reconcile oneself with him and taking pleasure in him and his energies; becoming like a child again on the spiritual level, i.e. toothless.

Archetypal principle: Mars-Mars.

Carpal tunnel syndrome

Physical level: Hand surfaces (honesty, openness), Thumb (unity), index finger (orientation), middle finger (leadership).

Symptom level: (above all in women between the ages of 40 and 50): due to pressure on the median nerve, weakening to the point of damage to the muscles of the ball of the thumb: thereby resulting in hindrance of the opposition work of the thumb, which is the basis of gripping and grasping: no longer being able to grip (grasp) properly (→thumb); no longer being able to knuckle down and grab hold of things; not being able to hold on to anything anymore: no longer coming to grips with life; difficulties in handling polarity; problems with sensibility of the palms of the hand and the first three fingers: having no feeling on (one's) hand, no more feeling for the things which one touches; no longer being touched, and instead being numb and without feeling; burning pains in the tendons of the arms, particularly at night, due to overly-tight wrist shackles: one feels like one's hands are tied (that they have become powerless and numb from being shackled with overly-tight bonds); danger of muscle degeneration in the case of long-term issues.

Handling: Practising letting go and loosening the firm grip; keeping one's hands off something; admitting to oneself one's lack of feeling with regard to relationships and contact with one's environment: relying more on oneself and one's own inner feeling, letting go of expectations on the external world (no longer grabbing hold, but instead letting [oneself] go); making oneself aware of the constrictive situation.

Resolution: Sensing the unity (thumb) behind the polarity and adjusting oneself to it as the last and highest goal of life.

Archetypal principle: Mercury-Neptune.

Cataracts

Physical level: Eyes (perspective, insight, mirror and window of the soul).

Symptom level: Dulled, blurred, veiled gaze, one does not (want to) see reality in its sharp focus; cloudy or overcast view of one's own life: drawing a dark curtain in front of truth and reality; due to the grey veil, the world loses its clarity, but also its painful sharpness; seeing "everything as grey and drab" and without contrasts: one sees the world the way one lives in it, i.e. without highs and lows; reassuring distancing from the surrounding world; pulling down the blind in order not to have to see anything one does not want to see; "not believing one's eyes", scales in front of the eyes; clouded, dulled gaze as the opposite pole to the shining eyes of childhood: bleak outlook; the twinkling stars of the eyes pale under the grey veil; occurs above all after reaching the midpoint of life, along with the fear of ageing and loss of attractiveness and power; the disease pattern causes one "to look old"; preference for security aspects rather than vitality.

Handling: Allowing the outer world to grow hazy, focussing one's gaze more sharply on the inner world; distancing oneself from the outer world in order to be able to devote oneself to the inner world; pulling down the

outer blind and ensuring order on the inside; transforming a bleak outlook into clear insight; exploring the question of what incorrect inner stance is clouding the clear outer view.
Resolution: Following the Christian bidding: "So then, because you are lukewarm, and neither cold nor hot, I will spit you out of My mouth"; insight instead of seeing through things externally, lifting the veil (of the Maya) and learning to see the truth; developing openness for the deepest sharpness and clarity within.
Archetypal principle: Sun/Moon-Saturn.

Catarrh

see Respiratory tract diseases, Cold diseases, Influenza

Cavernitis

see Penis, inflammation of the cavernous body

Cellulite

(also incorrectly referred to as cellulitis, although there is no inflammation; see also Connective tissue weakness)
Physical level: Skin (border, contact, tenderness), subcutaneous fatty tissue (overflow, excess reserves).
Symptom level: A fashion trend or fad to the extent that it refers to a phenomenon, which around the turn of the century before last was still not considered in any way as a disease, but quite the contrary formed part of the fuller-figured ideal of beauty of that time; nowadays, in contrast, the proliferation of fatty tissue on the thighs, rear, etc. does not fit in with the trim, taut and terrific ideal of our times; orange-peel skin phenomenon due to additional mild lymph blockage and →oedema formation; the feminine aspects of the figure are additionally emphasised and energetically

combatted (mostly with agents which only benefit the manufacturers, and have no effect on the phenomenon in the long term); with advancing age, gravity has a greater influence: flabby connective tissue reflects the inner state of letting oneself go; in combination with →obesity: abundance on the wrong level.
Handling: Homeopathically: acceptance of the archetypally feminine, gentle way of life, of weakness and softness, which become even stronger in the course of the ageing process; recognising yielding as an archetypally feminine life subject (instead of connective tissue weakness and simply letting oneself go); allopathically: weight loss and exercise, training and trimming down (towards the male figure ideal); also keeping fit on the intellectual level, setting the spiritual flow in motion; with advancing age, realising abundance on the levels of knowledge, wisdom and also material cushioning.
Resolution: Trusting oneself to the female life flow, staying in flow and reconciling oneself with one's own life theme.
Archetypal principle: Moon-Jupiter.

Cellulitis

see Cellulite (above)

Cerebral atrophy

(contraction of the brain mass, narrowing of the cerebral gyrus, enlargement of the ventricles [cavities], proliferation of the connective tissue, reduction of the ganglia cells, pigment accumulations)
Physical level: Brain (communication, logistics).
Symptom level: Shrinking back of the brain, particularly in old age: retreat of the spirit, emptiness on the physical instead of the spiritual level; enlargement of the cavities ("air-head, numbskull").

Handling: Transforming knowledge into wisdom in good time ("I know that I know nothing"); consciously planning and carrying out the process of retreat from the mid-point of life onwards; taking back the primacy of the intellect in favour of a richer life of emotions and feelings; consciously taking leave from the physical world: preparing oneself for passing over into the world beyond.

Resolution: Striving for emptiness on the figurative level (the Nirvana of Buddhism).

Archetypal principle: Mercury-Neptune.

Cerebral circulation disorders

(cerebral sclerosis; see also Circulatory disorders, Arteriosclerosis)

Physical level: Brain (communication, logistics).

Symptom level: Premature age degeneration with typical symptoms such as forgetfulness, concentration disorders, loss of performance, dizziness, headaches; in the advanced stage: softening of the brain, danger of →strokes and →dementia; insufficient supply of life energy to the central control headquarters; partial or general "cementing in" of the vital life flow to the central control headquarters, result: narrowmindedness; danger of isolation of the central switchboard and general performance errors, which can affect all areas of life; the memory and information retention capabilities are primarily affected; decline of performance capability in the (masculine) intellectual area; a female pole which has come up too short for (half?) a lifetime comes more to the fore because the aspects that drop out in this domain are usually more minimal: often it is more or less only the archetypally feminine which remains.

Handling: Concentration on the essential needs with regard to energy; restriction of the central control headquarters to what is absolutely necessary: now devoting more attention to the heart and stomach, whose energy has not yet been switched off by Fate, thus giving them both the chance to come to the fore; strict to highly stringent allocation of one's own energy for the highest level: reducing the energy wastage; recognising the isolation of the central control headquarters and its one-sided working orientation; voluntarily reducing intellectual memory and information retention work in favour of holistic perception and playful handling of the capabilities of one's central control headquarters; voluntarily devoting oneself to the archetypally feminine before one is left with nothing else anyway: fostering softness and adaptability; turning one's attention inwards.

Resolution: Realising (life) energy-saving solutions; living according to the principle of "the highest first" and recognising that the point of focus wants to shift from the brain to the heart and stomach; tackling what is really important and essential (feeling), instead of the "acting important" antics (of the intellect): discovering the feminine principle for oneself and living it out; preparation for transcendental worlds.

Archetypal principle: Mercury-Saturn.

Cerebral compression increase

see Cerebral compression syndrome (below)

Cerebral compression syndrome

(cerebral compression increase, Compressio cerebri)
Physical level: Brain (communication, logistics).
Symptom level: The cerebrum comes under pressure due to a process demanding more space, such as a haemorrhage, drainage obstruction of the cerebral fluid (liquor) or a quickly-growing tumour; the first sign is papilloedema: swelling and clouding of the entrance of the optic nerve into the retina; if this persists, it can lead to blindness.
Handling: Recognising in good time that one needs more room for central subjects related to the regulation of life; dealing more carefully with one's central control headquarters.
Resolution: Recognising that the central control headquarters have come under pressure and that one can no longer make heads nor tails of anything and is thus doing one's head in before the subject manifests itself physically.
Archetypal principle: Moon-Pluto.

Cerebral contusion

(more severe symptom of →brain concussion)
Physical level: Brain (communication, logistics), head (capital of the body).
Symptom level: The same as for brain concussion, although with the danger of permanent damage: rising up of repressed contents as a result of the severe concussion; previous thought patterns are shaken to the core; risking one's neck; running up against definitive limit(s); getting one's head snapped off; temporary retraction of the dominance of the switching control centre: regression into powerlessness (blacking out).

Handling: Voluntarily allowing the switching control centre extensive rest periods; granting oneself unconsciousness (insensibility) and blacking out (powerlessness); preferably allowing oneself to be shaken in one's thought world in good time.
Resolution: New beginnings.
Archetypal principle: Mercury-Uranus/Saturn.

Cerebral haemorrhage

see Stroke

Cerebral inflammation

(encephalitis; see also Meningitis)
Physical level: Brain (communication, logistics).
Symptom level: Struggle for the head issue, aggressive conflict over the (switching) control centre: to be or not to be.
Handling: Concerning oneself with the regulation of one's life courageously and in an open(ly offensive) way; taking on the struggle for survival and fighting it out with all one's resources; allowing oneself to be stimulated in central areas of life; having courage when facing challenges which affect one's vital nerve centre.
Resolution: Letting oneself get involved in all or nothing battles; courageous openness of the consciousness borders for revolutionary ideas and critical involvement with them.
Archetypal principle: Mercury-Mars.

Cerebral oedema

(see also Oedema)
Physical level: Brain (communication, logistics).
Symptom level: Build-up of water in the brain or between the structural elements of the brain: the spiritual element demands room and its rights

in central matters on the physical level; swelling of the brain: the world of thought (intellect) is over-inflated; mounting pressure on the brain: the head feels as if it is about to burst; headache, excess pressure, dizziness to the point of clouded consciousness and powerlessness (blacking out); dry retching: everything makes one continually want "to be sick", not being able to take in (absorb) or take on (accept) anything anymore, (wanting to) spew out everything; choked disk (papilloedema): reveals the pressure that the central control headquarters have come under, but also the disturbed, rigid view.

Handling: (after the life-threatening pressure has been treated allopathically on the physical level!): recognising that the (watery) spiritual element has been insufficiently integrated into one's thought processes and is now living itself out physically and blocking life; giving spiritual matters precedence over the intellect; conscious letting go instead of taking in (absorption); making oneself aware of the pressure which one has come under.

Resolution: Giving way instead of controlling; giving the soul room instead of just feeding the intellect.

Archetypal principle: Mercury-Pluto/Neptune.

Cerebral sclerosis

see Cerebral circulation disorders

Cervical cancer

(cervical carcinoma; see also Uterus, cancer of, Cancer)

Physical level: Mucous membranes (inner boundary, barrier) in the area of the cervix.

Symptom level: Occurring on the basis of a virus infection, frequently in younger women before menopause, after frequent →vaginal inflammations and frequent changing of one's sexual partner: chronic, unresolved conflicts in the sexual area, which tend to become malignant and bring one's whole life into question; can almost be regarded as a →sexually transmitted disease (e.g. never occurs in virgins [nuns]) since it is based on infections transmitted through sexual intercourse; often also affects women whose husbands frequently visit prostitutes, and then unload what they have brought with them at home; often occurring in women who are abused by their "dirty", "grubby" husbands; inability to protect oneself adequately against attacks and assaults; not being able to close oneself off properly; taking on board all worries, coldness, germs; hope of receiving love through sexual intercourse with changing partners; continuously activating the nest (womb) without any real chance of fertility; finding at least the taste of love in the orgasm, but ultimately only dirtying one's nest; connection with inadequate hygiene (foreskin smears [smegma]) since it is almost unknown in cultures where the men are circumcised.

Handling: Offensively addressing sexuality-related issues; recognising one's own over-stimulation in this area; learning to protect oneself against assaults and attacks from foreign interests on one's own sexual sphere; going one's own way, looking for love within oneself instead of in others; ensuring satisfactory sexual hygiene on the part of the partner instead of continually having to make (do with) cervical smears, which very frequently lead to incorrectly positive results; considering all the measures mentioned under →cancer: since cancer affects the complete organism, it must also be met across-the-board.

Resolution: Ensuring clean relationships (according to one's own standards); settling conflicts in the intimate area in one's own favour;

recognising the need to switch from the physical and therefore (life-) threatening level to the challenging, but life-saving mental-spiritual level, and relying in this realm on expansive growth; discovering love that transcends all boundaries, setting oneself above external rule and standards laid down by oneself or others, and living and expressing oneself solely in accordance with the obligations of one's own highest law.
Archetypal principle: Venus/Mars-Pluto.

Cervical carcinoma

see Cervical cancer (above)

Cervical dystonia

(torticollis spasticus; see also KISS syndrome)
Physical level: Neck (assimilation, connection, communication).
Symptom level: Leaning heavily to one side of the world (left or right) and turning away from the other; distorted, one-sided (world)view, not wanting to see the other half of reality; security/insecurity: unmasking of a demonstratively self-assured bearing, side-stepping unpleasant situations, looking the other way when it comes to conflict.
Handling: Accepting the physically-enforced, rigid position as a learning opportunity: initially overlooking the side being avoided and turning one's attention completely to the side that is within one's constrained field of view until the task lying here is (re)solved (homeopathic approach); having (re)solved this high-priority task, also setting one's sights on the other side (allopathic approach); learning to understand the different weightings of the left (feminine) and the right (masculine) sides; facing up to confrontations and looking the world straight in the eye.

Resolution: Finding the happy medium in the following point of view: the glass is neither half full nor half empty, but both half empty and half full.
Archetypal principle: Venus (neck)-Uranus.

Cervical inflammation

(cervicitis)
Physical level: Cervix (gate to the primordial cave of all beginning), mucous membranes (inner boundary, barrier).
Symptom level: Battle over the entrance to the feminine underworld, conflict over fertility and creativity.
Handling: Owning up to one's rage over one's partner; allowing oneself to be aroused by the struggle for the innermost portal; clearing up of rotten compromises in the area of fertility, questioning pseudo-solutions and replacing them with solutions which do justice to one's own plan in life.
Resolution: Courageous defence of one's own holiest-of-holies; clearly answering for oneself the question: "Who is allowed in here, and who is not?", and if necessary, courageously defending the decision to those in one's environment.
Archetypal principle: Moon-Saturn-Mars.

Cervical polyps

(see also Uterine polyps)
Physical level: Cervix (gate to the primordial cave of all beginnings), mucous membranes (inner boundary, barrier).
Symptom level: Mucous membrane outgrowths, which can also look out towards the mouth of the uterus; polyps, as guardians or policemen on the threshold of the most intimate area, can very easily cause →bleeding after sexual intercourse; on the

battlefield of the sexes, she waits with the "cudgel" for his "sword", but allows herself to be conquered and injured in the struggle: the female martyr.

Handling: Making oneself aware of one's inner vulnerability with every phallic contact; arming oneself appropriately on the level of consciousness; also playing out crazy out-of-the-ordinary ideas in the area of eroticism and sexuality.

Resolution: Intimacy lived out creatively.

Archetypal principle: Moon-Saturn-Jupiter.

Cervical vertebra displacement

Physical level: Atlas (pivot point of the upper storey), cervical vertebra (column) (being easily swayed, flexibility of the head).

Symptom level: The head aspect (main issue) is out of alignment; one's lookout point can no longer be manoeuvred freely (of pain): resistance to changes in direction; Atlas can no longer perform his task of bearing the (personal) weight of the world without pain; the head's load is no longer bearable: the pain limit has been overstretched; in the case of frequent dislocations: unconscious-opportunistic changes of tack "being easily swayed"; "having been hoodwinked".

Handling: Bringing things back into alignment; putting the most important and uppermost things right; committing oneself to a single direction instead of continually changing tack; making oneself aware of the unreasonable demands of one's head since it is now only possible to (always) keep one's head up with pain; laying it down from time to time and allowing oneself rest (breaks); setting one's head straight; voluntarily getting off the beaten track; taking new directions, e.g. allowing one's head to be turned in a loving way; in the case of those who are easily swayed: finding one's way to genuine flexibility and adaptability.

Resolution: Putting things right again oneself instead of having to have the spinal column put right; remaining aligned using one's own resources.

Archetypal principle: Venus/ Saturn-Uranus.

Cervicitis

see Cervical inflammation

CFS (Chronic Fatigue Syndrome)

see Burnout syndrome

Change of life complaints

see Climacteric complaints

Chickenpox

(see also Childhood diseases)

Physical level: Skin (border, contact, tenderness).

Symptom level: In addition to a number of minor general symptoms, an itching, spasmodically-spreading rash, whose papules turn into blisters and pustules, and then scab over; usually this heals up without scars if no secondary infection of the blisters takes place (danger in the case of immune defence suppression due to prior cortisone treatment): the breakthrough of the new takes place in stages and with great irritation.

Handling/Resolution: Allowing oneself to be stirred up and stimulated by new impulses; going beyond one's own limits in a courageous and open(ly offensive) way; aggressively and forcefully promoting new developments; arriving at the new stage and getting to the bottom of the new position; gaining a foothold.

Archetypal principle: Mars-Uranus.

Chilblains

(perniones)

Physical level: Skin (border, contact, tenderness).

Symptom level: Local chronic inflammation with signs of degeneration on the basis of extreme cold: exposing one's barrier and contact organ to chronic undercooling; long-term conflict with tendency towards dying off; danger of development of chronic ulcers.

Handling: Turning one's attention to one's own skin in a positive way; enjoying it as a protection, but also sensing the obligation to protect it in return; looking after one's own border (areas) with a sense of self-sacrifice, stimulating the supply of life (energy) (measures to promote circulation).

Resolution: Rugging up well when heading into icy situations: protecting oneself against emotional hostility in good time.

Archetypal principle: Saturn.

Childbed fever

(puerperal fever)

Physical level: Affects the whole organism.

Symptom level: Infection occurring after birth (miscarriage) with sepsis (originally caused primarily by doctors due to non-sterile working practices and today rare; clinics nevertheless still constitute a risk of infection due to their technology-intensive pre-natal and post-natal medicine, which makes use of electrodes, catheters and blood samples): life-threatening conflict in the childbed, generalised conflict over having children.

Handling: Entering into a life-and-death struggle with regard to the new situation; handling threatening conflicts over the new role courageously and in an open(ly offensively) way, and in this situation, also mentally-spiritually in order to relieve the body of the burden.

Resolution: Being prepared to deal with existential conflicts even directly after the birth when everyone wants to spare one any further strain, before the body takes over the conflicts instead.

Archetypal principle: Moon-Mars.

Childbirth problems

see Birth complications

Childhood diseases

(see also Inflammation, Skin rash)

Physical level: Various connections with different organs, above all the skin (border, contact, tenderness).

Symptom level: Many childhood diseases, such as measles, scarlet fever, rubella and chickenpox manifest themselves via the skin (→efflorescences), since symbolically something new is breaking through and indicating a development step; childhood diseases are infectious diseases, i.e. conflicts through which the child is challenged to undertake further leaps in maturity, respectively development; the child's own borders are brought into question from within and are finally broken through following the incubation period; sometimes children want to be left in peace and to remain in the dark while the subject itself is still in the dark; when the subject finally breaks through to the surface and the rash erupts outwardly on the skin, then the worst (of the new) has been withstood – the tension/uncertainty before the next step; according to R. Steiner, childhood diseases occur primarily as a result of the struggle between the genetic endowment and Ego forces (spirit) of the child. He assumes that, in the first seven years of life, the Ego must first create the body which really corresponds to the Ego, and which, given that the genetic endowment possibly may not suit it, first takes some forming. In keeping with this therefore, childhood diseases should not be suppressed, but instead the child should be effectively supported in its struggle (see also →vaccination damage).

Handling: (for parents and children): Accepting that new beginnings in life are almost always accompanied by crises (= dangers, opportunities, decisions) which want to be overcome; being open towards new developments; voluntarily calling one's own limits into question; being outgoing with regard to to new domains and levels of experience; being willing to face conflict and consciously reckoning with conflicts at the boundary (surfaces) since these are indispensable for growth.

Resolution: Undertaking courageous and conscious steps (also through conflicts and pain) into new territory; acting in an open(ly offensive) way with regard to one's own inner steps forward.

Archetypal principle: Moon-Mars.

Chlamydia infection

(see also Sexual diseases)
Physical level: Genitalia (sexuality, polarity, reproduction).
Symptom level: Bacteria settle in the cells and lead in the advanced stage of the disease to symptoms, such as adhesion of the Fallopian tubes, respectively →epididymis inflammation, →prostate inflammation and →infertility; later fulfilment of the desire to have children is blighted, respectively an unconscious resistance to the unborn child becomes apparent; sex as a performance sport or 'fashion drug' leads to a lack of inner fulfilment; taking in everything possible without differentiating.

Handling: In the partnership, honing in on the essential being of the partner instead of simply having sex; going into greater depth in sexuality; developing one's psychological

immunity; making a healthy choice; questioning the motives behind one's rejection of fertility and pregnancy.
Resolution: Recognising sex as a physical aspect of form, whose content would be spiritual love; search for meaning; listening to one's inner voice and heeding it.
Archetypal principle: Pluto.

Chloasma

see Pigment flecks

Choking (on food)

Physical level: Neck (assimilation, connection, communication), trachea (airpipe, exchange).
Symptom level: Misfortune; one's approach to processing the world is characterised by misunderstandings and mix-ups: "having something go down the wrong way", deceiving oneself, misunderstanding something; tending to get levels confused; naïve attempt to transform matter into mental-spiritual form; longing to suffuse matter with spirit and thus bring it into increased contact with the air element; wanting to transform oneself back into pure spirit: death.
Handling: Trying out unusual, creative approaches, taking new paths; learning to process the world with spirit and humour; enabling what one absorbs and processes to be suffused with spirit.
Resolution: Playing the game with the different levels in a creative way; switching from one level to the other, and knowing what one is doing in the process.
Archetypal principle: Uranus.

Cholangitis

(inflammation of the cystic duct starting from the intestines or the gall bladder; see also Gall bladder, inflammation)

Physical level: Gall bladder (aggression, poison and bile).

Symptom level: Offensive struggle in the domain responsible for discharging hidden aggressions.

Handling: Devoting oneself courageously and offensively to the discharging of old, and to some degree, stagnant aggressions.

Resolution: Coming clean with the letting go of pent-up aggressions.

Archetypal principle: Pluto-Mars.

Cholecystitis

see Gall bladder, inflammation

Cholera

(Asiatic cholera; see also Diarrhoea)

Physical level: Intestines (processing of material impressions).

Symptom level: Conflict over digestion, usually triggered by food that is contaminated (with cholera vibrions); fear, which is expressed in the form of severe attacks of diarrhoea ("being shit-scared", "shitting oneself/ one's pants"); impoverishment of the spiritual element (fluid loss caused by diarrhoea) threatens the life flow (circulatory collapse).

Handling: Open(ly offensive) struggle over processing/digestion: becoming aware of instances of self-deception in this area; confrontation with the dark sides (dirt) of what must be digested; letting out the spiritual aspect to the greatest possible extent, and bringing it into the light of consciousness; bringing restriction and fear to the level of consciousness; giving in completely to the fear, until it is transformed into expansiveness; subjecting oneself voluntarily to the total cleansing of the shadow world (in the figurative sense).

Resolution: Willingness to engage in conflict with regard to the shadow subjects, but also acceptance of the limits of one's own readiness for absorption and digestion; being in flow.

Archetypal principle:
Mercury-Neptune-Mars.

Cholesterol level, high

(basic problem: high stress level, which leads to injuries of the inner lining of the vessels as a result of blood pressure fluctuations; see also Hypercholesterolemia)

Physical level: Arteries (energy pathways), cholesterol (bandaging and sealing material of the body).

Symptom level: Attempt to protect oneself, to barricade all the cracks, to seal oneself off and clam up; overloaded energy pathways full of construction sites and repair crews: the flow of the life energy transports large quantities of sealing and patching material; danger of traffic bottlenecks (lumen reduction of the arteries), traffic jams (vessel closures) and gridlocks (total supply failures).

Handling: Searching for and sealing off leaky points in one's spiritual structure; protecting one's own network of nerves against overloading and the soul against lack of nourishment; switching conflicts in one's daily struggle for survival from the physical to the mental-spiritual level (e.g. exercises in expressing oneself verbally instead of the exercise of permanent tension and pressure in the arterial system); getting to the bottom of where, when and why one repeatedly restricts oneself; being armed and ready for all incidents (accidents) in the figurative sense; becoming aware of energy supply bottlenecks on the figurative level (with such increased traffic travelling at such a crazy speed, something is bound to come up short – e.g. [matters of] the heart); getting to know one's own sore (weak) points: giving oneself time to let the wounds heal; developing strong nerves (of steel); making the transport of patching material unnecessary by means of preventive measures: reducing the elevated tempo of life –visible in the increased pressure of life – by introducing measures to slow down the flow of traffic (artificial bottlenecks).

Resolution: Energy flowing calmly and in good time into the decisive areas (heart-related matters, inner progress [legs], all-encompassing insight [brain]).

Archetypal principle: Mars-Saturn.

Chondrodystrophia

Physical level: Bones (stability, strength).

Symptom level: Congenital ossification disorder which leads to dwarfism with a normal head and trunk, but with arms and legs that are too short; this handicap in the domain of physically conquering the world sensibly moves the focus of life to domains of intellectual-spiritual development.

Handling: Accepting one's smallness in the physical domain, learning humility, looking up, viewing the world from below, experiencing the world from the perspective of a child.

Resolution: Accepting oneself as an exception and becoming someone exceptional.

Archetypal principle: Saturn-Uranus.

Chorditis

see Laryngeal inflammation, Hoarseness

Chorea

see St. Vitus's dance

Chronic diseases

(see also Inflammation)
Physical level: The whole organism can be affected.
Symptom level: Bound energy, unclarified situation; prolonged conflict:

no real war, no real peace (→inflammation), rotten, lukewarm compromises; cold war; cowardice; fear of the consequences of acting, and of responsibility; fear of seeking out the decision; lack of courage/strength to make a decision: stagnation, static warfare; fear of sacrifices associated with a decision; permanent refusal to learn; frequently a phenomenon of advancing age, which appears on the scene when the shadow has not been addressed over a long period of time: situation of hopelessness (no further hope of healing [salvation], therefore, often resulting in embitterment to the point of spite and hatred [of life] as an expression of shadow energies).

Handling: Preserving and saving up energy on the figurative level (learning to budget); living under fire, holding out, sitting something out in the sense of Za-Zen; readily seeking consensus: finding one's centre, doing justice to both sides; getting off the beaten or dead tracks of life; sticking things out, learning to bear them; avoiding habitual reactions because this leads to perpetuation of the conflict (actio = reactio); risking the first step out of the vicious circle of one's habits; bearing the restrictiveness of the situation until, having reached its climax, it expands again; taking into account the opposite pole, which must also later be resolved (redeemed): making decisions (freeing the sword from the scabbard; Latin: dēcīsiō = 'a cutting off'); transforming potential energies into kinetic energies and vice versa (bringing movement back into a deadlocked situation; calming a hectic one): playing with energies; accepting responsibility: finding answers; developing empathy since the other side is also right (from its point of view); identifying the inner point of stagnation and making energetic attempts at bringing it back to life.

Resolution: Bearing responsibility for one's own decisions; finding the happy medium: harmony as a successful compromise between war and peace (the goddess Harmonia as the daughter of Venus – the goddess of love – and Mars – the god of war); consistent and persistent search for the (middle) path; acting by not acting: acting but being prepared to relinquish the fruits of one's actions in order to end the stagnation, but without tipping the balance to the other pole; recognition that great victories lead to great wars, and that remaining still helps one towards achieving inner peace; integration first of the one pole, then of the other; becoming whole/healed, becoming aware; staying power on the intellectual-spiritual level instead of on the physical level.
Archetypal principle: Saturn-Mars.

Chronic fatigue syndrome

see Burnout syndrome

Circulation problems

see Cardiovascular problems

Circulatory disorders

(see also Arteriosclerosis, Cardiac infarction, Claudicatio intermittens, Smoker's leg)
Physical level: Arterial blood vessels (transport routes of the life force).
Symptom level: Partial or general deficiency of supply to the tissue due to arteriosclerosis or other vascular diseases, strangulation of the dependent regions or organs: pains in the undersupplied areas as cries for help from the tissue; in the case of arteriosclerosis: "cementing in" of the life energy flow, hardening in the life flow.
Handling: Reduction of one's energy consumption, strict apportionment of one's own energy, ceasing to waste

energy, concentration on the essential with respect to energy; learning to call for help if something that is essential for life is lacking; learning to recognise that the essential aspects are coming up short in some areas.
Resolution: Living sparingly and modestly with regard to energy; genuine efficiency, concentration on the important and essential aspects; being able to accept help.
Archetypal principle: Mars-Saturn.

Clap

see Gonorrhoea

Claudicatio intermittens

(intermittent lameness, "window-shopper's disease" – so-called because sufferers frequently have to stand still – and often pretend to be window shopping; see also Arteriosclerosis)
Physical level: Blood (life force), blood vessels (transport routes of the life force).
Symptom level: Nothing (more) is moving forward and nothing (more) is on the way up in life; narrow limits, strong resistance; restricted mobility, minimal radius of action: "not getting far", "not going places".
Handling: Consciously letting go of ambition, fantasies about potential promotions and pretensions of making progress; not wanting to get anywhere; giving up the struggle: "taking smaller steps"; learning to respect the existing limits; accepting resistances as useful hints; forging new paths for the life force and extending old ones (training the blood vessels).
Resolution: Resigning in the sense of stepping back from previously-set objectives and high-flying dreams: surrendering oneself to the weakened flow of the life energy; drifting without aspirations or struggle; climbing down

from the Ego tower and relaxing with the aim of finding inner calm; turning around, returning home and arriving, instead of long marches and climbing to the top.
Archetypal principle: Mars-Saturn-Neptune.

Claustrophilia

(pronounced compulsion to shut oneself in)
Symptom level: Neurotic preference for restrictive situations and those of seclusion; striving to return to the womb and back into the first, primordial restrictiveness shortly before birth; paradoxical fear.
Handling: Making oneself aware once again of the security in the womb and the primordial sense of restrictiveness shortly before and during the birth and then experiencing this fully so that it can truly be left behind; ensuring adequate security and safety in life.
Resolution: Gaining basic trust through experiences of unity.
Archetypal principle: Moon-Pluto.

Claustrophobia

(see also Phobia)
Symptom level: Extreme fear of enclosed, restricted spaces: awareness of having no way out (hopelessness); reliving of the unresolved birth situation.
Handling: Processing of the birth trauma (e.g. through reincarnation therapy, breathing therapy); in addition to its restrictiveness, recognising the nourishing aspect of the womb; consciously letting oneself down into the depths of the fear and restrictiveness until they are transformed into expansiveness; discovering the positive aspect of closeness in terms of security and being held.
Resolution: Seeing all of life as a chain of births, which we must live through one after the other; after

every tight squeeze, once again adjusting oneself to the expansiveness which opens up a new outlook on life to us.
Archetypal principle: Pluto.

Claw hand

see Hand problems

Cleft jaw

see Facial clefts

Cleft lip

see Facial clefts

Cleft palate

see Facial clefts

Cleptomania

(compulsive tendency to steal)
Symptom level: Compulsive stealing, in which the focus is on the act of stealing rather than on actual possession (typically occurs without there being any need to steal).
Handling: Seeing through one's need to break the rules of ownership; leading a more exciting and riskier life; finding an earlier situation in one's own previous history that has to do with problems of possession (often a subject that has been brought along into this life); changing sides, for example, as a store detective, placing one's own desire to steal in the service of law and order and training detectives through one's own abilities.
Resolution: Overstepping limits and rules in the figurative sense; taking the things in life which one believes and which others believe one is not entitled to; allopathically: reconciling oneself to law and order, finding one's own inner order.
Archetypal principle: Mercury-Neptune.

Climacteric complaints

(menopause complaints; see also Hot flushes, Vaginal dryness, Female facial hair, Myoma, Involution depression)

Physical level: Genitalia (sexuality, polarity, reproduction), glands/hormones (control, information).

Symptom level: (Account) balance (symptoms) for the first half of life: the symptoms show the unresolved subjects as the organism continues to work on them: unlived femininity, anxiety over missing out, panicked mood, having a lot of catching up to do; 1. Hot flushes, hot flashes: the unlived aspects put the "heat" on and create fear; 2. Outbreaks of sweating: the "hot-blooded" woman; 3. dry, hot mucous membranes (→vaginal dryness): burning up with heat; 4. Flushes: attacks of →blushing, as with sexual arousal; 5. Irritability: challenging oneself to be lured in and stirred up by certain stimuli; 6. Being edgy: feeling inner unrest before setting off anew or making the turnaround; 7. Insomnia: not being able to sleep due to anticipation and anxious excitement; 8. Feelings of anxiety: feeling of restrictiveness (in one's chest) about the new, the breakthrough into new territory. The first four symptoms belong to the domain of the orgasm. They are, however, rather annoying if they occur when shopping, although they only appear on the scene if they have previously come up too short or if there is anxiety about now letting go of this phase; the second four symptoms could also be categorised under teenage behaviour. Frequent bleeding to give the pretence of fertility; tumoric growths/myomas as an unconscious desire for pregnancy; →depression to the point of suicidal tendencies.

Handling: Consciously flushing out the "hot-blooded" woman once again and bringing her (back) to life with the tendency to live it up completely, but also to complete life by wrapping things up; doing the little girl act once more before this phase is really let go; being fired up with enthusiasm and generating heat in the figurative sense: burning with passion for the forthcoming subjects; realising fertility on other levels; giving birth to things in the figurative sense; concerning oneself with the objective of the way, the Resolution and death: reading Books of the Dead, meditating on the "where from" and "where to" of the way.

Resolution: Instead of heatedness, finding warmheartedness and other hot topics, which now take priority; adjusting oneself to the new tasks and the spiritual homecoming: becoming a woman with the onset of the period, becoming a mother with its absence and with its definitive cessation becoming the Grand (spiritual) Mother; changing from the role of woman and mother into that of the Grand Mother and wise old woman; paying the outstanding bills (on figurative levels: "What have I left owing in the first half of life?") and devoting oneself to the new and grander subjects of the homecoming.

Archetypal principle: Venus/Moon (femininity)-Uranus (change)/Saturn (maturity).

Club foot

(pes varus; see also Hereditary diseases)

Physical level: Feet (steadfastness, deep-rootedness).

Symptom level: Severe deviation of the foot inwards (recessively inherited, affects twice as many young boys than young girls): handicap when walking; physical progress is brought into question; "development disorder": the club foot resembles the embryonic foot between the 5th and

12th week of pregnancy): being back-ward/left behind (often left behind in concrete terms due to the walking handicap); handicap, disfigurement: ungainly clumsiness instead of elegance.
Handling: Adjusting oneself to the task of slow but steady progress; going inwards instead of outwards (the club foot points inwards); consciously catching up on early development phases: placing inner progress above outer progress.
Resolution: Letting the challenge demand more of one in order to grow as a result of the demands.
Archetypal principle: Neptune-Saturn.

Club hand

see Hand problems

Clubbed fingers

see Hand problems

Coagulation disorder

see Bleeding tendency

Coccyx pains

Physical level: Coccyx (shock-absorber, protection of the pelvic bowl).
Symptom level: Having "fallen on one's behind" in various respects; painful changes in one's inner static equilibrium due to repositioning of one's life axis or a necessary re-alignment of one's inner balance, but without the corresponding changes taking place on the consciousness level: persisting in the old pattern causes pain; the spinal column cries out for help because it is no longer up to the new situation if the old stance is upheld.
Handling: Hearing the cries and inwardly listening to which direction the life axis wants to take; making an

effort to ensure the realignment of one's own life axis.
Resolution: Bringing one's own stance into accord with one's position in life so that one's life is brought back into alignment.
Archetypal principle: Saturn-Mars.

Co-dependency

see Helper syndrome

Coeliac

(see also Digestive complaints, Allergy)
Physical level: Small intestine (analysis, assimilation).
Symptom level: Allergy to gluten, the sticky element in grains which binds bread together: not wanting to assimilate the bread and butter of adult life, but instead aggressively struggling against it; war against what is greasy, slippery and slimy - the feminine pole of life; hostility towards one's body and life in general, the body and soul go their separate ways.
Handling: (for jointly-affected parents, whose problems are often reflected by the children): reconciliation with the aggression principle and the feminine pole of reality in the form of the slippery-slimy primordial swamp from which all life originates; reconciling oneself with one's own physicality; developing desire for the physical and making friends with one's own body.
Resolution: A vital life full of desire for the life-giving feminine principle.
Archetypal principle: Mercury-Pluto/Mars.

Cold diseases

(see also Influenza, Inflammation)
Physical level: Nose (power, pride, sexuality), neck (assimilation, connection, communication), lungs (contact, communication, freedom).
Symptom level: The current life situation leaves one cold, not being

able to warm to anything any more: getting (a) cold; it is not the cold conditions that cause us to become ill, but more so our conditioning to get (a) cold; catching/picking up the germ-inating elements (pathogens) one needs to play out the drama: "I've caught/picked up something"; conflict handling "being fed up to the eyeballs", "getting one's nose out of joint", "being in a huff"; retreat from the crisis situations of everyday life; "shutting oneself off"; building defensive walls out of tissues; keeping people and situations at arm's length: "Back off, I have a cold", being overloaded, desire to flee: "not wanting to hear or see anything more" (pressure on the ears; strained, tired eyes); "simply wanting to crawl into bed and pull the covers over one's head"; living out sensitivity: a splitting headache; restriction of communication: nose blocked, bronchia tending to close up, sore, clogged throat; refusal: "not wanting to swallow anything else"; defensive stance: "coughing up" what one really thinks of a person; feeling as if one has been through a punch-up and a screaming match: shattered state and hoarseness; sniffles, with the result that one does not have to get wind of anything else or put one's nose to the grindstone; hoarseness, with the result that one does not have to say anything else; inflammation of the tonsils, with the result that one does not have to swallow anything else; coughing, with the result that one can bark out one's opinion; catarrh of the tubes (blockage of the auditory tubes of the ears), with the result that one no longer has to pay attention to anything or lend anyone one's ear; cold also as a means of cooling oneself down after one has, for once, gone completely into the heat of the fray (fever); getting into the flow on a less refined level (sniffles).

Handling: Bringing something into flow, clearing up problems; flowing with life again, developing readiness for the transitions of life (spring and autumn) instead of using the body as a stage in substitute form for one's own spiritual situation at the transitional times of the year; preferably fasting and purging at the transitional times of the year instead of using a runny nose and coughing one's lungs out as a form of cleansing; cleansing rituals; shutting oneself off from others and coming back to oneself (turning inwards); becoming aware of what is leaving one so cold: allowing oneself to be stirred up by stimulating subjects, instead of falling victim to stirring elements in the form of pathogens; making room for oneself (in a conscious way), if necessary, also using aggressive methods ("coughing up" what one really thinks of others); opening oneself up again to the surrounding environment: being aflame with passion for the outstanding problems; living out one's enthusiasm; burning to deal with the upcoming tasks; battling one's way through life offensively and courageously, but where necessary, also in a slick and smooth (well-oiled), friendly manner; being headstrong in getting one's way.

Resolution: Being in the flow (of life): letting life overflow instead of one's nose.

Archetypal principle: oon (retreat, sliminess)-Mars (inflammation).

Cold haemoglobinuria

(a type of "cold allergy")

Physical level: Vascular system (transport routes of the life force).

Symptom level: So-called cold agglutinins (antibodies) attack one's own red blood corpuscles at low temperatures, and release their pigment material (haemoglobin) = haemolysis:

the lifeblood breaks down; danger of embolisms to the point of kidney failure and death; the "true blue"(honest) skin bares all showing its blue discoloration and lifelessness; cold causes the blood to break down: fear of cold.
Handling: Avoiding physical and spiritual coldness; ensuring that one stays nice and warm, both outwardly and inwardly; during cold snaps and spiritual ice ages, fighting a life-and-death battle to stop one's blood running cold; being aware at all times of the danger of the life flow coming to a standstill and the failure of all co-operative partnership mechanisms in cold situations.
Resolution: Living life fired up by enthusiasm; being on fire for one's own life subjects; being sparked off by ideas and living and loving with a fiery heart; being "hot to trot" for life and burning with passion for life.
Archetypal principle: Mars-Saturn.

Colic

Physical level: Various organs can be affected, most frequently in the area of the kidneys (balance, partnership), bile duct (aggression), intestines (processing of material impressions) and urinary bladder (withstanding and relieving pressure); see also in the related entries above.
Symptom level: Launching a field offensive against an obstacle in ever-recurring attack waves; exerting effort in a rhythmic fashion in oder to bear down on obstacles (attempting to expel them); labour pains similar to contractions, which usually help to give birth to a stone; extreme intensification of the naturally-occurring peristalsis in the relevant regions.
Handling: Using offensive muscle contractions to set in motion whatever is being held onto or that is stuck (repressed) and to get rid of it; managing to work out solutions through rhythmic ebbing and flowing actions instead

of through continuous effort: tackling blockages with ever-recurring efforts and exercises in letting go; letting go (in a painful way) of what is hindering one in life.
Resolution: Letting go of obstacles that are in one's way.
Archetypal principle: Mars-Uranus (Saturn = stones).

Colitis ulcerosa

(inflammation of the large intestine; see also Intestinal inflammation, Irritable colon)
Physical level: Large intestine (unconscious, underworld), blood (life force).
Symptom level: Great losses of water (spiritual fluid), salts (electrolyte as the salt of life), life energy (blood); civil war in the underworld with shadowy fronts: costly battle against oneself; auto-aggression: "busting one's ass"; being "an arse-licker" or "brown-noser" who "kisses ass" and "sucks up" to others in order to be everybody's darling; all hell has broken loose: magical blood rituals in the underworld milieu; sacrificial role; making a blood sacrifice (unconsciously sacrificing one's own vitality); working from the opposite pole: desperate attempt to cleanse oneself down to one's very lifeblood; dozens of voidings (enemas): obsessive compulsive washing on the lower level; the life force concentrates itself in the underworld; fear of self-realisation in one's own life and one's own personality; "sweating blood and water" out of great fear; continually "shitting oneself" is humiliating: feelings of embarrassment and shame; sacrificing one's own personal life in favour of symbiotic unity with another; an explosive happening when the dependency relationship is set in motion; being stuck in an early phase; the red, raw baby's bottom; not yet clean (potty-trained), needing nappies; the

mother, experienced as threatening and controlling, who demands submission; clinging on tightly to the mother; enforced symbiosis; fear of loneliness through self-responsibility; resignation, self-sacrifice, hopelessness; rotten compromises with respect to giving away and keeping things for oneself.

Handling: Showing genuine remorse instead of feelings of guilt (metanoia: Greek 'change of mind' [C.G. Jung]); courageous confrontation with one's own reluctant forces in the shadow (kingdom); being hard with oneself; making an effort in the struggle over the spiritual shadow issues; developing extensive willingness to sacrifice oneself (making one's own life force available); making binding commitments towards others; "oiling the wheels" to get relationships up and running; making oneself aware of the subject of dependency and independence, respectively the power of the soul and power over souls; recognising the restrictiveness in relationships and relating it to the fear of life (unprocessed birth trauma?); psychotherapy: seeing through and resolving the selling of the soul ("pact"), which binds one to the underworld – and thereby also discovering the "sunny upper world" (blood as an aspect of vitality); finding the way back to oneself; retreat into one's own realm: learning to respond to the demands (challenges) of Fate; loosening blood bonds with blood relations, and if necessary, re-establishing them on a voluntary basis.

Resolution: Offensive, courageous illumination of the underworld and the shadow; reconciliation with one's own magical roots; tough, inner struggles on the way to one's own self; readiness for sacrifice to the bitter end at the right point; consciously giving up power over other souls in order to let go and be free; realising the

great transformation using one's own power: metanoia.

Archetypal principle: Pluto-Sun.

Collapse

(flowing transition into shock; see also Heat collapse)

Physical level: Heart-circulatory system (heart = seat of the soul, love, feelings, energy centre); blood circulation (circuit of the life energy, supply and disposal).

Symptom level: Deficient flow of life energy to the central control headquarters: deficient circulation to the brain leads to acute collapse; paleness, outbreaks of sweating, the racing of the heart, shallow breathing: panic symptoms; the life energy plummets into the lower (legs) or inner (liver, intestines) region of the body and is then lacking in the seat of government and in the peripheral circulation; shortage of the feminine spiritual water in the central vascular system: deficiency in the brain and heart; a different reality which (obviously) was previously overlooked now breaks out (violently) and demands attention: those affected are partly out of their senses; the control centre switches off.

Handling: As emergency measures: putting the head in a low position, raising the legs, ensuring a supply of fresh air (oxygen), blood substitutes (plasma expander); giving preference to the central regions (such as the head and heart) as acute life-saving measures (= allopathic thinking); in the long term, giving the head a slightly lower priority in the supply of energy and attention (= homeopathic thinking); in the long term, aligning one's point of focus (i.e. central weighting) with the lower feminine pole and with the processing (digestion) of experiences; voluntarily coming into contact with the (ancient nature) god Pan; bringing the head

down from its high horse; resting (putting one's feet up); ensuring fresh communication (fresh air supply); also taking note of what is shocking; learning from shock experiences.
Resolution: Instead of collapsing (falling apart), voluntarily allowing oneself to fall (in the right place and at the right time); finding one's own life rhythm; ensuring a happy medium between demanding too much or too little of oneself, between the influence of feminine spiritual water and masculine fire energy; voluntarily and consciously adjusting oneself to the great letting go (at the end of life).
Archetypal principle: Sun/Moon-Uranus/Saturn.

Colon cancer

see Rectal cancer

Colour blindness

(achromatopsia)
Physical level: Eyes (insight, perspective, mirrors and windows of the soul).
Symptom level: Blindness to the diversity and colourfulness of life: nothing appears brightly coloured and joyful; seeing everything only in different shades of grey; attempt to level out differences; everything that would make life colourful is factored out, possibly for generations; in the case of red-green blindness: not being able to differentiate the colours of growth (red = the force of initiation and energy per se; green = nature and hope); red (energy of the human world) and green (energy of the plant world) are complementary colours, which complete and need each other – inability to distinguish between these two worlds; misjudging the difference between stimulation (red) and calming (green).
Handling: Recognising the monotony of one's own perception; recognising the danger of a colourless life; not

allowing oneself to be diverted from the actual tasks by the colourfulness of life; learning to see through everything as nuances of the same; consciously passing through what is grizzled/grizzly; recognising the colours of the world as an expression of what is lacking (every colour lacks its complementary colour for completeness, which is then expressed as white); specially for red-green blindness: learning to see energy and growth as a unity; learning to see the same basic force in the opposite poles of the complementary colours red and green, and recognising how they need each other; not allowing oneself to be seduced/ensnared by the play of colours of the Maya: meditation on the attraction of black-and-white photography.
Resolution: Recognising at all times the unity behind the polarity; in the depths of everything, recognising the oneness.
Archetypal principle: Sun/Moon-Saturn/Neptune.

Colpitis

see Vaginal inflammation

Coma

Physical level: Brain (communication, logistics).
Symptom level: Deep unconsciousness due to damaged brain metabolism; frequently marks the end of a long medical history; frequently the departure from life via a stage in the in-between area (kingdom) between life and death; extended preparation period of the soul for its journey through the bardo states into the beyond; sometimes an intermediate station (a period for stopping and turning back within) of the soul before it decides once again to return back to the dwelling place of the body.
Handling: (No longer actively possible for those affected; instructions for

family members): undertaking helpful supporting measures for the soul, which does indeed (still) fully perceive everything: e.g. playing masses, oratorios, requiems, readings from the Books of the Dead; rituals of transition; ensuring energy for the soul (Odic energy [Reichenbach], fresh flowers, burning candles) (caring attention is experienced in every form, whether as caring thoughts or physical presence).

Resolution: Inward readiness for the journey of the soul.

Archetypal principle: Saturn (as the Grim Reaper and guardian of the threshold)/Neptune (overstepping boundaries).

Commotio

see Brain concussion

Compressio cerebri

see Cerebral compression syndrome

Compulsive clearing of one's throat

Physical level: Larynx (expression), voice (tone [mood]).

Symptom level: Pre-announcing a contribution which then does not arrive; getting stuck, although one would actually like to say something for once; not being able to get a word in edgeways; asking for attention, searching for words; registering criticism without formulating it.

Handling: Owning up to the Ego problem behind it: one believes that one has something to say, but does not trust oneself to do so – usually based on the fear that it may not go down well (enough); ensuring an audience, (due) respect and attention for one's words; openly expressing constructive criticism.

Resolution: Using self-expression to ensure (earn) the scope that is one's due.

Archetypal principle: Mercury-Saturn.

Concentration disorders

Symptom level: 1. General: missing the point; having lost one's own centre; lack of focus and discipline; scatter-brained, all over the place, torn this way and that, concerning oneself with the non-essential; 2. In children: out of boredom or disinterest, not sticking to the matter at hand ("fidgeting" →hyperactivity); the natural reaction (disinterest) sinks into the unconscious and is treated as a disease pattern; resistance against compulsion to perform and adaptation to norms.

Handling: 1. Consciously letting oneself go; practising letting go in order to regain calm and composure; allowing oneself to be diverted to sensible alternatives; allopathically: mandala exercises for centring, Tai Chi from the centre, Za-Zen in order to find the Hara, the centre of the world of man (Dürckheim); 2. Individual support, bringing to life one's own interests, living life to the fullest through them; choosing a different form of schooling.

Resolution: 1. Searching for one's own centre, hitting the right point, zeroing in on the essential (= lifting of one's segregation); 2. Listening to the inner call, searching for one's own calling.

Archetypal principle: Saturn-Mercury-Neptune.

Conjunctivitis

(Conjunctivitis; see also Eyes, dryness)

Physical level: Eyes (insight, perspective, mirrors and windows of the soul).

Symptom level: Conflict between wanting to look more closely and shutting one's eyes; closing one's eyes to conflicts, not wanting to look the conflict in the eye (ostrich policy: sticking one's head in the sand); the tension between one's own way of seeing things and foreign points of view becomes inflamed in one's own eyes, and in this way, is written on one's face; often little confidence in one's own view of things.

Handling: Exposing childish avoidance strategies ("If I can't see you, then you can't see me") and at the same time allowing oneself phases of rest in order to release the tension in the eyes; being courageous about looking at things more closely; taking an offensive approach in confrontations; intentional, conscious looking away; learning to connect outer reality with inner reality.

Resolution: Looking life straight in the eye, with its conflicts; insight into one's own patterns; staring the ("ugly" and the "beautiful") truth in the face.

Archetypal principle: Mars-Sun/ Moon.

Connective tissue weakness

(see also Haematoma, Low blood pressure, Varicose veins, Striae, Thrombosis, Tear sacs)

Physical level: Connective tissue (connection, stability, binding commitment); it is mainly women who are affected.

Symptom level: Lack of stability, tendency towards giving way, lack of inner resilience and stability; living on a low flame; easily hurt, bearing a grudge (black mark) at the slightest prodding; lack of bonding and connective capabilities, non-binding character, low reliability; difficulty in giving form to mental-spiritual tasks; victim stance; wanting others to pull the chestnuts out of the fire; "weak connective tissue" today refers above all to female connective tissue, which although more yielding and adaptable is actually not so weak at all (consider the "weaker sex", which is also stronger and lives longer than the so-called stronger sex).

Handling: Learning to flow consciously with the current of life; conscious giving way: Tai Chi; using the outwardly saved life energy for inner processes; applying sensibility constructively (e.g. as an intuitive, empathetic educator, therapist, etc.); consciously applying "Panta rhei" ("everything flows"), remaining in movement and development; going about inner tasks with feeling and commitment; gladly making sacrifices instead of sacrificing oneself as a victim.

Resolution: Giving of oneself (devotion), trusting oneself; finding one's own direction and structure; softness of disposition instead of the tissue; working from the opposite pole: binding capacity and inner stability; giving support to everything that is hingeing and pulling on one.

Archetypal principle: Moon/ Venus-Neptune.

Constipation

(Obstipation; see also Travel constipation)

Physical level: Large intestine (unconscious, underworld).

Symptom level: Not wanting to give something up, clinging on tightly (excrement = money); no longer letting anything out, not disposing of anything (giving up): frugality/greed; inability to let go in the material domain; fear of being left without means; holding on to what must be given back to the world, and what is superfluous for oneself: burdening oneself with the unusable and withholding it from its actual determination; slowness: not getting completely over and done with digestion, "not getting one's shit together"; perfectionism: "Don't give me that shit" is taken too literally; being exaggeratedly careful: not "shitting" on anything or anybody; taking everything to heart; not allowing oneself an "I don't give a shit?"-attitude; letting out (one's opinions) too little; not "giving anybody any shit" even if they have deserved it; fear of letting unconscious matters (from the shadow kingdom) come to the light of day: being ashamed of one's own shadow sides; rejection of the deepest shadow; inability to leave spiritual impressions behind oneself; resistance: the conversion of old (excrement) into new (life) is boycotted; not taking part in the cycle of life: rigidity and slowness; dried out, hard life; draining the Plutonic underworld swamp out of fear (of the primordial feminine aspects). Possible inner attitudes: 1. The world is not worthy of receiving my treasures (in symbolic terms, the contents of the shadow world and kingdom of the dead are extremely valuable: "shitting" gold ducats like the gold-ass in the Brothers Grimm fairytale, etc.); 2. Possessing things is fun: lust for power through possession; greed (pleasurable sensations when holding back faeces, since there are many sensitive nerve endings in the rectum); 3. The rights of the rest of the world do not interest me (infantile power struggle on the potty).

Handling: Setting limits, but learning to hold on to what one still needs; learning to hold on tightly to dependable structures; owning up to one's inability to let go, and once one feels safe enough within one's limits, integrating the opposite pole and learning to let go; bringing unconscious contents to the surface: psychotherapy; getting to know and learning to accept the flow of life ("everything flows"); shadow confrontation: reconciliation with the dark and primordial feminine aspects; holding back the inner treasures that threaten to escape (learning to keep secrets to oneself);

developing more integrity, instead of gossiping about others.

Resolution: Finding the golden medium between the urge to retain or to pass on: learning the mutual interdependence between giving and taking from one's intestines; learning to acknowledge and understand the principle of "death and re-birth" – that everything in life is transitory.

Archetypal principle: Pluto.

Consumption

see Cachexia

Consumptiveness

see Pulmonary consumption

Contracture

(shortening, contraction)

Physical level: Possible at many points in the body.

Symptom level: Soft tissue shortening due to scar tissue contraction: unsuccessful processing of former problem areas; hardening as the remains and reminder of old battlegrounds.

Handling: Causing old scars to disappear through resolution of the underlying energies; processing former problem areas further: reducing the inferior tissue substitute (scar tissue); going to work on the old battlegrounds with consistency and strength.

Resolution: Completely working through and clearing up the old before it is finally left in peace.

Archetypal principle: Saturn.

Contusio

see Cerebral contusion

Contusion

(see also Accident, Work accident/ Domestic accident, Sport accident, Traffic accident)

Physical level: Joints (mobility, articulation), musculature (motor, strength), skin (border, contact, tenderness).

Symptom level: Badly bruising somebody (usually oneself): deceiving oneself in the assessment of a situation, a danger, etc.; acting as a buffer.

Handling: Bracing oneself for hard (painful) landings; arriving in reality with a bang.

Resolution: Correctly estimating the energies and dynamics acting in the game (of life) and being able to deal with them.

Archetypal principle: Mars-Saturn.

Convulsive attack

see Epilepsy

Cor pulmonale

(increased lung pressure)

Physical level: Lung vessels (contact, communication).

Symptom level: Coming under pressure in the communications area without noticing it (the clinical disease pattern produces hardly any symptoms) (first, interpret and deal with the basic problem in the lungs; e.g. →asthma); in the long-term view: going under from exhaustion (of the heart) (danger of [right ventricular] heart failure).

Handling: Owning up to the pressure one feels in the domain of contact and living up to it (the demands placed upon one); pouring one's heart out in good time; exchanging views on matters of the heart.

Resolution: Pushing oneself to the limits in relation to (matters of) the heart; wholeheartedly establishing (intact) connections between the inner and outer world.

Archetypal principle: Mercury-Pluto.

Corns

Physical level: Feet (steadfastness, deep-rootedness).

Symptom level: Showing where "the shoe is pinching"; certain areas of the head (reflex zones for the head are to be found in the area of the toes) have come under pressure; treading on one's own toes (standing in one's own way); attempt to armour weak points: every form of armour that is pushed too far, however, starts to hurt sooner or later.

Handling: First locate exactly where the pressure point lies (map of foot reflex zones); devising mental-spiritual measures of self-protection (shielding); confronting what is (op)pressing one; giving up the standpoint which is creating the counterpressure, or securing oneself with more substantive arguments; asking oneself where the shoe (of life) is pinching; stepping out in grand (grander?) style; affording oneself more freedom of movement for the feet (filling bigger boots); identifying more comfortable standpoints, where one can really take a stand.

Resolution: Being more generous with oneself; taking on more comfortable positions; making room for one's roots, granting one's "flippers" more room for movement

Archetypal principle: Neptune-Saturn.

Corneal inflammation

(Keratitis)

Physical level: Cornea of the eye (window pane of the eye, perspective, insight).

Symptom level: Conflicts over the uppermost level of seeing and recognition; having seen things which make one angry, and nevertheless having looked away; severe pains: feeling like screaming; conflict in the area of one's point of view, and as a result, the cornea often becomes clouded and limits one's clear vision;

ulceration is not uncommon: clouding one's window on the world; not wanting to see (or hear) anything more; putting up a barrier between oneself and the world; obstacles to seeing: no longer being able to see through things, clouded vision.

Handling: Critically confronting one's own point of view; being willing to struggle to see the light; admitting to oneself that one has serious problems with clearly seeing through (understanding) things; adopting other points of view; learning to see life through different eyes; putting distance between oneself and the world.

Resolution: Perspective and insight; struggling with one's own points of view in an open(ly offensive) way; turning away from the outer world and finding the inner light.

Archetypal principle: Sun/Moon-Mars.

Corneal ulcer

Physical level: Cornea of the eye (window pane of the eye, perspective, insight).

Symptom level: Wild growth on the uppermost level of seeing and recognition: something is growing directly in front of one's eyes that is distorting one's view without one being aware of it (so that the body has to make it apparent); one's own misdirected growth is distorting one's view; obstacles to seeing: certain areas of the field of vision are blanked out.

Handling: Allowing one's own view to grow; bringing those problems which are directly in front of one's own nose into one's field of view; admitting to oneself that one has serious growth problems with regard to clearly seeing through (understanding) things.

Resolution: Recognising and accepting one's own blind spots as potential points for growth.

Archetypal principle: Sun/Moon-Pluto.

Coronary insufficiency

see Coronary sclerosis (below), Cardiac infarction

Coronary sclerosis

(cardiovascular calcification; see also Angina pectoris and Cardiac infarction as possible consequences)

Physical level: Heart (seat of the soul, love, feelings, energy centre).

Symptom level: Giving the heart too little nourishment (energy, oxygen), strangling it by cramping together or "cementing in" the energy supply lines; constriction, fear (angina): oppressive situation: call for help by the left/female side; hardening, the feminine aspect has come up too short; a (process of turning to) stone in one's chest, heart of stone, starving heart; closed-heartedness, rigidity; blockage/hardening (of the flow) of the (heart) feelings; overvaluation of Ego forces and the dominance of one's willpower; a person striving for dominance/performance; fear of criticism and failure: victim of Ego forces and the desire for power; spasm and struggle over matters of the heart: (death) cramps of an already strangulated heart (in the case of infarction or areas close to it).

Handling: Making oneself aware of the deficient supply (strangulation) of one's heart (muscle) with (life) energy, time and loving attention; granting oneself rest; attuning one's life to one's heart; paying attention to the voice of one's heart: listening carefully to it, heeding and obeying its commands (its more tender stirrings); hearing the heart's calls for help in the cries of pain of the tissue (that is hungering for more loving attention = supply); crying in a heart-melting way; learning to release the build-up (of feelings); no longer turning one's heart into a skeleton closet: letting out and letting go of emotions; occupying oneself with the fear and the restrictiveness of the Ego and admitting to oneself that it takes first place in life even over matters of the heart; owning up to feelings of fear and hate; being rigorous and hard with oneself (with the Ego and its demands); finding one's own standpoints; concentrating on one's centre and on one's essence/the essential aspects in life; stopping to turn to inner peace before turning to the peace of the grave; recognising and accepting one's own weakness and vulnerability.

Resolution: Concentration on the heart, bringing one's own heart into the central point of focus in living (or dying), circling around the centre, dancing the dance around the centre; recognising the basic fear of losing oneself, but learning and recognising that one "merely" needs to lose the Ego in order to arrive at the centre; opening oneself to the needs of the heart; humility and concentration on the essential.

Archetypal principle: Sun-Saturn.

Corpus luteum cysts

(see also Ovarian cysts)
Physical level: Ovaries (fertility).
Symptom level: Following ovulation, the remains of the first nest are not given up, but in the case of a pregnancy, continue to grow; frequently disappears in the third month of pregnancy; being put more or less under pressure (depending on the size of the cysts) with respect to fertility and having children.

Handling: Addressing the problem of clinging tightly for too long to old attitudes about having children.
Resolution: Letting go of hindering traditions.
Archetypal principle: Moon-Saturn/Pluto.

Costal pleura inflammation

see Pleural inflammation

Coughing

(see also Respiratory tract diseases, Cold diseases, Influenza)
Physical level: Lungs (contact, communication, freedom).
Symptom level: Aggression which cannot be communicated in any other way and thus discharges itself physically; barking aggravated coughing, aggressive coughing fits, volleys of coughing; staccato coughing: keeping people at arm's length by coughing, aggressive defence; "coughing up" what one really thinks of someone; →whooping cough: the load of aggression that one is groaning and wheezing under; slight coughing as a means of clearing one's throat: indication that one would like to say something, but cannot get around to it.

Handling: Learning to state one's opinion to others verbally; making oneself aware of the load which the subject of aggression represents; developing more conscious means of expressing aggression: engaging in verbal dispute to the point of developing an effective conflict culture; cultivating conflicts; preferring to seek out the confrontation rather than burying the dispute; taking courageous paths; grabbing hold of red hot irons.
Resolution: Courageous, open(ly, offensive) conflicts.
Archetypal principle: Mars-Uranus (discharge), Mars-Mercury (aggressive expression).

C-Protein deficiency

Physical level: Lung vessels (contact, communication), blood vessels (transport routes of the life force).

Symptom level: C-Protein is one of the factors which keep the blood in fluid form, and thereby prevent →thromboses and →embolisms; this almost always congenital deficiency generally becomes noticeable first through shortness of breath (caused by →blood coagulation, which blocks the vessels of the lungs); this leads in the long term to exhaustion of the heart (muscle) with the danger of (right ventricular) heart failure.

Handling: Homeopathically: getting more out of the blood (the life energy); concentrating and intensifying the life energy; making more out of one's own energy; reducing contact and communication; self-reflection; developing one's own strength and joy for life; owning up to the pressure one is under in the domain of contact and giving way to it, less communication instead of less breath; allopathically: keeping one's life flow in motion, flowing with life; not turning one's heart into a skeleton closet, but instead pouring out one's heart in good time; physically: taking a blood-thinning agent (Marcumar).

Resolution: Placing one's focus in life on life energy and joy for life; making something out of one's own life energy and also showing this outwardly; keeping the life flow in motion, flowing with life; pushing oneself to the limits in relation to (matters of) the heart; wholeheartedly establishing (intact) connections between the inner and outer world.

Archetypal principle: Mercury-Saturn.

Crab-louse infestation

(pediculosis pubis; see also Sexual diseases, Itching)

Physical level: Secondary sexual regions (fertility, desire).

Symptom level: Itchy annoyance in the pubic hair region and sometimes the armpits, also very rarely the eyebrows; picked up through sexual intercourse; unresolved form of fertilisation (instead of passing on sperm organisms, other beasties are passed on instead); conflict in the area leading into the sexual underworld; resistance to the sexual domain (unconsciously) perceived as dirty, or to the partner or to sexual practices perceived as abnormal and perverse; self-chastisement.

Handling: Acknowledgement of one's own desires (perceived as dirty), which even in an impure (dirty) situation, know no bounds ("I'm itching to do it"); keeping the region of physical intimacy clean, finding clean solutions and playing areas for the corresponding desires and fantasies; preferring to let the fantasies wander in "dirty" depths instead; opening oneself up inwardly; preferring to internally run risks and overstep limits instead of allowing oneself to act without boundaries externally; developing a sex life that is full of life in a spiritual sense instead of picking up unpleasant life forms.

Resolution: Becoming more open on the decisive spiritual level, but on the other hand, recognising and safeguarding one's own limits outwardly; seeking and letting in stimuli that make one tingle on the mental and spiritual level; achieving challenging communication and fertilisation.

Archetypal principle: Pluto.

Cracked skin

(tears in the skin, chapping; see also Work accident/Domestic accident)

Physical level: Skin (border, contact, tenderness).

Symptom level: Cracks in the skin due to over-stretching or under-nourishing (excessively dry, chapped skin): exposing the outer border to too much violence and giving it too little loving attention; cracked skin and fissures at the anus (→anal fissures): (unconsciously) busting one's ass (for somebody or something); cracked, chapped corners of the mouth: running off at the mouth, talking oneself ragged; "having opened one's trap too wide".

Handling/Resolution: Becoming vulnerable in the figurative sense; approaching one's own skin with care: voluntarily opening one's borders to the outside under pressure and consciously expending the life force (blood).

Archetypal principle: Venus/ Saturn-Mars.

Cradle cap

(see also Skin rash)

Physical level: Skin (border, contact, tenderness).

Symptom level: The baby has problems at its borders: it does not feel sufficiently touched, but by means of the repellent rash tends more to ward off contact; being emotionally neglected; attempt to break through isolation; the baby has difficulties with the transition from being a water-based lifeform in the amniotic sac (scaly like a fish) into this world (of air): it wants to shed its skin, to burst with anger.

Handling: (for jointly-affected parents, whose problems are often reflected by the children): making the mother aware of (possible) feelings of inner aversion; allowing the child to receive plenty of physical contact (nursing), but also paying attention to where it is being smothered too much (emotionally and/or physically); enabling the child to get as much contact as possible at the contact surfaces of the skin as well as contact with other skin, as well as with air, wind, sun, water and earth, sand; (urine therapy).

Resolution: Offering the child and oneself contact and touch.

Archetypal principle: Saturn-Venus.

Cramps

(contractions of the muscles, without the control of the will and in rapid succession without any meaningful result; see also Calf muscle cramps)

Physical level: Musculature (motor, strength).

Symptom level: 1. Permanent cramps (tonic) = permanent tensions without (external) sense; 2. Cramps coming and going (clonic) = continual unproductive alternation between tension and release; strenuous efforts without (discernible) sense or purpose; hardening of the muscles due to exaggerated strenuous effort: e.g. →calf muscle cramps in people who are always on the go and who (often) do not succeed in making the leap to freedom; clinging on tightly to a situation which one cannot stand behind, which one cannot stand, which one does not want; the cramp then very successfully prevents one having to stand up to this situation any further, and clearly shows the previous hard adherence in the hardened musculature.

Handling: Undertaking strenuous efforts without expectation of any result; allowing discharges of tension which have no direct sense or purpose (e.g. as in orgasm or in therapy with connected breathing); transforming permanent tension into alertness and attentiveness; consciously building up tensions and bringing them to the point of discharge; alternating currents (tensions): exercises in switching polarity (e.g. arguing vehemently for 10 minutes in favour of a proposition, and then for 10 minutes against it); acting for the sake of (ritual) action (in Indian philosophy: acting by not acting), practicing the so-called "foregoing fruit" philosophy (Buddhist: Phala varja): making oneself independent of the anticipated fruits of one's work, yet still doing it with commitment and awareness.

Resolution: Recognising and acknowledging the build-up and release of tension as the natural opposite poles of the energy flow.
Archetypal principle: Mars-Uranus/Pluto.

Creutzfeldt-Jakob disease

(probably a human variant of "mad cow disease" [BSE = Bovine Spongiform Encephalopathy])
Physical level: Brain (communication, logistics), central nervous system (news service).
Symptom level: Transmitted by the body's own proteins (prions), which following their slightly-changed construction plan attach themselves to the nerve cells of the brain and force this plan upon it: the nerve cells die off and the brain becomes porous; transmission from brain to brain (operations, transplants); the transmission route from cattle to humans has not yet been demonstrated, but is probable (important in this respect: the feeding of infected sheep carcasses to cattle); the brain becomes porous like a sponge, shows deposits (plaques), and finally shrivels: death in coma; insomnia: no longer being able to find rest, no longer being able to "switch off"; headaches: "racking one's brains", no longer being able to find peace in one's head; signs of loss of motoric control: impairment of all further steps and movements; memory lapses even to the point of complete memory loss: opting out of all responsibility; feelings of numbness in the limbs: insensitivity from the inside outwards; mood fluctuations, outbreaks of aggression extending to depression: being a victim of one's own uncontrollable emotions; →hallucinations with paranoid tendencies: madness, no longer functioning in connection with this world, being tormented by one's own

inner images; disease patterns as a mirror for this society with regard to its treatment of animals.
Handling: (On the part of family members and society; for those affected, the disease pattern is to date without exception fatal): conscious palliative care and preparation for death; owning up to one's responsibility for Creation with all its sentient beings; preventing further steps in the inhumane direction with regard to the (ab)use of animals; seeing through the insensitivity of our times with regard to dependent creatures such as animals; opting out of the madness of our modern worldview (the crazy delusion that everything is doable, which for example, out of greed for profit results in sheep carcasses being foisted as feed onto herbivores such as cattle); admitting to oneself that, in the case of animals bred for slaughter, we also eat the stress and aggression produced in their life and death battle along with their meat; painting oneself clear pictures of the suffering of creatures tormented for human purposes; confrontation with dying in itself.
Resolution: Awareness of one's responsibility for the world and the beings living in it, willingness for transformation.
Archetypal principle: Pluto-Mercury, Mars (slaughter), Neptune (relinquishment).

Crohn's disease

(ileitis terminalis, inflammation of the small intestine; see also Anal fistula, Intestinal fistula)
Physical level: Small intestine/ileum (balance, analysis, assimilation).
Symptom level: Smouldering, creeping conflict in the area for processing reserves in the small intestine; (unconsciously) taking roundabout ways; creating tight situations; feeling oneself to have been cast aside, not

getting one's turn; symbiotic relationship pattern; shutting oneself off from the outside; low self-awareness; following traditional, established paths and patterns in life, getting stuck in accustomed habits; →Fistulas: Going new ways and taking ways out, but in a physical sense and via the back door (back passage), which in hindsight turn out to be even worse (too constrained, no sphincter [shut-off mechanism]).

Handling: Addressing the subject of hidden reserves and the retention of emergency reserves consciously and in an open(ly offensive) way; developing willingness to take (spiritual) roundabout ways; creatively and inventively trying out new ways oneself in the areas of digestion and the processing of life instead of making the intestines seek out new routes; adjusting oneself to tight situations: conscious restriction to the essential; ensuring more restricted and critical shaping of the passageway for what is taken on board or let in; building up a dependable contact to the outer world; setting up connections, creating binding commitments; seeking out and using new communications channels.

Resolution: Following new paths (of processing), accepting roundabout ways as part of the deal, overcoming tight situations; finding one's own way of digesting life.

Archetypal principle: Mercury-Mars.

Croup

Physical level: Larynx (expression, tone [mood]), neck (assimilation, connection, communication).

Symptom level: Conflict-laden swelling of the laryngeal mucous membranes due to diphtheria (croup) and other inflammations (pseudocroup); frequently amongst (city) children who are exposed to a particularly high level of environmental contamination

(and can therefore certainly no longer do justice to the needs of their body): war at (in) one's throat, "risking one's neck"; aggressive conflicts in the areas of the voice and swallowing; never being able to get one's fill: one throat gets fed up with minor battles and skirmishes, which become life-threatening because of their localisation; danger of suffocation: the neck swells shut; inner self-strangulation; no longer being able to cry out because of hoarseness and swelling; no longer being able to swallow because of pains in the area of the swelling; aggressive discharges: typical hoarse croupy coughing; things get a little too tight around one's neck, in fact, too tight to breathe; the connection between the head and body is in danger of being cut off completely.

Handling: (instructions for parents, who are jointly affected): learning to conduct conflicts in an open(ly offensively) way; waging war for survival, defending oneself; having out conflicts in the area of the voice and swallowing; learning to express and forcefully assert one's own opinion; bringing together the needs of the head and body.

Resolution: Getting rid of the aggressions that are at one's thoat by letting them out.

Archetypal principle: Mercury/Venus/Mars-Pluto.

Cruciate ligament rupture

(see also Meniscus injury, Accident)
Physical level: Knee joint (humility), ligaments (cohesion).

Symptom level: If the body is forced to perform movements for which it is not designed, the binds holding it together often tear; in the knee, the cruciate ligaments; typical →sport accident; pushing things too far with the result that one winds up "at the end of one's tether", not getting a grip on one's ambition; demanding the impossible and making the body pay for the mistake.

Handling: Demanding more of oneself mentally, and by all means, even demanding too much of oneself, preferring to expose oneself to trying tests which stretch one's thinking to the limit; bringing more mental instead of physical agility into the game of life or at least bringing one's mind into the sport.

Resolution: Positioning oneself skilfully in the game (of life); kicking over the traces with respect to joy for life and mental agility.

Archetypal principle: Saturn-Uranus.

Cushing's syndrome

(cortisone poisoning)

Physical level: The whole organism is affected.

Symptom level: Wrong priorities (first identify the basic problem, e.g. cortisone over-dosage, adrenal cortex tumour); disproportion in various measures: truncal obesity = scrawny extremities with an overly large body; feigned health: moon face with chubby cheeks (cherub face); feigned strength: bull-neck; personality alienation, spiritual changes (cortisone euphoria).

Handling: Concentrating on and strengthening one's own centre; striving for genuine health from one's own resources (inner doctor); improving one's mood from within oneself through activities which address the basic problem.

Resolution: Achieving one's own strong centre: the calm of the centre, from which strength flows.

Archetypal principle: Moon-Jupiter-Neptune.

Cyanosis

(blue discoloration of the skin; see also Mitral stenosis, Tricuspidal stenosis)

Physical level: Blood (life force), lungs (contact, communication, freedom).

Symptom level: Under-supply of the body's limbs: creeping away into one's inner self, thereby leaving the outer borders under-supplied, neglected and lifeless; invitation to surprise attacks and border infringements.

Handling: Learning to deal more sparingly with one's life energy; bringing one's inner self to life and re-solving inner issues; working from the opposite pole: after one's inner life is secure, coming out and taking care of the borders and contact surfaces to the outside world.

Resolution: Bringing the inner and outer worlds into harmony; creating harmony between one's own demands and those of the outside world.

Archetypal principle: Mars/ Mercury-Saturn.

Cysts

(see also Breast cysts, Ovarian cysts, Corpus Luteum cysts, Neck cysts)

Physical level: Various organs can be affected, e.g. ovaries (fertility), breast (motherliness, nourishment, safety and security, sensuality, desire), thyroid gland (development, maturity).

Symptom level: Self-encapsulating development; usually it is the spiritual element (water) which encapsulates itself, often triggered by spiritual shocks; growth along misdirected paths in the symbolic area related to the affected organ; unproductive secrets which threaten to burst into the open.

Handling: Creating room for one's own wayward development in the

affected domain; putting aside important things for oneself; learning to carefully guard (spiritual) secrets.
Resolution: Tolerance with regard to wayward developments; spiritual growth in the affected area.
Archetypal principle: Moon-Saturn.

Cystitis

see Urinary bladder inflammation

Cystopyelitis

see Urinary bladder inflammation, Renal pelvis inflammation

D

Dactylogryposis

see Flexion of the fingers and toes

Dandruff

Physical level: Scalp (skin = boundary, contact; head = capital of the body).
Symptom level: Shedding one's skin and casting it off; bursting out of one's skin with anger, wanting to get away.
Handling: Voluntarily giving up old layers; shedding one's skin in the sense of renewal.
Resolution: Bursting out of one's (old) skin and treading new paths.
Archetypal principle: Saturn.

Dark, fear of

see Nyctophobia

Daytime sleepiness

see Narcolepsy

Deaf-muteness

see Deafness (below)

Deafness

(see also Hearing, hardness of)
Physical level: Ears (hearing and obeying commands).
Symptom level: The outer world falls silent and no longer reaches one; sinking into a world without tone; in cases of early deafness, the ability to speak cannot develop, resulting in deaf-muteness: not being able to communicate in the conventional way, so the distance and gulf between oneself and the "others" becomes even wider; not being in synch with others, and not letting others share any part of one's own inner world; those who are not in synch with others, easily fall into discord: gruff, grumpy manner of some deaf people; wanting to/being forced to remain in one's own empire; shutting oneself off; the world appears absurd (Latin absurditas = 'deafness'); arming oneself against outside terror: keeping people and the world at arm's length; even after having rejected contact with the world, not wanting to pay attention to others and obey commands; no longer lending anyone one's ear, shutting oneself off from the vibrant world – forcing other people to shout at one.
Handling: Since the ability to listen to the outside world has abandoned one, finding other forms of shielding and protection; listening inwardly instead, paying attention to one's inner voice, which is never silent, and obeying its commands; pricking up one's ears on other levels; perceiving and following the compulsion to get closer to other people; consciously doing without communication and coming clean with oneself; based on the experience of being able to be alone, and ideally being able to be al(l)-one, re-integrating the opposite pole and turning oneself to the outside communicatively by means of sign language or special speech training.

Resolution: Recognising the call to seek the inner silence, which still exists behind one's inner voice; experiencing self-sufficiency and finding the solution in oneself, in one's own centre.

Archetypal principle: Saturn-Saturn.

Death, fear of

see Anxiety, Depression, Sleep problems

Debility

(oligophrenia; low-grade mental deficiency)

Physical level: Brain (communication, logistics).

Symptom level: Intellectually challenged, but often as if to compensate, a great depth of feeling and rich emotionality.

Handling: (For parents, carers): accepting the fate-ful intellectual limitation of the person concerned that Provide/nce has provided (German word for 'Fate' = Schicksal from schicken = 'to send' and Latin salus = 'health, well-being') and learning to appreciate their different developmental focuses (living life from the emotional sphere; attending to one's own emotional needs; happily restricting oneself to easy tasks).

Resolution: Penetrating into the older, more primordial domains of the human condition and the brain; living as an emotional person; carrying out easy and essential things with love instead of rationality.

Archetypal principle: Moon-Sun instead of Mercury-Saturn.

Deciduous teeth, retention

Physical level: Teeth (aggression, vitality), gums (basic trust).

Symptom level: The second seven-year cycle of life – from primary school to puberty, which serves for the preparation for adult life – drops out; knocking back a development step; remaining a baby face with one's baby teeth; the weapons of childhood do not measure up to the demands of adult life.

Handling: Taking the next development step, putting the Christian bidding of "becoming like a child" into practice, seeking one's inner child.

Resolution: Living the inner child; finding the golden child in oneself.

Archetypal principle: Mars-Moon.

Decubitus

(pressure ulcers caused by lying still for long periods)

Physical level: Skin (border, contact, tenderness); sacrum and coccyx, heel and all areas where the skin covers the bones without any padding.

Symptom level: Lack of movement leads to energy supply (circulatory) disruptions; the outer skin bursts open, and the raw flesh is laid bare: bedsores resulting from laying still for long periods.

Handling: Accepting the externally-imposed resting position and using it for inner movement and agility: flights of imagination, fantasy trips; inner journeys instead of thoughts about the hustle and bustle of the outer world; opening up the inner protective covers instead of the outer skin: doing justice to the inner world that has been exposed; becoming sensitive to all sensory stimuli (having a thin skin); standing behind and accepting one's own weakness.

Resolution: Achieving an inner world filled with life; dissolution of the boundary between the inner and outer worlds (becoming one with all); intellectual-spiritual preparation for the inner world, and then also for the world beyond – making the boundary easier to pass through: opening oneself up for the next step.

Archetypal principle: **Neptune** (opening)-**Saturn** (boundaries).

Deformities

(see also Aplasia)

Physical level: Almost all organs and areas of the body can be affected.

Symptom level: Congenital or acquired malformations, respectively organs or parts of organs that are missing: learning to deal with the fateful challenges or flaws that one has brought along into this life or become afflicted with, respectively learning to get by without what is missing.

Handling: Taking on and facing up to the challenges; recognising mis(s)takes as something that is missing and seeing the opportunity to acquire what is missing on other levels; developing the courage to be different (to proudly show what is lacking); sacrificing all possible forms of perfectionism; becoming modest in the sense of displaying modesty and humility in the face of the power of Fate.

Resolution: Recognising and acknowledging the healing that Fate (Provide/nce) has provided (German word for "Fate" = Schicksal from schicken = 'to send' and Latin salus = 'health, well-being'), which can and wants to help us to develop further.

Archetypal principle: **Saturn/ Pluto.**

Delirium

Physical level: Brain (communication, logistics) as the basis of consciousness.

Symptom level: Breaking down of the fortress wall between daytime consciousness and one's own deeper layers, e.g. due to →poisoning, the effects of drugs: unlived/unexpressed issues force their way in an uncontrolled manner through the intellect into consciousness; thrusting up from below of the shadow/the deepest dark side, which has been kept under too strict control for far too long.

Handling: Exercises which call the wall to the unconscious into question: voluntarily looking into new worlds (of consciousness); finding access to the shadow kingdom; taking unlived dreams and fears for real as well as taking them seriously; confrontation with them in a controllable way; conscious shadow therapy, which carefully penetrates the protective layer between the conscious and the unconscious spiritual levels in order to push on into deeper areas, and which gradually liberates the shadow aspects.

Resolution: Consciously using the exit and entrance to the shadow kingdom; shadow integration in the sense of the Jungian individuation process or reincarnation therapy: self-recognition; consciously accepting the relativity of our "real world".

Archetypal principle: **Neptune-Pluto.**

Delirium tremens

see Delirium, Alcoholism, Hallucinations

Delusions

see Hallucinations, Psychosis

Dementia

(see also Alzheimer's disease)

Physical level: Brain (communication, logistics).

Symptom level: Forgetting on a grand scale: what is temporally closer and more obvious is forgotten immediately, while the more remote past is forgotten more slowly; the central switchboard (the central computer) starts to break down; while the intellect disappears quickly, the faculties associated with experiencing emotions and feelings remain preserved for longer; all responsibility is given up (taking flight), and in fact, must be given up, since one is no longer in a condition to be able to perceive it.

Handling: Giving up the attempt to carry on as before; putting day-to-day matters on the backburner and devoting oneself to the process of coming to terms with the past; it is now only a matter of important relationships, the structures of life; the trivial matters should be ignored (forgotten): everything non-essential (concerning earthly aspects) eventually passes away; the essential aspect (one's spiritual development) remains preserved for a long time; asking the question: "What do I still owe (in) my life?"; placing a lower value on the intellect and reason, perceiving the world beyond the visible and taking it for real as well as taking it seriously; passing on the responsibility to the next in line in the generations; conscious withdrawal to the outbuildings (older parts) of one's mind instead of taking flight; retreat, homecoming.

Resolution: Accomplishing on the intellectual-spiritual level what remains restricted to the brain in the case of dementia: "I tell you the truth, unless you change and become like little children, you will never enter the kingdom of Heaven"; being modest in spirit, becoming simply mindful instead of simple-minded.

Archetypal principle: Mercury-Neptune.

Demineralisation

(mineral loss)

Physical level: Various organ systems and areas of the body can be affected.

Symptom level: Mineral deficiency: the salt of life is lacking; in the case of calcium deficiency: →osteoporosis; calcium and phosphate deficiency: →rachitis; iron deficiency: →anaemia, →iron deficiency anaemia; salt deficiency: →vomiting, profuse sweating.

Handling: Tackling the basic problem on the physical and spiritual level; determining what essential things one is lacking.

Resolution: Providing the salt in the soup of life.

Archetypal principle: Saturn.

Dental fistula

Physical level: Gums (basic trust).

Symptom level: Side passages and cul-de-sacs become preferred; choosing to take roundabout ways in conflict resolution rather than taking the straight and direct route; tendency to changing tack instead of direct confrontation.

Handling: Seeking other and better ways (out), e.g. (homeopathically): more courageous approaches, and often also (allopathically): more diplomatic ones.

Resolution: Finding one's own individual path of conflict resolution; "If you are in a hurry, take a roundabout way" (Eastern proverb).

Archetypal principle: Mars-Neptune.

Depression

(see also Winter depression, Manic-depressive disease, Post-natal depression)

Physical level: All levels of the body can be jointly affected; especially the brain (communication, logistics) in the form of an exaggerated protective reaction in a (stress) situation in which there appears to be no positive outlook.

Symptom level: Suppressed aggression/life energy, which – when directed against oneself – comes to light as →suicidal tendencies, →feelings of guilt or masked in the form of various symptomatic patterns (covert depression); lack of sense and meaning in life, lack of drive, lacking emotional connection to life; suppressed sorrow; suppression of the life energy at a turning point in life; fleeing from the pressure (de-pression in the sense of de-compression); inability to live and inability to die; unresolved (unredeeming) form of return (to God) on the path of life; blocked between rage and sorrow; fear of responsibility, playing dead; unresolved (unredeeming) form of preoccupation with dying (suicidal thoughts) and with the "dark" feminine archetype; regression to a deeper cerebral and development level: letting others care for one like a needy small child; release of tension on the wrong (physical) level: muscular strength declines because the muscles no longer build up any tone; constipation because the intestinal peristalsis becomes weaker; impotence and lack of passion because sexuality also lives from the build-up of tension; shallow breathing and reduced heart performance because the involvement with polarity also suffers on these central levels; inability to adequately let out (express) what is essential, leading amongst other things to a lack of drive (avolition), →fatigue, →lack of appetite, →insomnia, restlessness.

Handling: Attacking one's own defensive walls vigorously and forcefully (directing the fire of self-realisation against oneself); taking a closer look at one's own early traumas, processing them and letting them go; withdrawing oneself from the day-to-day pressure in order to find time for the essential (sense and meaning through contemplation, meditation = the conscious return to one's life centre); conscious turnaround measures in the sense of a resolved (redeeming) retreat in the direction of the centre of the life mandala; venturing into the realm of fear until, having reached the narrowest point of maximum restriction, the expansiveness of realisation opens up before one; learning to respond to the demands (challenges) of Fate; examination of one's own mortality (of the body) with respect to the immortality of the soul: Angelus Silesius - "So du nicht stirbst, bevor du stirbst, du auf ewiglich verdirbst" (= "If one does not die before one dies, one is damned for all eternity"; Tibetan/Egyptian Book of the Dead, Ars Moriendi (The Art of Dying) from The Middle Ages; daring to embark on the (heroic) journey into one's own underworld; conscious confrontation with classical dramas and tragedies; waking up to one's own needs for vital manifestations of life, pragmatic therapy: sleep-fasting (staying up all night, and then resetting the sleeping-waking rhythm); conscious confrontation, both with suppressed sorrow and also suppressed rage.

Resolution: Reconciliation with the rhythm of life: on the one hand with decay, dying and sorrow, and on the other, with rebirth and joy for life; finding the light in the darkness; following one's calling; finding one's own individual sense and meaning in life; following the path of individuation; moving into resonance with love.

Archetypal principle: Moon-Saturn (death)/Neptune (taking flight)/Pluto (pressure).

Dermatitis

(skin inflammation)

Physical level: Skin (border, contact, tenderness).

Symptom level: Conflicts over the border with the outside; confrontations in the area of contact.

Handling: In the case of disease patterns which lead to swellings and thickening of the skin, defending the borders courageously and in an open(ly offensive) way; in the case of disease patterns which lead to cracks, →rhagades (fissures) and other openings in the skin, opening up the borders courageously and in an open(ly offensive) way.

Resolution: Open struggle over the defence or opening up of the borders; successfully protecting one's skin.

Archetypal principle: Venus-Mars/Saturn.

Dermatomycoses

(see also Candidamycosis, Nail fungus, Athlete's foot)

Physical level: Skin (border, contact, tenderness).

Symptom level: Despite the protective shield provided by an acid layer, one's own border fortifications are occupied by brazen and freely-spreading foreign troops: being too weak to defend one's own skin (in the case of weakened state of immunity, e.g. AIDS or long-term antibiotic therapy); all non-living material can fall victim to the fungal infestation (fungi are saprophytes, which live on dead organic matter).

Handling: Opening up one's own borders in the mental-spiritual respect instead of defending oneself; making room for new and foreign elements and making them one's own instead of allowing oneself to be taken over by the foreign; yielding(being devoted) in relationships, but also learning to define one's own boundaries; dealing with the issue of freeloading; opening up one's own areas that are no longer used and consequently no longer needed, i.e. lifeless areas that have died off, to new and different life impulses; allowing oneself to get involved and dealing with stimulating matters at the outer contact surfaces in a courageous and open(ly offensive) way; concrete exercises: getting to know foreign elements and people; getting involved with what is foreign and confronting it critically in an open(ly offensive) way; taking in vital (living) nourishment, which the fungi cannot make use of, but which the body can transform into living structures; making oneself aware of the daily possibility of choice: either nourish the fungus with dead nourishment that has no nutritional value, or oneself with vital (living) nourishment.

Resolution: Allowing foreign impulses and life forms to get close to one's borders, getting to know them, accepting them, and integrating them into one's own life; also allowing in other views of the world; creating one's own living terrain (in consciousness) without dead areas.

Archetypal principle: Venus/Saturn (Haut)-Pluto (Pilz).

Dermatomyositis

Physical level: Skin (border, contact, tenderness), musculature (motor, strength).

Symptom level: Severe general illness with swelling and reddening of the skin, spreading muscle pains and gradual →atrophy of the musculature; no longer managing to feel good in one's own skin; conflicts over one's own borders and desires for contact; conflicts over (mental-spiritual) mobility.

Handling: Dealing with the definition of one's own borders, articulating one's desires for contact and courageously asserting them, or consciously withdrawing them; offensively marking out one's own scope for free movement, battling to determine the field of one's own influence.

Resolution: Taking courageous steps towards self-realisation in order to be able to feel good in one's own skin and about one's scope for free movement.

Archetypal principle: Saturn-Mars/ Neptune.

Dermoid cysts

see Teratoma

Deviated septum

Physical level: Nose (power, pride, sexuality).

Symptom level: One side is preferred over the other; inherent one-sidedness in life, either with emphasis of the left feminine or right masculine half: functioning better on one side (getting more air [life force - Prana]); one-sided flow of exchange and communication.

Handling: Preferring to be more involved with the favoured side (just like one's breath); initially putting aside the other side; reflecting and relying on one's strong sides.

Resolution: Using the strength which springs from one pole and thereby resolves it to bring the opposite pole into life: bringing oneself back into alignment.

Archetypal principle: Mars-Saturn/Uranus.

Diabetes

see Diabetes (mellitus)

Diabetes (insipidus)

(insipid diabetes)

Physical level: Kidneys (balance, partnership), urinary organs (waste water channels).

Symptom level: Inability of the kidneys to concentrate the urine as the basic problem: great quantities of spiritual energy (unconcentrated urine [close to water quality]) are lost; tremendous thirst for the spiritual (water of life).

Handling: Interpret and clarify the basic illness or problem (kidneys = balance, partnership); letting out the spiritual element: in the relationship area, letting go of energies and allowing them to flow; taking up much more of the spiritual element.

Resolution: Intensive spiritual exchange to unburden the body with regard to this subject.

Archetypal principle: Moon-Mercury.

Diabetes (mellitus)

(diabetes from the Ancient Greek for 'siphon' and 'sweet'. and mellitus from the Latin for 'honey')

Physical level: Pancreas (aggressive analysis, sweet enjoyment).

Symptom level: Several different forms can be distinguished 1. The possibly genetically-determined Type I: slow or sudden exhaustion of insulin secretion even to the point of complete insulin deficiency (IDDM = Insulin-Dependent Diabetes Mellitus, insulin-dependent or juvenile diabetes mellitus);

2. Type II, which is usually acquired due to an unhealthy lifestyle (→obesity), and is often non-insulin-dependent (NIDDM = Non-Insulin-Dependent Diabetes Mellitus); according to the WHO, the burgeoning epidemic of our times (along with obesity, which it often co-occurs with);

3. Gestational diabetes (GDM). a kind of "love diarrhoea" (love just goes straight through one): fear/ being scared shitless of love; not being receptive in matters of love (the cells do not open themselves to the glucose); often a desire to enjoy sweet things (love) and the good (sweet) life, coupled with the inability to accept love and let it in completely; not being able to absorb the sweetness of life, that is, not being able to let it in to one's innermost level (of the cells); not letting oneself get involved with love; unacknowledged desire for the fulfilment of love; tendency due to the inability to love to become a sourpuss (overacidity); not having learnt to give love; not trusting oneself/not having the courage to actively approach the domain of love; basic discord/dissatisfaction with life.

Handling: Recognising one's fear and restrictiveness with regard to matters of love; owning up to one's inability to allow love into one's innermost level (sugar into the cells); learning to avoid unresolved (unredeeming) levels of love, respectively shutting oneself off from them; experiencing closeness and distance more clearly and getting what is unloved off one's back in order to be able to let in enjoyment; setting one's own boundaries on the spiritual level and learning to say 'no'; working from the opposite pole: opening oneself up to love in the physical, mental and spiritual respect.

Resolution: Finding the happy medium between taking in and giving away; allowing emotional dependence instead of becoming dependent on insulin or dialysis on the physical level; recognising and living giving and taking as the two sides of love and reality; enjoying the sweetness of life in the figurative sense.
Archetypal principle: Venus.

Diarrhoea

(see also Vomiting and diarrhoea, Traveller's diarrhoea)
Physical level: Small intestine (analysis, assimilation), large intestine (unconscious, underworld).
Symptom level: Not (being capable of) absorbing what life has to offer, allowing opportunities and chances to slip by; over-abundance of (detailed) analysis and criticism, finding something wrong with everything, and not wanting to take in anything (voluminous small intestinal fits of diarrhoea); allowing impressions to slip through undigested; succumbing to one's fear and simply "letting things run their course" in the privacy and silence of the toilet /bathroom; the salt of life and the spiritual fluid of water are sacrificed in order not to absorb what one had pretended to like; existential fears, "being shit-scared" or "scared shitless", "shitting one's pants in fear"; fear of life; lack of flexibility (loss of fluid); unsuccessful desire for retention (tenesmus); regression to early childhood behaviour: "little shit", being entirely open and receptive like a child; cleansing, jettisoning of ballast (enema).

Handling: Taking a critical look at one's own critical tendencies as well; fasting; voluntarily and consciously not absorbing anything material; learning to consider things impartially, and to let some things pass through unchecked; developing willingness to sacrifice and learning to give (presents) voluntarily; facing up to the very depths of one's fear and thereby transforming the fear into expansiveness and openness towards one's existence; making room for one's inner child on the level of consciousness; letting go of excessive demands and tests of courage (→the traveller's diarrhoea of globetrotters); broadening oneself (one's mind), becoming flexible, letting things run their course; being honest ("dropping one's trousers") and admitting the pressure one is under.
Resolution: Allowing what must happen to happen; practising Uppekha (serenity): not giving a shit about the result; finding clarity and structure, discovering the core of one's own being.
Archetypal principle: Mercury (small intestine) - Pluto (large intestine) - Uranus (diarrhoea).

Diathesis, haemorrhagic

see Bleeding tendency

Digestive complaints

(see also Drum belly)
Physical level: Digestive organs (Buddhism: Bhoga = "consuming and digesting the world").
Symptom level: 1. Disorders with: Absorption of external impressions; 2. Differentiation between agreeable/disagreeable impressions (analysis); 3. Processing of impressions (assimilation); 4. Excretion of the indigestible.
Handling: 1. Openness and expansiveness in the absorption of external

impressions so that the body is not forced to absorb everything itself; 2. Focussed, properly-attuned analysis and differentiation of impressions; 3. Making good use of the absorbed impressions and information (starting from good selection of material and immaterial elements through good chewing [processing] and digestion to problem-free letting go); 4. Complete and rapid excretion of indigestible remains.

Resolution: Consciously taking for oneself what one needs for development, avoiding what is superfluous and harmful and willingly letting go of any remains.

Archetypal principle: Mercury-Pluto.

Diphtheria

(contagious disease, which in recent times has once again started to increase in frequency)

Physical level: Particularly the area of the throat (assimilation, defensive ring) and tonsils (police stations); due to the toxins, however, also damage to the heart (→myocarditis), circulation (→collapse) and nervous system (→paralysis).

Symptom level: Massive communications conflict; not being able to articulate one's needs, swallowing everything and not expressing anything; war over the entrance gate to the inside of the body; thick, inflamed coatings in the neck and throat: not being able/willing to swallow any more because of the pain; danger of extension of the conflicts to the heart: myocarditis = battle for the heart; to the nerves: paralyses = strike in the communications area; danger of circulatory failure: no longer taking part in the cycle of life; danger of shutting oneself off forever from polarity (life in this polar world) (death through suffocation); sweet-smelling mouth odour produced by the inflamed coatings which is specific to the illness:

tendency to sickly-sweet, phony communication.

Handling: Displaying readiness for combat at the admissions area (entry): "What should be let into my life, and what not?"; making oneself aware of how much swallowing hurts one, that one has swallowed enough and that one is no longer willing to do so ("I can't take it any more" = realisation and cry for help by the child); consciously closing up and shutting oneself off; consciously taking up the battle over matters of the heart; offensively defending communications and contact areas; actively dealing with polarity; learning to formulate one's own needs more charmingly and pleasingly, but nevertheless resolutely.

Resolution: Courageously waging the battle of life, risking conflicts over the sphere of admissions (entry); courageously deciding by oneself what one lets in; formulating and communicating one's demands on life in an appealing way.

Archetypal principle: Venus/ Saturn-Mars.

Discharge, Vaginal

(Fluor genitalis, leucorrhoea (Fluor albus); see also Vaginal inflammation)

Physical level: Vagina (commitment, desire).

Symptom level: Primarily often the result of incorrect or excessive hygiene (genital sprays, vaginal douching, tampons); usually the result of conflict (→inflammation) in the vaginal or womb area: the "debris of war" is disposed of in this way; bloody discharge: suspicion of life that is foreign to the body (mutation, →cancer) in this (subject) area; cleansing attempt of the sexual underworld, disgust due to the uncleanliness of the partner; having a blocked-up nose on the lower level (vaginal catarrh);

the possibly-repellent smell of the discharge reveals how much the situation stinks to the woman; the man can and should also note that a problem here "stinks to high heaven"; (unconsciously) making oneself unattractive; (wanting) to get rid of something (superfluous).

Handling: Forcing the processing/disposal of the fragments and debris of ongoing conflicts in the sexual domain into consciousness; if life energy is being discharged via this flow, searching as quickly as possible for forms of life that are alien to one's being in this subject area (and also, as always, seeking medical clarification!); keeping the sexual area clean (mental-spiritual clarity and purity); mustering the courage to send the partner off to wash before a visit on this level; bringing everything into flow again in the sexual area; coming out of one's shell.

Resolution: Consciously letting go of what is no longer needed (letting it flow away); ensuring order with regard to this sensitive issue (this sensitive area of the body).

Archetypal principle: Venus/Moon-Pluto.

Disgust

Physical level: Stomach (feeling, receptiveness).

Symptom level: Physical revulsion, pronounced rejection; fearful reminder of the transience of earthly things and one's own bond with the Earth; resistance with regard to decay and the return to Mother Earth.

Handling: Learning to articulate unwillingness; verbally giving vent to one's disgust; exercises aimed at recognising all Creation as transient.

Resolution: Acceptance of one's own physicality; reconciliation with one's own inevitable physical degeneration with advancing age and the decay of the body after death.

Archetypal principle: Pluto-Saturn.

Dislocation

(see also Accident, Work accident/Domestic accident, Sport accident, Traffic accident)

Physical level: Joints (mobility, articulation), musculature (motor, strength).

Symptom level: Putting oneself out of joint in order to still achieve something unachievable after all: "over-stretching oneself", "bending over backwards".

Handling/Resolution: Putting oneself out of joint on the mental-spiritual level in order not to overload the body.

Archetypal principle: Mars-Uranus.

Diverticulitis

(acute inflammation of intestinal pouches; preceded by →diverticulosis)

Physical level: Large intestine (unconscious, underworld).

Symptom level: On the basis of holding back and holding onto unconscious contents, many small conflicts occur in the area of the "hoarding" pouches of the intestines.

Handling: Open(ly offensive), courageous dealing with unconscious contents (aggressively carrying one's conflict readiness down into the darkest, most remote corners of the shadow kingdom); asking oneself what one is storing like a hamster in these "hoarding" pouches.

Resolution: Open(ly offensive) combat readiness with regard to one's own dark reserves.

Archetypal principle: Mars-Pluto.

Diverticulosis

(chronic existing pouch formation in the intestines)

Physical level: Large intestine (unconscious, underworld).

Symptom level: Small waste heaps in dark corners, "hoarding" pouches, money socks for "savings", toxic waste dump: need for security, frugality, restrictiveness, unacknowledged desire for hidden reserves; on the basis of holding back and holding onto unconscious contents, many small conflicts can occur in the area of the "hoarding" pouches (→diverticulitis).

Handling: Allowing oneself more reserves, including those that are superfluous, such as ballast materials in the diet; putting something aside in one's own house or at the bank instead of creating hiding places in the intestines; dealing with unconscious contents (looking into the dark corners of the unconscious) in an open(ly offensive) and courageous way: cleaning up one's own basement – the inner basement with psychotherapeutic intentions, the outer basement as part of a ritual.

Resolution: Coming to terms with one's own need for security and savings on the appropriate levels; finding security on other levels, e.g. through self-esteem.

Archetypal principle: Pluto-Venus.

Dizziness

see Balance disorders

Double chin

(see also Obesity)

Physical level: Neck (possession, connection, fear), chin (strong will, forceful assertion).

Symptom level: Claim to doubly-forceful assertiveness in the case of a prominent chin (e.g. Ludwig Erhard, the driving force behind the German economic miracle, famed for his multiple chins); physically-manifested insatiability: "never being able to get one's fill", claim to power, "puffing oneself up"; in the case of the opposite pole with a less prominent chin: allowing all will to become mired in soft fat; plump and cosy nature, weakness of will, softness, indulgence.

Handling: Doubling one's efforts and being pig-headed in pushing through one's will; satisfying the hunger at more demanding levels; carrying weight (importance) instead of becoming weighty; transferring the softness to more sophisticated levels: e.g. developing a soft, sympathetic heart; creating a soft, harmoniously-flowing connection between top and bottom.

Resolution: Creating an impression, having a strong will and carrying weight on the mental-spiritual level; defining oneself more clearly in the figurative sense, practising Bhoga (consumption of the world) and consciously consuming the karmic fruits.

Archetypal principle: Mars (forceful assertion)-Jupiter (abundance).

Double vision

See Seeing double

Down's syndrome

(Trisomy 21; previously commonly referred to as "mongolism" because of the Asian-looking slant of the eyes)

Physical level: In every cell nucleus, the 21st chromosome is doubled, creating an entirely different type of person (having too much of something central and basic); numerous deviations from the normal and usual brain development; connective tissue weakness with extreme over-extensibility of the joints; a range of outer indications such as hooded eyelids, transverse palmar creases of the hand, "sandal creases"; frequently heart defects.

Symptom level: Too much genetic substance: "less would be more"; mental handicap in the sense of intellectual disadvantagement, but often as if to compensate, great depth of feeling and rich emotionality; often a natural connection to the highest of all emotions – to love; weak extremities prevent the usual contact with the world: it is difficult to bring the world closer, moving forward (progress) is hindered and slowed down; work is restricted to simple tasks: usually unwillingness to perform; instead of maturation and differentiation, which allow one to increasingly take shape away from an original state of uniformity, remaining strongly underdeveloped and thus staying frozen in the collective form, diminished individuation; a new form of humanity: overall gestalt that is harmonious in itself, not actually handicapped; corresponds to a foetus having become capable of life (the "bun in the oven" was not fully "baked", not fully formed), the gestalt formation has remained at this stage of pre-configuration, diffuse, largely unstructured, the cognitive moulding/imprinting pressure is lacking; congenital acromicria = differentiation of the extremities of the body (nose, fingers, etc.) fails to materialise; →low blood pressure: low pressure behind everything; few goal-oriented actions, everything remains suspended for a long time in the process of carrying it out; speech: undifferentiated, unclear, indeterminate, inadequate conciseness; abstract thinking capacity – the pinnacle (highest point) of our thinking functions – is, like all other points, not fully formed; the world with all its differentiations remains locked away; the child (and also the adult) is hardly able to be self-reflective; of the three gestalt qualities – structure, quality and being – the structure is the most strongly affected by the regressive tendency, and these regressive tendencies become increasingly pronounced throughout the course of life. Handling: For the affected person (them)self-(evident): accepting the fate-ful intellectual limitation that Provide/nce has provided (German word for 'Fate' = Schicksal from schicken = 'to send' and Latin salus = 'health, well-being') and looking for other development priorities: living out of the emotional sphere, doing justice to (one's own) emotional needs, willingly letting oneself become involved with simple things and tasks, being allowed to remain a child for longer and enjoying the Moon principle. For affected parents, educators: a Down's child, like every (healthy) child, brings compensation into life (offsetting what is missing) with the tendency of bringing the family into balance; an intellectual focal point often acquires a counterweight: the magical world view of the Down's child; one's own attitudes and expectations are corrected: the child is not the image of its parents, but brings something with it that is completely its own; it is like neither of the parents, but has its own (Down's) family, whose other members it resembles, irrespective of race, even apes can be affected; it represents a much greater and unfamiliar task and challenge; a child from another kingdom ("mongolian") and another time (the dawn of humankind, life before development of the intellect); tasks that result from this: putting performance expectations into perspective; examining one's faith in one's own fate in life; recognising and accepting life as something which ultimately cannot be planned; showing reverence for all life: those who wanted an exceptional child get it (sometimes in this challenging way); those who wanted a child particularly urgently get a particularly childish one, which remains a child long beyond the normal time and should be able to expect the corresponding care.

Resolution: Accepting the mental handicap and turning it into an opportunity: willingly allowing oneself to be hindered in intellectual games; penetrating more deeply into the

older, more primordial domains of humanity and the brain; standing up for one's status of being outside the norm: being an outsider in a self-confident way; consciously living as an emotional person: opening up in the area of naïve, more primordial sensory perception; doing simple and essential things with love instead of with intellect: putting into effect the rule of the Benedictine monks "Ora et labora" ('Pray and work'); redeeming simplicity: closeness to unity is often maintained in the form of heart defects (→heart septum defects); following Christ's words "Blessed are the poor in spirit, for theirs is the kingdom of Heaven"; trisomy sufferers were regarded by the Aztecs as holy, probably because they interpreted their simplicity as direct affinity with the divine; even amongst us, after the initial shock, the children become to some parents their "angel", "sunshine" or "gift from Heaven".
Archetypal principle: Moon-Pluto, Mercury-Neptune.

Drooping belly

(see also Obesity, Fat belly; also used in gynaecology for the situation in which the mother's pelvis is too narrow and the child remains completely outside the pelvis, causing the stomach to droop downwards)
Physical level: Stomach (feeling, instinct, enjoyment, centre).
Symptom level: Finding oneself difficult to bear; simultaneously signalling power (the large paunch) and powerlessness (the heavy load that one is dragging around); taking pride in one's own weight(iness).
Handling: Integrating the mental-spiritual which has been taken in; allowing oneself the feeling of just letting it all hang out; conceiving ideas instead of looking like one has conceived due to overeating; letting one's own

weight(iness) hang out at levels that are less difficult to bear.
Resolution: Realising power, influence and weight(iness) on less physical levels.
Archetypal principle: Jupiter.

Drop foot

(pes equinus)
Physical level: Feet (steadfastness, deep-rootedness).
Symptom level: Arises when the feet are held in an overstretched position for a long time; the Achilles tendon can end up being permanently shortened in this way; those affected then have to walk on tiptoe: problems with one's stand(point), missing the point.
Handling: Consciously re-assessing and questioning one's own standpoints; becoming more careful in one's standpoints; stepping forward in a more delicate and elegant way (in the figurative sense); claiming less space for one's own position.
Resolution: Hitting the mark at the central point (in the mandala of life).
Archetypal principle: Neptune.

Drop hand

see Hand problems

Drug addiction

(see also Addictions, Pharmacomania)
Physical level: Particularly frequently the brain (communication, logistics) and the liver (life, evaluation, reconnection).
Symptom level: Seeking – Fleeing – Becoming hooked: stopping too early in one's search, respectively taking flight; remaining stuck on a substitute level (the word addiction comes from Latin addictus, pp. of addicere 'to deliver, award, yield, devote oneself'); inner emptiness; feeling of being inadequate, coming up short: seeking a substitute in drugs, numbing the

feeling of deficiency with these, using drugs to make oneself believe the substitute sensation is the actual objective; projection of the ultimate objective of unity onto something more easily reachable; dangerous attempts at finding shortcuts; attempt to make things very easy on oneself; assimilation of the substitute, which cannot be satisfying in the long term; taking a wrong path on the way to the objective; lack of frustration tolerance (not having learned to process defeats and deal with rejection); fear of new experiences; too much convenience (laziness), over-the-top expectations regarding one's own well-being, overly child-like or even childish attitude to life = too little longing for (spiritual) healing/ wholeness.

Handling: Making oneself aware of one's tendency to take inappropriate shortcuts; taking part in searching rituals: seeking a vision, meditation exercises: Zen, etc.; exercises enabling the definition of one's own goal in life; acquiring better frustration tolerance, e.g. through psychotherapy: recognising that only that which one achieves oneself through conscious effort has any transformational character (in colloquial speech: "No pain, no gain"); in therapeutic processes, letting oneself encounter the fear until it is transformed into expansiveness and courage; learning to stand up to things instead of backing down and taking flight; recognising that the greatest commitment is required in order to realise the highest objective (unity): learning to recognise that this is the actual objective in the states that can be brought about by taking drugs; impelling disillusionment to the forefront: recognising the illusory world (of a drug-induced high) for the illusion that it is; uncovering regressive tendencies (wanting to have something without paying the price); reviving one's original motivation for

taking drugs (longing to be one and feelings of unity).

Resolution: Understanding life as a journey, becoming a seeker again; discovering unity as the ultimate objective: perceiving meditation and religion (reconnection) as vehicles towards this objective.

Archetypal principle: Neptune.

Drugs – individual critique

(It should be borne in mind that in a society which has ceased to be a culture, and which has lost sight of the search, almost everything can become a drug, e.g. work, possessions, gambling, sex, etc.; →addictions)

1. Heroin

Symptom level: Total escape from the confrontation with the world; feeling of invincibility; dangers: enormous addictive potential, slide into drug-related crime,→ AIDS (due to infected needles), brain atrophy, degenerating to the level of a parasite (living off society or family members).

Handling: Daring to embark on the true heroic journey (heroine, heroes); undertaking more sensible attempts at becoming grown-up, adult and strong; learning to take back projections (e.g. holding the parental home, society, etc. responsible for one's own misery).

Resolution: Experiencing unity (through religious rituals) instead of fleeing from polarity via the "Golden Shot" (overdose).

Archetypal principle: Neptune-Pluto.

2. Alcohol (see also Alcoholism)

Symptom level: Double self-deception because it is a legal drug; typical escape drug (having a skinful); feeling that the world is well-rounded; softening effect: avoidance of the hardness of life; regression to the child level: lurching, babbling, clinging to the bottle; dangers: →Cirrhosis of the liver, nerve damage,→ Delirium, social decline.

Handling: Searching for other levels of experience, which, although more demanding in terms of effort, cater for the legitimate need for giving in (devotion), softness and roundness, openness, courage, joyfulness and ecstasy.

Resolution: Immersing oneself in the sea of unity, instead of going under and drowning in alcohol: spirituality (from Latin spiritus) instead of spirits.

Archetypal principle: Neptune-Moon.

3. Cocaine

Symptom level: Hunger for success and love; success is misunderstood as love; enormous, supernatural performance capability with elevated mood on stage, in bed and wherever one's own energy is not adequate (any longer); drug of top performers; used as a creativity booster in artistic circles; dangers: nervous breakdown, over-exploitation of body and soul.

Handling: instead of snorting one line after the other, bringing one's life into line; enhancing performance in a natural way: strenuous, but healthy fitness training; finding ways to attain one's own performance potential using one's own resources; learning that creativity can also be developed through hard work; learning to see through the misconception that applause and success have anything to do with love.

Resolution: Dealing conclusively with inner obstacles on the way to self-development by oneself; independent of success and artificial aids, becoming one with oneself and a loved one.

Archetypal principle: Neptune-Sun/Mars.

4. Amphetamine, Speed and other uppers (stimulants)

Symptom level: Increasing the speed of one's overall life feeling (more and more, ever faster, changing impressions); wanting to make more out of oneself and one's time (artificial performance enhancement); dangers: nervous breakdown, over-exploitation of body and soul.

Handling: Becoming more instead of living at a faster pace; experiencing more in the sense of going into things more deeply; natural performance improvement drawn from one's own resources.

Resolution: Experiencing a state of being, in which the highest speed and absolute calm are one.

Archetypal principle: Neptune/Uranus-Mars.

5. MDMA (Ecstasy, disco drugs)

Symptom level: Artificial ecstasy due to the release (pouring out) of all available serotonins into the synaptic gap; opening of the heart chakra in order to feel oneself in love (feeling of having arrived at the objective); form of spiritual masturbation; dangers: circulatory collapse with potentially fatal consequences when combined with vigorous exercise and not drinking enough (e.g. in techno-discos where Ecstasy is sometimes cheaper than mineral water).

Handling: Finding natural ways to open the heart: ecstatic love; letting oneself become truly involved in relationships (from heart to heart); living with a sense of community and solidarity.

Resolution: Through the process of loving another person, the world, experiencing oneself as one with all, peak experiences, experience of unity.

Archetypal principle: Neptune-Venus/Sun.

6. Valium and other (originally) medically-prescribed drugs (mother's little helper, sleeping pills, performance-enhancers, antidepressants); see also Pharmacomania

Symptom level: General: lightening of the mood, "being in better spirits", depending on the drug: suppression of day-to-day reality (Fluctin/Prozac = medication that belongs to the latest antidepressant generation of serotonin-resorption inhibitors, pharmacologically similar to Ecstasy, since the latter also increases the serotonin availability in the synaptic gap, just with lesser effect), lightening of the mood (Lexotanil), performance enhancement (Kaptagon), relieving anxiety (Valium); dangers: to a certain degree, high addiction potential; people affected are often lulled into a false sense of security because they have obtained their addictive drug from a doctor; increased suicidal tendency.

Handling: Learning to tackle the corresponding issues in a more sophisticated/effective way using one's own resources.

Resolution: Experiencing happiness using one's own resources; coping with life "the hard way" way using one's own resources and own commitment; considering obstacles as natural tasks and challenges along the path of life instead of refusing to accept difficulties and always immediately calling for help; looking first and foremost for the helping hand at the end of one's own forearm, and only then for the one from other people, and under no circumstances, the helping hand in chemical form.

Archetypal principle: Neptune-Mercury.

7. Cannabis products (hashish, marihuana)

Symptom level: Lulling feeling of safety and security; taking flight from harsh reality; increased sensibility for music and feelings; intensification of one's overall mood; artificial merriment (fits of foolish giggling, etc.); can loosen (stiff) tongues; low addictive potential, but danger of social disintegration, which is usually fancifully exaggerated; inner softening: becoming increasingly limp, lacking drive and a

will of one's own (in a negative sense) ("jellyfish-like existence").

Handling: Seeking security in interpersonal relations; developing more resolved (redeeming) communal rituals (the passing round of the joint is strikingly similar to the passing round of the peace pipe amongst American Indians and has a similar significance); increasing sensibility through alert awareness; exercises related to confronting reality; increasing the intensity of life in a natural way (e.g. through interesting work).

Resolution: Experiencing genuine security; also being able to see the wonders of life soberly and take pleasure in them.

Archetypal principle: Neptune-Neptune-Moon.

8. Psychedelic drugs (LSD, Mescalin, etc. – "hippie drugs")

Symptom level: Attempt to push forward into transcendence; breakthrough to other consciousness levels (hallucinations); search for the true inner reality; longing for initiation into the ultimate reality; sudden, unexpected break-ins, respectively breakthroughs into the unconscious extend even to the point of psychotic (shadow) experiences (horror trips); searching for adventure in the sense of becoming grown-up; dangers: only a very low addictive potential; practically no physical dependency; nevertheless, through the triggering of psychotic episodes, potentially permanent blockage of the access to one's own shadow via honest, and in the long term, more effective, but also strenuous paths.

Handling: Meditation exercises in order to arrive at results that are honest due to having been achieved from one's own resources and commitment; learning to be patient until one has reached the point where one is able to receive the gift of the longed-for experiences; psychotherapy in order to reconcile oneself

with the shadow, before it visits one unexpectedly in the form of a horror trip; meditation and spiritual exercises in order to experience one's own, and at the same time, collective Archetypal spiritual imagery in an honest and well-dosed way; for late hippies: seeking initiation into being grown-up. Resolution: Genuine initiation experiences.
Archetypal principle: Neptune-Uranus-Jupiter.

Drum belly

(see also Drooping belly, Obesity)
Physical level: Stomach (feeling, instinct, enjoyment, centre).
Symptom level: Overblown dignity; puffed up weightiness (importance); false foodstuff instead of healthy vital nourishment (fast food = animal feed for humans?); insufficient pre-digestion in the mouth, insufficient chewing: wolfing down food instead of eating a nourishing meal; dysbiosis (disharmony) in the intestines, which form one of the basic foundations of life for humans (according to F. X. Mayr, death lies in the intestines, which in any case is undisputed in symbolic terms [large intestine = realm of the dead of the body]).
Handling: Letting off steam; developing weight(iness) on the figurative level; when eating, making the change from ensuring pure survival to ensuring life and vitality; digesting life well from the very beginning: chewing thoroughly; ensuring harmony with one's own dark spiritual powers.
Resolution: Taking up the space which one needs to unfold inwardly; finding abundant fullness in fulfilment; reconciliation with the shadow.
Archetypal principle: Moon-Jupiter.

Drumstick fingers

see Hand problems

Ductus Botalli, open

(see also Heart defect, congenital)
Physical level: Heart (seat of the soul, love, feelings, energy centre).
Symptom level: Clinging to an earlier phase (embryonic situation in the womb is held onto): being on the wrong path with one's life force; refusing to enter into the unholy (damned)/unwhole (incomplete) state of polarity.
Handling: Submitting oneself to the game of opposites; practising exchange, communication along prescribed paths.
Resolution: First leaving the childlike situation (of the energy flow), before later reconquering it on a higher level and in the mental-spiritual respect ("Unless you change and become like little children ..." Matthew 18:3).
Archetypal principle: Sun-Moon.

Duodenal ulcer

(ulcus duodeni)
Physical level: Small intestine/Duodenum (analysis, assimilation).
Symptom level: Enormous ambition and the drive to get ahead lead one to tear oneself apart, for example, if one's aggressive addiction to criticism causes one to pick all thoughts to pieces down to the very last detail, and if in the battle over every last detail, one loses the overview; biting self-criticism; spreading a corrosive atmosphere around oneself; cry for nourishment and the feminine element.
Handling: Overcoming limits and sacrificing a part of the life force in the process; spoiling oneself with food; creating safety and security; allowing conscious regressions; declaring war on the intellect and its criticism-addicted efforts; living out passivity and surrender.
Resolution: Creating one's own nest for recuperation and regeneration.

Dupuytren's contracture

(see also Hand problems)

Physical level: Hand surfaces (honesty, openness), rarely also the tendon plate of the feet (mobility, progress, deep-rootedness), musculature (motor, strength).

Symptom level: Depending on which hand or foot is affected, this concerns the feminine (left) or masculine (right) way of understanding life; closed hand: no longer being able or wanting to take on anything; holding oneself back from being happy, failing to get a grip on life (the hand shows the cramped attempts); clenched fist: unconscious aggression, hostility; caginess, dishonesty: the open hand would be the honest one; the clutching hand ("closed-fistedness" - greed): no longer being open to life; no longer being prepared to grasp it (mentally or physically); fear, secretiveness; not being able to get a foothold.

Handling: Making oneself aware of the aggression and attempting on the figurative level to get a grip on life, to grasp opportunities and get a firm foothold on the Earth; owning up to one's dishonesty (with oneself or others); confronting one's own greed ("closed-fistedness"): learning conscious giving and taking; venturing into the narrow realm of one's own fear until it is transformed into expansiveness and openness.

Resolution: Owning up to the quality of one's handling of things; entering into life; harmony, the right hand (in German often referred to as die schöne Hand – 'the beautiful hand') results from war (Mars) and peace (Venus); making peace with the world.

Archetypal principle: Mercury-Pluto.

Dwarfism

(official definition: height below 150 cm; see also Stunted growth, and as the opposite pole - Gigantism)

Physical level: The whole body is affected in the full length of its "shortness"; glands (control, information).

Symptom level: Hypophysis, thyroid or gonad disorders (first clarify and interpret the basic situation); for example, reduced secretion of growth hormone as a result of thyroid gland hypofunction leads to little growth in height: standing out due to one's shortness; going under everywhere, keeping a low profile, disappearing, being overlooked; always being the smallest; feeling of having turned out too small for this world (everything is too big and too high); difficulties in finding clothes and shoes which fit: being permanently assigned to the child role (only children's sizes fit); difficulty in taking part in the auto-mobile society, because one cannot simultaneously reach down or reach up far enough to be able to look further ahead; not being able to get close to the important things, to attain them: having to permanently stretch and (over)strain oneself.

Handling: Accepting the task of Fate and also developing inner smallness to match the outer stature: learning modesty and the ability to take a backseat; accepting the inner child and resolving (redeeming) it: instead of struggling against being assigned to what is child-like, accepting and redeeming the wonderful sides of being a child; creating one's own smaller world for oneself: consciously learning to do without the big, wide world; learning to expand oneself and grow inwardly: after having accepted the outer smallness, also conquering the opposite pole: gaining stature inwardly.

Resolution: Learning to face up to one's (outer) smallness (also

inwardly): "small but mighty"; "good things come in small packages"; taking full possession of one's small body, filling it out and accepting it, and then growing beyond oneself in the mental-spiritual sense if one so desires; learning to keep a low profile and disappear also in the figurative sense (bringing together form and content): becoming a Nobody in the eastern sense or like Odysseus with the Cyclops (because Odysseus claimed to be Nobody, he was able to outwit the Cyclops).
Archetypal principle: Saturn (inhibition)-Uranus (singularity).

Dying, fear of

see Anxiety, Depression, Sleep problems

Dysbiosis

(imbalance between useful and pathological bacteria in the intestines)
Physical level: Large intestine (unconscious, underworld).
Symptom level: Disorder (destruction) of the co-existence (symbiosis) between the intestines and their natural bacteria cultures (symbiotes), above all due to antibiotic therapies: →digestive complaints, →flatulence, →diarrhoea.
Handling: Instead of fighting against the inhabitants of the large intestine with antibiotics, preferably going into battle against the dark subjects of one's own underworld with the weapons of light (consciousness); reconciliation of the opposing forces in the shadow kingdom: psychotherapy; conscious nourishment and active rehabilitation of a natural intestine environment; symbiosis control.
Resolution: Being in harmony with the other life forms which bring life to this particular body (microcosm) and that of the Earth (macrocosm).
Archetypal principle: Pluto.

Dyscalculia

(see also Learning disorders)
Physical level: Brain (communication, logistics).
Symptom level: Making systematic errors in the basic methods of calculation due to following a subjective logic; misunderstanding of the world of numbers with regard to quantities; inner chaos with regard to world order, the Harmony of the Spheres; in a world increasingly dominated by numbers, danger of making many miscalculations in life; not being willing/able to commit oneself to fixed values, rejecting masculine structures; fear of encrypted knowledge, number patterns and inscrutable, abstract worlds.
Handling: Finding out what one has a gift for, what one can bring to life, where other focal points lie in the area of talents that one has brought with one (such as in the area of feelings or aesthetic perception); countering the world of numbers, as applies for example, in the economy, with something uniquely one's own, something qualitatively different.
Resolution: Learning to grasp the essence of numbers in the Pythagorean sense; penetrating from quantity into quality; giving the world of numbers and the economy a soul.
Archetypal principle: Mercury-Saturn.

Dysentery

(see also Diarrhoea)
Physical level: Mucous membranes (inner boundary, barrier) of the large intestine (unconscious, underworld).
Symptom level: (Feverish) general mobilisation of the body against enemies that have forced their way into the underworld (dysentery bacteria = shigella); fear: "shit-scared", "having the runs" or "the trots", "shitting one's pants"; "being in a cold sweat" (bloody and slimy (mucoid)

diarrhoea): losing the water and salt needed for life; fleeing into the powerlessness of a blackout (circulatory collapse).

Handling: Courageously taking up the all-embracing and exhausting struggle over the shadow world with every available means; allowing oneself to be stirred up by shadow subjects instead of opening up the underworld to stirring elements in the form of pathogens; recognising one's own restrictiveness/fear and dealing with it consistently and with concentration; giving up essential, existential things; learning to give to the point of self-abandonment; voluntarily surrendering power.

Resolution: Conquering the shadow kingdom and illuminating it with the torch of awareness; transforming fear into consistency and discipline; carrying surrender to its ultimate consequence; laying oneself at the feet of the world; placing all power in higher hands and trusting oneself (to them).

Archetypal principle: Pluto.

Dysmenorrhoea

see Menstruation, painful

Dyspareunia

(pain during sexual intercourse; see also Bleeding after sexual intercourse)

Physical level: Vagina (commitment, desire).

Symptom level: Hot, dry vagina, occurs above all in the second phase of the cycle during which no fertilisation is to be expected; resistance towards a coarse, inept or egoistic partner: "he causes me pain"; rejection of sex which does not lead to procreation of a child; traumatisation of the floor of the pelvis following a birth, or due to rape or abuse; attempt to keep the wrong man at arm's length; alibi in order not to have to sleep with him or allow oneself to get involved with

him; fear of a penis that is allegedly too large.

Handling: Questioning one's fear of giving oneself to another and physical fusion; learning to open oneself up and trust in the masculine; ensuring varied and satisfying love play; learning to say 'no'.

Resolution: Overcoming polarity in the act of orgasm.

Archetypal principle: Venus-Mars.

Dysphagia

(swallowing disorder; see also Achalasia)

Physical level: Gullet (assimilation, defence).

Symptom level: On the basis of a physical obstruction of the passage in the oesophagus, or more frequently, primarily spiritual; unconscious rejection of absorption (of material impressions); choking on something: "taking something the wrong way".

Handling: Learning not to swallow everything, but instead to consciously shut oneself off to some things, to reject what does not agree with one.

Resolution: Taking other, unconventional ways in terms of digestion and one's processing of the world.

Archetypal principle: Venus-Uranus.

Dysphasia

(speech disorder, e.g. in the case of →Alzheimer's disease)

Physical level: Brain (communication, logistics).

Symptom level: Disorientation, losing the thread; having nothing more to say; no longer swinging in the same rhythm with others.

Handling: Dissociating oneself from conventional structures and rules; voluntarily relinquishing all power; attuning oneself to one's own rhythm.

Resolution: Introspection instead of outward orientation.

Archetypal principle: Mercury-Neptune.

Dystonia

see Vegetative dystonia

Dysuria

(disorder of urinary bladder evacuation; see also Anuria)
Physical level: Urinary bladder (waste water reservoir, withstanding and relieving pressure).
Symptom level: Letting go of the spiritual waste becomes more difficult or painful; occurs for example with →prostate enlargement; cramping together instead of opening oneself up.
Handling: Courageous holding back of old spiritual matters in order to finally process them once and for all; subsequent offensive letting go of the spiritual waste.
Resolution: Retaining that part of the spiritual element that is still necessary in order to truly be done with it.
Archetypal principle: Moon-Mars/Pluto.

E

Ear inflammation/ear pains

(see also Middle ear inflammation)
Physical level: Ears (hearing and obeying commands).
Symptom level: Aggressive conflict which is ignited by the issues of hearing, listening carefully and obeying; usually in children around the age of learning to hear and obey commands: "There are none so deaf as those who will not hear"; sudden onset of ear pain: cry for help from the hearing organ; fever: general mobilisation of the defensive forces of the body; hardness of hearing: not wanting to hear or obey: "I'm sick of hearing it"; perforation of the eardrum

with outflow of pus: discharge of the excess pressure from the middle ear cavity; lack of willingness to listen to someone, "to lend someone one's ear"; the poles of egocentricity and humility are out of balance.
Handling: (for jointly-affected parents, whose problems are often reflected by the children): waging aggressive, offensive conflicts over the subjects of hearing, listening carefully and obeying; throwing all available spiritual forces into the struggle over paying attention to commands; learning to obey – both one's own inner voice, but also outer voices; encouraging the closure (occlusion) of the ears to the outside world in favour of turning inwards; encouraging breakthroughs into new niches of consciousness; mastering the golden medium between forceful self-assertion and conforming.
Resolution: Being able to hear inner and outer voices and obeying them.
Archetypal principle: Saturn-Mars.

Ear noises

(tinnitus)
Physical level: Ears (hearing and obeying commands).
Symptom level: Unresolved, internalised stress: noise that has been taken inwards, "being up to one's ears in something"; alarm bells, warning sirens; not having put up a fight, wanting to (inwardly) sort/shut everything out by oneself; one's need for silence is finally made clear by means of the symptom.
Handling: becoming outwardly loud; upholding one's own standpoints, displaying aggressions; learning to listen carefully inwardly; giving in to the compulsion and listening to (one's own) inner tones (the "little voice in one's head"), making peace with it; giving in to the hardness of hearing that often accompanies the complaint and listening less to the

outside world; granting oneself outward silence, bearing the inner noise;
meditations for reconciling oneself
with the goal of becoming inwardly
and outwardly at peace.
Resolution: Granting the inner
voice an audience and obeying its
commands; relying on oneself; being
in harmony with the "inner" music,
which corresponds to the Music of the
Spheres and therefore divine music;
fulfilling the burning need for inner
peace by means of appropriate spiritual exercises; progressing along the
path of individuation.
Archetypal principle: Saturn-Mer-
cury/ Neptune.

Eardrum
inflammation

see Middle ear inflammation (which it
is always connected with)

Eating disorders

see Bulimia, Anorexia, Binge eating
disorder, Obesity, Depression

Eclampsia

(tendency to cramps and convulsions
during pregnancy, late gestosis; see
also Gestosis, High blood pressure,
Cramps)
Physical level: Musculature
(motor, strength), kidneys (balance,
partnership).
Symptom level: Severe fits of
cramping (battling) towards the end of
pregnancy (tonic-clonic cramps of the
skeletal musculature); high pressure
that the mother is under (→high blood
pressure); essential elements are
lost in the partnership (protein loss
in the urine); instead of gaining in
weightiness (importance), she gains
radically in weight; running away from
responsibility (losing consciousness);
danger of stealing away completely
and taking the child with her (fatal
danger to mother and child).

Handling: Risking the great struggle
over the birth; facing up combatively
to the new phase of life and undertaking all necessary efforts; perceiving
the pressure that one is under; owning up to how one's hopes have been
dashed in the partnership; making
oneself aware of one's own importance to the life of the child; withdrawing oneself, being there completely
for oneself and the child: giving the
pregnancy the top priority (healthy
eating and living).
Resolution: Bundling of all one's
strengths, concentration on what is
essential; experiences of unity (between the mother and child).
Archetypal principle: Moon-Pluto.

Ecstasy

(condition of great rapture, considered in psychiatry as pathological;
in reality, not only healthy, but also
close to enlightenment, ultimate deliverance, paradise)
Physical level: Brain (communication, logistics), the whole organism is
affected.
Symptom level: Ecstasy (from Ancient Greek ek 'outside or beyond'
and stasis 'standing still, immobility');
stepping away from stagnation; being
beside oneself, feeling, sensing and
going beyond all boundaries.
Handling: Consciously going with the
life flow; allowing moments of ecstasy
to flow together to form ever longer
periods of bliss.
Resolution: Resonating in harmony
with the energy of the universe, allowing oneself and others to be; all in
one – one in all.
Archetypal principle:
Uranus-Neptune.

Ectopia

(displacement of the mucous membranes and plate epithelium boundary
at the mouth of the uterus)

Ectopic pregnancy

Physical level: Mouth of the uterus (lower mouth).

Symptom level: Conflict between two types of skin/membrane; the mucous membrane of the uterus turns outwards from the inner area, resulting in contact bleeding during sexual intercourse and mucoid →efflux; conflict between the sensitive inner world and the rough outer world; problematic opening up of oneself to the outside; conflict over the desire to have a child; the inside pushes towards the outside and seeks confrontation.

Handling: Courageously coming out of one's shell, offensively expressing one's own desires (for a child); exploring the (unconscious) need for more intimate contact with one's partner; paying more attention to the lower body and the themes related to it; preferring to risk conflict with one's partner spiritually and with his sexual-erotic needs instead of transferring it to the physical level; but also refusing unwanted sexual availability (e.g. with the pill).

Resolution: Letting inner primordial feminine needs come to light and fulfilling them for oneself.

Archetypal principle: Moon-Uranus.

Ectopic pregnancy

(extrauterine gravidity)

Physical level: Usually the Fallopian tubes (fertility, the first slide of life), more rarely the ovaries (fertility), and very rarely the free abdominal cavity (safety and security).

Symptom level: Often a result of Fallopian tubes becoming blocked during youth (→adnexitis): youth problems burden the time of motherhood; as the main cause: also →endometriosis: femininity at an inappropriate level; blockages on the basis of conflicts (physically manifested in →inflammations, possibly due to contraceptive coils) which can extend across generations; the egg implants too early: impatience on the journey and in becoming pregnant, not leaving oneself (or the egg) enough time; fertility in the wrong place (outside the designated womb): misdirected creativity; double bind: on the one hand, wanting to become pregnant, and on the other, not giving the child enough room to live; giving the child (the new life) and oneself no chance; danger of bleeding to death from the pregnancy at the wrong level; in the case of a tubal pregnancy (tubal gravidity), danger of inner tearing (of the tube); is aimed at gaining outside aid (if no spontaneous miscarriage, an operation is often unavoidable).

Handling: Tearing oneself apart (inwardly) for one's desire (to have children); working from the opposite pole: learning patience with regard to one's own desires to have children; waiting for the right time and the right place (right partner?); clarifying unconscious resistances with regard to pregnancy; producing original fruits: being extraordinarily fruitful (fertile) in the figurative sense, spiritual fruitfulness (fertility) at unusual levels; letting the life force flow for a matter of the heart; learning to allow oneself to be helped; accepting help.

Resolution: Waiting for the right moment; going one's own, even unusual, creative ways; allowing one's complete heart energy to flow into a "child" (creativity); having children on other levels (in the figurative sense).

Archetypal principle: Uranus-Moon.

Eczema

(see also Skin rash)

Physical level: Skin (border, contact, tenderness).

Symptom level: Rebellion of the skin, e.g. against dangerous chemicals, but also because the contact (skin) with a dearly-beloved person or animal has been broken off; something from within breaks through the barriers to the outside; something that has been held back or suppressed until this point attacks the border of repression in order to come into view (into consciousness): fearful defence against a conflict pushing to the surface or something new that is transgressing one's boundaries; damage to one's (surface) integrity from inside; the appearance of the pure, honest skin is disfigured by something impure.

Handling: Letting what is inside come out and what is deep down below come to the surface; voluntarily opening one's inner borders to previously-suppressed subjects; allowing oneself to be pushed by repressed elements to greater openness; preparing and arming oneself for injuries from within, e.g. due to realisations rising to the surface; being vulnerable in the sense of sensitive.

Resolution: Impure, dark inner subjects are processed by allowing them to expand outwards and illuminating them with the light of consciousness.

Archetypal principle: Saturn/Venus-Mars.

Efflorescences

Physical level: Skin (border, contact, tenderness).

Symptom level: Skin problems accompanying →childhood diseases, such as measles, scarlet fever, etc.; efflorescences on the skin: something blossoms forth which has been unable to find room in the spiritual domain; the skin bears strange fruits; something comes to the surface in order to gain attention; lack of necessary skin contact with regard to caring attention, tenderness and love.

Handling: Allowing children a time-out period, during which what is bursting to the surface can spread out and also establish itself in consciousness; allowing what wants to get out to blossom in one's own being; showing

oneself in all one's creations and budding forms; exposing what is pushing to the surface and seeking to get out into the light of public view; voluntarily calling one's own boundaries into question and overstepping them of one's own accord.

Resolution: Living up to the new challenges; taking them on and allowing them to help one to push forward.

Archetypal principle: Saturn-Jupiter.

Ejaculatio praecox

(premature ejaculation, often before the penis has even penetrated the vagina; frequently connection with earlier →bed-wetting)

Physical level: Penis (desire, power).

Symptom level: Impatience: wanting too much too quickly; being over-aroused, overly wound up and letting the excessive tension (suspense) fall apart too quickly; prematurity prevents the development of desire on the part of the female partner: depriving her and oneself of the orgasm (the experience of unity); concealed aggression against the woman and unconscious revenge against her; fear of failure, which itself leads to failure.

Handling: Helping one's own creativity to come into play earlier and more quickly; practising conscious waste in other domains; learning to give (gifts) without speculating about potential success and reward: developing generosity and the ability to give freely; making creative investments in advance: allowing one's charm to bubble forth; consciously entering into the realms of fear and restrictiveness, as well as into fantasies of impatience and aggression and experiencing them; letting oneself go to one's heart's desire; working from the opposite pole: learning control in the sense of tantric ideas, but only after desire has been enjoyed freely and without reserve.

Resolution: Allowing oneself to be excited by one's own creative capabilities, and being able to bring these into play at all times; developing enthusiasm for many domains of life and allowing inner arousal to swell.

Archetypal principle: Mars-Uranus.

Ejaculation, premature

see Ejaculatio praecox (above)

Elbow inflammation

see Rheumatism

Elbow pains

see Tennis arm/Tennis elbow

Elephantiasis

(thickening of the skin caused by lymph blockages in the subcutaneous fatty tissue, particularly of the limbs; aspect of the opposite pole to truncal obesity caused by an excess of cortisone)

Physical level: Subcutaneous connective tissue (protection, insulation).

Symptom level: Looking like an elephant: being plump, putting oneself forward in a clumsy way, heavy, lethargic movements, hindered forward progress; problem showing oneself without inhibitions; compulsion to keep oneself covered.

Handling: Building a strong protective wall to the outside, developing a thick skin: no longer allowing everything to come so close to one; learning to screen oneself off; breaking down one's own sensitivity; no longer allowing everything to get under one's skin; learning to defend oneself verbally; putting on a stronger appearance: learning to radiate strength and power; broadening out; gaining weight(iness); strong arms want to bring the world closer; strong legs to conquer it: tackling these subjects in the figurative sense: conquering the world for oneself (particularly frequent amongst women during menopause).

Resolution: Filling up the space that is one's due (e.g. filling the role of the "grand"mother; giving one's own personality more weight; finding calm and composure in oneself (and behind the thick armour of skin).

Archetypal principle: Moon-Jupiter.

Embolism

(e.g. →lung embolism, cerebral embolism; see also Blood clot)

Physical level: Blood (life force), blood vessels (transport routes of the life force).

Symptom level: Hardening of what has been set loose, congealment of what is flowing; sluggish, rigidified vitality solidifies and forms blockage material: obstruction of a channel of the life energy; (self-) hindrance of the life (flow), stopping it above all in the communications area (lungs); putting obstructions and blockades in one's own way; →circulatory disorders in the relevant dependent area.

Handling: Crystallising and extracting something from the flow of life, making something enduring out of it; bringing things to the point of materialisation; allowing oneself more time; slowing down the tempo of life; breaking up the well-established chain of energy supply of the organs/life themes (affected by the embolism); looking after these regions in a new way and with more attentiveness (e.g. after a stroke [cerebral embolism], getting to know the paralysed side of the body again in an entirely new way – in the same way that the supply of blood to the affected opposite hemisphere of the brain must take place by following completely new paths).

Resolution: Life flow; materialisation of ideas and plans.

Emesis

see Vomiting/Nausea, Pregnancy
complaints

Emotion, lack of/ deficiency

see Depression

Empty nest syndrome

Symptom level: Fledglings who have
flown the nest are inwardly not set
free and allowed to head off into life;
severe feelings of abandonment lead
amongst other things to →depres-
sion; falling into a vast emptiness.
Handling: Extending the concern for
one's children to other and ultimately
all children; giving up overprotection
in favour of a second "catch-up" birth,
in which the children are also let go
of in the social sense; developing
independent perspectives for a fulfilled life; filling empty rooms with new
contents.
Resolution: Gratefully accepting and
going through the natural stations
along the path of life; becoming the
Grand Mother/Grand Father; as
"grand"-parents, recognising and
accepting all children as one's own
"grand"-children; loving all children as
the preliminary stage of comprehensive love of thy neighbour (loving all
people).
Archetypal principle: **Moon-Saturn.**

Encephalitis

see Cerebral inflammation

Endangitis obliterans

see Smoker's leg

Endocarditis

(inflammation of the endocardium)
Physical level: Heart (seat of the
soul, love, feelings, energy centre).
Symptom level: Unresolved conflict
in the interior of the heart; aggressive
struggle over the centre of life; being
shaken awake; letting one's heart be
gripped with courage instead of gripping at one's heart in pain.
Handling: Consciously regulating
matters of the heart; decisively
fighting out conflicts; facing up to the
struggle over one's own centre in an
open(ly offensive) and courageous
way; waking up to matters of the
heart and paying attention to them.
Resolution: Courageously fighting
out the decisive struggle in one's own
centre (lion-heart).
Archetypal principle: **Sun-Mars.**

Endocardium, inflammation

see Endocarditis (above)

Endometriosis

(endometrium located outside the
normal dispersal area, e.g. in the vagina, Fallopian tubes, urinary bladder,
in the free space of the abdominal
cavity; also caused by medical inter-
ventions such as curettages).
Physical level: Endometrium (womb
= fertility, security; mucous membrane = inner border, barrier).
Symptom level: (Unconscious)
femininity in the wrong place; one's
own natural rhythm is forced upon
problematic areas (cyclical occur-
rences where they do not belong);
the side effects of femininity occurring
on the wrong level are uncontrollable
(disposal of the waste products of
the cyclical breakdown and renewal
of the mucous membrane are often
only possible surgically); deranged
(= out of place) femininity (typically

feminine activities in an unfitting domain) forces the opposite pole into play ("high-action" surgical medicine as a typically masculine form of manifestation); pain during intercourse indicates conflicts in this area; infertility as a common consequence: femininity on an inappropriate level leads to the blockage of primordial feminine fertility (→ectopic pregnancy).

Handling: Taking femininity to other, unaccustomed levels; extending one's own natural rhythm to other areas of life; problematising and reflecting on the side effects of one's own feminine strength; bracing oneself for the fact that the emphasis of the one pole also always forces the opposite pole onto the scene.

Resolution: Finding new areas to unfold one's own femininity.

Archetypal principle: oon, Uranus.

Endometritis

(endometrium inflammation)

Physical level: Endometrium (womb = fertility, security; mucous membrane = inner border, barrier).

Symptom level: Possible side effect of foreign bodies, such as contraceptive coils; conflict over the nest for one's own children (endometrium); aggressive conflict over the basis of one's own fertility.

Handling: Grappling with the basis of one's own creativity in an open(ly offensive) way; coming to grips with it with respect to forming a nest for one's own children.

Resolution: Fertility.

Archetypal principle: Moon-Mars.

Endometrium inflammation

see Endometritis (above)

Enteritis

see Intestinal inflammation

Enteritis necroticans

see Gangrenous enteritis

Enuresis

see Bed-wetting

Epicondylitis

see Tennis arm

Epidemics

Physical level: In the individual, all parts of the body can be affected; act as a mirror for the consciousness of the collective.

Symptom level: Epidemics are limited in time and with regard to geography, while pandemics spread out over one or more continents: fates shared by the masses which confront many people with the same pattern of tasks, although the reaction to these nevertheless remains largely individual; radioactive irradiation of various parts of the Earth could be regarded as a modern epidemic: admittedly, this is of course not an infection in the classical sense; nevertheless, we are wantonly conjuring up a fate to be shared by the masses.

Handling: The aspects that these similar patterns of fate have in common reveal tasks typical of the times: just as consumption had its heyday, and before it, cholera and plague, the main problems nowadays are →AIDS and →radioactive irradiation.

Resolution: Doing justice to the tasks that are revealed in the disease patterns in terms of archetypal principles; for the disease patterns that are currently a threat due to the unresolved feminine pole (cancer, AIDS, radiation), an essential form of resolution (redemption) would be metamorphosis: radical transformation, respectively metanoia - repentance in the sense of a change of heart.

Archetypal principle: Pluto.

Epididymis, inflammation

(epididymitis)
Physical level: Epididymis (fertility, maturity).
Symptom level: War in the storehouse of the semen; struggle for masculine fertility; danger of infertility in the case of unconscious prolonged conflict (chronic →inflammation).
Handling: Consciously addressing the issues of procreation, starting a family and reproduction in an open(ly offensive) way; struggling inwardly for mature masculinity.
Resolution: Courage to create something new (new life); fulfilling the necessary prerequisites for this purpose.
Archetypal principle: Moon-Mars.

Epididymitis

see Epididymis, inflammation (above)

Epiglottis inflammation

(epiglottitis)
Physical level: Epiglottis (switching point between the respiratory and alimentary tract).
Symptom level: Conflict feared in childhood at the forking of the ways (switching point) between the air passage and food passage; refusal to deal with the discord between material and verbal communication with the outer world (e.g.: "Should I simply swallow everything or protest?"); danger of things going down the wrong way.
Handling: Offensive conflict over the discord between the world of thought and material assimilation: giving children the courage to say what they really want to eat (swallow); ensuring that nothing goes down the wrong way or that they do not catch word of what they still cannot stomach.

Resolution: Learning to courageously shut one's mouth when one has taken in (swallowed) too much; blocking the passage when one is fed up; striving offensively for the ability to distinguish properly; learning to courageously distinguish between the realms of air and earth.
Archetypal principle: Mercury-Mars.

Epilepsy

Physical level: Brain (communication, logistics), nerves (news service).
Symptom level: Discharge of powerful inner (electrical) tensions; all fuses blow simultaneously in a major attack (grand mal) – comparable to an earthquake or medical electric shock therapy; inner blockage discharges itself in convulsive battle waves: being completely beside oneself; exploding: the attack is like an offensive that starts from within a besieged fortress (the patient becomes offensive and abusive); the excess energy that has flowed into the body is expended in waves of convulsions, followed by extreme exhaustion (the organism recovers from the high-voltage experience); in the long term, the excess voltage results in substantial damage to the network of power lines, i.e. the nerves; biting one's tongue: being lock-jawed; preferring to "bite one's tongue" or even "bite it off completely" rather than letting things out of the unconscious shadow kingdom; foaming at the mouth: with rage or high tension; (uneven) struggle between two worlds; bursting of the dam, which brings into motion those aspects of one's being/the shadows that have been held back; paroxysmal break-in of the other world/powerful supernatural forces: being violated by something overpowering; in earlier times, epilepsy was also known as Morbus sacer ('the holy disease') because those affected were thought to be under the influence of a higher

power, which used to be referred to as possession; ecstatic proceedings break into the day-to-day world, presaged by an aura (this is how Dostoyevsky describes his epileptic fits, which he would not have missed for anything in the world): too immense for the soul, which flees for its life (parallels in the Bible, where the direct sight of God is described as being too immense for anyone to endure); unresolved attempt to let oneself go and fall (falling sickness); often over-conformist and anxious to be considered as "normal" at any cost; holding back substantial tensions until they explode; poor connection to one's own dark sides and little flexibility (even a change in lighting conditions from bright to dark can provoke attacks).

Handling: Letting the tensions out and truly living them; letting oneself fall; letting go across-the-board; intensive breathing therapy to the point of corresponding discharge; orgiastic discharges (e.g. in the sense of all-embracing orgasms); striving for peak experiences; making oneself aware of the twilight zone – the intermediate realm between different levels of consciousness; giving in to the struggle between the worlds; voluntarily making contact with the other side/world (in the sense of development of psychic access to the transcendental domain); taking on the task of being a border-crosser between the worlds.

Resolution: Maintaining consciousness when stepping over into transcendental domains; being on a firm footing with the other side.

Archetypal principle: Uranus.

Epiphora

see Tear production, excessive

Epistaxis

see Nosebleed

Erysipelas

(Ignis sacer , St Anthony's Fire)

Physical level: Skin (border, contact, tenderness).

Symptom level: Flare-up of the skin that is sparked by streptococci and spreads via the lymph ducts (red streak and suspected →blood poisoning): aggressive confrontation on one's own skin, conflict over one's borders and contact with the outside; the disease pattern shows how endangered the outer borders are and how much pain is being caused by contact in the affected area; sharp demarcation line between the area of conflict and the healthy zone; the war zone is painfully swollen to the extreme and also draws the subcutaneous cell tissue in its wake; general mobilisation of the body's immune defences with temperatures over 40 °C, but this is often not sufficient to prevent the spreading of the disease pattern (Name: Swine Erysipelas/ Erysipeloid of Rosenbach, actually describes the milder subsidiary form); life-threatening if the battlefield spills over to inner organs.

Handling: Mobilising all of one's forces for the conflict in order to restrict it to the outer area; allowing oneself to be stirred up and letting these irritations get under one's skin instead of opening up the outer skin to irritants in the form of pathogens; waging spiritual conflicts instead of leaving the body at the mercy of a material war.

Resolution: Voluntarily opening up the outer borders and accepting confrontations with foreign life impulses at the contact surfaces; readiness for deeper-reaching conflicts and high powers of (mental-spiritual) integration in order to better protect the body in its necessary maintenance of (structural) integrity and the setting of limits.

Archetypal principle: Venus/
Saturn-Mars.

Erysipeloid of Rosenbach

see Erysipelas (above) (= more
severe form of Erysipeloid of
Rosenbach)

Erythrodermia

(see also Blushing)
Physical level: Skin (border, contact,
tenderness).
Symptom level: Intense blushing
over large skin surfaces (may be
due to →leukaemia or secondary
→psoriasis or →eczema): the skin
becomes a red flag, an irritated
surface: burning with the desire for
contact; intensive itching triggers the
need for scratching (scratching =
forceful opening of the border of the
skin); formation of dry, flaky skin on
the affected areas: peeling skin surface makes the border easier to pass
through.
Handling: Granting oneself stimulation of the skin; opening one's own
borders from the outside and making
them easier to pass through; giving
signals visible from afar, which simultaneously warn (red traffic light) and
fascinate (red beacon).
Resolution: Paying attention to one's
own borders with the world: vitalis-
ing and opening them and making
them more sensitive/ easier to pass
through.
Archetypal principle: Venus-Mars.

Erythrophobia (fear of blushing)

see Phobia

ESME (Early Summer Meningo-Encephalitis)

see Cerebral inflammation, Meningitis

Eunuchoidism

Physical level: Gonads (fertility) and
secondary genitalia (fertility, desire).
Symptom level: Absence of secondary genitalia because of deficient or
completely lacking gonad function,
which can lead to →gigantism and
also →obesity: rejecting the development into a man (unconsciously and
at a late stage).
Handling: allopathically: timely hormone therapy; scaling back one's
claims to manhood, developing and
nurturing the feminine (anima) sides
and the inner child.
Resolution: Realising one's own soft,
feminine characteristics; putting the
masculine on the back burner; living
childishness on the spiritual level
(open and spontaneous like a child).
Archetypal principle: Uranus.

Ewing's sarcoma

(see also Cancer)
Physical level: Bones (stability,
strength).
Symptom level: The bone tissue
degenerates and forms extremely
malignant connective tissue tumours.
Handling: Finding one's own path
and taking it courageously and offensively with respect to one's own
structure and strength.
Resolution: Self-realisation in that
domain whose symbolism is particularly addressed by the localisation
of the tumour; finding one's own
structure (which corresponds to one's
own being).
Archetypal principle: Saturn-Pluto.

Exhaustion

see Burnout syndrome, Depression

Exostosis

see Ganglion

Exsiccosis

(dehydration; a danger particularly in children)
Physical level: The whole organism is affected; every cell loses water.
Symptom level: Loss of water (spirit) from all cells; the life energy becomes more sluggish (thickening of the blood); the strength of one's heart (muscle) declines; the (skin) surface becomes wrinkled, looks old: unconscious desire to make oneself scarce?
Handling: acute, allopathically: becoming aware of one's own condition of drying out and drying up (withering); taking in more of the spiritual element (water): drinking; long-term, homeopathically: putting the spiritual element on the back burner in favour of dry, sober considerations; letting the life flow run its course more calmly; giving emotions a lower priority; behaving in a more adult and mature way; developing into a drier character with an eye for the essential.
Resolution: Only when the water has been emptied out can one identify the reason (a ship goes into dry dock for repair): penetrating through to the essential, being more sober.
Archetypal principle: Saturn.

Extrasystole

see Heart contraction

Extra-uterine gravidity

see Ectopic pregnancy

Eyes, dryness

(see also Conjunctivitis)
Physical level: Eyes (insight, perspective, mirrors and windows of the soul).
Symptom level: Embittered eyes without tears (opposite of bright,
radiant eyes); the feelings have been extinguished or no longer show themselves in the eyes, the emotions have dried up; dry (emotionless) point of view, soberness; lack of tears = lack of spiritual expression (pain, sadness, rage, joy); the drying up of the eyes, the drying up of the source of tears means the female spiritual element (water) comes up short; suppression of crying; the mirror of the soul threatens to become dull; the bright eyes dry out; one's radiance (anima) starts to wane; very common problem in this day and age, since the eyes are endangered by working with computer screens/staring, dry rooms/working environments and over-straining.
Handling: Looking at things in a consistent and concentrated way: developing a dry, focussed, emotionless gaze; developing a transpersonal point of view without entangling oneself in emotions; learning to look deeper in addition to just visually perceiving things: developing inner vision.
Resolution: Having a clear view for the essential; experiencing sober dryness as a form of concentration on the essential; ultimate objective working from the opposite pole: reconciling male sight with female insight.
Archetypal principle: Sun/Moon-Saturn.

Eye floaters

(mouches volantes)
Physical level: Vitreous humour of the eyes (eyes = insight, perspective, mirrors and windows of the soul).
Symptom level: Tensions in the vitreous humour (glassy gel of the eyes), particularly in the case of people who are short-sighted (→short-sightedness), lead to cloudy, erroneous perceptions; perception of veils and blurred wafts of mist against a light background; illusions

in perception: the inner world is taken for the outer.

Handling: Learning to distinguish between (one's own) inner and outer problems: learning to recognise the splinter in one's own eye for what it is and not taking it for "the beam in the eye" of others; moving outwardly instead of feigning movements inwardly; learning to acknowledge and accept the incompleteness of one's own view.

Resolution: Perceiving the veil in front of one's own eyes and consciously incorporating it into one's view of the world; developing inner mobility; animating one's view of the world.

Archetypal principle: Sun/Moon-Neptune.

Eye movement, involuntary

see Nystagmus

Eye problems

Physical level: Eyes (insight, perspective, mirrors and windows of the soul).

Symptom level: Problems with (in) sight and perspective, conflict over seeing the light; unwillingness to look at one's own life; fear of looking forward; fear of the future.

Handling: Perception exercises: learning to visualise; working on one's own perspective on life.

Resolution: Paying attention to visual perception, and the apparent reality.

Archetypal principle: Sun/Moon, Mercury.

Eyes, puffy

Physical level: Eyes (insight, perspective, mirrors and windows of the soul).

Symptom level: Not being able to open one's eyes, not wanting to look

closer; not wanting to see the world and one's own situation in the world; no longer being able able to just watch or look on; "looking old/foolish": looking unwell/bad, being over-burdened; something is weighing down one's eyelids: desire to close one's eyes (to something); →weariness (of life), unwillingness to take a close look at one's own situation (one's own life); fear of looking forward; fear of the future.

Handling: Closing one's eyes and resting; learning to turn a blind eye to things; recognising and becoming aware of one's own excessive demands; taking a good look at one's own perspective on life.

Resolution: Allowing oneself peace and quiet, and time for recovery; recognising who or what is weighing down one's perspective on life.

Archetypal principle:Sun/Moon, Saturn.

Eyes, rings under

(see also Tear sacs)

Physical level: Eye frames (for the mirrors and windows of the soul), connective tissue (connection, stability, binding commitment).

Symptom level: The rings mark someone for whom things are not going well; reaction to a stressful life: being bleary-eyed, tired, worn out; in the case of kidney problems, grey rings make one look old (and grey) (inadequate filtration); in the case of liver problems, yellow to brown rings indicate processing and detoxification problems, and give a lethargic appearance; bluish rings make the face look somewhat regal and jaded.

Handling: Consciously facing up to the subjects which are burdening one's life: from the balance in relationship matters to detoxification; living up to the high expectations.

Resolution: Transforming oneself from someone who is marked

to someone who is marked by distinction.
Archetypal principle: Sun/Moon-Saturn.

Eyelid inflammation

see Lid inflammation

F

Facial clefts

(harelip, lip-jaw-palatine-cleft)
Physical level: Face (visiting card, individuality, perception, façade).
Symptom level: Lateral cleft lip (harelip) most common, otherwise central cleft lip and facial cleft; a defect in the middle of the face: being marked, but not marked with distinction; being in any case an outsider and distanced from the norm; fateful task which one has brought along with one and which longs for resolution; difficulty, with an open cleft lip, of becoming a well-rounded personality; problems with coming-of-age and being able to speak for oneself if one's mouth cannot be closed completely and causes problems when one opens it.
Handling: Accepting one's specialness and consciously accepting oneself as marked (with distinction) by Fate (e.g. frequently found amongst shamans); after surgical covering up of the physical defect, striving for spiritual closure of the defect in the area of sensuality; practice in matters of maturity (i.e. speaking for oneself): verbally practising defending one's own skin; taking over self-responsibility, wherever opportunities present themselves.
Resolution: Reconciliation with the fateful task of being marked (with distinction); making something special

out of oneself: becoming the unique person that only each individual can be.
Archetypal principle: Saturn-Uranus.

Facial erysipelas

(see also Shingles)
Physical level: Face (visiting card, individuality, perception, façade).
Symptom level: A long-suppressed conflict becomes impossible to overlook and makes itself felt, explosion of a time-bomb; enormous resistance to a central area of life becomes clear on the mirror of the face: "it is written all over one's face"; something got under one's skin or got on one's nerves a long time ago; fear of breaking out, forth and open; the flame of holy wrath (Ignis sacer); being marked (with distinction) (temporary mark of Cain); the blossoming of a rose, unfolding oneself (self-development) on an unresolved (unredeeming) level; connection to shame in blushing (over a long time period).
Handling: Allowing the repressed things to come to the surface and into the light; depending on the affected part of the face, dealing with the suppressed feminine (left) or masculine (right) energies; expressing what up until now has been left unsaid; no longer beating around the bush, but instead doing without flowery language; bringing one's own true being into bloom, letting things in the background and the depths blossom forth; learning to stand up for one's own erotic desires and fantasies.
Resolution: Openness and lack of floweriness; letting the core of one's own being blossom.
Archetypal principle: Venus-Mars.

Facial nerve paralysis

(facial paresis)

Physical level: Face (visiting card, individuality, perception, façade), nervus facialis (mood, identity).

Symptom level: Being torn to pieces at a deeper layer of existence: "one is forced to pull a face"; the two faces of a person are revealed, one-sidedness becomes apparent; the (outer) façade collapses, the mask (mimicry) spirals out of control; one can no longer save face: showing one's true face (grimace, scowl); the soul is torn this way and that: "two souls in one breast" (Goethe); letting it all hang out in a single stroke; the (shadow) side that one has let slide comes to the fore: satanic duality; longing for the darker side of one's personality; the opposite pole to the credo of "just keep smiling"; resignation: the drooping corners of the mouth, the drooping eyelids.

Handling: Allowing oneself to be touched/affected on one's other side; confronting the other, previously-concealed side: discovering and dealing with areas of one-sidedness; depending on which side is affected, coming to terms with the dark feminine (left) or the dark masculine (right) pole; letting it all hang out more often and bringing the other side of one's own being to the fore; giving way to one's withdrawal tendencies and giving way to relaxation and rest; giving up self-control and pulling oneself together again and again before one's façade (the face) is torn apart; standing behind one's divided self; voluntarily letting the mask fall; owning up to the resignation of parts of one's own being instead of always pulling oneself together; letting it all hang out and resting before it tears one apart.

Resolution: Open display of one's own being behind the façade; doing justice to both sides of one's own being; finding the centre in oneself between building and releasing tension; laughing and crying again, arguing and making up: the laughing face of the Harlequin which, standing in the middle of the polar world as a distinct outsider, is neither orientated to any norms nor interested in any façade.

Archetypal principle: Uranus-Neptune-Pluto.

Facial paresis

see Facial nerve paralysis (above)

Faecal vomiting

(see also Vomiting/Nausea, Intestinal paralysis)

Physical level: Gullet (assimilation, defence), large intestine (unconscious, underworld).

Symptom level: Unwillingness to accept (one's circumstances in) life: "being up to one's neck in shit"; ruminating over old, already long-outdated odds and ends; giving up unresolved issues in completely the wrong way; handling matter the wrong way round; extremely unresolved variant of the resurrection from the kingdom of the dead.

Handling: Owning up to one's (previously-unconscious) stance towards one's own circumstances in life; consciously breaking loose from the old and the dead; practising definitively taking leave and letting go; leaving material aspects in their place; not allowing them to force their way into the higher levels of life; conscious work on one's shadow.

Resolution: Seeing through the cycle of living and dying as a process of metamorphosis and protecting oneself against forceful interference and influence.

Archetypal principle: Pluto.

Fainting

(e.g. with epilepsy, low blood pressure, circulatory deficiency)
Physical level: Brain (communication, logistics).
Symptom level: Attempt to flee from responsibility, avoidance manoeuvre; beating a hasty retreat; no willingness to face up to a situation/problem.
Handling: Consciously letting go of claims to power; penetrating into the depths of other dimensions.
Resolution: Placing the power in higher hands: "Thy will be done."
Archetypal principle: Neptune.

Fallen arches

see Flat feet

Falling sickness

see Epilepsy

Fallopian tubes, inflammation

(Salpingitis; see also Ovaries, inflammation, Ovaries, suppuration, Fallopian tubes, suppuration, Adnexitis)
Physical level: Fallopian tubes (fertility).
Symptom level: Conflict over the conveyance of fertility; injury of the feminine capacity for absorbing things.
Handling: Offensive and courageous discussion of any potentially-unfulfilled wishes to have a child; owning up one's own rage against the man; allowing oneself to be stimulated by creative projects.
Resolution: Forging paths for fertility and creative expression on all levels of one's being.
Archetypal principle: Moon/Mercury-Mars.

Fallopian tubes, suppuration

(pyosalpinx; see also Fallopian tubes, inflammation, Ovaries, inflammation, Ovaries, suppuration, Adnexitis)
Physical level: Fallopian tubes (fertility).
Symptom level: Conflict over the conveyance of fertility; frequently the result of an ovarian inflammation; the slide into life is blocked with the debris of war (pus).
Handling: Open discussion of one's desire to have a child; turning one's attention to the feminine pole; opening oneself up to creative projects.
Resolution: Conveyance of creative impulses.
Archetypal principle:
Moon-Mercury/Mars.

Fat belly

(see also Obesity)
Physical level: Stomach (feeling, instinct, enjoyment, centre).
Symptom level: The folds of fat protect and conceal: in this case, the genitalia, just as the folds of (a loin) cloth cover our nakedness; protection against dirtiness and defilement; fleeing behind excess weight due to comfort-eating and baby-fat; not wanting to face up to the lower body and its needs: emphasis of the stomach is reminiscent of a child's stomach; the stomach makes one sexually neutral and therefore harmless; often combined with soreness: conflict over motherhood; the stomach as a symbol of pregnancy.
Handling: Addressing one's own sexuality and shame(facedness); protecting oneself against unwanted sexual approaches on extended levels; recognising the attempt to remain untainted, and reassessing whether there are not perhaps more effective methods for achieving this in consciousness ("becoming like children"); not restricting Jovian fullness to mountains of fat.

Resolution: Fulfilment instead of (physical) fullness; more resolved (redeeming) aspects of shamefacedness (sensibility); conscious ascesis (as an art of life).
Archetypal principle: Moon-Jupiter.

Fat embolism

(see also Embolism)
Physical level: Blood (life force), blood vessels (transport routes of the life force).
Symptom level: Due to a traumatic event (bone fracture, major stomach injury), droplets of fat get into the bloodstream, where they cause blockages (first interpret the basic trauma): fat as the symbol of over-abundance and excess reserves leads to obstruction of the energy supply; excess at inappropriate levels; suffering due to one's own excess reserves; blockage of a channel of the life energy; obstruction of (the flow of) life; supply (circulatory) disorders in the relevant dependent area.
Handling: Making oneself aware of the (problematic) role of one's own excess reserves and over-abundance; allowing oneself more time; slowing down the tempo of life; breaking up the accustomed processing of the life subjects (organs) (affected by the embolism) and bringing it onto a new level; looking after these subjects/regions in a new way and with more attentiveness, e.g. getting to know the paralysed side of the body again in an entirely new way after a stroke [cerebral embolism] – in the same way that the supply of blood to the affected opposite hemisphere of the brain must take place by following completely new paths.
Resolution: Allowing oneself to be slowed down in the tempo of life by the over-abundance that one has achieved; peaceful and creative life flow.
Archetypal principle: Saturn-Jupiter.

Fatigue

(see also Spring fever, Burnout syndrome, Depression, Sleep problems)
Physical level: Starting from the brain (communication, logistics), the whole organism is affected.
Symptom level: Lack of energy and strength to the point of being tired of life; expression of resistance (with regard to one's own work, partnership, family, life situation, etc.); sign of wasted energy (over-expending, sacrificing oneself) or an energy leakage (e.g. as the result of a central rotten compromise [= trouble brewing from a central hotspot (lesion) in the sense of chronic exhaustion] or due to an unresolved life crisis).
Handling: Granting oneself pockets of time for regeneration, and above all for reflection, in order to identify and consciously process the precise point of resistance, waste or leakage; plugging energy leaks through the resolution of unresolved crises and the clearing up of rotten compromises and hotspots (lesions) that have developed as part of recent conflicts; recognising energy wastage and consciously remaining generous when giving, but also practising taking (regeneration); seeing through the spiritual backgrounds of different forms of resistance and learning to understand and accept the (Archetypal) principles concealed in them.
Resolution: Being more peaceful and finding peace within oneself, reconciling oneself to finding one's final peace and the great letting go; allowing oneself sound sleep and thorough regeneration; slowly awakening in sleep in order to become the Awakened One.
Archetypal principle: Saturn-Neptune.

Fatigue paralysis

see Myasthenia

Fatty heart

see Heart, fatty degeneration

Fatty hump

(see also Hunchback, Fatty neck)
Physical level: Fatty tissue (over-flow, excess reserves), back (strenu-ous effort, uprightness).
Symptom level: Rucksack full of reserves which is dragged through a burdensome life (→obesity); becom-ing crooked (dishonest) under the weight of one's own excess.
Handling: Owning up to the burden-some ballast which one is dragging along through life; clarifying the question of what is on one's back and hanging like a millstone around one's neck.
Resolution: Learning to bear one's task and what one wants to take from life with genuine humility.
Archetypal principle: Saturn-Jupiter.

Fatty liver

Physical level: Liver (life, evaluation, reconnection), fatty tissue (overflow, excess reserves).
Symptom level: Expansion due to high demands in the processing of excess (usually alcoholic spirits); initially useful growth, but soon only fatty mass accompanied by a loss of function; misjudgement of what is useful or harmful/poisonous; excessiveness in one's intake: stor-age – actually a subordinate task of the liver –becomes, in this case, an overblown function dominating all others; overblown desires for expan-sion, overly high ideals, delusions of grandeur; loss of energy and potency as a corrective for excess; neglect of ideological subjects.
Handling: Expansion in areas of philosophy and religion instead of on the liver level; addressing ideological things spiritually instead of with al-coholic spirits ("In vino veritas" is not enough); expecting a great deal of oneself on the mental-spiritual level; finding more resolved (redeeming) levels of storage: even the financial cushions in one's bank accounts pro-vide more security than the padding of the liver; being more economical in the expenditure of energy (also sexual energy).
Resolution: Finding the right mea-sure: "The dose makes the poison" (Paracelsus); trust.
Archetypal principle: Jupiter-Jupiter.

Fatty neck

(Submental or cervical mass, see also Fatty hump, Obesity)
Physical level: Neck (strength, vulnerability).
Symptom level: Pretence of a strong neck: hidden behind the mountains of fat lies wimpishness; inability to pull one's cart out of the mire when it be-comes stuck; soft, sluggish immobility due to limited capacity for bearing heavy loads, but giving a strong im-pression; often a thick-skinned owner overall.
Handling: Owning up to one's need for help; developing genuine strength instead of just the illusion; developing Mars-like strength from the Jovian ex-cess: becoming a beast of burden in the figurative sense and pulling one's cart out of the mire.
Resolution: Genuine weightiness (importance); strong self-confidence.
Archetypal principle: Venus-Jupiter.

Fatty stool

(steatorrhoea)
Physical level: Pancreas (aggressive analysis, sweet enjoyment) or liver (life, evaluation, reconnection).
Symptom level: Either a problem of the pancreas (lack of enzymes for digesting fat) or the liver (lack of the bile acids necessary for digesting fat) or caused by taking medications such as Xenikal; voluminous, often stinking

stools: no longer digesting fat, no longer being able to get the most nourishing element out of life; no longer being able to deal completely with excess.
Handling: Consciously letting the excess pass one by; becoming easily satisfied, being modest, cutting back.
Resolution: Taking in only the essential, doing without everything excessive and lavish.
Archetypal principle: Mercury/Pluto-Jupiter.

Feet, sweaty

see Sweaty feet

Female facial hair

(see also Hirsutism, Climacteric complaints)
Physical level: Face (visiting card, individuality, perception, façade).
Symptom level: Male element (animus) that has come up too short; the cosmetic defacement is aimed in the direction of the opposite pole, thus showing one's true face: the concealed masculine hardness; desire for willpower and forceful assertiveness.
Handling: Directing attention to the masculine pole (animus); bringing the existing feminine (Moon) path into harmony with one's own masculine (Sun) elements in order to do justice to both sides of one's own soul; realisation of the animus principle; integration of the opposite pole on the spiritual level instead of on the physical level; standing behind one's own characteristic traits that stand out; consciously breaking out of the mould of feminine norms.
Resolution: Developing the inner man (animus), demonstrating typically masculine characteristics such as forceful assertion, decision-making capability and the ability to act; becoming one with the opposite spiritual pole: the alchemic wedding of polar opposites.

Archetypal principle: Moon-Sun, Venus-Mars.

Femoral neck fracture

Physical level: Bones (stability, strength).
Symptom level: Being overbearing: "There's no fool like an old fool"; ignoring age/fatigue: overstepping natural (age) limits; overly wild, daring leaps; taking excessively dangerous youthful paths: remaining too focussed on forward progress in the external sense; breaking up of a rigid form and stance.
Handling: Treading more gently, living more peacefully: adopting "More haste, less speed" as one's motto; distancing oneself more and more from the fast-moving, external (youthful) life; accepting the (life) situation; refraining from taking on too much; finding one's bearings in one's life design and taking on one's tasks in accordance with the mandala: in the role of the Grand Mother or Grand Father, progressing along one's path with the dignity and serenity of age; exploiting the "follies" of the old fool to the fullest in the mental-spiritual respect; taking the load off the motoric area; daring to make great leaps over deep clefts in the spiritual sense instead of demanding too much of oneself physically.
Resolution: Transforming hubris into humility ("pride goes before a fall"): calmly progressing along one's path with an attitude of mindfulness and humbleness (in the face of Creation) instead of wandering all over the place like a gypsy; contemplation of the essential.
Archetypal principle: Jupiter (thigh)/Saturn (bones) Uranus (rupture).

Fermentative dyspepsy

(see also Diarrhoea, Flatulence)
Physical level: Large intestine (unconscious, underworld), rectum (underworld).
Symptom level: Disorders in the digestion of carbohydrates lead to fermentation in the large intestine; typical developmental path of the illness: rejection of aggression often leads to a vegetarian diet (not wanting to harm any animal); a wholefood vegetarian diet, however, requires particularly good, aggressive use of the weapons in the mouth (teeth); otherwise, indigestible chunks get into the large intestine, which becomes a witches' cauldron of billions of inhabitants from hell, who now cook up their special brew: fermentation and the corresponding build-up of gas (aggressive bellyaching [complaining]; "raising a stink against someone"); burbling fermentation diarrhoea: seething with (suppressed) aggression (rage); "shitting one's pants", "being shit-scared"; not being able to digest the sweet things in life (carbohydrate = sugar), but instead turning them into explosive fuel for the underworld; being forced to drop one's pants.
Handling: Addressing one's own aggression problem; making decisions: chewing things over thoroughly or making a stink?; owning up to one's fear and getting to the very bottom of it where it can transform itself into expansiveness; letting oneself get involved with the sweet sides of life in an open(ly offensive) way.
Resolution: Recognising aggression as a fundamental force of nature and consciously letting oneself get involved with its opposite pole – Venus (enjoyment); being honest with oneself with regard to aggressive forces.
Archetypal principle: Mars-Pluto.

Fetishism

(see also Perversions, sexual)
Symptom level: Sexual arousal through contact with parts of the body and objects (e.g. [red] shoes, underwear); narrowing down of the triggering of sexual arousal; imprinting in the sexual-erotic area for untypical triggers; separation of form (sexuality) and content (love); fear of people, objects appear less dangerous.
Handling: Conscious (psychotherapeutic) return to the starting point and moment of the narrowing down of arousal and reliving the defining imprinting event; clarifying, understanding and thereby reconciling oneself with its symbolism; meditating on the meaning of fetishism in the spiritual sense; extending the capacity for arousal again via the secondary genitalia to the primary genitalia.
Resolution: Keeping in mind and pursuing the goal of one's path in life to recognise God's loving Creation in everything.
Archetypal principle: Uranus-Venus.

Fetopathy

Physical level: Possibility of congenital deformities at almost all levels of the body.
Symptom level: 1. For the affected person (them)self-(evident): accepting the fate-ful intellectual or physical restriction limitation that Provide/nce has provided (German word for "Fate" = Schicksal from schicken = 'to send' and Latin salus = 'health, well-being') and looking for other development priorities; doing justice to one's own accentuated, often emotional needs; willingly letting oneself become involved in possible simple tasks and work; being allowed to remain a child for longer and enjoying the Moon principle; 2. For affected parents, educators: handicapped children, like healthy children, bring compensation into life (offsetting what is missing)

with the tendency of bringing the family, which is a small cosmos in itself, into balance: a one-sidedness of whatever sort thereby often acquires a counterweight; one's own expectations and ideas are corrected: the children are often less the image of their parents, but bring with them something that is completely their own and unexpected; the child represents a much greater and fully-unexpected task and challenge.

Handling: Putting one's own performance expectations on the child and oneself into perspective; examining one's faith in one's own fate in life; recognising and accepting life as something which ultimately cannot be planned; recognising the growth and healing components in one's own fate; reverence for (all) life: those who wanted an exceptional child (sometimes) get it; those who wanted a child particularly urgently (sometimes) get a particularly childish one, which remains a child long beyond the normal time, and requires corresponding care.

Resolution: Accepting the handicap and recognising the opportunity it offers; learning to do simple and essential things with love instead of with rationality or skill: recognising the rule of the Benedictine monks "Ora et labora" ("Pray and work") as an opportunity.

Archetypal principle: Moon/Saturn-Pluto.

Fever

(see also Inflammation)
Physical level: Affects the complete organism.
Symptom level: Being fired up on the physical level instead of in consciousness (the fever of passion); general mobilisation (of the armies) of the body in the fight against the invasion by foreign intruders (bacteria, viruses): generalised conflict which affects the whole being; with every degree of fever, the combat strength increases by more than double (with a corresponding increase in the metabolic rate): fevering towards a solution, anticipation/tension reaches a fever pitch; boiling with rage, stewing in one's own juices; letting (irritating) problems go up in flames; sign of a healthy immune resistance, the worse symptom is the inability to run a fever; high fever in childhood (in connection with the corresponding →childhood diseases) shows the initially still present enthusiasm for facing up to conflict on the physical level (on the spiritual level, this is represented by such things as phases of defiance, fits of rage, lust for adventure, recklessness and childish curiosity).

Handling: Dealing with conflicts in an open(ly offensive) way in one's mind/spirit; training combat readiness on the level of consciousness (rapid-fire comebacks, sharp, darting tongue, striking (crushing) line of argumentation, etc.); fanning the fire of enthusisasm; loving/working/acting in a feverish way.

Resolution: Making decisions: freeing the sword from the scabbard (Latin: dēcīsiō = 'a cutting off') and striking out; letting oneself get involved (in conflicts); facing up to the struggle (of life).

Archetypal principle: Mars.

Fever blisters

see Herpes labialis

Fever convulsions

(particularly in children; see also Fever)
Physical level: Skeletal musculature (motor, strength).
Symptom level: Cramped and tense general mobilisation in the battle against an enemy invasion; fevering towards a solution with excessive combativeness; losing all perspective

due to feverish and tense expectation; fighting for one's life with dogged (lock-jawed) tension.

Handling: Mobilising all forces in the battle over the decision (crisis); tackling things with highly-strung combat readiness; putting the intellect on the back burner and pitching all one's forces into the battle.

Resolution: Facing up to the battle courageously and bravely, and struggling for one's survival (one's life).

Archetypal principle: Mars-Uranus.

Fibroadenoma

see Breast nodes, benign

Fibromatosis

(growth-like proliferation of the connective tissue of various organs)

Physical level: The whole organism can be affected.

Symptom level: Suppression of the essential by the non-essential (connective tissue proliferation along with suppression of the specific organ tissue); the servants take over power (excessive proliferation of the connecting helper (auxiliary) cells with shrinkage of the specialists: the civil servants are now in charge); danger due to the dropping out of the corresponding (organ) subject.

Handling: Granting more importance to the non-essential subsidiary matters on the level of the organ subject; paying attention to the intermediate aspects; recognising the value of the surrounding odds and ends; taking binding commitments seriously, learning to appreciate what bonds and binds; putting binding commitment before performance.

Resolution: Recognising that the body and life essentially consist of many small things and steps, and appreciating the value of these: "The journey is the destination."

Archetypal principle: Mercury-Jupiter, Saturn.

Fibromyalgia

(see also Auto-aggressive/ Auto-immune diseases)

Physical level: Musculature (motor, strength), connective tissue (binding commitment, stability).

Symptom level: Great fear of changes, looking out for danger (extreme caution) and looking after (oneself) (being extremely considerate), hardly risking anything new; being overly intimidated by movement (of the mental-spiritual kind), preferring to cling to the fearful situation that one is used to rather than risking fruitful attempts at breaking out of the familiar "vale of tears"; mindset of negative expectations ("nothing will do any good anyway"); possible symptom of an →amalgam poisoning (tick bites have also been blamed, but ultimately, what actually triggers it is still unknown); muscle pains if Mercury has accumulated in the sheaths of the muscles (fascia) and the nerves supplying them; joint pains, also due to the accumulation of Mercury in the joint capsules: mental-spiritual mobility is called into question, long lines of transmission and grit in the works ("false rheumatism"); the conversion of inner impulses into external activities no longer functions very well or only accompanied by pain; mild to medium →depression, →insomnia.

Handling: Recognising the blockages on the level of mental-spiritual mobility and communication (in effect, corresponding to the blockages of the connective tissues, which connect everything to everything else); reassessing one's relationships, taking back projections; putting an end to mobbing: fighting back, quitting one's job.

Resolution: Preferring to withdraw oneself from the outer world, reducing one's outward movement; forcefully mobilising inner strengths; giving a new framework to one's own

movements in one's inner and outer life; paying keen attention to one's own binding commitments.
Archetypal principle: Mercury/Mars-Pluto.

Finger joint inflammation

see Rheumatism

Fingernails, brittle

Physical level: Fingernails (claws, aggression).
Symptom level: The claws become blunt and break; sign of defenceless-ness and the inability to use one's "claws" to get what one needs.
Handling: Restraining oneself, exposing oneself less; disarmament, scrapping the obsolete weapons; waiting until what one wants comes along instead of aggressively and offensively "clawing" one's way to it.
Resolution: Allowing peace to return to one's relationships with the surrounding world, making peace, finding inner peace.
Archetypal principle: Mars-Saturn.

Fingertips, chapped/cracked

Physical level: Fingers (getting a grip on the world).
Symptom level: (Bleeding) →cracked skin on the fingertips: repeated outbreaks of conflicts in areas requiring a subtle touch and sensibility when dealing with the surrounding world; lack of a subtle touch (instinctive feeling) leads to persistent pains in day-to-day life.
Handling: Giving overdue conflicts space in one's consciousness and daily life; having out conflicts in one's handling of the world; facing up to painful experiences in the figurative sense and allowing old wounds to

heal: finally giving things a rest, letting (house)work rest.
Resolution: The subtle touch (instinctive feeling), sensibility.
Archetypal principle: Mercury-Mars.

Fishskin disease

see Ichthyosis

Fissures

see Cracked skin

Fistula

(connection between various hollow organs or the way to the outside, but also a surgically-inserted tube [gastric fistula for nourishment, intestinal fistula as an artificial outlet]; see also Anal fistula, Intestinal fistula, Urinary bladder fistula, Dental fistula)
Physical level: Various organs can be affected.
Symptom level: Looking for ways out, roundabout ways, secret paths; dangerous actionism; misdirected attempts at repair; attempts at improvement which bring nothing but disadvantages; reworking of Creation (and of the body) which endangers both the former and the latter; danger of spreading troubling matters (pathogens) into areas where they do not belong and thus become dangerous.
Handling: Looking for ways out in the mental-spiritual area; taking new, unconventional paths; transferring matters to other areas in multifaceted ways; risking improvements, but also checking them for their quality; dealing with and resolving conflicts over letting go courageously and in new ways.
Resolution: New ways of disposal; unconventional ways of letting go; creative improvements and re-orientations.
Archetypal principle: Mercury-Uranus.

Fits

see Epilepsy

Flail joint

Physical level: Joints (mobility, articulation).
Symptom level: Instability in the area of articulation, as well as in relationships and other connections (from family bonds to business connections); lack of control in movement; increased mobility, but at the expense of reliable control.
Handling: Loosening up and becoming more relaxed in one's connections and with regard to one's binding commitments; relying more on one's own control and initiative; extending one's radius of spiritual movement.
Resolution: Learning to uphold connections in a laid-back and looser form; extending one's span of spiritual movement and relying on one's own inner control as outer control becomes less and less important.
Archetypal principle: Mercury-Uranus.

Flat feet

(see also Splayed feet)
Physical level: Feet (steadfastness, deep-rootedness).
Symptom level: Problems with one's stand(points); the arch of the foot has been walked flat, the complete sole of the foot now lies on the ground even when not under stress; fallen arches as the preliminary stage (flattened longitudinal arch, feet turned inwards, ankles standing out on the inside; when viewed from behind, it can be seen that the transition from the calf muscle via the Achilles tendon to the heel now bends to the outside = skew foot; weakness of the foot musculature due to a lifestyle with too little exercise and too little walking barefoot as the cause): incorrect transmission of force when walking and standing; in the case of flat feet, this leads to the collapse of the (typically human) longitudinal arch: overloading, imbalance between the loading and load-bearing capacity (weakness of the tendons or obesity); no longer being poised for action (flexible) on one's way through life; diminished foothold: slipping and sliding on the surface of the Earth; false grounding which can given no real foothold; heavy-footed skidding over the Earth since genuine deep-rootedness is lacking, but at the same time, a strong unconscious desire for security; loss of differentiated standpoints; freely shiftable standpoints: not (wanting to) be tied down; unfounded/unfathomable lifestyle, groundlessness.
Handling: Giving up standpoints which are too firm and rigid; making oneself aware of "shallow" standpoints and positions; starting to glide smoothly; consciously allowing oneself to be carried along by the flow of life; swimming along in the river of life using one's own "flippers"; being open on all sides and flowing along; developing flexible standpoints; rising up in order to arrive at differentiated standpoints; elevation of the flat feet (with the help of inlays) aims at breaking loose from this earthbound life.
Resolution: Giving in to the free flow of one's own energy: playing the game of life in the world ("Thy will be done"); swimming through life like a fish in water; working from the opposite pole: putting down genuine roots.
Archetypal principle: Neptune.

Flatulence

(see also Drum belly)
Physical level: Large intestine (the unconscious, the underworld), rectum (the underworld).
Symptom level: Often on the basis of intestinal flora that have been destroyed (cause: anti-biotics [= against life], fast food, etc.): Aggression gone

astray: being a "stinker", "raising a stink with someone", "letting off steam (via the back door)"; keeping unpleasant people away by "fuming"; driving others away with one's own stink bombs; "hot air" from the rear; letting off steam instead of constructive energy; invaluable energy disappears out the back door; lack of power for spiritual integration; having assimilated things which do not agree with one, but instead stink to high heaven.

Handling: Relieving pressure in good time; learning to express oneself aggressively, fuming; showing to what extent one feels that something stinks, and how one wants to raise a stink against it: developing courage for direct confrontation.

Resolution: Learning to consume and digest the world (practising Bhoga); processing everything immediately in its correct time and place.

Archetypal principle: Pluto.

Flea infestation

Physical level: Skin (border, contact, tenderness).

Symptom level: Severely itching bite areas betray the diagnosis, regarded as very embarrassing; since it is seen as a sign of unhygienic living conditions, it has been strongly tabooed; unacknowledged conflicts over one's own borders; unacknowledged problems with cleanliness and closeness to other people.

Handling: Letting oneself be stimulated and tempted; consciously seeking closeness, offensively opening one's own borders.

Resolution: Voluntarily giving away one's own life force to others.

Archetypal principle: Pluto.

Flexion of the fingers and toes

(dactylogryposis)

Physical level: Fingers (getting a grip on the world), toes (foothold).

Symptom level: Developing clawed hands and feet: manifestation of greed and avarice coupled with neediness, and of the search for a stable hold where currently a good foothold is lacking.

Handling/Resolution: Owning up to the basic situation and ensuring satisfaction of one's needs; creating for oneself inner and outer (backing) support.

Archetypal principle: Mercury-Saturn.

Fluor albus

see Efflux

Fluor genitalis

see Efflux

Flying, fear of

(see also Anxiety, Phobia)

Symptom level: Fear of crashing down; fear of leaving the (mother) earth, of losing one's grip, fear of flying off the handle; fear of: high flying; fear of cramped spaces (the cramped space of the body of the aircraft can evoke associations with the cramped space in the mother's body (womb) in the time shortly before birth).

Handling: Planting one's feet firmly on the ground, and from this safe basis, developing confidence in the air element; leaving the safe ground of what is familiar, the habitual; allowing oneself flights of the imagination and developing openness for fantasy journeys; re-living one's own birth trauma (with psychotherapeutic help) and thereby reconciling oneself with it.

Resolution: Recognising falling and crashing down as primordial human themes (the fallen angel, Lucifer's fall) and making oneself aware of these as continually threatening dangers which one simply has to live with.

Archetypal principle: Saturn-Uranus.

Foehn disorder

(see also Sensitivity to changes in the weather)

Physical level: The whole organism can be affected.

Symptom level: Pressure changes between air fronts in the atmosphere trigger a great variety of symptoms; weather fronts emphasise the imbalance of a situation; weather is nothing more than the balancing out of atmospheric imbalances; these are strongly sensed, internally rejected and combatted in the form of corresponding symptoms; headaches: combatting changes in one's mind; excessive irritability, nausea: feeling sick of everything, reacting to changes with unwillingness; fatigue, feeling exhausted (weather-beaten): responding to changes with resignation; general lethargy: new developments induce passiveness; →depression to the point of →suicidal tendencies: feeling downcast.

Handling: Instead of fighting against changes in (weather) conditions, taking them on as a mental challenge; letting oneself be stirred up by external stimuli; meeting changes with willpower instead of unwillingness; taking an offensive stance and facing up to what is new instead of allowing oneself to be overcome by it; developing self-confidence and inner strength so that, working from this basis, one can meet changes in internal and external weather conditions in an active and open(ly and offensive) way in keeping with the motto: "There is no such thing as bad weather, just unsuitable clothing and unfitting attitudes"; becoming sensitive to collective mood changes.

Resolution: Approaching the changes (transformations) in the weather openly: understanding changes in the weather as a symbol of the continually-changing life flow; figuring out and accepting "everything flows" (Heraclitus) as a universal law; transforming the basic passive attitude of "hopefully nothing will happen" into the active "hopefully quite a lot will happen and development will progress forward".

Archetypal principle: Moon/Uranus/Neptune.

Foetor ex ore

see Halitosis

Folliculitis

(pimples; see also Puberty acne)

Physical level: Hair follicles and sebaceous gland openings of the skin (border, contact, tenderness).

Symptom level: Something has got under one's skin and is smouldering there; a deep-seated conflict is gaining access to consciousness (venting itself) by forcing its way upwards to visibility; volcanic development: what is brewing and bubbling in the depths in terms of tension and charge becomes visible on the (skin) surface and waits for discharge and eruption; a (symbolic) message breaks through the (skin) border.

Handling: Voluntarily paying more attention to issues which have gotten under one's skin and have not been processed; giving way to issues forcing their way up from below; facing up to discharges and eruptions of inner energies in an open(ly offensive) way and helping them to advance; opening up borders (of consciousness); questioning accepted norms; enabling contacts; ensuring exchange.

Resolution: Making the breakthrough; leaving one's own boundaries behind.

Archetypal principle: Mars-Uranus (eruption)/Neptune (flight)/Pluto (volcano).

Food poisoning

see Botulism

Foot-and-mouth disease

(stomatitis epidemica; see also Stomatitis aphtosa)

Physical level: Oral mucosa (boundary between inside and outside), hands (grasping, gripping, ability to act, expression) and feet (steadfastness, deep-rootedness).

Symptom level: →Aphtosa epidemics primarily affect livestock, but can also spread to humans: blisters break out on the lips, the inside of the mouth and the hands and feet, which are painful and which eventually heal again accompanied by fever (the name sounds much worse than the actual disease pattern); conflicts in the area of assimilation, getting a grip and being deeply rooted; the connection to the world of contrasts is painfully brought into the focal point of attention.

Handling: Feverishly striving for clarification of the relevant conflicts.

Resolution: Courageous and offensive conflict over one's connection to the world.

Archetypal principle: Moon-Mars.

Foot oedema

(see also Oedema)

Physical level: Feet (steadfastness, deep-rootedness).

Symptom level: Build-up of (spiritual) water makes one's standpoint more difficult to bear; water drags one down into the lower feminine domain; the feet act like two anchors, which hinder movement and progress more than helping it.

Handling: Allowing spiritual aspects to flow into one's own positions and standpoints; voluntarily concerning oneself with the lower feminine domain; coming more to rest inwardly; finding firm standpoints and positions; reading the Oedipus (= swollen foot) myth.

Resolution: Discovering one's own task area and putting down roots there; contemplation; also arriving at the lower, feminine part of one's own being.

Archetypal principle: Neptune.

Foot pains

Physical level: Feet (steadfastness, deep-rootedness).

Symptom level: The roots are hurting and cry out for help, deep-rootedness causes pain: having problems with being firmly anchored in life, being painfully threatened right down to one's very foundations; difficulties in standing up for oneself, finding and stepping forward with one's own secure and undisputed standpoint; painfully experiencing that one has not yet found one's place (in life), that one's current standpoint or place in life is causing one pain.

Handling: Directing energy into the issue of deep-rootedness; working on one's own standpoints with commitment and painful callousness towards one's own person; anchoring oneself in life with offensive strength.

Resolution: Finding and taking up one's place (in life) firmly and with courage.

Archetypal principle: Neptune-Mars.

Foot problems

see Foot drop, Flat feet, Splayed feet, Hallux valgus

Foot-sole warts

(see also Plantar warts)

Physical level: Feet (steadfastness, deep-rootedness), sole of the foot (deep-rootedness, grounding).

Symptom level: Wart = outgrowth from the shadow kingdom, which can be made to disappear by magic (conjuring); message from the shadow world, which puts pressure on one's own standpoints; "trampling around" on one's shadow without recognising its meaning: "the thorn in one's own flesh", painful grounding, painful standing and understanding, painful deep-rootedness, problematic relationship with Mother Earth.

Handling: Recognising that one "is standing" on a shadow, which is based on the occult; making oneself aware of the occult side of one's existence: illuminating the magical shadows; clarifying in which contexts the warts are bothersome/what they hinder one from doing; treading more gently; learning to step forward, even under difficult conditions; learning a more careful handling of the Earth and one's own roots; learning to stand up for oneself even in painful situations; asking oneself where the shoe (of life) is pinching.

Resolution: Also being able to take in painful impressions; developing growing understanding (for painful situations); acknowledgement of one's own shadow world which one is standing on.

Archetypal principle: Neptune-Saturn/Pluto.

Foot sprain

(see also Sprain)

Physical level: Feet (steadfastness, deep-rootedness).

Symptom level: Having made a hard landing; taking overly large leaps, putting one's foot in it, missing the mark; contact between the world of thoughts and reality is not running harmoniously and is following dangerous paths.

Handling: Admitting to oneself when one has put one's foot in it and missed the mark; making oneself aware of faux pas (= false steps) in order to learn from them; providing better safeguarding for spiritual leaps and high flying; striving for more outer calm while maintaining inner mobility.

Resolution: Large leaps must be adapted to one's own stability (stepping out in grand style = grand-hearted (generous) style in order to attain more security); keeping one's feet planted firmly on the ground, despite intellectual high flying: "Raising one's head to the Father in Heaven, with one's feet firmly rooted in Mother Earth" (Indian proverb).

Archetypal principle: Neptune-Uranus.

Foreskin, narrowing of

see Phimosis

Forgetfulness

Symptom level: Losing sight of what is close at hand; not wanting to retain anything; turning away from the world, locking oneself away from it.

Handling: Consciously heeding the call to let go of what has been forgotten; (dysfunction of the short-term memory): gaining an overview of one's life design and heeding the call to detach oneself from day-to-day matters; (dysfunction of the long-term memory): coming into the moment; coming to terms with unconscious needs; recognising and loosening up perfectionist demands on oneself.

Resolution: No longer bearing grudges, forgiving; arriving in the flow of the moment; recognising the grace in forgetting (Lethe, the river of the Underworld, is the place of oblivion and therefore of cleansing); practising being oblivious to all those around one and living more intuitively.

Archetypal principle: Mercury-Neptune.

Fracture

see Bone fracture

Freckles

(ephelides)

Physical level: Skin (border, contact, tenderness).

Symptom level: Reaction to sunlight without any particular pathological significance in people with strawberry-blonde hair and fair skin; are an attribute of youth which give the face a cheeky, alert and brazen look, especially around the nose (Pippi Longstocking); "A face without freckles is like a sky without stars".

Handling: Living up to the outwardly cheeky impression; freely and frankly taking what life has to offer.

Resolution: Living one's own life even if still a child or young adult.

Archetypal principle: Mercury-Uranus.

Frigidity

(literally: coldness; see also Orgasm problems, Listlessness)

Physical level: Genitalia (sexuality, polarity, reproduction) of the woman; in men, the same situation is rarely diagnosed as frigidity, although most men are frigid, and do not contribute any fluid to the smooth functioning of sexual intercourse. The prostate would be quite capable of doing this, although it is rarely called on to do so because of the brevity of sexual intercourse which has become so usual in western culture. In principle, it would be enough if just one of the partners produced lubricating fluid, or to put it another way: for a man who was healthy in this respect, there would be no frigid woman.

Symptom level: Leaving the main region of desire high and dry or not even awakening it (Sleeping Beauty, who is forever waiting to be awakened by a kiss from her Prince Charming); sex leaves her (or him) cold and constricted; constriction = fear of opening oneself up to sexuality (because of extremely negative experiences, such as rape or adverse attitudes towards sexuality); lack of warmth and the slimy-moist climate of fertility and enjoyment; drying up in terms of enjoyment, not granting oneself (and one's partner) anything; fear of animalistic urges and (feminine) lack of control; sober dryness instead of juicy slipperiness: nothing glides smoothly any more in this respect, instead the region is jammed up and painful; masculine politics right in the middle of feminine homeland (desert instead of swamp, Saturn instead of Moon); fear of death = orgasm (=death of the Ego, the Me-You boundary is dissolved), loss of control; fear of one's own femininity (or lubricious masculinity), of one's own desire and unleashed (exuberant) wildness, fear of the threateningly aggressive masculine aspect (the devouring feminine aspect); fear of giving oneself to someone and letting go, of ecstasy; clinging to the Self/ Ego: desires for dominance; fear of performance; failing due to pressure to perform: fear of not being the super seductress (the super stud), of being compared with previous partners; clinging to (being trapped in) the intellect; flinching away from the feminine (masculine) role; denigrating sexuality as dirty: leaving the dark lower cave high and dry; Oedipal problems (of the woman): not wanting to be unfaithful to one's own father; feminine compensation: becoming a successful (career) woman instead of a woman on all levels; punishing oneself and one's partner through the painfully dry situation (e.g. for tactless or exaggerated wishes inappropriate to the situation; frequently amongst women who, for too long, have been putting on an act for their partner, and sometimes for themselves, or who have been forced into sexuality or had to force themselves into it); not yet being mature enough for mature sexuality (in the case of young girls or late bloomers), who have not yet made the step towards becoming a woman); in men, the fear of being regarded as a "softy" if they openly display their gushing feminine characteristics and contribute something to the smooth running of the situation..

Handling: for women: understanding and accepting the essence of one's own femininity: seeing through sober thinking, dry humour and objective arguments – as belonging to the masculine pole – without denigrating them; recognising and acknowledging the soft, watery, atmosphere that is pregnant with emotion as belonging to one's own feminine pole; ensuring sufficient safety and security to be able to truly give oneself to another; restraining oneself and consciously and emphatically rejecting what one does not enjoy: finding oneself and discovering for oneself one's own needs; consciously being prudent and cool on levels where this makes more sense than in the sexual area: becoming sober and dry in certain areas of life; working from the opposite pole: exercises in letting go, meditation; exercises in which one lets oneself fall into the (feminine-spiritual) water, classifying desire as essential to life (and survival) instead of cutting off the (spiritual) water from it, learning to enjoy it; arranging the poles properly: allowing the (feminine) Yin and (masculine) Yang to come into their own at their proper places; recognising (dis) composure as a virtue; admitting to oneself one's own juicy thoughts and fantasies; recognising ecstasy as a right in life, which we are entitled to, from the ecstatic-oceanic feelings in the womb to the orgiastic experiencing of music, sport or sexuality; making friends with one's own masculine strengths in order to find one's way back to the soft, feminine side; getting to know and apply one's own masculine assertive strength: knowing and making it understood in an open(ly

offensive) way that the woman does not simply have to be lying at the ready; discovering the 'no' in sexuality in order to be able to say 'yes' in more suitable situations with one's whole heart and one's whole being; bringing the suppressed back into view; switching off and outwitting the overpowering intellect; learning (for one's own sake) to act out orgasms so well until they really happen; working from the opposite pole: defrosting the fridge as a conscious ritual (Milton Erickson); for men: discovering one's own feminine side and allowing it to flow into the sexual encounter; contributing something to the spiritual experience of unification; involving one's own soul (water, the flowing element) in sexuality.

Resolution: Relinquishing the 'Self' in the orgasm as a preliminary exercise for the final great relinquishment and the great orgasm with Creation (= cosmic consciousness); addressing the subject of dying as the ultimate form of giving oneself to another and surrender of the Ego.

Archetypal principle: Venus-Saturn/ Pluto.

Frontal sinus inflammation

see Sinus inflammation

Frostbite

Physical level: Particularly the extremities (fingers, toes, ear lobes, tip of the nose).

Symptom level: Extreme lack of caring attention (undercooling) leads to dying off of the extremities of the body; letting oneself partially die off due to the lack of movement and inner warmth; being frozen (in one's reactions).

Handling: Allopathically: Warmth and movement (rubbing, kneading); Homeopathically: Applying cold (rubbing oneself with snow); making oneself aware of one's coldness towards oneself: the extremely chilly type; becoming emotionally cooler (more controlled, more considered), reflecting on the consequences; freezing = slowing down: winter wants silence and calm from us, not racing around in the world that lies frozen under the snow (burial shroud); paying heed to one's own limits and extremities; not challenging Fate, but warming to the pointers (hints) that are at one's fingertips.

Resolution: Considering in advance the consequences of how one handles things; taking into account the characteristic qualities of the prevailing season; giving time what it demands more coolly and in a more controlled way; realising the diamonds of complete clarity and structure within oneself (inner silence instead of outer rigidity); taking care of oneself.

Archetypal principle: Saturn.

Fungal diseases

see Candidamycosis, Dermatomycoses, Pityriasis versicolor, Nail fungus, Athlete's foot, Vaginal mycosis, Inflammation

Funnel chest

Physical level: Rib cage (sense of self/Ego, personality).
Symptom level: Limiting of the personality, of the room that it is allowed to take up; oppression of the heart and the (wings [lobes] of the) lungs; "turning one's heart into a skeleton closet" (in the concrete sense).
Handling: Limiting oneself in matters of the heart and communication in a prudent way, not taking on too much; using the available room for the unfolding of one's personality.
Resolution: Cultivating self-restraint and modesty.
Archetypal principle: Saturn.

Furuncle

(hair follicles deep in the skin; carbuncle = several furuncles in contact with each other; see also Abscess, Folliculitis)
Physical level: Skin (border, contact, tenderness).
Symptom level: A conflict-laden subject (e.g. great rage) has penetrated (deep) under one's skin without being processed, and threatens to explode (carbuncles: a group of subjects); as always, the location of the occurrence reveals the level: e.g. in the genital area: a sign of rage and disappointment with regard to unlived sexual "volcanic eruptions"; on the buttocks: sign of resentment at not being able to forcefully assert oneself; deep-seated conflict (e.g. unresolved resentment) gaining access to consciousness (venting itself) by forcing its way upwards to visibility; volcanic development: what is brewing and bubbling in the depths in terms of tension and charge breaks through to the (skin) surface; a breakthrough, a breakout, the discharge of a (symbolic) message across the (skin) border.
Handling: Allowing oneself to be stirred up down to one's very depths by agitating subjects; voluntarily and offensively paying greater attention to deep-seated subjects which have got under one's skin and have not been processed ; making way for agitating subjects forcing their way up from below; having it out with discharges and outbreaks of inner energies in an open(ly offensive) way; opening up the borders (of consciousness); questioning norms; enabling contact; nurturing courageous exchange.
Resolution: Achieving breakthroughs, offensively and courageously growing beyond one's own limits.
Archetypal principle: Mars-Uranus, Neptune, Pluto.

G

Galactostasis

see Milk accumulation

Gall bladder cancer

(see also Cancer)
Physical level: Gall bladder (aggression, poison and bile).
Symptom level: Suppressed, unrealised aggression which, deep below the surface, has become bitter, poisonous, and due to a long build-up of the backwater, dangerously insidious, begins to go its own ways, to run riot in the body, and in this way, to realise itself after all; having strayed so far off track from one's determination in life with regard to the storage area and reservoir of aggression that the forces that have been unlived for too long strike out on their own initiative and go on a physical ego trip in the form of degeneration.
Handling: Making oneself aware of one's own excess bile; consciously allowing the corresponding, long-suppressed mental-spiritual forces to come to the fore in order to relieve the body of the burden; whatever is allowed to be acted out on the stage of our consciousness becomes unimportant on the stage of our body and is then often dropped from the programme; courageously ensuring relief in the storage area of profound, hidden aggressions: letting suppressed, toxic aggressions run their course into consciousness; offensively letting out (expressing) one's own excessive bile (nevertheless, experiencing something does not necessarily mean living it out); adopting all the measures mentioned under →cancer: since cancer affects the complete organism, it must also be met across-the-board.

Resolution: Returning to one's own inherent path, and not allowing one's own self-realisation to be hindered anymore by built-up, stagnant aggressions; recognising the necessity to switch from the physical and thus (life-)threatening level to the challenging, but life-saving mental-spiritual level, and relying in this realm on expansive growth; discovering love that transcends all boundaries, setting oneself above external rule and standards laid down by oneself or others, and living and developing oneself solely in accordance with the obligations of one's own highest law.
Archetypal principle: Pluto-Pluto.

Gall bladder, inflammation

(cholecystitis, see also Cholangitis)
Physical level: Gall bladder (aggression, poison and bile).
Symptom level: Offensive battle in the storage area of profound, hidden aggressions; suppressed, unlived aggression deep below the surface becomes bitter, toxic, and due to having been held back for a long time, dangerously insidious; with its (physical) outbreak, this form of aggression becomes painfully clear; an excess of offensive bile breaks out (physically).
Handling: Facing up courageously to the reservoir of old, stagnant aggressions; offensively restoring the connection to the original formative situation for this aggression.
Resolution: Coming clean with one's pent-up aggression before it directs itself against oneself.
Archetypal principle: Pluto-Mars.

Gall stones

(see also Stony concretions, Biliary colic)
Physical level: Bile ducts and gall bladder (aggression, poison and bile).

Symptom level: Congealed energy, petrified aggression, above all within the framework of family-related constraints (suffered most frequently by married women with children); poisonous, profound aggression which causes an energy backlog; giving birth to unlived biliousness, solidified poison; concentration of those (rage and anger) outbreaks which one has denied oneself for a long time.

Handling: Expressing and living out aggressive energy via verbal attacks and concrete actions; emphatically enjoying the fullness, spice and luxury of life; forceful movements and loud cries ease the birth of gall stones; when practised early enough, these can also make them superfluous; everything which keeps the above matters in flow is preventive.

Resolution: see Biliary colic.

Archetypal principle: Pluto/Saturn-Mars.

Ganglion

(Bible cyst)

Physical level: Occurring at the joint capsules (joints = mobility, articulation) or the synovial membranes of tendons (the binding cords which everything hinges on).

Symptom level: Connective tissue-like growth (jelly-filled cyst), which occurs due to mucoid degeneration of connective tissue; although of little pathological significance, it can occasionally be bothersome: harmless growths which, in the worst case, may be optically displeasing.

Handling/Resolution: Surgeons of the old school used to solve the problem by striking the ganglion, often with a heavy book such as the Bible (hence the name Bible cyst), which burst the cysts and cleared up (resolved) the problem: violently banging one's fist on the table to put an end to the growths; letting striking aspects grow (out of oneself).

Archetypal principle: Jupiter-Mercury-Saturn.

Gangrene

(necrotic tissue which decomposes through a process of self-liquidation; see also Circulatory disorders, which are the basic problem)

Physical level: Extremities of the limbs (mobility, activity), intestines (processing of material impressions), lungs (contact, communication, freedom), oral cavity (mouth = absorption, expression, maturity – speaking for oneself).

Symptom level: Life withdraws itself from certain areas of the body, just as one's consciousness was previously withdrawn from the corresponding subject areas; one allows part of oneself to decay by cutting it off from the life flow; often connection with resentment, which is symbolically associated with the decaying part of the body. 1. Dry gangrene: desiccation (mummification); being mummified (drying up) while still alive; 2. Wet gangrene due to bacterial decay: rotting alive; stinking breakdown of one's own organism.

Handling: Consciously giving up certain subjects which are no longer current, and withdrawing oneself from these areas; allowing them to die internally (e.g. progress if the feet are affected); reserving one's remaining life energy for the essential, central subjects(e.g. [matters of] the heart); asking oneself: What is rotten in my life? What stinks about it? What in fact stinks to high heaven?

Resolution: Inner calm; reconciliation; recognition that everything earthly is transient and perishable; dying in order to live.

Archetypal principle: Pluto-Saturn.

Gangrenous enteritis

(Enteritis necroticans)
Physical level: Intestines (process-ing of material impressions).
Symptom level: Dying off of parts of the intestinal wall, which are cut off from the circulation, e.g. as the result of constrictions (in the hernia sac, due to adhesions), formation of →throm-boses: the lively (vital) digestion of life is partially impaired or drops out completely; rotting of the areas that have died off: something is rotten with one's processing of life.
Handling: Leaving those areas alone which are none of one's business; excluding certain things from one's processing; concerning oneself only with what one has actually been given to digest.
Resolution: Digesting one's own kar-mic fruits; processing life only to the extent that it concerns oneself.
Archetypal principle: Mercury/ Mars-Pluto.

Gas gangrene

Physical level: Skin/subcutane-ous tissue (boundary, contact, tenderness).
Symptom level: Secondary war: on already existing battlefields (open wounds); the actual fatal aggression breaks out; poisonous gases devel-oping in the struggle complete their destructive work; sepsis: flooding of the complete system with (bacterial) toxins; danger of collapse of the central supply structures: circulatory collapse; conflict over life and death: high death rate.
Handling: Exercising caution with theatres of war that have not yet been swept clean, properly dealt with or cleared up; keeping an eye on the toxic by-products of warlike conflicts; courageously and offensively deal-ing with and clearing up unhealed wounds; learning to deal with the toxic side-effects of conflicts; allowing oneself to be affected by these ef-fects, which can easily become the main problem.
Resolution: Courageously allowing oneself to get involved with life-and-death issues conducted with all avail-able means.
Archetypal principle: Mars-Pluto.

Gastric bleeding

see Stomach ulcer

Gastric catarrh

(gastroenteritis; see also Diarrhoea)
Physical level: Stomach (feeling, receptiveness), intestines (processing of material impressions).
Symptom level: Upsetting one's stomach: taking the wrong thing on board (e.g. something containing bacteria or salmonella); fear symp-tom: diarrhoea ("shit-scared", "shitting one's pants").
Handling/Resolution: Instead of stirring things up by taking dangerous pathogens on board, tackling the processing and digestion of volatile subjects instead.
Archetypal principle: Moon-Mercury-Mars.

Gastric juices, deficiency

see Achylia

Gastritis

see Stomach mucosa, inflammation

Gastro-cardial symptom complex

see Roemheld's syndrome

Gastroenteritis

see Gastric catarrh

Gastroptosis

see Stomach, descended

Gaucher's disease

see Lipid storage diseases

Genital warts

(Condylomata acuminata; infection with condyloma virus)
Physical level: Skin surface (boundary, contact, tenderness), particularly in protected, moist areas: genitalia (sexuality, polarity, reproduction) and anus (entrance and exit of the underworld).
Symptom level: Harmless, small, cleft-, cauliflower- or cockscomb-shaped growths (at most cosmetically disturbing in large numbers).
Handling: Also granting oneself small harmless playful pursuits (in the affected areas); allowing "small things" to grow which serve no purpose, have no use and do no damage, but represent something that is one's own; also affording oneself idle, pointless pursuits; harmless conflicts in the affected areas.
Resolution: Playful expression of growth possibilities; creativity and harmless, playful conflicts in the intimate area.
Archetypal principle: Venus-Mars-Pluto (warts).

Gestational diabetes

see Diabetes mellitus

Gestosis

(short for gestation toxicosis = [poisoning], symptoms occurring during pregnancy which are caused by problems in adjusting to the new [hormone] situation; see also Oedema, High blood pressure, Glomerulonephritis)

Physical level: Affects the complete organism.
Symptom level: Being under unbearable pressure; unconscious rejection of the pregnancy; struggle against the pregnancy on various levels (preclampsia: →eclampsia, hepatoses: →liver diseases); inability to adapt oneself to the new situation of being a twosome.
Handling: Adjustment to pregnancy and motherhood: rituals related to becoming a woman; learning to think and plan for two, but not eating for two: controlling weight gain (12 kilograms as a guideline figure); gaining weightiness only in the figurative sense (in the partnership and society); conversations with the unborn (via the inner voice); trying to become the mother of a family, founding a family, finding social security.
Resolution: Reconciliation with the new (life) situation, with being a woman and becoming a mother.
Archetypal principle: Moon-Uranus.

Gigantism

(according to orthodox medicine, but [due to →Puberty, premature] long-since outdated definition: height of over 180 cm for women and 190 cm for men; see also Dwarfism as the opposite pole)
Physical level: The body is affected over its whole length.
Symptom level: The increased secretion of growth hormone caused by a tumour of the front lobe of the pituitary gland leads to increased growth in terms of height (although there are many people over 190 cm in height who certainly have no such tumour); attracting attention due to one's size, standing out everywhere, always being the biggest (greatest); feeling of being too big (great) for this world (everything is too small; difficulties in finding clothes and shoes which fit).

Handling: Matching one's outer greatness by developing inner greatness; also standing out in the extended sense (bringing together form and content); at the same time, also relating to the next, greater (transcendental) world.
Resolution: Standing up for one's (outer) greatness (internally as well); filling out the great body in the mental-spiritual sense.
Archetypal principle: Jupiter.

Gingivitis

see Gums, inflammation

Glans, inflammation

see Balanitis

Glaucoma

Physical level: Eyes (perspective, insight, mirror and window of the soul).
Symptom level: Painful vision under great pressure (often from emotional wounds and disappointments from long ago); what one had to view in the past puts one under pressure; veiled vision, veiled gaze; hindered circulation of the aqueous humour: too little spiritual exchange in the background; weighed down by unshed tears; the unshed, pent-up emotions create pressure and threaten the eyesight; often coupled with old resentment and the inability to forgive oneself and others; rigid tunnel vision: inflexible point of view, seeing the world as if wearing blinkers; being fixated on details, obstinate; having (seen) enough; one's overview and broad vision are lost: one's own (world) view comes under increasing pressure if the basic conflicts are not dealt with; danger of going blind in the case of untreated glaucoma attacks: giving way to the pressure and being forced to look inwards.
Handling: Placing emphasis on looking (more closely) (inwardly?); making one's own (point of) view softer and seeing things in a more forgiving light; intensifying spiritual exchange, e.g. getting back in touch with old emotional contents that have been stored away (e.g. sorrow); feeling the pressure of unshed tears and giving way to it, opening up the spiritual floodgates and safety release valves, letting off pressure; concentrating one's gaze on the essential, blocking out the non-essential; looking potential opponents squarely in the eye; direct, straightforward, intense gaze; reducing one's overview of the material world in favour of deeper insight; realising the pressure that one's own world view has come under and weighing up the consequences; counteracting the danger of going blind through voluntary introspection.
Resolution: Gaining insight into one's own depths; tunnel vision into the depths; seeing through the world; developing one's own world view; obtaining insight into transcendental levels.
Archetypal principle: Sun/Moon-Pluto.

Globus feeling

see Throat, lump sensation

Glomerulonephritis

(kidney inflammation, inflammation of the renal corpuscles)
Physical level: Kidneys (balance, partnership).
Symptom level: Often conflicts rising up from the urinary bladder (letting off pressure), which then spread in the interior of the kidneys from the renal pelvis to the specific kidney tissue (glomeruli); irritating matters (e.g. in the form of streptococci from the urogenital tract) can also make their way up out of the lower shadow kingdom into the upper areas of the partnership and the balancing of contrasts; in the case of acute glomerulonephritis

(conflict in the renal corpuscles at the filters), irritations also come from the throat area (conflicts in the area of the tonsils: war over swallowing things), from the sinuses (being chronically sick to the eyeballs of things), tooth abscesses (aggression conflict) or from scarlet fever (heated struggle in relation to a development crisis); general mobilisation of the body's own war machinery (high fever) and battles that shake one to the core (attacks of the shivers) in connection with the themes of balance of the inner contrasts and partnership; difficulties in letting go of the spiritual element (hindered, painful urination); important materials (for relationship dramas) and other subject matters are lost in the (spiritual) waste water flow (loss of protein in the urine); failure of the filter system to differentiate and distinguish: important matters/ problems are no longer recognised as one's own and are lost (the filter systems are damaged due to the war in the renal corpuscles [glomerulus]); danger that (sham) harmony on the surface will become sign-ificantly apparent as inner disharmony: a prompt to also enter into disharmony externally (dispute, conflict), with the aim of achieving genuine harmony; danger of chronification and transition into →kidney insufficiency; being severely scarred and disappointed by relationship problems; living at odds with one's feelings in order to sustain a partnership beyond its due time and to reflect the outward appearance (pretence) of a healthy marital life.

Handling: Voluntarily allowing shadow subjects from the domain of the balancing of contrasts and partnership to rise up from below in order to critically process them (together) in consciousness as they wrestle with each other; making oneself aware of how easily unresolved conflicts from other areas (e.g. issues such as assimilating and letting in [throat area];

underlying aggressions [tooth-root ulceration], chronic frustrations [sinusitis] or development crises) can penetrate into the partnership area and cause problems here; throwing all one's strength into the conflict, even to the point of risking being shaken to one's very foundations; also letting go of and letting out important things and subject matters in order to relieve the body of them and to be able to retain the protein important to (survival in) life; expanding the pores of one's (consciousness) filter and no longer keeping (back) everything for oneself: learning to give and give away freely; admission that matters of vital importance will be lost in this conflict, and should in fact be let go; recognising the explosive potential of the issue of balancing contrasts and keeping one's centre (safe), and making oneself aware that otherwise one's life can end up in danger.

Resolution: Genuine harmony (bringing the contrasts into balance); addressing those matters which; for example, must be kept in play in the partnership in an open(ly offensive) way and letting go of other matters: giving and giving away freely; offensively and courageously addressing the subject of partnership in the widest sense, and working on balancing the contrasts; knowing that occasional imbalances cannot be avoided; placing the focus on retracting projections.

Archetypal principle: Venus-Mars.

Glossitis

see Tongue inflammation

Goitre

(struma, usually on the basis of iodine deficiency; struma with normal glandular function; see also Thyroid gland hyperfunction, Thyroid gland hypofunction)

Physical level: Neck (assimilation, connection, communication).

Symptom level: Persistent striving for possession; insatiable greed, being tight with money; tendency to store away things like a hamster/ to hoard things/to snatch whatever one can: "never being able to get one's fill"; unacknowledged bid for possession/power along with unconscious greed, which cut one off from life; puffing up one's hackles with anger ("being eaten up by something", being worked up/ruffled), because one does not get what one wants; oppressive anxiety weighing down on the soul; (being able to take on) connectivity to the Earth; conservative immobility; hunger for energy, activity and change; knotted nodes in the struma: unresolved knotty problems which are still hanging around one's neck and which want to be cleared up; hot nodes put one under pressure, run one off one's feet and set one's heart racing (due to the fact that these activate hormones, and thus also one's metabolism); in contrast, cold nodes cause little agitation (due to lack of energy), but on the other hand, are all the more dangerous (→thyroid cancer).

Handling: Acknowledging and owning up to one's own need for security and power; safeguarding oneself in the figurative sense in order to free one's head of the issue and thus be able to move the neck freely again; finding other places for storing possessions (piggy-bank, bank account, brain for one's intellectual possessions, heart for one's emotional experiences); getting a feeling for how possessions and all the things hanging around one's neck are hindering one and using this to bring about relief.

Resolution: Getting rid of surplus and superfluous possessions to save one's neck.

Archetypal principle: Venus-Pluto.

Gonarthritis

see Knee joint inflammation

Gonorrhoea

(clap; second most common and oldest sexual disease, see also Sexual diseases)

Physical level: Originating from the genital region (sexuality, polarity, procreation), untreated gonorrhoea can drag many areas of the body into its wake.

Symptom level: Massive conflict originating from the domain of sexuality: (festering) discharge (from the urethra or vagina) transports the debris of war out of the body; the letting go of spiritual waste is experienced as a burning challenge: irritation and burning sensation when passing water (above all in men, women are often almost without symptoms); once inflamed, tendency for the conflict to escalate initially to the complete genital area before invading the vagina, womb, Fallopian tubes or prostate; later also the joints (mobility, articulation), pericardial sac (protective wall), costal pleura (rib cage lining), and muscles (motoric system); the conflict frequently prevents later pregnancies (sterility in women due to the Fallopian tubes sticking shut, "gumming up the works").

Handling/Resolution: see Sexual diseases.

Archetypal principle: Venus-Pluto.

Gout

Physical level: Initially the smaller, and later also the larger joints (mobility, articulation).

Symptom level: Disorder of the (uric) acid disposal, resulting in massive excess acidity; waste disposal problem in the domain of aggression; excess acidity in the whole landscape of the body (hyperuricemia = too much acidic (acerbic), aggressive energy in one's life flow); becomes partic-ularly apparent in the big toe joint (podagra): every step is hindered by pain; one becomes bogged down – "a sitting " (both in concrete terms and in life); painful conflicts in one's smaller field of movement, which later spread to one's overall mobility; deposit-ing of acerbic, condensed combat energy in the areas of articulation: articulation is painfully blighted by congealed aggressive energy; unre-solved problems condense painfully at particular points (gout nodes = tophia); unresolved nodes of acidity (acerbity) thrust their way painfully into consciousness; (uric) acid in the energy supply system condenses at the weak points, and in this way, shifts them into consciousness; blockage of all activity in the muscular domain: progress is hindered or com-pletely thwarted; inability to bring the masculine pole (acidity) to a resolved level (to keep it in solution): often domineering instead of manly, rage instead of strength (earlier a disease of the ruling class); being bent out of shape over one's own situation, but only rarely prepared to change some-thing substantial with regard to the basic spiritual situation; being rigidly walled-in in one's basic pattern; being tormented to the extreme by the (gout) needles (of uric acid crystals) in one's flesh, but still being inflexible enough to prefer to stay sitting in a sulk, rather than bringing movement into the life flow and one's pent-up emotional world: presenting the typ-ical picture of "someone stuck in a rut"; difficulties with accepting help.

Handling: Conscious holding back of aggressive waste products from the course of the day in order to process these further: it is precisely what has caused the annoyance that must be digested; conscious transformation of the aggressive energy: rapid-fire re-sponses, willingness to deal with con-flict, lively manifestations of life with regard to oneself; bringing the mas-culine pole in one's own being to the point of (re)solution; courage to carry the conflicts from one's closer domes-tic area into one's wider environment (instead of, for example, drowning them every evening in a glass of wine or beer); consciously feeling how one's freedom of movement is being hindered by one's unlived conflicts in order to allow oneself to get involved with them after all; linking aggressive problems to certain points and deal-ing with them in an open(ly offensive) way; using the enforced external rest to ensure more inner movement; grappling combatively with one's own unlived, unexpressed and unresolved nodes; inner retreat, instead of re-treating into every bar.

Resolution: Inner progress; inner development; courageously dealing with the inner conflicts and articulat-ing them combatively (waging holy, healing war with one's own Ego).

Archetypal principle: Jupiter-Mars/ Saturn.

Greenstick fracture

(see also Bone fracture, Accident)

Physical level: Bones (stability, strength).

Symptom level: Harmless, partial fractures (usually in children): inter-ruption of the previous way of life, which was characterised by too much activity and movement; deviation (kink) in the course of life; structural change; breaking up of rigidity; change from the norm; unwillingess to bend; attempt at kicking up a stink; overstretching things, pushing a development too far; overlooking the end of a development; enforced rest before the development can go on.

Handling: Taking a break from the development thus far; stopping along the way; settling down, "not doing things at breakneck speed"; going beyond one's mental-spiritual limits;

re-alignment, helping what is new to break through.
Resolution: Daring to live and re-garding life as a challenge; bringing variety into one's firmly-established track in life.
Archetypal principle: Saturn-Uranus.

Greying

(see also Age-related symptoms)
Physical level: Hair (freedom, vitality).
Symptom level: Resignation, cutting back on things, worrying ("giving one-self grey hairs"); fright, fear of death, dread; the variety of the colours of life pales under the grey veil, which makes almost all people equal; grey temples suggest experience; the wis-dom of the grey-haired (tribal) heads.
Handling: Conscious retreat towards rest; like the youth in the Brothers Grimm fairytale - going forth and learning to shudder with fear (the last and most important transition in life) and thereby overcoming the fear once and for all; switching to the dark side of life; having experiences which are still open-ended.
Resolution: Greying in wisdom: transforming knowledge into wisdom.
Archetypal principle: Saturn.

Guilt, feelings of

(see also Allergy, Depression)
Physical level: Consciousness prob-lem, which like →fear creates a broad basis for symptoms of disease.
Symptom level: Having become stuck.
Handling: Asking oneself what debt one owes to life so far ("What is over-due?"); re-examining one's expecta-tions of oneself and the world.
Resolution: Self-responsibility; becoming the unique person that only each individual can be; for-giving oneself and others (Christ consciousness).

Archetypal principle: Saturn.

Gums, bleeding

(see also Gums, inflammation)
Physical level: Gums (basic trust), blood (life force).
Symptom level: Injured basic trust and trust in oneself; exhaustion: "a toothless tiger", "being down in the mouth".
Handling: Helping oneself to de-velop basic trust and trust in oneself; making up for missing basic trust; ensuring regeneration of one's own powers; building a nest for the weap-ons of the mouth; taking care not only of one's own weapons, but also of their basis; creating a good founda-tion for vitality.
Resolution: (Basic) trust, experi-ences of unity (meditation, spiritual exercises).
Archetypal principle: Moon-Mars.

Gums, contraction

see Parodontosis

Gums, inflammation

(Gingivitis; see also Gums, bleeding, Inflammation)
Physical level: Teeth (aggression, vitality), gums (basic trust).
Symptom level: Inflammatory red-dening of the complete surface of the gums, frequently occurring during puberty and pregnancy, but also in the case of →poisoning; conflicts over a lack of basic trust become clear on the surface: at transitional periods in life is a symptom of taking stock; lack of willingness to crack hard nuts or put up a fight; conflict over one's su-perficial vitality; can be an indication of impending rootlessness (as a pre-liminary stage of →parodontosis).
Handling: Helping oneself to develop trust (in oneself); making up for missing basic trust; courageously en-suring the regeneration of one's own

powers; creating a reliable regeneration basis for vitality.
Resolution: Developing (basic) trust; having experiences of unity (meditation, spiritual exercises).
Archetypal principle: Moon/Neptune-Mars.

Gynecomastia

(development of female breasts in men, frequently around the middle of life)
Physical level: Breast (sense of self, personality); mammary glands (motherliness, femininity).
Symptom level: 1. False: purely due to fatty deposits; 2. Genuine: growth of mammary gland tissue; female development in a physical sense instead of mental-spiritual development in the direction of the anima; effeminate habitus, effeminacy on the physical level instead of in consciousness.
Handling: Allowing the feminine pole to grow in consciousness; occupying oneself with nourishing tasks; nourishing (brain)children in the figurative sense.
Resolution: Blossoming of the feminine part of one's own soul.
Archetypal principle: oon.

H

Haemangioma

see Strawberry marks

Haematemesis

see Blood, vomiting

Haematocolpos

see Bleeding blockage

Haematuria

(blood in the urine)
Physical level: Kidneys (balance, partnership), urinary tract (waste water channels).
Symptom level: Life force/vitality is lost through the (spiritual) waste water (first clarify and interpret the basic problem).
Handling: Being more generous with one's vitality; directing life force into the tributary of the soul and learning to flow with it or let it go.
Resolution: Allowing one's vital force to gush out.
Archetypal principle: Mars-Moon.

Haemolysis

see HELLP syndrome, Cold haemoglobinuria

Haemophilia

(passed on by women, but occurring almost only in men; see also Bleeding tendency, Hereditary diseases)
Physical level: Blood (life force).
Symptom level: x-chromosomal hereditary lack of stabilisation capabilities of the life energy: danger of bleeding to death; the life energy runs away at the slightest provocation: danger of loss of vitality, →fatigue, feebleness; external bleeding, but even more dangerous, internal bleeding (e.g. bleeding of the joints: any vigorous movement can already prove too much; →bleeding of the gums: the bed of aggression is particularly sensitive and endangered); having to be particularly careful with the valuable life blood: having to control one's own vitality at every turn and keep it in check; blood transfusions correspond to borrowed vitality, which only holds out for a short time; life task of avoiding all aggression and any injury (having to get by on the physical level without the Mars principle); having to live under the

sword of Damocles of an early death and recognise what is essential on non-physical levels; having to bleed (= pay) for an inherited history.
Handling: Taking the legacy of the past seriously and processing it internally; learning to allow one's own life force to flow generously and to give away energy (strength, money, time, etc.) as a gift: exercises in letting go; learning to accept help; accepting that one is reliant on foreign influences/ people; becoming vulnerable on the spiritual level; religious awareness rituals (e.g. Za-Zen, Vipassana); exercises in renunciation of force: practising meekness ("Blessed are the meek, for they shall inherit the earth"); consciously learning to appreciate the preciousness of time and life energy: meditation on the principle of "death and rebirth"; voluntarily making sacrifices before they are claimed forcibly; shifting life to the figurative levels since everything physical is threatening.
Resolution: Letting go of the demands of the Ego; recognising the gift of life as the special something that it is: regard for (all) life; reconciliation with the uncertainty of our existence and the certainty of death (Tibetan/ Egyptian Book of the Dead).
Archetypal principle: Mars/ Saturn-Pluto.

Haemorrhage, violent

(sudden haemorrhaging of large quantities of blood from a bodily orifice, e.g. anus, vagina, mouth)
Physical level: Basic problem in the intestines (processing of material impressions), womb (fertility, safety and security), lungs (contact, communication, freedom), oesophagus (food pipe, nutrition supply).
Symptom level: Gambling with one's own life blood; losing large quantities of life energy in a rush; acute threat

to life due to loss of vitality: blood sacrifice; an event that scares one to death.
Handling: Using one's vitality for surprising projects; using large quantities of energy without reservation; giving in freely to surprises that suddenly take one by storm; addressing the definitive loss of the life force.
Resolution: Achieving extraordinary feats with one's own life force; reconciliation with one's own mortality; acceptance of death as the final station in life.
Archetypal principle: Uranus-Mars.

Haemorrhoids

(both internal haemorrhoids [at the mucous membrane border] that are invisible from outside and external haemorrhoids that are visible; see also Thrombosis)
Physical level: Rectum (underworld), anus (exit of the underworld), blood vessels (transport routes of the life force).
Symptom level: 60-80 % of adults in Germany suffer from haemorrhoids; →connective tissue weakness is frequently the basis, but it is only with the advent of additional strain in the sense of unconscious, unmanageable pressure (e.g. pregnancy) that this leads to an outbreak; a sedentary way of life also weighs one down (being stuck, not getting ahead), →obesity, chronic →constipation; becoming mired in bogged down situations, being held fast and tied up in knots in the hopeless twists and turns of family entanglements that constrict life and block the ways out: tendency to look for solutions via the back door (back passage); feeling oneself hemmed in, e.g. like soldiers who cannot get out (of their ways), but are trapped in the (uniform) pattern of the military, or like pregnant women who feel themselves ensnared and bound (up) by the pregnancy; the life energy

runs off behind one's back (bleeding); the water of life seeps away from (the) behind (wetting oneself); irritation at the rear exit (itching); pent-up vitality: the life force (blood) gets bogged down, congeals and forms an obstacle or barrier to the rear exit; sitting on one's knotty problems instead of clearing them up: sitting something through or sitting it out; quashed energy; being a slacker; only being able to express oneself in roundabout ways in the form of one's knotty problems; bloody conflict over giving (a) way; a shut-off mechanism of the rear exit: things backfire on one; not being able to kick butt (forcefully assert oneself); avoiding a tight squeeze (by squeezing together one's butt cheeks instead), putting one's tail between one's legs; authority conflicts that are below the belt line; betrayal of one's own rights in life; in the case of bleeding haemorrhoids: sweating blood and water, one's lifeblood runs away behind one's back, energy is released from below and behind instead of from above and forwards.

Handling: Making oneself aware of the bottling up of the life energy, feeling the (spiritual) knotty problems that one is sitting on and making oneself aware of the pressure that one is under; owning up to one's tendency to hold things back and to be backwards in being forward with one's own vitality and one's criticism of the constricting situations; recognising concealed aggressions and consciously putting them to use and into practice; retaining energies for oneself and making use of them for oneself; consciously dealing with one's conflict over the holding back of the life energy; critically questioning the barricades at the rear exit; allowing the energy to flow again (surgeons used to lance the nodes in earlier times); being upright, standing up for one's own interests and being straightforward; taking a look at what

one is "busting one's ass" for; letting off the identified pressure, clearing up knotty problems.

Resolution: Holding back necessary vitality for oneself and one's own path in life; working from the opposite pole: free-flowing vitality.

Archetypal principle: Pluto.

Hair loss

(Alopecia, loss of head hair, baldness)

Physical level: Hair (freedom, vitality).

Symptom level: Moulting; paying for something past: "losing fur in the fray"; having to make sacrifices: "letting feathers fly", "a close shave that doesn't leave one unscathed"; in the past, people were shorn in order to humiliate them (in the same way as women who consorted with the enemy and witches); allowing too little of the new to grow back; loss of the (lion's) mane: loss of power, influence and vitality; when one gets fleeced, one is then exposed and naked and feels oneself as though rubbed raw; self-punishment; regression into the hairless period of early childhood: "a bald head as smooth as a baby's bottom"; thinning out of a magnificent head of hair: the primordial forest (of the unconscious) becomes thinned out; in the case of soldiers: sign that they have been robbed of their own freedom and power and subjected to the power of another; in the case of nuns and monks: sign that they have subjected themselves voluntarily to a higher power, and that they have chosen to relinquish their own insignia of freedom and power; sign of simple-mindedness: "not having a lot up top"; biochemically an indication that male hormones significantly outweigh female ones.

Handling: Questioning old structures, letting go of what is old/outmoded, making way for the new; bidding farewell to certain patterns of thought; paying off old debts (including those to oneself); asking the question: "What do I still owe (to myself)?"; admitting to oneself that too little of the new is breaking through, things are not progressing anymore (in life), and that one's spiritual progress has been brought into question; voluntarily sacrificing freedoms which, in the meantime, have become a hindrance; admitting and accepting the loss of freedom; recognising tendencies towards self-punishment and complying with the inner demands instead of paying the price (in the form of hair loss); baldness: rediscovering one's own childlike nature at a higher level; thinning out and becoming aware of the primordial forest of the unconscious.

Resolution: Coming clean with the past in order to allow new impulses and forces to sprout; making a conscious sacrifice of the hair: consciously giving up external freedom and power (a cloistered life).

Archetypal principle: Sun-Uranus/ Pluto.

Special forms of hair loss (Symptom and handling level)

1. Spot baldness (alopecia areata): facing up to deeply-rooted unconscious sorrow and grief (e.g. through the loss of siblings who died at a young age) (rending one's hair in pain, tearing one's hair out), consciously grieving, belatedly making up for missed grieving rituals; detaching oneself in a delimited area from structures that have outlived their usefulness; solving clearly-delimited problem spots by paying the price or letting feathers fly with regard to freedom and power.

2. Hair loss similar to a monk's tonsure in men: preferring to open oneself up to higher spheres.

3. Receding hairline: opening oneself up more fully to philosophical aspects and spiritual things.

4. High forehead: opening up room for spiritual worlds; bringing the spiritual aspect of one's own life into the foreground.

Hair loss, complete

(complete loss of all body hair; relatively new disease pattern, to date only observed in women)

Physical level: Head hair (freedom, vitality), body hair (animalistic strength).

Symptom level: Being naked and laid bare, exposed without protection (to everyone's gazes); no longer being able to hide anything, compulsion to the greatest possible openness; need for withdrawal; unconscious desire to break off contact with the surrounding world (throwing off all feelers and antennae); showing shame and being shamelessly open; loss of face in public due to completely open honesty; baldness as at the beginning of life; shedding one's skin, moulting: attempt at renewal.

Handling: Allowing oneself the freedom to withdraw; giving up superficial contacts and reflecting more on oneself; creating complete openness without regard to power and influence in the outer world (head hair); showing naked honesty and defenceless openness in the erotic respect (pubic hair) – to the point of shamelessness.

Resolution: Regaining child-like openness; making oneself independent of the outer world; rediscovering one's own childlike nature at a higher level; finding a new identity, new beginning.

Archetypal principle: Moon-Venus.

Half-vision

see Hemianopsia

Halitosis

(Foetor ex ore)

Physical level: Mouth (absorption, expression, maturity – being able to speak for oneself), digestive tract (Buddhism: Bhoga = "consuming and digesting the world").

Symptom level: Locate and interpret the source of the bad breath: mouth/teeth, cleft tonsils, stomach, intestines; neck as Hell's Gorge (the gateway to Hell): Hell stinks to high Heaven; causing a stink for others: keeping them at arm's length (unconscious desire to distance oneself); avoiding erotic-sexual encounters: inhibitions about kissing on the part of one's partner; unconsciously wanting to scare off any possible suitors; rotten attitudes and indecent thoughts that people turn their nose up at escape from one's lips with a corresponding vapour trail; blazing a trail of bad breath; allowing others to get wind of one's true colours - the foul message precedes one.

Handling: Consciously getting to the bottom of one's hell: dis-tinguishing/ex-tinguishing impure intentions in the aggressive domain of the bite, in the nest of the stomach or the depths of the shadow kingdom; consciously establishing and maintaining distance using more sophisticated means; coming to terms with one's own erotic-sexual intentions.

Resolution: Ensuring clean conditions in the oral domain.

Archetypal principle: Venus-Pluto.

Hallucinations

(illusions, perceptions without external stimuli)

Symptom level: Perceptions taken for real or images (imaginings) which others do not (cannot) share: visual = seeing things; acoustic = hearing voices; olfactory = sensing smells; tactile = detecting touches; taste hallucinations.

Handling: Taking all perceptions for real and taking them seriously; paying attention above all to the inner ones: those who listen carefully to their own inner voices at the right time and have faith in their inner visions do not need to go to the psychiatrist because of them; concerning oneself with inner perceptions; recognising the function of inner visions and voices as important to (survival in) life (if dreams are suppressed for one week in a sleep laboratory, everyone develops hallucinations); ensuring adequately long REM (Rapid Eye Movement) sleep phases; making oneself aware that every creation is based on stored inner images (musical creations are based on stored inner melodies); learning to decode the meaning of the inner information before the pressure behind it becomes too great; from time to time, taking spiritual reality for real; taking (on) inner reality as truth; consciously learning to imagine: e.g. being able to see inner visions with one's eyes open is one of the training objectives in Tibetan Buddhism and in various occult-based orders.

Resolution: Recognising that every perception we take for real always originates first from the inside; paying attention (respect) to one's own inner perceptions in good time.

Archetypal principle: Neptune.

Hallux valgus

(X-position of the big toe in the case of →splayed feet)

Physical level: Toes (foothold), feet (steadfastness, deep-rootedness).

Symptom level: Big toe crossed over the others, along with a fallen frontal arch of the foot, ball formation: deviation from the straight and narrow, hindrance of the smooth, rolling motion of the foot; usually caused by overly-narrow and pointed shoes: the roots and therefore also one's deep-rootedness are hindered; distorted concepts in one's head: the deviation from the straight and narrow (directness) makes itself painfully felt.

Handling: Recognising problems with one's deep-rootedness; preferring to lose one's grip on reality in the figurative sense; striving to elegantly put one's best foot forward in more natural ways rather than in tight, high-heeled shoes; making oneself aware of the tightly-confined living space of one's own roots; stepping back a little and living more modestly, consciously restricting oneself; learning to see through one's own crooked ways; accepting one's own deviation from the norm: consciously going unusual ways.

Resolution: working from the opposite pole: creating room for one's roots; ensuring better conditions in order to be able to put down roots at all, as well as to grow and feel comfortable; willingness to be deeply rooted in order to be able to grow towards Heaven.

Archetypal principle: Neptune-Uranus.

Hand problems

(see also Dupuytren's contracture, Rheumatism, Flexion of the fingers and toes)

Physical level: Hands (grasping, gripping, ability to act, expression).

Symptom level: 1. Monkey paw (paralysis of the musculature of the ball of the thumb, the thumb falls into line with the fingers): difficulties with getting a grip (grasping);

2. Drop hand (the hand can no longer be opened due to paralysis of the nervus radialis): the open hand stands for honesty, peaceful intentions;

3. Claw hand (over-extended knuckle joints and bent middle and end joints due to paralysis of the nervus ulnaris: claw, predator's hand): lacking functionality, but looking threatening and dangerous; coarse, undifferentiated approach to life;

4. Club hand: due to the fact that the nervus radialis is lacking; the hand looks inhuman, daemonic, dishonest, suspicious or at least untrustworthy;

5. Drumstick fingers or nail clubbing (swelling, particularly of the end phalanx of the fingers, due to an insufficient supply of nutrients as a result of chronic heart and liver diseases; compare the desperate swelling of the shoots of trees threatened by forest dieback): the under-supplied extremities attempt to build up supplies in advance, thereby giving the fingers a club-like, inelegant appearance.

Handling/Resolution: Admitting to oneself that one cannot get a grip on life in this way; taking on board and taking seriously the particular approach to life being expressed by the hand and accepting the corresponding learning task, which naturally leads one to the the opposite pole: the monkey grip encourages us to embrace rather than grab at (grasp) things, and this therefore becomes the special task; in the case of the drop hand, it is a matter of recognising one's own dishonesty and hostility, as well as accepting honesty and openness as a challenge; the claw and the club hand want to reach (out to) things roughly, but must learn differentiation and sensitivity as the opposite pole.

Archetypal principle: Mercury.

Hands, sweaty

see Sweaty hands

Handicaps

see Deformities

Hardening

see Sclerosis

Harelip

see Facial clefts

Hashimoto's thyroiditis

see Thyroid gland inflammation

Hay fever

(see also Allergy)
Physical level: Nose (power, pride, sexuality), lungs (contact, communication, freedom), bronchia (connecting channels between the inner and outer world).

Symptom level: Fear of sexuality, animalistic instinct, fertility, love; resistance to these areas of life through the dangerous battle against representatives of these themes, such as blossom pollen (male plant seeds) and other seeds (grasses, hay); aggressively shutting oneself off from these symbols: the nose almost swells shut, the bronchia almost swell shut; fear of the potential power to conceive life; build-up of aggression, which is let out at every (symbolically-suitable) opportunity; heavily armed defence system, armed to the back-teeth against fertility symbols with guided weapons (antibodies).

Handling: Owning up to (unconscious) restrictiveness and resistance with regard to the sexual-erotic area; recognising in the pollen the representatives of the feared themes; learning to acknowledge and appreciate aggression as one of the basic forces of life; making oneself aware of one's own possibilities and putting them to use and into practice in life; directing one's own pent-up aggression towards rewarding goals; taking a closer look at the escalation of one's armaments and learning to see oneself as aggressive(ly inhibited); discovering one's unlived or unlively sexuality and tackling the subject anew; taking up the battle regarding one's own desires and capacity for love in an open(ly offensive) way.

Resolution: Discovering Eros (the god of love) as the child of Venus (the goddess of love) and Mars (the god of war, energy and combat strength) and doing justice to him.
Archetypal principle: Mars-Saturn/Pluto/Neptune.

Headaches

(see also Migraine)
Physical level: Head (capital of the body).

Symptom level: Blocking one's first (thought) impulses at the head level; living out something in one's head which belongs elsewhere; attempt to overcome emotional and feelings-related subjects by racking one's brain instead; 1. High- or excess-pressure situation: over-emphasis of the upper, masculine pole; "brain-boxes" are particularly affected: the "blockhead" who feels as rigid, solid and square as the world of "four" that the problem originates from; mental overload/top-heaviness, neglecting the heart as the second centre; detachment from the lower pole/body; reconnection [re-ligio(n)] to one's own roots is missing; safeguarding of the Ego, "one's head spins" (with ideas and thoughts); the pushing through (of one's initial impulse) causes splitting headaches; banging one's head against the wall: "Where there's a will, there's a way", the head as a battering ram; wanting to control too much, everything should fall in line with my way of thinking; being headstrong and pushing through one's own ideas, great strength of will; claim to power, forcing one's way through; overestimating oneself: "taking an idea into one's head and setting one's mind on it", "letting something go to one's head"; pain as a warning against faulty reasoning: "racking one's brains" naturally hurts, "beating one's brains out", "braining someone", "a pounding headache"; strong pressure to perform, excessive mental strain: ambition, thinking of one's career, perfectionism; critical climb to the top. Forehead pain (behind the forehead lie the frontal lobes of the cerebrum = rational thinking): confronting life; bravely fronting up to life; the heavily-furrowed brow of the defiant person reveals the tension and effort of this stance, which is painful in the long run. Temple pains, both sides: feeling as if clamped in a vice, between a rock and a hard place, being able to move neither forwards nor backwards, being stuck, in a tight squeeze; Pounding: life is beating on the door to sound the warning of a confrontation or struggle. Pains at the back of the head (in the rear area of the head lies the cerebellum = theme of balance in life): still "keeping something at the back of one's mind" (making a mental note in the sense of holding onto a grudge); region of unresolved problems and unsettled accounts, which want to be settled and thus make their presence felt in the form of pain. Pains in the centre of the head: shutting oneself off from enlightenment from above, not letting in any flashes of inspiration from above, experiencing pressure from above and feeling weighed down, "having someone come down on one like a ton of bricks".

2. Situation of depression or low pressure, insufficient blood flow: blurred thoughts, no longer being able to "wrap one's head around things" or see through them: being a "blockhead"; deceiving oneself: dizzy "feign"ting spells; not being master (mistress) of the situation.

3. Due to feeling chronically sick to the eyeballs of everything: being snuffy and in a huff (→sinusitis), one's head feels like lead.

Handling: Trusting one's first impulses; living out at the heart, gut or muscle level whatever does not belong in the head; 1. Finding the solution instead of searching for it; becoming aware of the overestimation of the masculine pole; once again feeling the pressure that one is holding out and thinking under; learning to see through the Ego in its narrow limits and desires; recognising "always-more-of-the-same"-style thinking as offering no way out; learning to hold the Self in high esteem instead of overestimating oneself in the sense of overemphasising the Ego; counteracting one-sidedness through inclusion of the female pole; letting go of the narrow-mindedness of "I want", of ambition, thick-headedness and being stubbornly headstrong after one has seen through these; remembering one's roots (lower pole/ feet); relieving the strain on the head: allowing fantasies and playful thinking to develop; courageously taking the first steps into new areas; making decisions (freeing the sword from the scabbard; Latin: dēcīsiō = 'a cutting off') and forcefully asserting these , respectively oneself.

2. Finding intuitive solutions; consciously doing things in the more creative and non-conformist left-handed way.

3. Fasting; jettisoning ballast; rearing up with one's head held high.

Resolution: Creating harmony in the demands between the head, heart and gut; being head of the show on non-intellectual stages as well; moving forward with a clear head.

Archetypal principle: Mars.

Headlouse infestation

(pediculosis capitis)

Physical level: Head (capital of the body), hair (freedom, vitality).

Symptom level: One's own capital city (head town) is settled by foreigners, brazen intruders who "trample all over one"; the louse sticks its eggs (nits) to the roots of the hair: irritating troublemakers settle in one's own underbrush, stirring things up and making a public nuisance of themselves; sign of inadequate hygiene, of being unkempt, and therefore often resulting in shame; nevertheless, nowadays also frequently found in well-groomed kindergarten and schoolchildren who often stick (their heads) close together: something disgusting, a "creepy-crawly" jumps across, "Pass the parcel".

Handling: (Homeopathically:) becoming livelier, allowing more life to come into one's own capital city (head town); (allopathically:) maintaining distance, ensuring a clean environment, improving hygiene, cutting back and cleaning one's own antennae better; use of poison, combing out the pests; setting oneself apart.

Resolution: Better and clearer communication; letting oneself get involved in life in different ways; offering living space to life; creating a home for lively vitality; allowing things to "dance around in one's head" in the positive sense and dancing along with them; spawning new ideas and life impulses.

Archetypal principle: Pluto-Mars.

Hearing, hardness of

(hypacusis; see also Senile deafness, Deafness)

Physical level: Ears (hearing and obeying commands).

Symptom level: The outer world gradually retreats from one acoustically: in elderly people, a sign of unresolved tendencies, such as unwillingness to bend or give way: not wanting to hear (or see) anything more; the body does what the person fails to do: it withdraws itself from the day-to-day business; unresolved form of retreat into one's own world; loss of adaptability and flexibility; declining willingness to listen to commands; no longer willing (or able) to lend anyone

one's ear; the outside world becomes less important; one becomes less accessible, and thereby unconsciously distances oneself.

Handling: Recognising and acknowledging the call of Fate to turn oneself away from the outer world towards the inner world; no longer listening to and obeying commands outwardly; learning to trust one's inner voice.

Resolution: Listening carefully to one's own inner voice and obeying its commands.

Archetypal principle: Saturn-Saturn.

Hearing, sudden loss of

(see also Hearing, hardness of, Ear noises)

Physical level: Ears (hearing and obeying commands).

Symptom level: Abrupt, suddenly striking (often unilateral) failure of one's hearing ability in a life situation of excessive external demand (stress) through situations or people; one ear is switched off, the receiver is hung up with regard to the surrounding world, and one is thrown back on oneself and the inner world; hardness of hearing betrays the declining willingness to listen to orders (obey): "Are you deaf?"; "not wanting to pay attention anymore", "being up to one's ears with things to do"; unresolved form of retreat into one's own world: the symptom pushes the world away from the person affected; switching off one's hearing on the inner level; often →ear noises: the outer voices are drowned out by the inner soundscape.

Handling: Preparing oneself for sudden decisions (to retreat); cutting out listening to others (outside voices) and instead learning to listen to the commands of one's inner voice; distancing oneself from the hectic environment (and toxic load) of the (outer) world, before Fate takes it all away.

Resolution: Once again making use of the ability to be all ears; listening carefully inwardly and trusting and obeying one's (own) inner voice.
Archetypal principle: Saturn.

Heart anxiety

see Heart problems

Heart asthma

see Asthma cardiale

Heart block

see AV block

Heartburn

(see also Belching, acidic)
Physical level: Stomach (feeling, receptiveness).
Symptom level: Not displaying one's aggressions openly and instead overshooting the mark with acid production in the stomach - the nest of childhood and security: acting like a sourpuss and being offended; inability to consciously handle resentment: swallowing resentment; auto-aggression: hard self-criticism, immediately placing the blame on oneself; burning desire for life.
Handling/Resolution: Learning to express aggressions in more conscious ways.
Archetypal principle: Mars.

Heart contraction, premature

(extrasystole)
Physical level: Heart (seat of the soul, love, feelings, energy centre).
Symptom level: One's own centre has fallen out of step; wanting special treatment; inability to subordinate oneself to a higher idea; having one's own way in central matters.
Handling: Consciously dropping out of the prescribed role and placing

central demands on distinctiveness and originality; giving up plodding along in a rut and letting something new spring to mind; living individuality; kicking over the traces, stepping out of line, living out "eccentric" (off-centre) ideas and creative flashes of inspiration.
Resolution: Finding one's own (unique) rhythm; standing up for one's own (unique) nature.
Archetypal principle: Sun-Uranus.

Heart defect, congenital

(see also specific defects)
Physical level: Heart (seat of the soul, love, feelings, energy centre).
Symptom level: Central life tasks that have been brought along with one; defect in one's own centre: something central is missing; not being completely adjusted to life in the polar world: (unconscious) rejection of taking part in the cycle of life; not being decisive enough in wanting to remain (in the world); being reliant on foreign, external help.
Handling: (for the parents and the later adult): adjusting oneself to old tasks that have been brought along into this life or helping those affected to make this adjustment; going in search of what is missing in the centre; involving oneself in life in the world of polar contrasts without losing sight of the centre and the actual meaning of life; recognising the necessities that are part of the cycle of life: choosing either life-threatening shortcuts (short circuits) or a life-sustaining longer way along prescribed paths; consciously deciding in favour of this world; learning to accept external help.
Resolution: Consciously giving oneself over to the cycle of life with its necessities and compulsions; it is only through the resolution of polarity that access to unity emerges; "Whatever

you do, do it with your whole heart"
(Confucius).
Archetypal principle: Sun-Saturn/
Pluto.

Heart degeneration

(myodegeneratio cordis)
Physical level: Heart (seat of the
soul, love, feelings, energy centre).
Symptom level: The heart- specific
tissue is replaced by inferior connective tissue: hardly any work gets
done anymore; one's place in life is
merely held onto without really filling
it out completely; one's life centre
gives up; the powers of the heart are
exhausted; the conflicts consuming
one's power of resistance remain in
the background.
Handling: Giving in from the centre
outwards; maintaining one's place in
life without (great) expectations; becoming aware of the overdue central
transformation (metamorphosis); preparing oneself spiritually for the final
letting go of matter.
Resolution: Loving and feeling
without regard to norms and limits;
preparation for the opening up of
oneself for and the return to the home
of the soul.
Archetypal principle: Sun-Uranus.

Heart failure

(Cardiac insufficiency, see also Senile
heart)
Physical level: Heart (seat of the
soul, love, feelings, energy centre).
Symptom level: The heart cannot
cope anymore – it is no longer able to
deal completely with the challenges
(demands) required of it; the will to
live comes to a standstill in the heart;
unconscious "I (the heart) can't go
on"; the central point of life gives up;
giving up at the central point of life;
a series of emergency measures
precedes the collapse: expansion,
working overtime (increased heart
rate), water retention (reduces the

volume of blood) = mobilisation of the
last reserves; the collapse is accompanied by: a back-up of fluid into the
lungs (in the more frequent case of
left-side heart failure) or in the body
in the case of right-side heart failure
(e.g. after persistent →asthma): the
spiritual (water element) becomes
backed up, and can no longer be kept
in circulation; in the case of a back-up
into the lungs (→lung oedema), those
affected face the threat of suffocating,
respectively drowning in their own
spiritual fluid; failure with regard to
one's central life theme or conscious
bailing out of the chaos, taking flight;
bowing out of polarity: ultimately, the
end of every life is accompanied by
cardiac arrest since the heart can
no longer go on under the given
circumstances.
Handling: Expansion of the capabilities of one's own heart; opening
oneself more extensively for the
broad flow of the life energy and life;
getting to know the dual nature of
every task: facing up to it as long as
it makes sense to do so, but also recognising the right moment for giving
up: surrendering oneself to one's fate;
concrete spiritual exercise: fasting
therapy in order to give the physical
heart the chance to get back into (its
original) shape and become more
expansive in the figurative sense.
Resolution: Big-heartedness;
remaining calmly in one's centre
(being at home in oneself), and from
this starting point, opening up and
expanding (one's horizons): giving
oneself up to Creation and becoming
one with all; finding (final) peace; surrender: from "My will be done" to "Thy
will be done".
Archetypal principle: Sun-Neptune.

Heart, fatty degeneration

(lipomatosis cordis)
Physical level: Heart (seat of the
soul, love, feelings, energy centre).

Symptom level: Not admitting to oneself the full weight of one's centre and its central life themes; emphasising the weight befitting the centre in a heavy-handed way; the well-insulated/isolated heart packed in cotton wool (fat = best insulation for retaining warmth and preventing shock): screening against the stress of life.

Handling: Consciously granting more weight to the heart; admitting to oneself the weight(iness) of one's central heart(-related) matters; directing enthusiasm into one's heart; becoming rich and magnanimous (big-hearted) in the figurative, spiritual sense (instead of physically fat); learning to protect and defend one's heart in the figurative sense and screening oneself off from dangerous threats using conscious measures; insulation/isolation in the sense of withdrawal into one's own, essential being (hermitage).

Resolution: Making one's centre into a place of safety.

Archetypal principle: Sun-Jupiter.

Heart flutter

Physical level: Heart (seat of the soul, love, feelings, energy centre).

Symptom level: On the basis of toxic heart damage (glycosides), →cardiac infarction, →lung embolism, electrical accidents, etc.: the heart rhythm goes haywire, being all in a flutter over matters of the heart (muscle); impulses which concern the life centre go around in circles; great turbulence in one's heart without any result; absolute chaos with regard to the information in the life centre – a condition only very briefly compatible with (survival in) life; heaving and surging of the heart, which cannot find its way (rhythm): rearing up (death struggle) of the centre; the pounding of one's heart at every opportunity calls it into one's consciousness; fear of tackling

life-and-death issues that revolve around love.

Handling: Allowing oneself to be all in a flutter due to a racing heart at the right time; allowing oneself to be turned this way and that by the heart and following its twisted, illogical paths; giving in to the (superficial) chaos of feelings; discovering the background to the feelings; allopathic and life-saving method: waking up to life; using strength to overcome the fear of life; making decisions which restore the proper hierarchy in the heart (medical defibrillation disempowers all centres in order to help the first one [the sinus node] back to power); returning to the hierarchy: discovering the highest first, i.e. the true order which lies behind our visible world; being united with regard to a single impulse centre and one (paramount heart's) desire, i.e. deciding in favour of life.

Resolution: Recognising and accepting hierarchy as the dominance of the holy: deciding to put the highest in first place.

Archetypal principle: Sun-Uranus/Neptune (Chaos).

Heart muscle degeneration

see Heart degeneration

Heart muscle inflammation

see Myocarditis

Heart neurosis

Physical level: Heart (seat of the soul, love, feelings, energy centre).

Symptom level: Compulsion to continually observe one's heart and to subordinate one's life completely to the physical needs of one's heart: protective stance; over-emphasis of the body while overlooking the soul:

everything revolves around the heart, but only on the physical level; continually listening to one's heart while neglecting one's (spiritual) centre; listening to one's (physical) heart, but without obeying its commands; fear of the breakdown of the Ego; fear of exploding; need to cling on tightly, separation anxieties, symbiotically-close partner relationships; fear of not being complete by oneself; panicked fear of dying; aggressive tendencies towards an overpowering force which constrains the heart (often the mother figure); fear of heartlessness (in the physical sense).

Handling: Shifting the heart back into the centre of life in the spiritual respect; transferring the heavy weight of loving attention from the physical to the spiritual heart; becoming "capable of love": showing loving inclination towards a person; confronting the powers of one's Ego; letting go of the inner domineering mother figure; freeing oneself from dependency; becoming aware of aggression, particularly of the aggressive desire for liberation; setting out on the path to find and live out one's Ego; involvement and reconciliation with the subject of death; psychotherapy.

Resolution: Showing courage (lion-heart); moving away from the implosion to the explosion; obeying the stirrings of one's heart, living in a more heartfelt way; task of the small personal Ego in the great sea of cosmic awareness.

Archetypal principle: Sun (heart)-Pluto (compulsion).

Heart pacemaker

Physical level: Heart (seat of the soul, love, feelings, energy centre).

Symptom level: Mechanical strike-breaker: predictable beat in the heart – in contrast to one's own unpredictable rhythm; robot in the centre of life; taking flight from the unreliability of the heart; reliability is placed above lively vitality; having originally realised too little of one's unique character and individuality.

Handling: Recognising how much of what is dead and mechanical has already taken possession of one's own life; addressing the poles of rhythm and beat, respectively the lively (unreliable) heart and the non-living (reliable) machine.

Resolution: Elevating one's goal to living instead of just surviving; encouraging joy for life.

Archetypal principle: Sun-Uranus (technology).

Heart pain

see Heart problems

Heart phobia

see Heart neurosis

Heart problems

(stabbing pains (in the chest), heart-focussed anxiety, heart pain, racing heart)

Physical level: Heart (seat of the soul, love, feelings, energy centre).

Symptom level: Stabbing pains in the heart: stabbing pains in one's emotional centre as an important signal; heart-focussed anxiety: momentary feeling of constriction in matters of the heart, being stuck tight (uptight) in heart-related issues; heartache: love pangs; the heart cries out for loving attention; racing heart: life/fate runs the heart off its feet; galloping, rapidly coursing, racing feelings; heart problems in general: be(com)ing ill due to one's centre; spiritual derailment in a central area that touches one's centre of life.

Handling: Learning to listen to one's heart and to follow it; tracing the source of the stabbing pains, and finding out who is guiding the knife; tracing the source of the fear in

restrictiveness and airing the secret; allowing oneself to be moved in terms of the heart, increasing the speed of the life flow.
Resolution: Consciously placing the heart in the centre of one's life and following it (at least in heart-related matters).
Archetypal principle: Sun-Saturn/Uranus/Mars.

Heart, racing

see Heart problems

Heart rhythm disorders

(see also Heart contraction, Tachycardia)
Physical level: Heart (seat of the soul, love, feelings, energy centre).
Symptom level: Sudden breakings in the general order of life/the heart, derailments from the normal balanced pace; one no longer trusts oneself to be carried away by the emotions; only wanting to listen to one's head; being orientated too much towards reason and norms; allowing too little room for emotions; not being in synch with one's own rhythm.
Handling: Allowing breaks in the accustomed order; voluntarily taking the leap out of the balanced pace of normal life again and again; consciously being eccentric (= off-centre) now and again, stepping out of line, kicking over the traces (using Carnival, Mardi Gras, etc.); learning "to listen to one's heart" as well as one's head: voluntarily giving room to one's emotions and feelings and contrasting them to the normalised behaviour.
Resolution: Allowing oneself to be stirred out of one's peaceful state of composure by emotions and feelings; openness to the breaking in of irrational feelings; searching for one's own rhythm and living independently of all norms.

Archetypal principle: Sun-Uranus.

Heart septum defects

Physical level: Heart (seat of the soul, love, feelings, energy centre), heart septum (threshold in our centre between this side and the beyond).
Symptom level: The necessary final step into polarity is not taken, the single heart from the time in the womb does not properly divide itself into the two chambers: always remaining close to unity (continual closeness to death); remaining stuck in an earlier development stage; not wanting to let go of unity/the paradisiacal state in the womb; difficulties in adjusting to polarity; not managing the step into duality; holding on to the tried and tested becomes an obstacle in life.
Handling: Reconciling oneself with the past in order to then let go of it; learning to grow beyond tried-and-tested things from the past; making oneself aware of the compulsions and necessities of the polar world and accepting them; learning from the handicap of the situation (using disease as a path): living more calmly, with more orientation towards inner steps than outer performance, etc.; accepting being an outsider (in matters of the heart) in the positive sense.
Resolution: Continually maintaining unity as the ultimate goal in consciousness; consciously taking leave of Paradise, but carrying within oneself the certain knowledge of a later return.
Archetypal principle: Sun-Uranus.

Heart, too small

Physical level: Heart (seat of the soul, love, feelings, energy centre).
Symptom level: Insufficient challenge, lack of exercise; heart palpitations at every opportunity call the heart into consciousness; feeling (too)

little courage/strength/love/emotion; faintheartedness, weakness; opposite pole: big, wide-open heart; hardly being able to rely on the strength of one's heart; disorders in regulating one's circulation: not being able to take part actively and offensively in the circulation (cycle) of life.

Handling: Taking greater care of one's own heart (e.g. self-help instead of exaggerated willingness to help others), demanding less of the heart in the figurative sense and also looking after the physical heart, e.g. through gentle exercise training; doing something for the heart, its strength, its emotions and feelings, not only in dreams, but also in concrete terms; directing one's attention to the heart at every opportunity; sensing its needs and also creating a (physical) basis for them; learning commitment.

Resolution: Concentration on the matters that are close to one's own heart; giving in to the needs of one's heart; living out longings; genuine modesty in the sense of self-denial; allopathically: taking heart and allowing it to grow beyond oneself in the direction of expansiveness, openness and courage.

Archetypal principle: Sun-Saturn.

Heart valve insufficiency

(tricuspidal insufficiency; see also Heart defect, congenital)

Physical level: Heart (seat of the soul, love, feelings, energy centre).

Symptom level: Sisyphus task in the middle of one's life; the forward flow of one's life progression is bought at the cost of significant setbacks; tendency to regression; problem of retreat; lack of backing in life; lack of ability to distinguish (oneself); essential divisions (of the blood flow) are not possible: work must be performed aimlessly.

Handling: Conscious taking back of the life energy; learning to withdraw back to oneself; conscious regression; developing openness also for one's own setbacks; learning to shut one's trap, to say 'no'; asking oneself what is missing.

Resolution: Consciously taking on the Sisyphus situation as a life task; reconciliation with the life that is constantly taken back again and again.

Archetypal principle: Sun-Saturn.

Heart wall dilation

see Aneurysm

Heatstroke

(sunstroke)

Physical level: Brain (communication, logistics), spinal cord (data highway).

Symptom level: Dizziness to the point of delirium, brain damage extending to cerebral haemorrhages: dropping out of conscious responsibility; the life energy leaves its prescribed paths and blocks the "government work" of the central control headquarters: "frying one's brains out in the sun"; extreme effect of the sun fire element on the head leads to the flight from responsibility (sunstroke): the head, capital city and seat of government (brain) of the body closes down functioning and lays down its office; in extreme cases, death due to paralysis of the respiratory centre or cardiac insufficiency; the exchange with the polar world is shut down; death due to one-sided emphasis of the fire element.

Handling: Applying the sun fire energy on the figurative level as enthusiasm, commitment and being fired up for things, and avoiding the extremes of the actual sun; granting the government headquarters voluntary breaks more often, long before it comes to a blockade of the whole capital city;

allopathically: learning to deal with fire in the right measure.
Resolution: Reconciliation with the (Sun-)fire element.
Archetypal principle: Sun/ Mars-Uranus.

Heat syncope

(see also Collapse)
Physical level: Blood circulation (circuit of the life energy, supply and disposal).
Symptom level: Collapse of the circulation under extreme, extended exposure to heat: due to the enlargement of the blood vessels of the skin, they draw in too much blood, leaving a shortage in the central control headquarters of the brain; too much spiritual water vanishes completely from the body due to perspiration or to the peripheral areas of the body due to enlargement of the blood vessels of the skin; excessive demands on the feminine spiritual element of water as a result of excessive exposure to the masculine fire element : too much fire – too little water; too much of the spiritual element (water) is given off to the outside under the strong masculine influence of fire, with the result that one comes up too short oneself.
Handling: acute allopathic approach: ensuring correction of the imbalance: cool shade, supply of water; long-term homeopathic approach: involvement with the fire element and its effects, discovering more resolved (redeeming) levels such as fiery enthusiasm, inner fire, etc.; bringing the spiritual element to the surface, instead of physically giving off water.
Resolution: Finding the happy medium between the flooding in (influence) of feminine spiritual water and the masculine fire energy; balance of the four elements in one's life.
Archetypal principle: Sun-Moon.

Heavy metal poisoning

(see also Amalgam poisoning, Lead poisoning)
Physical level: Nerves (news service).
Symptom level: Blockage of the system of basic regulation with symptoms similar to →rheumatism or even →multiple sclerosis: the basic overall tone in the organism is no longer in harmony; there is (dangerous) grit in the works; blockage of the physical control circuits: the interplay between the individual departments functions increasingly poorly; →nervousness, hypersensitivity, forgetfulness, states of exhaustion, intestinal problems, such as →constipation, fungal infection; vegetative problems ranging from →headaches to →insomnia.
Handling: Careful flushing out of the toxic materials; learning to confront the surrounding world effectively: reasonable adaptation to the prevailing conditions of life while at the same time showing respect for one's environment; allowing things through more easily: not taking everything personally, not putting on every shoe that fits; transforming physical (over-) sensitivity into emotional sensibility.
Resolution: Learning trust, taking leave of the pure, wholesome world: taking concrete steps towards healing of one's immediate inner and outer world.
Archetypal principle: Mercury/ Uranus-Saturn/Neptune.

Hebephrenia

("adolescent craziness", disorganised schizophrenia)
Symptom level: Most malignant form of →schizophrenia, usually beginning with puberty, can progress without any delusions or hallucinations to gradual breakdown of the personality; idiotic behavioural patterns that

cannot be taken seriously: the clown, Jack-of-all-trades, great joker, who creates an alarmingly good to over-the-top mood; for the other family members, an unbearable lightness of being; also has an overbearing effect; compulsive wisecracking; unquenchable desire for silly patterns of behaviour, never-ending foolishness, idiotic mannerisms; often mad(ly) comic ideas, brilliant(ly bold) flights of fantasy that are intoxicatingly hectic and bubble forth with genius-like speed: frittering life away in a ridiculous way; loss of one's centre and all centring: jokes and mocking comments cover up for a time the destruction of the life centre; getting stuck clinging to childish role patterns far past the right time, and often then, for all time.

Handling: Consciously departing from parental/educational norms at an early stage and developing the courage to have one's own identity; finding ways of becoming an adult (puberty rituals); acknowledging all the different elements of one's soul that are struggling for supremacy in one's own heart ("Two souls dwell, alas! in my breast" [from Goethe's Faust]); allowing oneself to be different even if that means being more laid-back, off-the-planet and happy-go-lucky; following one's own inspired ideas and adjusting oneself to a high speed of life and high flexibility; integrating centring exercises into one's life in good time: Tai Chi as a philosophy of life, i.e. letting all movement come from one's centre; seeking conscious contact with one's own centre; the whirling dance of the dervishes, dancing the waltz in order to practise centring, making pottery on the rotating potter's wheel: using the centre of the pot to find contact with one's own centre; as an opposite pole, exercises in grounding: hearty eating, earthbound life, physical work.

Resolution: Bearing one's own lightness of being and also possessing the necessary discipline to often showcase the talents of one's genius for good effect(iveness)

Archetypal principle: Moon-Uranus/Pluto.

Heel spur

Physical level: Heel (weak point).

Symptom level: Painful (bone) outgrowth at the point for putting one's foot down firmly; often unbearable pressure complaints when putting one's foot down: coming under pressure in the area of one's own standpoints; signs of wear and tear at the vulnerable point of the heel.

Handling: The symptom forces one to physically not put one's foot down so firmly (to tread more gently): being lighter of foot and floating through life, instead of trampling; learning to step up to things with offensive strength even under pressure; allowing one's own structure to grow – if need be – even with pain; proving oneself under pressure; continuing to stand up for oneself and move forward; becoming aware of one's Achilles heel (the weakest point) and being able to stand behind it.

Resolution: Growth in the area of one's own weak points, respectively right or left standpoints.

Archetypal principle: Neptune-Jupiter-Saturn.

Heliosis

see Heatstroke

HELLP syndrome

(complication in pregnancy, short designation for bleeding tendency [Haemolysis = disintegration of red blood cells], liver problems [Elevated Liver Enzymes = increased liver enzymes] and low thrombocyte count [Low Platelet Counts])

Helper syndrome

Physical level: Liver (life, evaluation, reconnection), blood (life force).

Symptom level: Total breakdown of almost all systems in the mother, impending extinguishing of the pregnancy and the life of the mother, escalation with respect to →eclampsia and →gestosis; severe coagulation disorder with far too few blood platelets causes the life force to flow away inwardly; the inner wounds can no longer be patched up; highly serious liver problems also disturb the coagulation system even to the point of causing the liver to rupture ("being fit to burst"): lack of meaning in life and life force; possibly demanding too much of the liver as a detoxification organ due to harmful substances from the surrounding environment: overloading it with superfluous and dangerous elements.

Handling: Allowing the life force to flow inwards; looking after oneself (in energetic terms), giving of oneself completely for the new life; looking after one's own re-ligio(n) (from Latin religāre 'to bind, tie again'), finding the meaning of (one's own) life.

Resolution: Applying life energy, giving of oneself completely; making sacrifices; discovering meaning in life.

Archetypal principle: Moon-Jupiter/Pluto.

Helper syndrome

(co-dependency)

Physical level: Consciousness problem.

Symptom level: Sacrificing oneself for others, and thereby – without being aware of it – projecting one's own problems onto others and only being able to deal with them in this way; pushing one's own needs far into the background; living for others without noticing that this still only has to do with oneself; apparently selfless dedication even to the point of making this a career choice: behind this in the shadow lurks one's own longing for rescue; looking after the needy and addicts in order not to have to confront oneself with one's own dependency and neediness (false helper).

Handling: Recognising one's own neediness in the needy, seeing one's opposite as a mirror and using it for one's own development.

Resolution: Becoming one with everything: "loving thy neighbour as thyself".

Archetypal principle: Neptune-Venus.

Hemeralopia

see Night blindness

Hemianopsia

(half-side blindness)

Physical level: Eyes (insight, perspective, mirror and window of the soul), crossing point of the optic nerves (light cables).

Symptom level: 1. Homonymous hemianopsia (the left or right half of the vision in both eyes fails in the event of damage to the optic nerves behind the crossing point): the feminine, respectively masculine side of reality can no longer be perceived, while the other side remains completely untouched;

2. Heteronymous hemianopsia: blinkered vision (the outer areas, the peripheries of the field of view are lost in processes that affect the chiasma – the crossing point of the optic nerves): going through life as if wearing blinkers; living a small-time, narrow-gauge existence;

3. Rare form of heteronymous hemianopsia (in the event of processes which simultaneously encompass the sella turcica from both sides and put pressure on the outer fibres of the optic nerves responsible for the central areas of the field of view): the centre of things can no longer be

perceived, loss of the centre, inability to concentrate on central matters.
Handling/Resolution: 1. Resolving the remaining side of reality with its tasks, and in that way, regaining the opposite pole and the bilateral view of the world; 2. Concentrating on the remaining central matters, and from the awareness of what is essential, gradually broadening one's circle of vision again; 3. Approaching the concerns of life in a less target-oriented and more laid-back way; letting go of thoughts of efficiency; "The journey is the destination." as a learning task.
Archetypal principle: Sun/ Moon-Saturn.

Hemicrania

see Migraine

Hemiplegia

see Stroke

Hepatitis

see Liver diseases

Hereditary diseases

Physical level: The whole organism can be affected.
Symbolism: Continually-recurring learning task within a family; family fate, family karma: continuing the tradition and/or elevating the pattern of one's forebears to a more resolved (redeeming) level.
Handling: Reconciling oneself with one's family history, assuming one's place and one's role and making the best of it; growing into the task and possibly also growing beyond it (usually better for promoting development than rebellion, which is linked to the danger of falling into the opposite pole).
Resolution: Consciously integrating oneself as a link in the chain of one's forebears and accepting the task

handed down with respect to its Resolution and redemption.
Archetypal principle: Pluto-Saturn.

Hermaphroditism

(androgyny; genuine hermaphrodites are extremely rare; in the more frequent pseudo-hermaphroditism, the secondary and primary genitalia are not in accord with each other)
Physical level: The complete organism, but above all, the genitalia (sexuality, polarity, procreation).
Symptom level: The gonads of the one sex and the secondary sexual features of the other sex put those affected completely between two stools; on the outside, (one's own) nature puts on the appearance of the sex for which the appropriate equipment is missing; however, over the course of life, those affected increasingly develop in the direction of their inner sex.
Handling: Experiencing in oneself both sides of human existence and helping each of these to their own; Yin and Yang, reconciling the feminine and masculine with each other: solving the task, which normally arises more strongly with the onset of menopause, throughout one's whole life instead.
Resolution: Consummating the alchemic wedding of the feminine and masculine in consciousness.
Archetypal principle: Uranus.

Hernia

(see also Inguinal hernia, Umbilical hernia, Hiatus hernia, Intestinal incarceration)
Physical level: Various areas such as the groin (vulnerability) and stomach (feeling, instinct, enjoyment, centre).
Symptom level: Competition between two domains: disregard of boundary and ownership ratios in which neither wins; establishing

false and unsuitable relationships, over-stretching oneself; overriding sensible limits instead of steadfastly holding faithfully to basic principles; having grappled with matters that are too difficult, having overreached oneself; danger of strangulation (strangulated hernia) of the foreign organs that have been trespassed upon; aggressive conflict, war involving sudden invasion; break-ins occur at weak points (in criminology as in the organism).

Handling: Overcoming boundaries between separated areas; enabling breakthroughs into unfamiliar areas; break with what is traditional and conventional; overriding externally drawn boundaries, enabling exchange: learning to occupy space, but watching out for invasions; tackling weighty subjects; taking on a great deal (on the mental-spiritual level); handling new incoming subjects intensively; identifying areas in which it is worthwhile to overstretch oneself; respecting one's own fragility and weak points (groin, navel, diaphragm passages).

Resolution: Intensive intellectual exchange that transcends boundaries: taking new paths in intellectual-spiritual areas and allowing the insights gained to burst forth; connecting bordering subjects in one's mind; arriving at seemingly-impossible connections; having a great deal of confidence in one's binding commitment on the intellectual -spiritual level.

Archetypal principle: Uranus-Mercury/Venus/Moon (depending on the area of the body concerned).

Herpes genitalis

Physical level: Genital region (sexuality), labia (curtains of the treasure chamber).

Symptom level: (Unconscious) conflict (pressure) ignites itself in the sexual area; fear of defilement/ impurity; feelings of disgust; shame and → feelings of guilt (for having a fling on the side); self-punishment (for having an affair): marking oneself or letting oneself be marked, with the associated compulsion to show one's true colours; encrusted attitudes with regard to sexuality; punitive superego; ambivalence of desire and the feeling of guilt: the withheld fire raises (fever) blisters; hindrance of desire and further sexual intercourse (pain, contagious infection); "unclean", unacknowledged desires cross one's lips (Latin: labia).

Handling: Opening oneself up to exciting experiences in the sexual area, in which shadow elements can also come to the surface and cross the border of consciousness; giving way to the burning needs: igniting the fire in the area of desire; exploring one's own shadow realm; getting to know one's own taboo zones; recognising and addressing one's own unconscious ideas of cleanliness on the different levels; respecting the need for forgiveness in order to take the weight (of guilt) off one's mind; living as if in a fever instead of developing fever blisters.

Resolution: Openness in the sexual area for new experiences; stepping beyond one's own boundaries and pushing forward into shadow areas.

Archetypal principle: Venus/ Pluto.

Herpes labialis

(fever blisters)

Physical level: Mouth (absorption, expression, maturity – being able to speak for oneself), lips (sensuality).

Symptom level: Conflict in the area of sensuality: the lips swell up, showing the unconscious tendency towards burgeoning sensuality (unacknowledged desire); feelings of disgust; resistance to kisses and intimacies: warning potential partners using deterrents and repulsion;

ambivalent message: "Look at my swollen lips, but do not touch me"; deep disgust about one's own unfathomable depths; the unspeakable and unmentionable crosses one's lips in coded form: herpes blisters bubble to the surface instead of speech bubbles (the lips swell up); fear of the primordial slime/swamp: something which one dreads wants to come out; unclean thoughts cross one's lips physically instead of verbally; disfigurement as disguise; fear of infection: punishment for "unclean" thoughts; fevering towards something, being under stress (champing at the bit and foaming at the mouth); weak resistance: not being able to properly defend one's own skin; risking a fat lip for being cheeky; letting saucy, suggestive things spring from one's own lips; suppressed, unarticulated rage and deep disgust alike raise blisters.

Handling: Allowing the repulsive aspects in one's own being to break forth in controlled doses; letting one's own shadow issues rise up into consciousness; getting to know one's own dark desires; accepting sensuality instead of disfiguring it; letting unspeakable things cross one's lips, risking a fat lip for being cheeky: raunchy jokes and hot topics; reducing one's resistance to so-called unclean desires; relying more on physical rather than spiritual resistance.

Resolution: Courageously allowing even hot, risqué topics to cross one's lips; letting one's own sexuality blossom.

Archetypal principle: Venus/Moon-Mercury-Pluto.

Herpes zoster

see Shingles

Hiatus hernia

(see also Reflux oesophagitis, Rupture)

Physical level: Diaphragm (border).

Symptom level: No clear separation any longer between the upper masculine and lower feminine half of the body; break between the polar domains; repression of the anima and resulting invasion by the suppressed feminine pole; allowing what has already been assimilated in the stomach back into the foodpipe: enabling backsliding.

Handling: Allowing the upper and lower, masculine and feminine, to mutually penetrate each other so that the body is freed from this task; giving the anima free scope to unfold and enough room so that the body does not have to play out first its confinement and suppression and then the illegal act of liberation (hiatus hernia); opening oneself up to conscious regressions.

Resolution: Connection between the upper and the lower, the animus and anima.

Archetypal principle: Mercury-Uranus.

Hiccupping

(singultus; particularly common in children; in general of little pathological significance, but nevertheless annoying)

Physical level: Diaphragm (border).

Symptom level: Break in the normal life flow; brings the seat of the spiritual forces (in ancient times believed to be in the diaphragm) back to mind: convulsive discharge of tensions of the soul; unadmitted sobbing or suppressed laughter; directs attention to the act of swallowing: "having swallowed too much", "poor sucker", "having had something go down the wrong way"; reversal of the act of swallowing: something comes back up on the communications level (cf. also protective warding off spells: finding out who is thinking of one so that it stops); feeling of being at the mercy of one's body, becoming aware of one's powerlessness over inner processes; becoming the butt of jokes made by unaffected people who are witnesses to the problem: becoming a laughing stock.

Handling: Ensuring humorous and offbeat interruptions in the daily grind of life; letting go of what is pressing on one's soul and stirring it up (to make leaps and bounds); helping oneself to move forward in leaps and bounds instead: not shying away from ideas and flashes of inspiration that may be a little offbeat; in keeping with protective warding off spells that are part of folk medicine: somebody is thinking of one, so find out who it is and it will stop.

Resolution: Escaping the monotonous daily grind with humorous impulses and mental leaps.

Archetypal principle: Uranus.

High blood pressure

(hypertension)

Physical level: Blood (life force), blood vessels (transport routes of the life force).

Symptom level: Blood pressure = energy/bloodstream resistance/vessel wall phenomenon; being permanently under pressure and permanently overstimulated: "putting oneself under pressure"; continually living in close proximity to conflict without being able to find a solution; not facing up to things; continual exam stress situation and readiness for defence; tense basic situation full of nervous expectation and inner agitation; unresolved authority conflicts; suppressed hostility; chronic inner need; persistent, apparently insurmountable worries; taking flight into a frenzy of activity on the outside, distraction; repressed aggression; self-control on the physical level; blockage of activity on the level of physical functioning; attempt to control everything; the external world is considered more

important than oneself, which quickly makes criticism a problem; wanting to prove through performance who one is, respectively what a good person one is; communication problem: dishing out (criticism) rather than sharing (ideas and thoughts), rapid-fire retorts as if from a pistol (rather than real answers), tendency to contradiction.

1. Blood pressure leading to a reddish complexion: feeling oneself to be irreplaceable, wanting to be involved in every thing; a boastful stirrer, motto: "I am needed everywhere!";

2. High blood pressure leading to a pale complexion: superhuman control; permanent life struggle in a cage (formed by the vessels); behind the façade, a tense and highly-strung person;

3. High blood pressure in old age: bogged down (channels of) communication.

Handling: Instead of holding out permanent pressure, seeking the decisive conflict; putting all one's strength into its offensive solution; identifying and tackling the authority problem; standing up to enemies; ceasing the frenzy of activity in favour of the one decisive battle; courageous, offensive living; genuine inner self-control; control of one's own emotions in order to make use of them in a well-targeted way (no longer turning one's heart into a skeleton closet); release of tension after the confrontation; fostering communication: fast, rapid-fire comebacks at the right point, otherwise preferring to listen; recognising the wisdom of the saying "talk is silver, silence is golden"; consciously catching one's breath and letting go when exhaling; owning up to one's desire for recognition.

1. Recognising the desire to flee in one's own furious hustle and bustle; relieving pressure (at the right point);

2. Seeing through one's own suppression, then once again bringing

pressure to the surface in order to finally let it out at the decisive point; 3. Letting one's heart speak.

Resolution: Declaration of one's own power; facing up to the pending confrontation; applying pressure to get the deadlocked situation back into motion again; concentration on essential points (often matters of the heart); taking an inward look at one's own heart subjects instead of projecting them outwards; growing beyond oneself on other levels.

Archetypal principle: Mars-Saturn.

Hip joint diseases/ pains

(see also Arthrosis, Rheumatism)

Physical level: Hips/hip joints (making strides).

Symptom level: Steps forward (progress), and in fact, every single step is painful: striding/stepping forward is hindered or prevented, getting ahead in life is brought into question; great strides, and certainly great leaps, are no longer possible with ease; deadlocked situation; feeling of having become rusty.

Handling: Owning up to one's own lack of flexibility, to the pain caused by any steps forward; consciously sensing the effort of will required by every step; resigning oneself to the enforced rest; acknowledging that steps forward and movement in general are difficult to bear; taking inner steps instead of outer ones.

Resolution: Inner journeys: being outwardly calm, and taking large steps inward; accepting and appreciating one's own age.

Archetypal principle: Jupiter-Saturn.

Hip joint luxation

(dislocation of the upper end of the thigh bone from the socket in the hip bone)

Physical level: Hips/hip joints (making strides).

Symptom level: Articulation in terms of steps forward (progress) is hampered enormously (on the basis of retarded development of the skeletal system): waddling gait like a duck, which allows one only slow steps forward (progress); making strides is hindered or prevented, getting ahead in life is brought into question; great strides, and certainly great leaps, are no longer possible with ease: the legs find it difficult to carry the body; the burden of life becomes very difficult to carry (bear); elegant steps forward (progress) are hindered or prevented; emphasis of polarity: one goes deep into the left and the right pole (with every step).

Handling: Giving oneself time to mature in structural areas (in the same way that medicine immobilises the hip joint in order to give the hip socket time to catch up developmentally); coming to terms with the basic problems in matters of taking steps forward (progress); understanding one's comic-looking gait as a symbol and recognising where similar behaviour exists in the figurative sense; allowing oneself time for development; getting ahead leisurely and in one's own, albeit unusual manner and style; owning up to one's own inflexibility; resigning oneself to the enforced smaller radius of life in concrete terms; acknowledging that external steps forward are difficult to bear and adjusting oneself to inner steps; letting oneself get deeply involved in the highs and lows – the ups and downs of life.

Resolution: Instead of taking long, strenuous external paths, preferring to seek inner paths; using the relative calm of the outer world in order to progress further inwards.

Archetypal principle: Jupiter.

Hirsutism

(masculine hair growth in women; see also Female facial hair)

Physical level: Hair (freedom, vitality).

Symptom level: Cosmetic disfigurement in the direction of masculinisation (hairy, animal-like appearance): neglected masculine elements that have been pushed back into the shadows and now want to gain the upper hand; the masculine part of the soul (animus) spreads throughout the body; excessive amount of male testosterone: problems in becoming pregnant; if the animus comes up too short spiritually during menopause, the masculine pole frequently manifests itself in this physical way; masculine pubic hair: unacknowledged phallic-aggressive streak in the sexual area; female facial hair: desire for willpower and forceful assertiveness ("being a real man", "being man enough to wear the pants in life"); single chin hairs (in German, often referred to as Hexenhaare = 'witches' hairs' because witches were typically portrayed with hairy warts): a prompt not to overlook one's own dark sides; great need for protection; a "hair-raising" man's man, a "bristly" wildcat who is able to bite back.

Handling: Discovering and developing the masculine pole; integration of the opposite pole on the spiritual rather than the physical level; accepting and living out the animalistic part of the soul (the bristly beast); helping one's own will to break through, earning respect for oneself, showing one's bristles (being defiant).

Resolution: Living up to one's own life pattern and bringing it into harmony with the universal life pattern of the mandala, which from the middle of life at the latest, envisages the conquest of the parts of the soul belonging to the opposite pole: what takes place in consciousness, however, does not need to be acted out once again on the physical stage of the body; becoming one with the opposite spiritual pole.

Archetypal principle: Mars-Uranus, Pluto.

Hives

see Urticaria

Hoarseness

(to the point of losing one's voice [aphonia])

Physical level: Larynx (expression, tone [mood]).

Symptom level: Rough, toneless voice: symptom of many diseases of the larynx from inflammation to paralysis of the vocal cords and even to the point of tumours; embattled voice (inflamed larynx), aggravated, over-stretched vocal cords: not enough calmness in the voice; conflict over one's voice, e.g. not having the confidence to voice one's opinion, to forcefully assert oneself; when accompanied by inflammation: rage over not standing up enough for oneself and for the overall tone of one's life, as well as rage over sacrificing oneself and one's own interests for the sake of outward impressions; attempt to hush something up; irritated tone; not standing behind one's own utterances with one's whole being (unconsciously distancing oneself from one's own utterances with parts of one's personality); having roared, but not created an uproar with one's whole voice (whole effort); no voice = having no say (voting rights), disempowerment, disenfranchisement; no longer having to say what one thinks (because one no longer can): unacknowledged disinclination to speak, to raise one's voice; croaky voice in the attempt to go on speaking despite the hoarseness (overestimating one's own importance?): irritation due to buzzing around too much;

the voice does not come from the heart or the gut, but instead from the overworked throat: no resonance in the body; strained voice = strained overall tone (mood); exhausted voice = exhausting situation; in the case of →influenza: being hoarse from all the unsaid things; having neglected to "cough up" what one really thinks of someone, to splutter with rage, to raise one's voice and to scream out the aggressions; being compelled to whisper (secrets can only be passed on by whispering).

Handling: Learning to tone things down, consciously sticking one's neck out (stirring things up) and thereby getting ahead; getting to know one's reservations with regard to one's own utterances in order to be able to voice them more in accord with the full force of one's own voice; learning to scream out in synch with one's own inner roar; screaming out all of one's own inner roar; during the period of hoarseness, when screaming out is not yet possible, following the compulsion to speak more softly, and learning to be quiet; with the deepening of the voice due to the hoarseness: task of combining this with deeper levels of one's own being, of giving the voice better grounding, creating more resonance for it in one's own body and therefore also in the world; allopathically: learning to fight with one's voice; raising one's voice, letting oneself (one's own demands) be heard, and also sometimes striking harsher tones; learning to help set one's voice to rights for one's right to voice (voting rights).

Resolution: Only those who can scream out everything they have to scream about can also hush up their total silence.

Archetypal principle: Mercury/Saturn.

Hodgkin's disease

(lymphogranulomatosis; see also Cancer)

Physical level: Lymph node system (defence).

Symptom level: Wild and ruthlessly rampant growth in the immune defence centres; having strayed so far off track from one's inherent developmental direction with regard to defence that the body must now bring it to the point of expression on its own initiative; the mental-spiritual growth in this area has been blocked for so long that it now forges a path in the body in an aggressive, random and ruthless way and helps the unlived energy to express itself on the physical stage of the body; the cancer realises physically in the area of defence that (turnaround) which would be spiritually necessary in the corresponding area of consciousness.

Handling: Opening oneself up in the area of defence to one's own wild ideas and bold fantasies, courageously allowing them to grow and flourish without control; learning to defend oneself more creatively and committedly without boundaries and respect; thinking back to early dreams of one's own life and one's own readiness to attack; bringing these (back) to life and putting them into practice with wild decisiveness; having nothing more to lose and courageously tackling one's own life; putting all one's forces at the disposal of this new programme in the sense of a general mobilisation (attacks of fever); allowing oneself to be challenged; attacking the borders and itching to stir them up; living in a way that is bristling with excitement; allowing the domains of life philosophy and re-ligio(n) (in the sense of 'reconnection', from Latin religāre 'to bind, tie again') to grow and increase in importance (swelling of the liver); at the same time, also increasing

the regeneration of the life force (swelling of the spleen); considering all the measures mentioned under →cancer: since cancer affects the complete organism, it must also be met across-the-board.
Resolution: Discovering love that transcends all boundaries, setting oneself above external rule and standards laid down by oneself or others, and attacking and defending in accordance with the obligations of one's own highest law; recognising the necessity to switch from the physical and thus (life-)threatening level to the challenging, but life-saving mental-spiritual level, and relying in this realm on expansive growth with respect to courage, reconnection and renewal of the life force.
Archetypal principle: Mars-Pluto.

Hollow back

Physical level: Spinal column (dynamics and hold, uprightness).
Symptom level: Compensation employed by the broken child/adult (→round back); hollowness of the compensating stance that one has dragged through life; wanting to make things right for everybody: feigned uprightness.
Handling: Learning to be straight with oneself from the inside out/to stand up for one's own needs instead of adopting a particular stance; re-discovering the broken child underneath the impressive pseudo-uprightness; also learning to make it right for oneself.
Resolution: Inner posture (uprightness) as the basis for one's outer bearing.
Archetypal principle: Saturn (spinal column, uprightness) Neptune (appearance).

Hordeolum

see Stye

Hormone disorders, female

(see also Ovarian insufficiency)
Physical level: Ovaries (fertility) or hypophysis (central control).
Symptom level: Not being able to find one's own rhythm, dropping out of rhythm, not being able to follow regulations (regular cycles), going one's own way in matters of femininity.
Handling: Accepting unusual paths of femininity, living out one's creativity; breaking loose from outside (social) ideas and compulsions.
Resolution: Finding and making one's own individual lifestyle a reality; finding time for oneself and using it.
Archetypal principle: Moon/ Mercury-Uranus.

Hospitalism

1. Spiritual and physical disorders of children during longer stays in hospital.
Physical level: Different areas can be affected.
Symptom level: Signs of deprivation with regard to letting out (expressing) feelings, in particular being deprived of love; typical are, for example, rocking movements, through which children set themselves into a cradling rhythm in order to get a sense of themselves and have a calming effect; often downright falling into a trance (fleeing from the unbearable reality); to some extent, serious self-harm, such as banging one's head against a wall in order to be able to get a sense of oneself and still feel something; begging for attention – even aggressive attention if there is nothing else to be had.
Handling/Prevention: Maintaining regular, dependable contact with the child under all circumstances: in the case of younger children, the mother should stay with them in the hospital;

encouraging dependable contacts between caregiving personnel and children and between children amongst each other.

Resolution: Maintaining the family situation in the hospital or providing other comparable security.

Archetypal principle: Moon-Saturn.

2. Hospital- specific infections, triggered by particularly resistant pathogens which are often virtually cultivated by the indiscriminate use of antibiotics.

Physical level: Inflammations (conflicts) in widely differing areas.

Symptom level: The sickbed makes one sick; clinic-specific conflicts cultivated in hospital inflame the weak points of the patients; unconscious conflicts over the hospital situation which have slid down into the body.

Handling: Critically disputing the need for hospitalization and the stay there; battling with the hospital or its representatives for one's health in an open(ly offensive) way.

Resolution: Wrestling for one's release from the sickening environment.

Archetypal principle: Mars-Pluto.

Hot flushes

(see also Climacteric complaints)

Physical level: Blood circulation (circuit of the life energy, supply and disposal).

Symptom level: The organism continues to work on unresolved subjects: unlived femininity ("a hot-blooded woman"); something unlived and forbidden makes one "hot"; sexual "hot flushes"; fear of missing out on something: having come up too short, and now offensively taking every opportunity to catch up on what has been missed out on; panicked mood: having missed out on something and now no longer being able to be over and done with it.

Handling: Courageously owning up to the missed opportunities; catching up on what can be made good; facing up to one's own inner heat; getting over and done with one's (life) tasks instead of allowing oneself to be done in by them: checking off internally what is past and gone; living out intellectual-creative fertility with a blazing heart on figurative levels: awakening the fire of enthusiasm for a subject/project in oneself, developing commitment; heat = fire subject: recognising the fire (still unsatisfied drives = Mars) that is making one break out in a sweat for what it is, and transforming it into the fire (of the sun), which alludes to the heartfelt warmth and the enthusiasm of the blazing heart.

Resolution: Changing the archetypal principle from Moon to Sun; warm-heartedness coming from inside, instead of (quickly passing) flushes of (superficial) heat; giving in to the gentler and deeper experience of the time of life that is now approaching.

Archetypal principle: Moon-Mars-Venus-Sun.

Hunchback

(extreme curvature of the thoracic spinal column to the rear [kyphosis])

Physical level: Spinal column (stability and dynamism, uprightness).

Symptom level: Penitent posture; being bowed by life/fate; "crooked as a dog's hind leg"; by having one's gaze forced downwards/to the Earth, one is forced to humbly acknowledge one's own origin: the sky is not the limit; being humiliated; being compelled to meet everything and everyone humbly: having to look from bottom to top; hardness towards oneself; swelling in the area of the neck ("stooped with sorrow"): unexpressed sadness.

Handling: voluntarily doing penance where needed; learning respect for Mother Earth; learning to meet people with humility: learning to serve;

learning to look upwards (to God?) with humility; being rigorous and strong towards oneself; dissolving and clearing up hardened elements with tears. Resolution: Starting from the humiliation of the external posture, allowing genuine humility to grow as an inner attitude.
Archetypal principle: Saturn-Saturn.

Hydatiform mole

(Mola hydatiformis; see also Pregnancy, false)
Physical level: Womb (fertility, safety and security).
Symptom level: Pregnancy consisting only of vesicular placental tissue: plenty of placenta (Latin: 'flat cake') but nobody who wants to live off it; not wanting to take reality for real; the egg and the semen are so severely impaired that the bad fruit that results from them eats into the surrounding tissue like a cancer, thereby greatly endangering the woman: dangerous creativity which pays no attention to content and sense, being blind to oneself in a way that is threatening.
Handling: Developing a sense for what is do-able.
Resolution: Letting productivity flow into constructive channels.
Archetypal principle:
Neptune-Moon.

Hydramnion

(excess of amniotic fluid)
Physical level: Womb (fertility, safety and security).
Symptom level: Offering too much of a good thing with up to 10 litres of amniotic fluid instead of one litre, pushing the watery-spiritual pregnancy situation too far, surrounding the child with too much of a protective layer; not allowing anything or anybody close to the child; danger of over-distension of the womb with the consequence of →birth complications: premature contractions; attempt

to be prematurely rid of the unbearable problem which the pregnancy has become; frequent occurrence in women with →diabetes mellitus: problem with (motherly) love and the (spiritual) amniotic fluid.
Handling: Adjusting oneself much more to the pregnancy on the spiritual level; giving the child far more loving care and attention in a spiritual sense, protecting it even better and surrounding it with spiritual energy; ensuring relief of the burden.
Resolution: Surrounding the child with oceanic feelings of unity, giving much more inner room to the pregnancy.
Archetypal principle:
Moon-Neptune.

Hydrocele

(accumulation of water in the mucous membrane fold of the testicle or spermatic cord)
Physical level: Testicles (fertility, creativity).
Symptom level: The spiritual element thrusts itself forcibly into the area of procreation and creativity; the testicle swells up due to the invadion of spiritual fluid: bursting/breaking in of water (hydrocele) into the field of masculinity; the feminine element forces its way into masculine territory: feelings flood the area of creativity – drowning it, so to speak; enormously exaggerated demands in the area of procreation (greatly-enlarged testicles).
Handling: Voluntarily allowing far more spiritual energy to flow into the area of creativity and sexuality; consciously giving the subjects of masculinity, procreation and creativity more room.
Resolution: Combining the soul with masculinity and sex with loving, soulful feelings.
Archetypal principle: Moon-Mars.

Hydrocephalus

(Water on the brain)
Physical level: Brain (communication, logistics).
Symptom level: The expansion of the spiritual water areas inside the brain results in the degeneration of the brain substance (due to pressure) and enlargement of the skull (basic problem in the case of tumours; first clarify the cause of the excessive liquor production): the enlarged head as a symbol of power and influence ("big-head"); the shrunken, restricted brain as a brake on the intellect; the intellect (cerebrum area) comes under spiritual pressure; the squeeze is put on it and it is thinned out.
Handling: In the course of one's further life: creating space for the soul in the area of the seat of government – the central control headquarters for pushing all the buttons and calling the shots; allowing the head, which has been extended by the spiritual dimension, to expand beyond its limits, making an impression; reducing and giving a lower priority to the intellectual part of one's own being in favour of spiritual needs.
Resolution: Connection of the spiritual with the intellectual, of feelings and reason, while giving precedence to the soul.
Archetypal principle:
Moon-Mercury-Neptune.

Hydropsy

see Oedema

Hypacusis

see Hearing, hardness of

Hypalgesia

see Insensitivity to pain

Hypasthesia

see Insensitivity to pain

Hyperacidity

see Acidosis

Hyperactivity

(in children: see Hyperkinesis)
Physical level: Nerves (news service).
Symptom level: Pent-up activity which discharges itself at the wrong point.
Handling: Sport, artistic activity; bringing movement into previously-lifeless areas so that calmness can set in where it makes sense; recognising the state of being innerly wound-up and highly-strung as the result of inhibited movement impulses (like the wound-up balance spring of a clock).
Resolution: Finding one's calling and losing oneself in it.
Archetypal principle: Mars-Uranus.

Hyperacusis

(hypersensitivity to sound, nervous acuteness in hearing)
Physical level: EMars/hearing (hearing and obeying commands).
Symptom level: Suddenly reacting oversensitively to normal sounds; feeling oneself disturbed by even the smallest sounds.
Handling: Learning to rely on one's true perceptions; prompt to listen more closely, pay careful attention, and to heed and obey appropriately; working from the opposite pole: becoming loud oneself and screaming out what is unbearable.
Resolution: Listening closely and obeying (one's own inner voice or suggestions from outside); in pregnancy: communicating with the child via one's inner voice even before the birth.

Hyperalgesia

see Over-sensitivity to pain

Hypercholes-
terolemia, inherited

(congenital tendency to a high cholesterol level; see also Cholesterol level, high)

Physical level: Arterial vessels (energy supply), cholesterol (bandaging and sealing material of the body)

Symptom level: Exaggerated attempt to equip oneself from the very beginning with too much bandaging material in order to protect oneself against leakages and seal oneself off; the bandaging material, which the flow of the life energy transports in excessive quantities, becomes a problem; every even minor construction site in the life energy pipelines (vessels) becomes built up further into a major construction site because there is so much building material available in abundance; this in turn results in highly over-stretched energy pathways full of construction sites and repair crews on all levels; increased danger of traffic bottlenecks (reduction of the diameter of the arteries), traffic jams (vascular closures) and total gridlock (complete breakdown of supply).

Handling: Recognising the over-strained provision situation on the physical level and choosing instead to transfer it to the mental-spiritual level; concerning oneself with protection and shielding on the figurative level; looking for areas where one is starting to crack up and taking appropriate steps on the figurative level; protecting one's own nerve system against overload; making oneself aware of conflicts in one's daily struggle for survival, and developing conscious strategies in this respect; getting to know one's own sore (weak) points: allowing oneself time to let the wounds heal; developing strong nerves (of steel).

Resolution: Replacing excessive bandaging material production and transportion with preventive measures on the figurative level: reducing the tempo of life by restraining traffic; creating artificial bottlenecks.

Archetypal principle: Saturn.

Hypergalactia

see Breast milk production, excessive

Hyperhidrosis

(increased secretion of sweat; see also Sweaty feet, Sweaty hands)

Physical level: Skin (border, contact, tenderness).

Symptom level: Continuous anxious sweating; sweating (blood and) water; being continually bathed in sweat; sweaty, wet, cold hands, which show no willingness for contact, and whose greeting is neither warm nor heartfelt; cold (sweaty) feet: basic fear, insufficient deep-rootedness; sweating = bleeding = bleeding dry (to death), i.e. losing life force; sweating with exertion: permanently and unconsciously over-exerting oneself; sweating due to heat: continually (unconsciously) being hot (for something); continuous cleansing attempt by the body from all pores; loss of spiritual fluid.

Handling: In the case of cold sweating: making oneself aware of the fear; in the case of hot sweating: bringing one's inner heat and highly-charged sexuality into consciousness; checking for signs of over-exertion and exerting oneself consciously.

Resolution: Letting oneself get so deeply involved in one's primordial fear that it is eventually turned into expansiveness.

Archetypal principle: Saturn (restriction, exertion)-Mars (heat).

290

Hyperinflation (of the lungs)

see Pulmonary emphysema

Hyperkeratosis

see Keratosis, Acanthosis

Hyperkinesis

(psychogenic, uncontrolled stormy outbreak of movement), "hyperactive children", Attention-Deficit Hyper-activity Disorder [ADHD], Attention Deficiency Syndrome [ADS], see also Concentration disorders)
Physical level: Skeletal musculature (motor, strength), consciousness.
Symptom level: Overabundance of movement; pressure to perform, chaotic sensory overload and spiritual unrest run riot physically; "Sturm und Drang" ("Storm and Stress") period on the physical level of the body; lack of natural (life) rhythms; hyperactive children as a reflection of our erratic modern life; involuntary caricature of a self-assured life in the here-and-now; being "out of it" after having "kicked off" all social life; those affected are troubled by themselves and the world, for which they are too jumpy, spontaneous and often also too intelligent; with their divergent "ideas", they become a provocation for parents and bourgeoi-sie society; in the alternative scene, highly prized as "indigo children"; the fidgety child is nowadays "treated" by traditionally-accepted medicine with amphetamines (Ritalin), which in their effect are similar to the drug Ecstasy (MDMA, also an amphetamine).
Handling: allopathically: ensuring physical exhaustion (sport, work); counteracting the prevailing trends of the over-demanding, aggressive and egoistic, performance-based society within one's own family; conscious handling of determination and control by others; setting limits; giving one's attention; homeopathically: making oneself aware of the spiritual unrest and lack of well-roundedness; even allowing room for the modern trends and letting them exhaust themselves, which in turn also leads to exhaus-tion; using high-tech computers and the modern world of sports in order to draw out new ideas and create new challenges, which fascinate children on the brink of overload; making use of the possibilities of this "erratic and crazy" time, which prac-tically demands equally erratic and crazy answers; allowing one's own rhythm; finding one's own talents; following one's own calling; accept-ing one's own individual nature and non-conformity.
Resolution: Creating inner move-ment in order to take the load off the body; concentration on the essential.
Archetypal principle: Mars-Uranus.

Hypermastia

(abnormal enlargement of the breasts)
Physical level: The female breast (motherliness, nourishment, safety and security, sensuality, desire).
Symptom level: Over-the-top fem-ininity; excessive emphasis of the nourishing feminine aspect in the body; possibly compensation for a corresponding deficit in conscious-ness; often no need at all to nurse and provide for children or to nourish men in an erotic way; often a feeling of shame due to the large breasts: not being able to face up to one's own femininity in its full extent, danger of →postural defects if the attempt is made to conceal the breasts; signal effect on men, especially those with mother problems: large breasts trigger high expectations with regard to nourishment, security and being held; associations with a big heart and corresponding big-heartedness

(generosity) and willingness to bare all (permissiveness): "being well-stacked", "having plenty up front", which is emphasised by the traditional, tight-fitting dirndl dress and supposedly invites men to "take a peep", "milk bar".
Handling: Owning up to one's own signal effect and learning to stand behind it: accepting the situation, respectively the gift of (one's own) nature and learning to handle it; recognising and accepting the demonstration of femininity as a task; recognising and living the abundance of one's own natural leanings.
Resolution: Being "master (mistress)" of the situation, and consciously using the effect of one's image on others; consciously experiencing oneself as having been given a gift, and consciously giving gifts.
Archetypal principle: Jupiter-Moon.

Hypermenorrhoea

see Menstruation, too heavy

Hyperosmia

(heightened sense of smell)
Physical level: Nose (power, pride, sexuality).
Symptom level: Reference back to archaic times; checking things out by smell (e.g. a sure way to good nutrition); heightened alertness in pregnancy and other situations: being able to better protect oneself and one's ward by being good at catching wind of things; having what or who "stinks" pointed out to one in a drastic way.
Handling: Learning to take things for real (perceive) more consciously, following one's instincts; falling back on the old levels of orientation; recollecting one's human inheritance; checking whether one can stand the smell of somebody (which is much more conclusive than finding them attractive from the physical point of view).

Resolution: Having a good nose that can be relied on and that is taken seriously in the selection of people and food, as well as in catching wind of dangers; in pregnancy: catching wind of dangers to oneself and the child in good time.
Archetypal principle: Pluto (connection with primordial instincts).

Hypersensitivity to sound

see Hyperacusis

Hypersomnia

see Narcolepsy

Hypertension

see High blood pressure

Hyperthyreosis

see Thyroid gland hyperfunction

Hypertrichosis

(whole-body hair, hairy people, Werewolf syndrome; see also Hair loss as the opposite pole)
Physical level: Skin (border, contact, tenderness), body hair (animalistic power).
Symptom level: Whole-body hair: the person "has gone (back) to the dogs": phylogenetic regression; virilisation syndrome: exaggerated masculinisation, which lends a dangerous, animalistic appearance; the memory of one's own history and origins triggers deep rejection; for those in the surrounding environment, one becomes a reflection of their shadow.
Handling: Reconciling oneself with one's own animal origins; recognising and taking on the animalistic side of one's own being; sensing the drives and deeper instincts; learning to take them for real and to appreciate them; learning to confront what is causing

anxiety about one's own appearance; becoming a (complete) man on the level of consciousness.
Resolution: Conscious resolution of the subject of masculinity.
Archetypal principle: Mars.

Hyperventilation

(attempt by the organism at self-healing; generally mistaken by traditionally-accepted medicine as a symptom of illness; used in various therapies as a means of expanding consciousness)
Physical level: Lungs (contact, communication, freedom).
Symptom level: The organism is flooded with life energy (oxygen, Prana) and loses waste residues (carbon dioxide) in abundance: in this exaggeratedly-clean situation, all sorts of impurities come out which hinder one's own development: one's birth pattern may be manifested, but also sexual problems or those related to holding on too tightly may become apparent; coldness, unlived sorrow and joy are discharged; due to the overblown exchange/hyperventilation (overloading with Prana = life energy), cramps can occur: restriction = fear; adopting the embryo position if one's birth trauma has not yet been processed and takes this opportunity to force its way to the surface; attempt by the organism to free itself from a restrictive or fearful situation; stirring up too much wind [venting] (about nothing?) (Latin ventus = 'wind').
Handling: Continuing to breathe and intensify the process until, at the deepest point of the fear (greatest feeling of restriction in the body), deliverance/liberation – the breakthrough into expansiveness – can take place; pressing ahead with the struggle for deliverance/liberation from the primordial fear (often corresponds to the primordial restrictiveness of the birth process); flooding oneself with (breath) energy in order to flush out the energy blockages; allowing oneself, through an abundantly great amount of wind, to be taken to the depths of one's own problems (often into the restrictiveness of the birth trauma), and then into expansiveness when one has become sufficiently aware of the restrictiveness.
Resolution: Finding deliverance/ liberation under one's own steam through intensified exchange with the world (deeper breathing); letting a breath of fresh air into one's life; allowing oneself to be intoxicated by the abundance of the Prana (life energy): sensing one's own limitlessness and ecstasy: soaring beyond all limits on the wings of the swinging momentum of life's breath.
Archetypal principle: Mercury-Mars.

Hypochondria

(fear of illness/disease; see also Heart neurosis)
Physical level: Consciousness problem (hypochondrium: actually the upper lateral region of the abdomen below the lower ribs, which the →malaise is frequently projected onto).
Symptom level: so-called hypochondriac patients suffer from pathological delusions (of grandeur?) and easily let everything get under their skin and be a dig in the ribs; due to continual concern about their own health, the body is observed with painstaking meticulousness: everything continually revolves around their own life, but only around the physical instead of around the spiritual; the fear of death is projected onto the body, with the result that patients are afraid of dying from all sorts of different symptoms.
Handling: Giving increased care and attention to the relevant subject behind the organ under observation; looking after one's own health in the mental-spiritual respect; reconciling oneself with one's own mortality:

study of the various Books of the Dead, but also the relevant passages in the Bible; taking the threat to life seriously in a wider sense: as humans, we are unholy and mortal, which is why we need "a saviour" to accompany us on the descent into the kingdom of the dead or shadow kingdom; occupational illness of many doctors which is exacerbated by the body-fixated focus of their traditional medical training: their own issues can then be processed in the form of a projection on the patients.

Resolution: Recognition that man is, in fact, basically ill, but in a deeper sense: he lacks the other half – the shadow – above all, in the spiritual respect; concerning oneself with the integration of the shadow with all its fears; reconciliation with death.

Archetypal principle: Mercury-Saturn.

Hypogalactia

see Breast milk production, deficient

Hypoglycemia

(low blood sugar level)

Physical level: Metabolism (dynamic equilibrium).

Symptom level: fall in the blood sugar level: too little sweetness and love in the lifeblood, too little nourishment for life; the feeling of vitality is based on the sweetness (glucose) in the lifeblood: if it is lacking, →panic breaks out; trembling, outbreaks of sweating: fear of coming up too short; feeling knocked out (exhausted); sadness: not getting what one needs; burning hunger for (unlived) life: hunger for life and love; a racing pulse wants to run the person affected and their heart off their feet: the heart pounds home its right to love (glucose).

Handling: Admitting to oneself the lack of sweetness and love; making clear to oneself that one has too little

(of the spiritual) to live on; following one's own restriction and fear to their very depths in order to reach the expansiveness that lies behind them; directing the burning hunger at worthwhile objectives; providing the heart with what it needs to live in terms of caring attention and love.

Resolution: Taking in (perceiving) and living one's own vitality in more resolved stirrings: partaking in (benefiting from) the sweetness of life and love and enjoying it.

Archetypal principle: Saturn-Venus/Moon.

Hypomenorrhoea

see Menstruation, too light

Hypophysis insufficiency

Physical level: Hypophysis (pituitary gland; harmony and adaptation at the highest level)

Symptom level: Far-reaching collapse of hormonal control; symptoms depending on the hormones that drop out: menstruation problems, such as amenorrhea (→menstruation, absent); no lactation (→breast milk production, deficient) due to lack of prolactin; no growth/stunted growth due to the lack of somatotropin (growth hormone - HGH); →diabetes insipidus due to lack of the stress hormone cortisol.

Handling/Resolution: In accordance with individual symptom patterns (see relevant entries); overall: living a less planned and ordered life.

Archetypal principle: Mercury-Saturn.

Hypotension

see Low blood pressure

Hypothyreosis

see Thyroid gland hypofunction

Hypotrichosis

(deficient hair growth)
Physical level: Hair (freedom, vitality); the whole body is affected, above all, the head.
Symptom level: The cause is genetic predisposition or the taking of medications (cytostatics); reduced defence of one's own borders due to lack of hair; low radiant aura (individual hairs as antennae); low power and strength; unconscious openness to contact and touch.
Handling: Seeking out for oneself other forms of protection, radiating strength and power; recognising and taking on innocent, child-like aspects of one's own personality.
Resolution: Becoming more open and defenceless, meeting the world and others more directly.
Archetypal principle: Mars-Saturn.

I

Ichthyosis

(Fishskin disease)
Physical level: Skin (border, contact, tenderness).
Symptom level: Excessive flaking of the skin with simultaneous lack of sebaceous gland and sweat production: shutting oneself off to the point of armouring oneself against the outer world; frequently beginning in early childhood, and more rarely, also even before birth: task that has been brought along with one in life.
Handling: Finding other ways to secure the borders, consciously arming oneself against all the dangers of the world.
Resolution: Finding security in one's own skin, within one's own four walls, at home, in this world or in God, respectively finding God in oneself.
Archetypal principle:
Saturn-Neptune.

Ideas, flight of

Symptom level: Ideas no longer follow the accustomed, strictly-rational logic, but run off in free association, at rapid speed, in a disorganised sequence and without concentration; a disjointed, completely-uncontrolled chain of thoughts rises up unchecked from the unconscious; the flight of ideas gets on the nerves of so-called "normal people" because the thought scraps are simply spit out too quickly and too illogically, just as they pop up from the depths of the unconscious: the symptom betrays the great demand for control exerted by the industrialised society; the closeness to the free association used in psychoanalysis shows its closeness to the unconscious, which psychoanalysts can approach in this way; the inability to flight of ideas in overly well-adjusted people betrays the opposite pole, but is not attributed any importance as a disease in our "performance-based society".
Handling: Consciousness exercises aimed at making oneself aware of the inner monologue, which is often just as irrational in order to calm it down as the long-term objective; courage to acknowledge one's own illogical depths and the mad rush of the flow of life and ideas; being of one mind (agreeing) with the flow of thoughts: learning to observe it; learning control over oneself and one's own depths; consciously turning one's attention to one's own unconscious; learning to fish ideas out of the flow and to bring them to realisation; exercises for the centre: mandala painting, meditation, Tai Chi, etc.
Resolution: Finding the happy medium between total lack of ideas and being inundated with them, between total control that is hostile to life and being carried away by sweeping chaos.
Archetypal principle:
Mercury-Uranus/Neptune.

Ileus

see Intestinal blockage

Ileus, paralytic

see Intestinal paralysis

Illusions

see Hallucinations

Immobility

see Apraxia

Immune deficiency

(see also Inflammation, Allergy)
Physical level: Immune system (defence).
Symptom level: Exaggerated defence at the level of consciousness; opening up the body to (different) stimulating elements in the form of pathogens instead of allowing one's consciousness to be stimulated; locking oneself away to an excessive degree, saying no to everything; inability to open oneself up inwardly; struggling excessively (against something).
Handling: Learning to put up a fight on the physical level against things that are hostile to life: using measures that toughen up and increase one's immune defence capacities (from "Kneipp" hydrotherapy to "inner smiling"); love as an act of letting in; opening up borders (the Ego) for the "You"; becoming one.
Resolution: All-embracing love; spiritual openness grounded in strength; openness wherever this is possible (in consciousness); defence wherever necessary (in the body).
Archetypal principle:
Mars-Neptune-(Saturn).

Impetigo

(itching, suppurating blisters, particularly in children, pregnant women and women in childbed)

Physical level: Skin (border, contact, tenderness).
Symptom level: Suppurating blisters and pustules, which by itching make one bristle to scratch them open; these then scab over: cleansing action of the body (pus = debris of war); pus (boils): (symbol of) uncleanliness forces its way to the surface; scab formation: unclean relationships manifest themselves; contact problems: bristling irresistably to open up one's borders and come into contact with one's own depths; border problems: unlived energies blaze a trail up out of the depths and give rise to unsightly blossoms on the surface; the now repulsive skin rejects its erotic function and turns it into the opposite by repelling others (pregnant women and women in childbed can keep thereby the partner at arm's length in this inconspicuously conspicuous way); deterrence by means of weakness instead of by strength: making oneself unattractive; on the face: a hideous mask instead of the (silky-)smooth façade; not being able to save face, the ability to "put on a brave front" is lost; leprous outcast appearance: casting oneself out and down (exposure and degradation).
Handling: (also as advice for jointly-affected caregivers): living in way that is more stimulating, itching to be stimulated and stirred up by what life has to offer; letting out and confronting the unclean matters; (aid in) opening up the borders, ensuring stimulating contacts; consciously keeping whoever or whatever currently does not suit one at arm's length; ensuring room and opportunities for retreat.
Resolution: Openness to the strange, unfamiliar and original budding imperfections, which grow in one's depths and pine for consciousness; being at home in one's own skin, feeling comfortable: playing one's own tune when it comes to

securing one's borders and the need for contact and doing this under one's own direction and at one's own pleasure.

Archetypal principle: Saturn/Venus-Mars.

Impotence

(see also Listlessness)

Physical level: Genitalia (sexuality, polarity, reproduction), consciousness problem.

Symptom level: Fear of death = orgasm, loss of control; fear of one's own masculinity and aggression; inability "to make a stand like a man"; fear of performance; failing under the pressure to perform: fear of "not being able to get it up", of being a limp-dick softie and a failure; fear of engulfing feminine forces (Freudian fear of castration); fear of being trapped (subject of →vaginism: a lot of talk about more or less nothing, the fear is related less to the physical than to the social level); clinging tightly to (being trapped in) the intellect; avoiding a tight squeeze by backing out, being repressed, putting one's tail between one's legs and ducking out; giving way, becoming soft (in coming to grips with the battle of the sexes); revenge on the female partner: not being a real man for her, not satisfying her; irrationally placing the female partner on a pedestal, not wanting to defile her as a Madonna; devaluing sexuality as something dirty: not wanting to place one's proud sceptre into the dark grotto; Oedipal problems: not wanting to be unfaithful to one's own mother; lack of creativity: not being able to spawn any testimony to oneself; lack of confidence in oneself and in the future; frequently external attempts at compensation: becoming a big man on the social level because one cannot get up the little man; often due to shocking experiences in the sexual area; nowadays often a reaction to comments from self-confident women: "If that was it, then that was it, goodbye!" or "I'm not the jealous type, feel free to go and practise a little more"; difficulties of modern young men facing the dilemma of the double bind: having to remain cool on the one hand because romance is "mega-out", and on the other hand, successfully managing such a "red-hot iron" as the first night of passion.

Handling: Recognising that virility needs the feminine aspect as a basis (inner calm and released tension [parasympathic condition] result in better bloodflow to the genitalia); exercises in letting go: meditation, allowing oneself to fall into the (feminine-spiritual) element of water; making friends with one's own soft, feminine sides in order to be able to stand up again for the masculine forces; in older men: too much softness is a call for empathy and spirituality to be given more room on the mental-spiritual level; getting to know and love one's own phallic strength: knowing that a man is not and does not always have to be able to perform; learning to yield to the feminine: exercises in the water, Samadhi tank; working from the opposite pole: giving in to one's own phallic strength; involvement with one's own body (sport, yoga, etc.); allowing what has been repressed to become visible; switching off and tricking the intellect; paying attention with regard to over-compensation: a strikingly-large number of financially-potent men suffer from potency problems in bed: they strut their stuff to the whole world because they were not able to strut their stuff to their wife/a woman; puffing oneself up instead of him; in such cases, having a powerful position in society compensates for physical powerlessness (societal power which arises in this way is dangerous for the sufferers themselves and for society because it must continually [and demonstratively] be reaffirmed and re-proven).

Resolution: Developing joy for one's own feminine, soft side and the masculine, hard strength and enjoying both (in physical terms, one after the other, but in the spiritual respect, also simultaneously).

Archetypal principle: Mars-Saturn.

Inability to read

see Alexia

Inappetency

see Appetite, lack of

Incontinence

(loss of control over the closures [sphincter muscles] of the body)

Physical level: Urinary bladder sphincter muscle (urinary bladder = withstanding and relieving pressure), anal sphincter muscle (anus = entrance and exit of the underworld).

Symptom level: It is no longer possible to withstand and overcome any pressure at all, everything empties itself spontaneously; the desire to control everything is thwarted on the physical level; the repression mechanisms are strained to their limits; urine (waste water of the soul) overflows, and due to muscular weakness of the bladder sphincter, cannot be held back (anymore): the spiritual flood is released physically instead of in the figurative sense; the spiritual element, pushed back into the shadows, overflows; attempt to flee from what is bearing down on one: "pissing off"; letting go too quickly and without control; stools are released without control due to weakness of the anal sphincter muscle: shadow contents are released spontaneously and physically instead of in the figurative sense, the underworld rises to the surface; regression to childhood

level (the cycle is closed at the wrong level): nappies (diapers) come back again; relapse into the time before acquiring the capacity for control; life without restraint; no longer being able to hold oneself back; having lost one's (backing) support in the life flow; after the change of life: finding no (backing) support in life anymore: the new life perspective does not yet provide any support; clinging on tightly to the outlived womb(anly) mother role; after a pregnancy: not yet having managed the transition back to the new state of being alone (in one's own body), seeking and not yet finding spiritual support (in the new mother role); in this case, also being stuck in the womb(anly) mother role.

Handling: Giving up control; learning to let go; urine: allowing the (waste) water of life to flow freely; allowing the soul to run over/overflow; getting back into flow; flowing spontaneously with the water of one's life (flow); stools: learning to let go of the material; bringing movement and flow into the shadow kingdom; letting money flow and taking pleasure not only in its coming, but above all, in its flowing on.

Resolution: Becoming like children again, who allow everything to run its course without control and live in the moment without worrying.

Archetypal principle: Moon-Pluto.

Incubation period

(not a symptom, but important in the case of →inflammation)

Physical level: Immune system (defence).

Symptom level: The time between the penetration of the pathogens and the recognisable manifestation of the disease as a result of the defensive measures of the immune system: reaction-free interval at the beginning of conflicts, in which the defence system sizes up the situation and produces its guided weapons (antibodies) against any bacteria in the weaponry forges and armament factories of the bone marrow.

Handling: Preparation for the battle, war, conflict; adjusting oneself to the struggle: whetting the blade, gathering arguments; allowing the body rest so that all forces are available for the defence.

Resolution: Recognising the mobilisation as the basis for a successful field campaign and following it through with the corresponding awareness.

Archetypal principle: Mars.

Infantile jaundice

(newborn jaundice, kernicterus; massive breakdown of the red blood corpuscles, frequently in cases of premature birth; see also Jaundice)

Physical level: Liver/hepatitis (life, evaluation, reconnection), blood (life force).

Symptom level: Immature blood metabolism; faster decay of the carriers of the life energy (red blood corpuscles) than they can be replaced and broken down: decay of vital strength at the beginning of a life which was often begun too early; overloading; not yet being able to deal completely with one's own existence and the waste residues of one's life energy; still insufficient liver function: lack f adjustment to independent life; not yet being up to the rough world of contrasts.

Handling: Giving the maturing processes time; transfer of external life energy in the form of sunlight (light therapy), if necessary and in rare cases, also by means of blood replacement.

Resolution: Taking one's time to commit oneself to life.

Archetypal principle: Moon-Jupiter.

Infantile paralysis, spinal

(poliomyelitis)

Physical level: Stomach (feeling, receptiveness), intestines (processing of material impressions), breathing (exchange, law of polarity), muscle system (motor, strength).

Symptom level: The disease pattern (which most probably due to vaccination has become rare in our society) can express all possible stages of non-compliance, from being slightly in a huff to full departure from the polar world (respiratory paralysis); muscle cramps in the neck and back area: conspicuous resistance to bending one's neck; unwillingness to subordinate oneself and show humility; paralyses (which come on suddenly and usually overnight); tremors and muscle weakness; jaw muscle weakness, changes in one's voice, difficulties in swallowing, respiratory paralysis: the tremors reveal fear, the paralyses of the jaw muscles the reluctance to continue chewing things over; paralysis of the swallowing process makes it clear that those affected have swallowed enough; long-term effects: disabling deformations of the skeletal muscle system; depending on the handicap, the deformations amount to acceptance of the life task expressed by the disease pattern: walking handicaps enforce slower and more conscious steps forward (progress); handicaps in the area of the spinal column place the central focus of life on the subjects of uprightness and straightforwardness; imposing one's will on others through the disease pattern; controlling and manipulating others through one's own weakness.

Handling/Resolution: Every (apparent) humiliation by Fate calls for Resolution in the form of humility; the greater the task, the more wonderful and satisfying when it is nevertheless resolved.

Archetypal principle: Saturn-Neptune.

Infantilism

(mentally and physically remaining in an earlier development stage)
Physical level: Genitalia (sexuality, polarity, reproduction).
Symptom level: Remaining stuck in a childish development stage (first clarify and interpret the basic problem): rejecting development; instead of later again becoming like a child, simply remaining a child in the first place; shunning the definitive entry into polarity: the differentiation between the brain and genitals fails to take place.
Handling/Resolution: (for the jointly-affected parents/carergivers): taking on the task sent by Fate: living in line with the hint given and concerning oneself intensively with the childish development stage; resolving (letting loose) the realm of childhood: enjoying life in the here and now.
Archetypal principle: Moon-Saturn.

Infarction

General term for the degeneration and dying off of tissue (→necrosis); see also Cardiac infarction

Infection

see Inflammation

Infertility

(sterility; see also Ovulation, absent)
Physical level: Genitalia (sexuality, polarity, reproduction).
Symptom level: 1. Society in general: decline in the sperm count over the last 50 years to half the previous level (from 100 to 50 million/cm3) as a result of stress, environmental pollution; in addition to the reduction in quantity, similar development in terms of quality (more immobile and deformed sperm, →akinospermia, necrospermia): gentle form of extinction; the wealthier the nation, the more serious the decline in fertility (environmental toxins can be confirmed both in the follicle and in the seminal fluid). 2. In relation to affected individuals: unconscious resistance prevents the letting in or letting oneself become involved with a soul; methods of resistance: overwork, which is connected with a lack of vital sperm; stress inundation, which can also prevent conception; deep unconscious fears, which are so restrictive that no soul can pass the bottleneck; much ado with little effect: fruitless efforts; exposure of dishonest motivations (attempt to bind the partner by means of a child); fear of binding commitment and responsibility; overly rigid life planning that is stuck in a rut (fixation) appears to scare off the soul; failing as a giver of life; inability to procreate: not being able to create life, generate offspring; not being receptive.
Handling: 1. Owning up to one's own situation with regard to demanding too much of oneself in the spiritual and ecological respects; fertility (productiveness) is declining; in industrialised nations, things are going downhill both quantitatively and qualitatively; preferring to take back harmful developments that are making us sick than continuing to take down the entire community. 2. Becoming clear about one's true motivations: one should really only decide to have a child if one is prepared to gratefully receive any child with any task it may bring with it; clarifying one's priorities: what comes first and has top priority: the desire to have children, one's career/work or one's life planning?
Resolution: 1. Becoming more modest overall and on figurative levels (finding ideas, solutions for the pressing problems in the ecological and health respects: "more is less"). 2. Preparing oneself in line with the

motto: "Thy will be done"; being open
to the fact that we get what we wish
for or something more important,
which we perhaps cannot immediately understand; consciously existing
for oneself and becoming blessed
for one's own sake alone instead of
through a child.
Archetypal principle: Moon-Saturn/
Pluto.

Inflammation

(infection, inflammation; see also Lesion, Incubation period)
Physical level: Can affect the entire
organism and be caused by external
influences (micro-organisms such as
fungi, viruses, bacteria or injury) or by
the body's own irritants.
Symptom level: Inflammation (-itis)
= conflict having become material,
war, aggression: "boiling with rage";
the spark igniting the powder-keg,
a smouldering conflict flames up
or is re-ignited, "fire in the hole",
"throwing a firebrand into a house",
something goes up in flames, fuel
for conflict brings something to the
point of explosion; new challenges,
new impulses penetrate through the
defences of the consciousness border
and stir things up ("War is the father
of all things", "What is causing such
a heated reaction?"); those who do
not allow their consciousness to be
stimulated will instead unconsciously
open their physical borders to stimuli
in the form of pathogens, the stronger
the spiritual defences, the weaker
the physical equivalent: an inflamed
(infected) person puts up too little
defence in a spiritual sense; modern
hostility towards life: liveliness (vitality) is combatted with antibiotics (anti
= against, bios = life); chronic conflict
(→lesion): rotten compromises,
permanent frustration, merely a half-
hearted struggle that one no longer
really believes in.

Handling: Allowing the discharge of
what has built up; opening oneself
up to a stimulating conflict instead
of turning the body into a battlefield;
risking confrontations, fighting out
conflicts, grabbing hold of red hot
irons; making decisions, releasing
bound energies; relinquishing one's
defences against new impulses for
one's consciousness, strengthening
the defences: promoting increased
awareness, risking transformation,
sacrificing old outlooks, letting old
habits die a natural death, risking
leaps in maturity and development,
taking back projections; reconciling
oneself with all forms of life.
Resolution: Basically acknowledging
the inherent conflict-based nature of
being human; living courageously
with conflicts; bravely tackling things
on the mental level; loving one's
enemies.
Archetypal principle: Mars.

Influenza (infections)

(see also Respiratory tract diseases,
Cold diseases, Avian influenza)
Physical level: Head (capital of the
body), nose (power, pride), neck
(assimilation, connection, communication), lungs (contact, communication, freedom), musculature (motor,
strength).
Symptom level: One's life situation
leaves one unmoved and cold; shutting oneself off and no longer being
able to warm to anything: getting (a)
cold; catching/picking up the germ-inating elements (influenza viruses) one
needs to play out the drama; shutting
up, closing off the gateways of the
senses to the outside: "being fed up
to the eyeballs", "being in a huff";
letting one's neck puff up; retreat
from the crisis situations of everyday
life: building defensive walls out of
tissues, creating a field of illness;
keeping people and situations at
arm's length: "Back off, I have a cold";

overload, desire to flee: hearing and seeing give out on one: "not wanting to hear or see anything more, simply wanting to crawl into bed and pull the covers over one's head"; rejection of further social contact: "not wanting to swallow (let in) anything more" (swollen tonsils aggressively block the passageway); defensive stance: "coughing up" what one really thinks of a person; feeling as if one has been through a punch-up and a screaming match: shattered state and hoarseness; restriction of communication: blocked nose and throat – fed up to the gills (with phlegm), bronchia tending to close up to the point of blockage of all (gas) exchange with →lung inflammation (communications conflict on the deepest level), but one for which one has to supply one's own germ-inating elements (usually bacteria) to stir things up; being shaken to the core by the defensive struggle (attacks of the shivers); cleansing efforts on the physical level.

Handling: Owning up to one's disinterest and lack of enthusiasm for one's life situation; shutting oneself off from the outside, setting boundaries, keeping one's inner space free; voluntary withdrawal from external activities, actively keeping external demands at arm's length; offensively closing the locks oneself against further influence (inflow), making clear that one is no longer prepared to accept (to swallow) the situation (the previously-existing conditions); giving vent to things; aggressively defending oneself in an open(ly offensive way): "coughing up" one's real opinion to adversaries; creating room for oneself; facing up to the challenges/the struggle; actively earning the shattered feeling and the hoarseness; rejecting any further exchange (communication) of the type up till now; letting oneself be shaken up by the struggle over the improvement of one's life situation; living

out sensitivity (a splitting headache: "don't touch me"); clearing up unclear situations; the attempt, which is doomed to failure, to banish the subject from the world through vaccination shows how little this well-meant prevention strategy can achieve.

Resolution: Being in the flow; clearing up problems that have become stuck/phlegmatic; bowing to the characteristic qualities of each season (the great influenza epidemics in autumn and winter force us to allow ourselves a rest which we do not take voluntarily, although everything around us at these times clearly suggests taking a "winter sleep").

Archetypal principle: Mars-Neptune.

Inguinal hernia

(see also Rupture)

Physical level: Stomach (feeling, instinct, enjoyment, centre), groin (vulnerability).

Symptom level: Being overbearing; having taken on matters that were too difficult to bear, having over-stretched oneself (e.g. when breaking loose from old customs/traditions or separation from children), bursting one's performance limits, demanding too much of oneself; not being able to hold out as much as one believes; being more delicate than one assumed; ignoring one's own weak points; having ended up on the wrong path; archaic emotional forces push their way into the sexual sphere; competition between two areas: disregard of boundary and freehold relationships, in which neither wins; danger of strangulation of the infringing foreign organs; aggressive conflict, war with sudden invasion.

Handling: Tackling subjects which are weighty in the figurative sense; taking on a great deal (on the mental-spiritual level); learning to more realistically estimate one's own potential in terms of what one can carry (bear); learning to make allowance for one's own weak points (limits); re-examining one's own paths in the domain of primordial emotional stirrings and sexual ambitions; overstepping borders in the figurative sense; bringing previously-separated areas into contact to the benefit of both sides; setting oneself above externally-drawn boundaries , enabling exchange; processing newly-emerging (incoming) subjects intensively and in an open(ly offensive) way; venturing to tackle subjects of (spiritual) weight; giving more freely and becoming more open.

Resolution: Fostering intensive spiritual exchange across borders; connecting subjects in one's mind that lie close together; courageously entering into binding connections; trusting oneself to be capable of quite a lot of binding commitment in a mental spiritual sense.

Archetypal principle: Venus-Mars.

Inhibition

see Anxiety

Injury

(see also Aggressiveness, Accident, Work accident/Domestic accident, Sport accident/injury, Traffic accident, Trauma, Amputation, Bite injury, Brain concussion, Greenstick fracture, Bone fracture, Paralysis, Nasal bone fracture, Muscle tear, Contusion, Bruising, Skull fracture (base of the skull), Whiplash, Burns, Poisoning, Dislocation, Sprain, Irradiation)

Physical level: All areas of the body can be affected.

Symptom level: Calling the (structural) integrity of the organism into question; something foreign penetrates the borders of the body and damages them, along with potentially deeper-lying structures: e.g. Cut wounds: having fleeced (deceived) oneself, cut corners; being cut off from communication, severing ties, a rift; Injuries due to striking blows: having shut oneself off (in advance) from striking arguments, being struck down by something; Injuries due to high impacts, bruises: having been bruised (maliciously deceived), without realising it; repression.

Handling/Resolution: Exerting oneself more strenuously on the mental-spiritual level, and if necessary, putting oneself out of joint or "bending over backwards" in order not to overload the body and in order to preserve its borders - preferably going beyond one's own limits in the figurative sense instead of forcing the body to do so; making a cut and coming clean with oneself; voluntarily allowing foreign elements into one's own awareness and integrating them instead of getting a "punch in the face"; willingly opening oneself up.

Archetypal principle: Mars-Uranus.

Insensitivity to pain

(hypasthesia = reduced sensitivity to touch, hypalgesia = diminished sensitivity to pain, analgesia = no sensitivity to pain, anaesthesia = no sensitivity to pain, total numbness)

Physical level: Skin (border, contact, tenderness).

Symptom level: reduced sensitivity to pain to the point of total insensitivity (numbing = anaesthesia); insensitivity with the tendency to blunted feeling: nothing can touch one physically or emotionally; insensitive reactions to the point of complete rigidity of reaction; hiding, entrenching oneself in one's own inner world: drawing in all outside antennae, drawing back into one's snail shell, creeping away into one's tortoise shell.

Handling: Consciously not allowing oneself to be knocked off balance or to lose one's inner calm; conscious withdrawal inwards: self-sufficiency.

Resolution: Remaining true to one-self, living in a centred way, at peace with oneself; perceiving the outside world in the role of an uninvolved witness; eastern attitude of "acting by not acting".
Archetypal principle: Saturn/Venus-Neptune/Saturn.

Insomnia

(problems with falling asleep, staying asleep; see also Sleep problems)
Physical level: Usually a conscious-ness problem, often combined with →depression; sleep disorders, but also on the basis of organic disease patterns (e.g. heart, prostate or blad-der weakness, or muscle cramps, hot flushes) or due to age (changes in the sleep pattern in advanced age) as well as the issue(s) concealed behind the consciousness problem.
Symptom level: Fear of loss of con-trol, giving oneself up completely and committing oneself to the unknown when going to sleep; not being able to let go of the day, because one could not completely get over and done with it – with the day, with life in general; feelings of guilt which prevent one from relaxing and letting go; loss or change in rhythm (→age-related symptoms, senile insomnia); being torn from one's sleep by an unfin-ished issue (usually unremembered dreams); lack of trust in the feminine pole; over-emphasis of the masculine pole of rational thought: too much life energy (blood) in the central control headquarters (brain), which therefore cannot switch off and come to rest; overly strong Ego identification: Sleep = Death (Thanatos, Death, is the brother of Hypnos, Sleep); call to wake up in the spiritual sense (Bud-dha = The Awakened One).
Handling: Bringing the day to a proper close and being completely over and done with it on the con-sciousness level: recognising what needs further processing, crossing off what can no longer be changed; identifying and tackling the conflict in daily spiritual image journeys; solving problems which pop up again and again, and which threaten and call one's night-time life into question; consciously allowing oneself to be stirred up until one can again sleep in peace; waking up more to the night - the feminine side of our 24-hour day; discovering enjoyment in letting go; exploring the pleasures and enjoyments of the female pole of life; consciously experiencing the transi-tion from the active (masculine) to the passive (feminine) side of the day, and for example, celebrating it with an evening stroll, welcoming the twilight; consciously bringing the day to a close (e.g. by making use of a good-night ritual, such as prayer, keeping a diary, mandala painting, meditation, etc.); bringing every day to a close as though it were a life (taking Sleep seriously as the little brother of Death); contemplation of transience and Death; working allopathically from the opposite pole: switching over from the left to the right hemisphere via meditation, concentration on one's breathing, mantras, etc.; in the case of sleep disorders, using the relevant sleep-disturbing symptom to help one to wake up to the issue(s) involved; allowing stirring subjects into con-sciousness and getting over and done with them.
Based on the above description, some useful aids for falling asleep include the following:
1. Counting up to 100 and back again, counting flocks of sheep or clouds in the sky until the intellect switches off out of boredom, and one can then sink gently into a state of sleep; 2. Koan method: attempting to solve an intellectually-insoluble task using the intellect, e.g. listening to the clapping of one hand (from the Rinzai-Zen tradition); 3. Schiele

footbaths or Kneipp hydrotherapy (in order to entice the blood away from the head); 4. Satisfying and physically-exhausting sexual intercourse before falling sleep; 5. Falling asleep rituals, such as reviewing the day once again on the level of inner imagery; guided visualisations (instructions for both in Dahlke: "Inner Journeys").
Resolution: dividing up one's daily work so that it is manageable; reconciliation with the dark side of the day and reality; consciously accepting things that have remained uncompleted: letting go of perfectionism; waking up to reality and one's own spiritual life; discovering Night and Death as life themes.
Archetypal principle: Moon-Pluto (falling asleep); Moon-Saturn (staying asleep).

Intercostal neuralgia

Physical level: Rib cage (sense of self/Ego, personality), ribs (safety, protection, adaptation).
Symptom level: The rib cage becomes painful; neuralgiform pains in the areas between the ribs: the place of protection of the heart (feeling) and lungs (exchange) is stirred up; the place of self-identification that one points to when saying "Me" is threatened (from outside); the bony cage for the heart and lobes of the lungs cries out for attention.
Handling: Questioning the armouring of one's feelings and the exchange function (or letting it be called into question); allowing oneself to be challenged (stirred up) in one's Ego area; admitting to oneself that exchange and flexibility in one's Ego area are painful and approaching this field attentively and cautiously; allowing calm to return.
Resolution: Bringing quiet attention and conscious rest to the cage of the inner wings (lobes of the lungs) and feelings of the heart.

Archetypal principle: Sun-Saturn.

Intermenstrual bleeding

(metrorrhagia)
Physical level: Endometrium (protective sheath of fertility), genitalia (sexuality, polarity, reproduction).
Symptom level: Insufficient hormone secretion (oestrogen) causes the build-up of the mucous membrane in the womb to be aborted and prevents implantation (nesting) of the fertilised egg or even ovulation; waste of life energy at the wrong point, with the accompanying threat of →anaemia.
Handling: Taking care of oneself; lining one's own comfortable nest; becoming aware of the pattern of rejecting things prematurely (impatience).
Resolution: Expending less of one's energy for external things and outsiders and allowing more life energy to flow into the centre of one's own circle of life; allowing an active everyday schedule to be broken up by phases of rest.
Archetypal principle: Moon-Uranus.

Intertrigo

(skin soreness, chafing)
Physical level: Occurs between areas of skin that lie close together (skin = boundary, contact, tenderness): between the scrotum and inner thigh, in the armpits and anal folds, between the upper thighs and under the breasts.
Symptom level: Rubbing oneself sore at one's own intimate border areas; close contact with oneself leads one to be rubbed raw (spiritually); occupation of these sore spots by foreign intruders; weeping of the sore spots: spiritual water "seeps" out of the intimate areas.
Handling: Becoming more open and courageous in the intimate contact area; voluntarily becoming more

sensitive and receptive at one's own borders; letting out the spiritual element in the intimate, intrapersonal area; voluntarily assimilating new, foreign ideas into intimate areas of life; working from the opposite pole: leaving room to breathe between the partners, maintaining distance.

Resolution: Finding the happy medium between the different areas of one's own being with respect to closeness and distance.

Archetypal principle: Venus-Saturn.

Intervertebral disc prolapse

(see also Sciatica)

Physical level: Intervertebral discs (female pole of the spinal column), spinal column (dynamics and hold, uprightness).

Symptom level: Excessive existential pressure: the soft, female element is pinched between two hard male elements and trapped; the female pole is "in a tight squeeze", it is pressed (oppressed?); inner pressure forces its way out; over-burdening (e.g. as compensation for a lack of self-assurance, feelings of smallness and inferiority): taking on too much, over-burdening oneself too much, over-stretching oneself; the pressure gets on one's nerves; the soft, female pole gets on one's nerves (is cut away during operation); the life axis is out of alignment: spinal cord and intervertebral disc displacements, deadlock; humiliation (being forced to lower oneself) if lacking (moral) uprightness: "crooked as a dog's hind leg"; breaking one's back for the security of one's livelihood, the family; exaggerated uprightness in the form of self-righteousness: "a stick-in-the-mud"; search for recognition.

Handling: Placing the central focus on the soft, female aspect of one's own existence; consciously carrying (bearing) the burden of existence;

consciously perceiving the pressure one is under; forcing emphasis on the female aspect, allowing one's own female side to come into consciousness; experimenting with the life axis – the central focal point of life; finding another orientation; when things are out of joint, putting matters back into alignment, setting things right; using the rest and relaxation forced by the symptoms for inner flexibility and reflection; giving way to the inner pressure.

Resolution: Integrating the alternation of hardness and softness as well as the build-up and release of tension into one's life; honesty, activity and uprightness; humility instead of humiliation; unconditional love instead of compulsion to perform.

Archetypal principle: Moon-Saturn.

Intestinal blockage

(ileus; see also Crohn's disease)

Physical level: Small intestine/ileum (balance, analysis, assimilation), large intestine (unconscious, underworld).

Symptom level: Strike blockade; shutting down: "life can't go on like this", "I'd rather be dead than go on like this"; overload (e.g. too much of the wrong thing at the wrong time and without preparation); unclarified conflict perceived as hopeless; the flow of life is obstructed by too many smouldering conflicts (as in Crohn's disease): "I get too little, and there is too little in what I do get"; mechanical ileus: caused by tangible, concrete blockade; having taken in something too bulky, having bitten off more than one can chew; paralytic ileus: caused by intestinal paralysis; feeling paralysed and putting a stop to the digestion of life; self-boycott.

Handling: No longer just taking part; learning to restrict oneself in time and also to refuse things where necessary; using the many problematic

issues in order to slow down the tempo of processing and take breaks; stopping the throughflow of impressions: allowing oneself more time and preparing oneself better; learning to wait patiently for the right moment ("good things take time"); questioning oneself about the greatest impediment in the processing of the (one's own) world: taking a snapshot of one's own life situation.
Resolution: Digesting life calmly.
Archetypal principle: Mercury/Pluto-Saturn (blockage).

Intestinal cancer

see Rectal cancer

Intestinal fistula

("illegal" connection of the intestines to the surface of the body or to another hollow organ; see also Crohn's disease)
Physical level: Intestines (processing of material impressions).
Symptom level: Shadow issues taking roundabout ways or wrong paths; shadow contents force their way into the light of consciousness via spectacular and unusually-problematic routes, thereby risking wars and conflicts; forming dangerous connections in the underworld; trying dangerous shortcuts (escape routes).
Handling: Integration of the shadow instead of the attempt at avoidance (escape routes): bringing the shadow into the light in an unusual and creative way; envisaging risky ways of processing the shadow; trying to shorten the way courageously and in an open(ly offensive) manner (instead of taking roundabout ways); also looking for shadow issues in completely unexpected areas.
Resolution: Reconciliation with the dark domains of one's own existence, while taking into account their individual characteristics.

Archetypal principle: Pluto-Uranus-Mercury.

Intestinal fungus

see Candidamycosis

Intestinal incarceration

(see also Hernia)
Physical level: Intestines (processing of material impressions).
Symptom level: A part of the intestines becomes blocked, thereby crippling the complete digestive tract; no longer being able to absorb the tasks and karmic fruits which ripen for one on one's way; life can no longer be digested; quite the contrary, it is in fact acutely threatened; deathly silence in the stomach, spiritual dead-end.
Handling: The acute threat to life requires immediate surgical intervention; not letting anything new in, not letting anything out, lodging a total stop; coming completely to rest.
Resolution: Becoming independent and self-sufficient, withdrawing oneself, maintaining distance from the turmoil and (information) exchange of social life; finding one's inner self without needing or serving the outside world.
Archetypal principle: Mercury-Saturn.

Intestinal inflammation

(see also Colitis ulcerosa as a particularly serious form of intestinal inflammation, Irritable colon)
Physical level: Small intestine (analysis, assimilation), large intestine (unconscious, underworld).
Symptom level: Conflicts with digestion (of the world), in particular: with analysis and assimilation (differentiation and acceptance) = small intestine area; with the journey to the

underworld = large intestine area; aggressive conflict over what is to be taken into or let go of from the body; overly careful and anxious confrontation in one's consciousness.

Handling: Courageous struggles over the matters that should be let in; offensive confrontation with shadow subjects (in the case of →colitis ulcerosa); courage to adapt to the given life circumstances; openly having it out with conflicts over saying 'yes' and 'no' (digesting also means separating the chaff from the wheat, and learning what is good and what is bad for one).

Resolution: Consciously and in an open(ly offensive) way letting oneself in for with what has been "let in" and swallowed; courageously going about the journey through the shadow kingdom.

Archetypal principle: Pluto-Mars-Mercury.

Intestinal influenza (Intestinal catarrh)

see Intestinal inflammation

Intestinal paralysis

(paralytic ileus; see also Intestinal blockage)

Physical level: Small intestine/Ileum (balance, analysis, assimilation), large intestine (unconscious, underworld).

Symptom level: Passive strike on the intestinal front: the intestines stop all work and movement; cessation of the serpentine movements (peristalsis) due to the effects of poisoning; shutting down: "things can't go on like this"; attempt to force a change in the working conditions; the flow of life through the shadow world is obstructed: back-up of the shadow aspects to the point of being thrown up; faecal vomitting: the shadow world cannot be processed and pushes its

way to the entrance instead of the exit; the shadow spews to the surface, the situation makes one want to be sick.

Handling: Taking genuine breaks in the processing/digestion of the world; no longer just taking part; learning to refuse things; granting oneself rest; withdrawing oneself from polarity from time to time; taking a holiday now and then with regard to the processing of impressions; stopping the inflow (influence) of new shadow material: taking a time-out and giving oneself time to reflect; proceeding forcefully with new forms of processing; bringing up the shadow in an unusual way: spitting out instead of jamming in.

Resolution: Absorption and processing of life are in rhythmic harmony.

Archetypal principle: Mercury (small intestine)/Pluto (large intestine); Neptune (paralysis).

Intestinal parasites

Physical level: Intestines (processing of material impressions).

Symptom level: Hosting freeloaders (parasites), weight loss e.g. as a result of tapeworm infestation; loathing and fear ("opening up a can of worms", being eaten alive by worms, reminder of the end of the body); feeling of being internally infested; "being possessed" on the level of the underworld; having to feed uninvited guests; unconsciously feeling oneself to be the victim of exploitation.

Handling: Devoting oneself on the mental-spiritual level to the themes of the shadow kingdom; discovering what is going wrong with one's digestion of life, where the "can of worms" or other "guests" are; addressing the issue of "exploiting and being exploited"; consciously nourishing dependent, weaker beings (creatures) in one's environment in order to relieve one's own inner world of the burden; consciously restricting oneself (fasting often also physically starves out the parasites).

Resolution: Allowing others (other beings) to coexist with one, cultivating love for others; issuing conscious invitations; becoming a patron; developing a feeling for one's own needs and the needs of other living beings; reconciliation with one's own underworld.

Archetypal principle: Mercury-Pluto.

Intestinal polyps

(polyposis intestinalis)

Physical level: Mucous membranes (inner boundary, barrier) of the large intestine (unconscious, underworld).

Symptom level: (Benign) growths in the underworld (in the unconscious); possibility of losing life energy to the underworld via these growths (bleeding); large polyps can obstruct the transport in the underworld (→intestinal blockage); danger of degeneration and becoming malignant (polyposis, →intestinal cancer).

Handling: Making oneself aware of one's own tendency to growths (excesses); taking indications of uncontrolled growth in the shadow kingdom seriously: asking oneself what could be growing in one's own underworld; allowing creations of the shadow kingdom to rise up into consciousness; considering the question of suppressed dark sides; taking into account the danger of degeneration of shadow subjects into uninhibited ego trips before it is too late (therapy) and forging one's own paths of consciousness raising and illumination; voluntarily giving up life energy to the underworld in the sense of awareness and consciousness raising in this area; taking transport blockages into account in the case of shadow contents and working on these.

Resolution: Creative handling of the shadow; allowing growth in the domain of the underworld: recognising that growth is only possible through the integration of shadow elements; retraction of projections, recognition that it is not only others who afford themselves the luxury of evil excesses (malignant growths) and running off the rails.

Archetypal principle: Pluto-Jupiter.

Intestinal problems

Physical level: Small intestine (analysis, assimilation), large intestine (unconscious, underworld).

Symptom level: Problems with the digestion of life.

Handling: Learning to integrate more consciously = adopting the foreign, making it one's own.

Resolution: Digesting the world; processing one's karma (Buddhism: Bhoga = "consuming and overcoming the world") instead of rejection and attachment.

Archetypal principle: Mercury, Pluto.

Intestinal prolapse

see Anal prolapse

Intoxication

see Poisoning

Involution depression

(see also Depression, Climacteric complaints)

Symptom level: Mental stagnation after the middle of life; mentally-spiritually not getting the process of coming back and coming home in the second half of life underway: the body has to step in to fill the gap and increasingly has to tackle the process of involution (decline); disregarding the opportunity for voluntarily turning back and turning within oneself in the middle of life; concerning oneself too little with the objective of life: the resolution in death.

Handling: Pausing to take stock in the time around the middle of life: re-consideration with regard to one's path and direction in life; from the middle of life onwards, placing one's central focus on the aspect of turning back to home and turning within; occupying and reconciling oneself with the resolution of life: the letting go in death; acknowledging the transience of matter and thus also of the body.

Resolution: Voluntarily slotting oneself into the overall life design – the cycle of life or mandala – and following the archetypally-prescribed path.

Archetypal principle: Saturn.

Iris, inflammation of

(iritis)

Physical level: Iris (shutter of the camera of the eye).

Symptom level: Conflict over opening and closing the shutter ("What should I photograph, and what not?"), insufficient flexibility in adjusting to the prevailing light (and life) conditions; not standing behind one's eyes and their perspective; painful view of things; problems with exposure to light ("How much light should I let into my images/my life? How much light should I grant myself, both in the concrete and figurative sense?"); desire to close one's eyelids in order not to have to see anything more; one's desire to look and listen has faded.

Handling: Becoming aware of one's possibilities for shutting one's eyes to certain things; aggressive confrontation with regard to the images seen; learning to cope offensively with the powers of light; giving oneself "(time) frames" in which the eyes can close in peace; admitting to oneself when things are going badly.

Resolution: Choosing freely which impressions one wants to let in or shut out.

Archetypal principle: Sun/Moon-Mars.

Iritis

see Iris, inflammation of (above)

Iron deficiency anaemia

(see also Anaemia, Demineralisation)

Physical level: Blood pigment (colour of the life force).

Symptom level: →Fatigue, exhaustion, feebleness and general energy deficiency; the energetic strength of iron is lacking: the "red" power of attack and new beginnings is unable to make its mark.

Handling: Getting by largely without masculine energy, making oneself independent of it; carrying on gently, calmly and in a relaxed way without any gripping, spectacular new impulses – doing what must be done; trusting and yielding to one's own rhythm; taking over responsibility for one's own individual life flow; consciously choosing an energy-conserving and modest way of life with regard to energy consumption.

Resolution: Mastering one's life with calm composure (in Buddhism: keeping the wheel in motion, not out of rapture, but simply because it must turn); following the prescribed paths in one's own unmistakable and steady way; commitment.

Archetypal principle: Mars-Neptune.

Irradiation

(see also Accident)

Physical level: The complete organism can be affected right down to its very depths, depending on the type of radiation.

Symptom level: From burns to the skin to genetic damage due to the high energy of ionising radiation: having deceived oneself (been "burnt", "had one's fingers burnt"): having let oneself get involved too closely with something dangerous; playing with (atomic) fire and paying the price (in technology and medicine); the splitting of the atom (nuclear fission) is a classic symbol for polarity; splitting leads to duality and ultimately to distress (Latin: "pulling in opposing directions") and des-pair; initial immune defence reactions of the organism, early damage: radiation dermatitis and radiation sickness; later damage: →cancer, →leukaemia, genetic damage, radiation fibroses (rampant growth of connective tissue).

Handling: Choosing to act more offensively with the fire of the spirit and daring to make oneself clearly aware of dangers; becoming more critical; allowing oneself to get involved in heated confrontations; letting oneself be impressed to the very core; making a clear decision as to whether one wants to deepen the rift or work on unity; accepting the consequences of one's own actions and being clear about the fact that the first option will ultimately lead to despair, and the latter option to becoming one with oneself and with Creation; making clear to oneself that one is living in a threatening environment, respectively that one is endangering oneself – this also applies for therapy attempts with ionising radiation; avoiding the danger whenever possible; in medical applications, always weighing up the questionable benefits against the definite damage.

Resolution: Taking up and taking on one's place in Creation; in the case of radiation therapy, fighting side-by-side with the high-energy radiation (on the level of inner imagery) against the cancer.

Archetypal principle: Pluto.

Irritable colon

(see also Constipation, Diarrhoea, Nausea, Stomach cramps)
Physical level: Intestines (processing of material impressions),
particularly the large intestine (unconscious, underworld).

Symptom level: Constipation and diarrhoea show from both sides the problem with letting go and the general fear of it; nausea: lack of reconciliation with the present life situation, one's own life leaves a nasty taste in one's mouth; stomach cramps: overstretched, strained efforts; wanting to digest life properly and get a grip on it with all one's might and exaggerated force, which naturally does not work (on the physical level); pains: cries for help from the unconscious, the shadow world; these show that things cannot go on like this, that help is necessary, and that the area of digestion (of nourishment and life) needs more attention.

Handling: Practising letting go on different levels; acknowledging one's constriction in the digestion of one's own life subjects; straining to manage the tasks of life and to digest the challenges; approaching the processing tasks forcefully; consciously assuring oneself of the necessary help.

Resolution: Consciously practising Bhoga (Buddhism: consuming the world), learning to digest life, letting life into oneself and consciously facing up to it with all its tasks and challenges.

Archetypal principle: Pluto-Mercury.

Ischaemia

(circulatory deficiency), see Cardiac infarction, Arteriosclerosis

Ischialgia

see Sciatica

Itching

(pruritus; see also Skin rash, Pruritus vulvae)
Physical level: Skin (border, contact, tenderness), the exact localisation shows the level of the problem.

Symptom level: When one is itching for a fight, the itching makes one want to scratch oneself, thereby tearing open the border to the outside with one's fingernails – the remains of the claws; even if this leads to blood being shed, it will generally relieve the itching; being challenged to have it out: "itching to do something", "it's no skin off my nose"; reaction to a stimulus (sexuality, aggression, affection) which stimulates/arouses and is experienced either as alluring or provocative; unsatisfied desire: lustfulness/lasciviousness (see titles of cheap sex films); love of life, passion/ inner fire/fury thrusting to the surface, "bristling with excitement" = being open; scratching the surface of a stimulating subject = airing the secret.

Handling: Consciously and courageously opening up one's borders; letting things pass through more easily, letting inner things out and outer things in, thereby allowing the life force to flow; voluntarily allowing oneself to be challenged to have things out: life, one's own situation and the situation of the world should be allowed to make one's skin crawl and to itch to change things; facing up to one's own curiosity and trusting oneself to follow up on what one finds stimulating; consciously absorbing the many stimuli and allowing oneself to be lured out of one's shell; becoming more responsive; allowing oneself more.

Resolution: Scratching at the surface in consciousness for as long as necessary until one knows what one is itching and stirred up to do, and what burning issue is ablaze in one's soul; living courageously and openly and trusting oneself to give way to stimulations and enticements so that these enticements can be transformed into enjoyment of life.

Archetypal principle: Venus/ Saturn-Mars.

J

Jactation

see Twitching of the limbs

Jaundice

(icterus; see also Infantile jaundice, Liver diseases/ Hepatitis)
Physical level: 1. Gall bladder (aggression, poison and bile); 2. Liver/ hepatitis (life, evalution, reconnection); 3. Blood metabolism (life force).
Symptom level: 1. Energy blockage: Blockage of the outflow related to the profound, hidden, corrosive and soft-soaping bile energy; poison and bile builds up; 2. Lack of power to distinguish (oneself): struggle over the laboratory of the body; the right balance is under threat: the toxicity of all excess; 3. Disintegration of the carriers of the life energy faster than they can be replaced and broken down; yellow (a component of the green colour associated with envy) in the face: non-vital, lacking lively vitality or energy, jaded.
Handling: 1. Learning to control one's profound and hidden bilious energy; 2. Risking aggressive conflicts over questions of life philosophy; courageously battling for one's philosophy of life; critically coming to terms with one's own personal right balance; 3. Consciously renewing the basis of the life energy; allowing things to simmer down and turning one's attention inwards.
Resolution: 1. Both holding back the bilious force, but also allowing it to flow when required (function of the gall bladder): conscious handling of this form of energy; 2. Finding the sense and meaning of one's own life and establishing one's own personal balance within it; 3. Recognising

and accepting the eternal process of change, also of the life force.
Archetypal principle: . Pluto-Jupiter, 2. Jupiter-Mars, 3. Saturn-Jupiter.

Jaw luxation

(dislocation of the lower jaw)
Physical level: Lower jaw (weapons store), chin (strong will, forceful assertion).
Symptom level: Originates from opening one's trap too widely when yawning or from excessive effort when biting; standing around gawping with one's mouth agape: shooting one's mouth off, being a big-mouth; pushing things too far; doggedly biting off more than one can chew.
Handling: Making oneself aware of one's own expectations with regard to assimilation and expression; learning to open one's mouth (in the figurative sense); becoming a mature person in the sense of being able to speak for oneself and obtaining one's share in life; biting off one's own (corresponding) chunk of the cake (of life): ensuring that one is up to the mouthful, and can not only assimilate it, but also digest it.
Resolution: Maturity; modesty, but also avoiding false modesty: not biting off more than one can chew, but still getting one's fill; opening one's mouth, but not being a big mouth and opening it too wide.
Archetypal principle: Mars/ Saturn-Uranus.

Jetlag

(→malaise after crossing time zones during intercontinental flights)
Symptom level: Unconscious resistance to (situational) changes; demonstration of greater flexibility than actually corresponds to one's own being; lack of grounding and empathy in new situations.
Handling: Landing after a period of high-flying; learning to come back down to earth; bringing one's own high demands on flexibility into harmony with the physical reality; recognising that the soul needs time to catch up with the body, and cannot keep pace with flying; pragmatic procedure: immediately taking on the new rhythm on landing in the destination country, and in countries, such as Italy and the USA, where it is available without prescription, taking 2 mg/ tbl. of melatonin before the first period of sleep.
Resolution: Living in the here and now.
Archetypal principle: Uranus-Saturn.

Joint diseases

Physical level: Joints (mobility, articulation).
Symptom level: Becoming fixated on something, stretching something beyond the limit, going too far; bruising (alienating) someone, coming down hard on them, beating them into shape; putting oneself out, pushing things too far, bending over backwards; being overstretched, uptight or twisted.
Handling: Being upright in something, standing up for something; going beyond one's own limits; forcefully fending someone off; giving someone a good tongue-lashing; setting things back in order, putting them straight or right; doing exercises in building up and releasing tension (Jacobson training).
Resolution: Properly facing up (adjusting oneself) to things; knowing one's own limits and expanding beyond them; articulating oneself according to one's own capabilities.
Archetypal principle: Mercury-Jupiter (overstretching)/Saturn (stiffening)/ Uranus (clenching)/Pluto (bruising).

Joints, inflammation

see also Rheumatism

Joints, stiffening of

see Ankylosis

K

Kaposi's sarcoma

(cancer of the skin or subcutaneous connective tissue; see also [Skin] cancer, Aids)

Physical level: Skin (border, contact, tenderness), subcutaneous connective tissue (protection, insulation).

Symptom level: Degeneration in the border and contact area or in the area of connections, stability and commitment: e.g. connections/contacts which do not suit one in the deepest core of one's own being, but still receive energy; wild and ruthlessly rampant growth in this subject area; having strayed so far off track from one's inherent development path in this domain that the body helps the (forgotten/repressed) issue to express itself; the mental-spiritual growth in this area has been blocked for so long that it now forges a path in the body in an aggressive and random way; the cancer realises physically that (turnaround) which would be be spiritually necessary in the corresponding area of consciousness; one's instability becomes visible (in the tissue).

Handling: Opening oneself up in the area of contact and relationship to one's own outlandish ideas and bold fantasies and courageously allowing them to grow and develop without control (by others); consciously taking over control and responsibility oneself; thinking back to early dreams and one's own forms of expression in this respect; bringing these (back) to life and putting them into practice with wild decisiveness; in the certainty of having nothing more to lose, mustering courage for one's own self-realisation/one's own path; considering all the measures mentioned under →cancer: since cancer affects the complete organism, it must also be met across-the-board; discovering cancer as a form of perverted love (overcoming all limits, stopping at nothing, not fearing death): doing justice to love as the content of all sexuality.

Resolution: Providing expression for oneself instead of allowing the body to speak up (for itself); recognising the necessity to switch from the physical and thus (life-)threatening level to the challenging, but life-saving mental-spiritual level, and relying in this realm on expansive growth; discovering love that transcends all boundaries, setting oneself above external rule and standards laid down by oneself or others, and living and developing oneself solely in accordance with the obligations of one's own highest law.

Archetypal principle: Venus/Saturn-Pluto.

Keratitis

see Corneal inflammation

Keratosis

(see also Psoriasis, Corns)

Physical level: Skin (border, contact, tenderness).

Symptom level: Pathological cornification/hardening of the skin (e.g. localised in the case of callus formation, preliminary stage of →basalioma): armouring of the outer border; attempt to secure and shut oneself off from the outside; development of one's own suit of armour, one's own fortress (construction).

Handling: Learning to protect oneself against over-extension - both general and localised; creating security in the figurative respect; learning to protect

oneself and feel comfortable in one's own skin.
Resolution: Defending one's own skin even without outer armour, such as through spiritual armament.
Archetypal principle: Venus/Saturn-Saturn.

Kernicterus

see Infantile jaundice

Kidney, artificial

(see also Kidney, contracted)
Physical level: Kidneys (balance, partnership).
Symptom level: Lack of willingness to actively solve one's problems with real-life partners; overwhelming desire for freedom and independence; search for the ideal partner who does not bring along any demands of his/her own; the machine (artificial kidney) is the only partner which makes no demands of its own (at least from the spiritual point of view).
Handling: Reassessing one's level of expectation in questions related to partnership to determine whether such expectations simply boil down to the effective thwarting of every real partnership; examining one's desires for freedom and independence with respect to whether they stand in the way of decisive life subjects; learning to accept one's own imperfection, as well as that of one's partner; taking to heart the Pygmalion (or My Fair Lady) myth of the perfect female partner and drawing the consequences from it: recognising in good time when one's own expectations are so high that everything is leading towards an artificial substitute (artificial kidney); seeing through the associated dependencies resulting from the mechanical solution in good time.
Resolution: Recognising the difference between lifeless perfection (of the machine) and the lively imperfection and vitality of human partners;

conceiving life as a school, in which we continually receive new possibilities (partners) and can repeat individual classes more or less as desired; a school, in which the outer limits are far more expansive than in the schools devised by people, but also a school, in which in cases of complete refusal (to learn), there is also the threat of serious consequences.
Archetypal principle: Venus-Saturn.

Kidney cancer

(see also Cancer)
Physical level: Kidneys (balance, partnership).
Symptom level: Aggressive destruction of kidney cells with the tendency towards causing the kidney functions to collapse: having strayed too far off track in the area of partnership and harmony; not finding one's own identity with regard to one's relationship with others; not being able to adequately set one's boundaries (cancer runs rampant across all boundaries); not being able to safeguard one's own domain, one's own realm; degeneration in the domain of balancing out contrasts, respectively the partnership: wild and ruthlessly proliferating growth that has run off the rails; having strayed so far off track from one's inherent line of development with regard to relationships and the reconciliation of the opposite poles, respectively true harmony (as the golden medium between war and peace), that the body has to help the (forgotten/repressed) issue to express itself; mental-spiritual growth in relation to this subject has been blocked for so long that it now manifests itself in the body in an aggressive and random way; the cancer realises in the subject area concerned that (turnaround) which would be spiritually necessary in the corresponding area of consciousness.

Handling: Courageously and aggressively getting a grip on one's own notions of partnership and the harmonisation of opposing forces and allowing these to flourish without regard to what is normal and prescribed by society; not allowing oneself to be hindered, but instead going one's own way offensively and boldly; as far as partnership, relationships and reconciliation of contrasts are concerned; radically calling into question the old customs and traditions that have been passed down to one, and if necessary, ruthlessly destroying them; should one's desire to put the blame on others persist, questioning one's own projections (above all, those in the partnership area); (re)vitalising early dreams of one's own goals/wishes and aspirations in the domain of partnership and the balancing/harmonisation of the opposing poles and putting these into practice with wild decisiveness; in the certainty of having nothing more to lose, mustering courage for self-realisation/one's own path; not making any further rotten compromises, but instead standing up for oneself; in relationships, expressing what one needs and wants and what one is prepared to give; making the return to one's point of origin and reconnection to one's own roots into central themes of life; opening oneself up to the immortality (of the soul) and striving for omnipotence in unity as the goal of all life; considering all the measures mentioned under →cancer: since cancer affects the complete organism, it must also be met across-the-board.

Resolution: Breaking with old partnership and relationship notions, as well as methods for reconciliation of the contrasts, which are actually foreign to one's own being; offensive struggle for one's own purpose and meaning (in life); ensuring expression for oneself in the mental-spiritual area instead of allowing the body to speak up for itself; recognising the need to switch from the physical and therefore (life-)threatening level to the challenging, but life-saving mental-spiritual level, and relying in this realm on expansive growth; taking back projections (e.g. ceasing to make the partner responsible for one's own life); discovering all-embracing love that transcends all boundaries, setting oneself above external rule and standards laid down by oneself or others and living and expressing oneself solely in accordance with the obligations of one's own highest law.

Archetypal principle: Venus (kidney)-Jupiter/Pluto (cancer).

Kidney, contracted

(nephrosclerosis, hypertensive nephropathy)

Physical level: Kidneys (balance, partnership).

Symptom level: Hardening of the fine kidney vessels leads to increased blood pressure (this is a sensible attempt by the body to still direct enough blood through the kidneys despite the vascular constriction): those affected are under pressure (often in the partnership); in later stages, there is a loss of protein as in the case of →nephrosis and ultimately the danger of →kidney insufficiency and shrinkage of the kidneys: materials (and matters) that are essential for life are lost; one's centre and harmony can no longer be upheld.

Handling: Making oneself aware of the pressure that is cropping up in one's interpersonal relationships; being able to (allow oneself to) let more pass; giving more freely under the increasing pressure, letting go more.

Resolution: Admitting to oneself in good time when one can no longer succeed alone in finding the golden medium and living in harmony; asking for help sooner rather than later.

Archetypal principle: **Venus-Saturn.**

Kidney degeneration

see Nephrosis

Kidney, descended

see Kidney, floating

Kidney distension

Physical level: **Renal pelvis (first collection basin of the spiritual waste water).**

Symptom level: **The overflow builds up due to an obstacle in the outflow channel: a blockage prevents the letting go of old spiritual issues; initially still repairable, but later danger of hydronephrosis.**

Handling: **Recognising what is hindering the letting go of old spiritual matters; making clear to oneself that one is putting oneself under pressure in this way: identifying the pressure; physically removing the blockage and accepting it in the figurative sense.**

Resolution: **Forcefully tackling the issues of harmony in one's partnership and harmony in life; putting oneself under pressure to get down to the essential.**

Archetypal principle: **Venus-Saturn.**

Kidney failure

see Kidney insufficiency

Kidney, floating

(Descended kidney)

Physical level: **Kidneys (balance, partnership).**

Symptom level: **Due to weakness of the tissue that the kidneys are suspended in, the kidneys hang down loosely when standing with resulting pains and blockages in the blood vessels and urinary tract: the subject of partnership easily comes apart at the seams; this leads to blockages in** the energy flow and in the disposal of (spiritual) water as well as being painful.

Handling/ Resolution: **Concerning oneself with the issues of balance and partnership, as well as taking things more slowly; allowing oneself time for the supply of energy and the letting go of old spiritual energies; adjusting oneself inwardly to pain and conflicts in this area.**

Resolution: **Consciously taking unusual paths in the partnership.**

Archetypal principle: **Venus-Uranus.**

Kidney gravel

see Kidney stones

Kidney inflammation

see Glomerulonephritis

Kidney insufficiency

(kidney failure to the point of uraemia)

Physical level: **Kidneys (balance, partnership).**

Symptom level: **Loss of performance, →fatigue: no longer being able to or wanting to do anything; loss of appetite and listlessness: one's lust for life has disappeared; itchy skin (urea): wanting to open one's borders in order to let out what is building up inside; respiratory distress: threatening to choke on one's own waste products; diarrhoea: attempt at detoxification (the body's own enema); relentless vomiting: attempt to get rid of what is weighing one down; water and salt balance disorders: no longer being able to keep the water and salt of life in the right relationship to each other; build-up of urea: suffering from one's own waste; skin haemorrhages: one's lifeblood runs away; declining vision: no longer being able / willing to look closely at things; drowsiness to the point of coma: tendency to pass over to the other side.**

317

Handling: Opening all the floodgates and detoxifying oneself by all possible means: skin, intestines, stomach (vomiting); admitting one's own unwillingness to oneself, and that in one's innermost core, one no longer has any desire for this life; recognising that further repression will not achieve anything (not even greater peace): giving in in the sense of yielding; at the stage of incipient uraemia: giving way and reconciling oneself to the departure from this side and the (sMoon-to-come) arrival on the other side; before one starts falling asleep more and more, clarifying to what extent those left behind should fight for one's own life (artificial kidney, transplantation).

Resolution: Admitting to oneself that the body can no longer be saved by one's own efforts; making one's peace with this world, which one can still fight to remain in by means of dialysis or a kidney transplant, or which one leaves behind, as well as with the people that one was attached to, and with God.

Archetypal principle: Venus-Neptune/Pluto.

Kidney stones

(see also Stony concretions, Colic)
Physical level: Kidneys (balance, partnership).
Symptom level: Piling up of matters which should have been let go of a long time ago: outlived issues, above all, hardened, stony feelings and emotions from the problem area of harmony and partnership block the flow of development and cause a build-up of the backwater; spiritual stirrings easily become set in stone at this point because the thought of letting them out stirs up anxieties that this would change the relationship irrevocably; grit (gravel) in the workings of the partnership; petrification of subjects from the partnership and harmony area which can no longer be kept in solution and thus precipitate: unresolved, hardened problems; reacting in a hard-hearted, stony way: turning to stone in the face of the relevant problems; salts (the material that most stones are made of) represent a merging of the basic (feminine) and acidic (masculine) forces, and as such, are something completely new and neutral that is capable of combining these extremes; nevertheless, salts are concentrated and have a preserving effect (e.g. salted herring); in other words, they preserve the problems – not in a live form, but instead in a petrified state – thus preserving them for eternity; turning into a rigid pillar of salt (like Lot's wife, who turned back): no longer flowing along in a forward-looking way in the stream of life; stones as the catalyst for →colics, which launch a field offensive against the obstacle in ever-recurring waves of attack, similar to the contractions associated with labour, in an attempt to give birth to it, accompanied by the corresponding labour pains.

Handling: Making oneself aware of the issues which have become set in stone and which are blocking the flow of development; recognising the grit in the workings of one's own relationships; crystallising out unresolved elements in a spiritual sense instead of physically; confronting the corresponding energies with consistency, clarity and hardness; becoming aware of the matters which one could not keep in (re)solution and which are hanging around the relationship like millstones; trying to get rid of (expel) what can no longer be brought to the point of (re)solution; consciously trying to get over and done with certain matters that one is oversaturated with: it is precisely those matters in which one has reached saturation point that should not be suppressed, since these will become embodied and cause trouble; daring to take the plunge and move away from the old; keeping the feminine and masculine forces in one's own game of life in a balanced state of (re)solution, and creating something new and qualitatively neutral from them, which unites both sides within itself; using partnership as a catalyst for one's own development; orientating oneself forwards in the flow of life; setting things in motion (→colic): considering hindrances as tasks which have to be overcome (if need be, preferring to precipitate conflict rather than precipitating stones).

Resolution: Using concrete ideas about how to deal with the relevant matter as a means of preventing the formation of concretions in the corresponding organ; willingly and consciously working on the relationship; opening oneself up and becoming receptive for love and harmony, and the reconciliation of the contrasts; remembering that two contrasting people can produce something completely new and unique if they really join forces ("The meeting of two personalities is like the contact of two different chemical substances: if there is any reaction, both are transformed." C.G. Jung).

Archetypal principle: Saturn-Venus.

Kinetoses

(travel and movement sickness; see also Balance disorders)

Physical level: Balance organ in the inner ear (balance sensor).

Symptom level: Travel sicknesses are based on unwillingness to commit oneself to the journey: one "feigns" something to oneself in this respect (leading to dizzy "feign"(t)ing spells); typical progression: different, contradictory and even mutually-exclusive items of information arrive at the control centre (brain) from the sensory organs; for example, in the case of seasickness: the eyes report that everything is at rest, the balance organ reports rolling movements: the dizzy"feign"(t)ing spells reveal the deception: someone is not willing to commit fully to the sea; airsickness: unwillingness to commit to the air and to flying with all its possibilities; nausea and dizziness when a passenger in a car: unwillingnes to commit to the drive, not looking beyond to a sufficient degree; in general: experiencing oneself as being on unsteady ground; not feeling oneself in one's element; being neither here nor there, but instead between different worlds and between two stools; movements that are too fast for one's own consciousness; not being able to believe one's eyes; feeling like one wants to be sick (in this situation).

Handling: Bringing the conflicting information into accord, e.g. in the case of seasickness: going out on the deck of the ship and consciously perceiving the movement of the water or closing one's eyes to exclude them as a source of error; trusting the unsteady ground/the foreign element, yielding to it; adjusting speed and shifting it down a gear to correspond to one's own processing speed, or in the case of amusement rides at fairgrounds, increasing one's processing speed; developing a secure inner stance to the situation; being open to misperceptions of the eyes.

Resolution: Surrendering oneself to the situation and the respective element.

Archetypal principle: Neptune.

KISS syndrome

(Kinematic Imbalances due to Suboccipital Strain; see also Cervical dystonia as the extreme form)

Symptom level: The atlas and axis are not sitting correctly on top of each other, asymmetrical use of arms and legs, the head does not sit properly

on the shoulders and has to be set straight; the head aspect has no reliable basis; generally triggered by a difficult birth (ventouse birth, forceps delivery of twins, emergency Caesarean section, breech presentation, carrying over term, restrictiveness in the womb, →birth complications).
Handling: Setting the head straight by means of osteopathy, cranio-sacral therapy; courage for one-sided developments.
Resolution: Setting one's head straight in the figurative sense and bringing it into a well-balanced position, finding one's centre.
Archetypal principle: Saturn-Uranus.

Knee joint inflammation

(see also Rheumatism)
Physical level: Knee joint (humility).
Symptom level: Inflammation caused by pulmonary consumption, syphilis or gonorrhoea pathogens that are transferred via the blood: conflict over the subject of humility resulting from one's own vitality and based on a more widespread general conflict, whose subject results from the basic illness (see the entries in question.).
Handling: Courageously and offensively confronting one's own stance towards humility.
Resolution: Learning to handle one's own vitality and resolving the subject of humility.
Archetypal principle: Saturn-Mars.

Knee pains

Physical level: Knee joint (humility).
Symptom level: The strongest bones, and thus the strongest structures of our life, meet at the knee: the thigh bone (femur) and the lower leg bones of the shinbone (tibia) and calf bone (fibula); sensitive contact point, which is optimised by means of a

circular 'washer' (the meniscus); symbolises the connection between the traditional way of one's forebears and one's own attitudes to life, which must both be in harmony in order to make good forward progress along the path of life; the ideal connection of both requires, amongst other things, a great deal of humility, and can bring one to one's knees or force one to one's knees; it can be painful to be at ends with one's own tradition because one is already deeply divided; it will, however, be unbearably painful in the long term to deny one's own path.
Handling: Confronting oneself courageously and offensively with diverging demands on the path of life; if in doubt, placing oneself decisively on one's own side, and addressing one's inner stance to humility; genuine humility can solve everything – what is false, put-on or taken on for the sake of peace will sooner or later scream out to the heavens above and express itself in the form of pain.
Resolution: Transforming humiliations into genuine humility.
Archetypal principle: Saturn-Mars.

Knock-knees

see Part 1, Leg shape

Korsakow's syndrome

(see also Alcoholism, Alcohol psychoses, Addictions)
Physical level: Central nervous system (news service).
Symptom level: Late stage of →alcoholism, which is then triggered by even the smallest amounts of alcohol; desire for confabulation: the wildest stories emerge from the shadow kingdom without being controlled by a guiding golden thread; for this reason, substitute threads are continually spun, with which those affected enmesh themselves ever more deeply in

their insane worlds (often madly wild stories); everything becomes unimportant, irrelevant and inconsequential: loss of one's own history due to the gradual and complete decay of the memory.

Handling: Opening oneself up voluntarily and in good time to the inner kingdoms of fantasy and freely-flowing images; spinning the guiding golden thread through the labyrinth of one's own spiritual images at an early stage; getting to know and illuminating the shadow kingdom in good time and of one's own free will; making something constructive out of the stories of the inner kingdoms: releasing them from one's soul by writing or narrating them; learning to let go of one's own individual history in favour of the overarching collective interconnections: discovering model examples in one's own depths.

Resolution: Becoming a Holy Fool instead of making a fool of oneself.

Archetypal principle: Uranus-Neptune.

Kyphosis

(Curvature of the thoracic spinal column to the rear; normal in a mild form), see Hunchback

L

Labyrinthitis

(inflammation of the labyrinth system in the ear, e.g. in the case of middle ear inflammation)

Physical level: Ears (hearing and obeying commands).

Symptom level: Aggressive struggle over the (correct) stance towards the world and spiritual balance; →balance disorders: falling out of inner balance; states of dizziness:

deceiving oneself, dizzy "feign"ting spells; →vomiting/nausea: the situation makes one want to be sick, wanting to let everything just spew out (to get rid of it); increasing hardness of hearing: not wanting to hear anything more, no longer wanting to listen carefully and obey.

Handling: Having out the conflict over one's stance towards the world in an open(ly offensive) way: allowing oneself to be stirred up by stirring matters; struggling in a committed way to maintain one's own balance; standing by the fact that one has left one's centre instead of deceiving oneself and clinging tightly to positions which are no longer valid; consciously and combatively getting rid of (spitting out) what is outdated in order to make room for the new.

Resolution: Carefully listening inwardly (spiritually): obeying one's own inner voice and facing up to the stirring challenges of new situations with courage and full of combative enthusiasm in order to find the stance (to life) that is now appropriate.

Archetypal principle: Venus/Saturn-Mars.

Lactose intolerance

see Milk, intolerance

Large intestine, inflammation

see Colitis ulcerosa

Laryngeal cancer

(cancer of the vocal cords; see also Cancer)

Physical level: Larynx (expression, tone [mood]), vocal cords (expression, speech).

Symptom level: Fear is clamping one's throat shut: sinister fear, which is squeezing out life; terror leaves one speechless; degeneration in the communication area; wild and ruthlessly rampant growth in the area of the voice; having strayed so far off track from one's inherent development path with regard to speech and self-expression that the body has to help the (forgotten/repressed) issue to express itself; the mental-spiritual growth in this area has been blocked for so long that it now forges a path in the body in an aggressive and random way; the cancer realises physically in the domain of speech that (turnaround) which would be spiritually necessary in the corresponding area of consciousness.

Handling: Opening oneself up in the domain of speech to one's own outlandish ideas and bold fantasies, courageously allowing them to grow and expand; thinking back to early dreams and forms of expression; bringing these (back) to life and putting them into practice with wild decisiveness; in the certainty of having nothing more to lose, mustering courage for one's own self-realisation/one's own path; considering all the measures mentioned under →cancer: since cancer affects the complete organism, it must also be met across-the-board.

Resolution: Providing expression for oneself (in terms of content) instead of allowing the body to speak up for itself; recognising the need to switch from the physical and therefore (life-) threatening level to the challenging, but life-saving mental-spiritual level and relying in this realm on expansive growth; discovering love that transcends all boundaries; setting oneself above external rule and standards laid down by oneself or others, and living and developing oneself solely in accordance with the obligations of one's own highest law.

Archetypal principle: Mercury-Pluto.

Laryngeal inflammation

see Hoarseness

Laryngitis

see Hoarseness, Croup

Lead poisoning

(see also Heavy metal poisoning)

Physical level: All types of tissue are affected, but in particular, lead deposits in the bone system (stability, strength).

Symptom level: Severe →anaemia due to blockage of the bone marrow, damage to the vessel walls to the point of attacks of →angina pectoris, nerve paralyses; the structure of one's own life is endangered: danger of forfeiting all vitality, the flow of vitality is disturbed right down to the central areas (heart blockages, that is, the heart is cut off from the energy supply = strangled); dead, ashen appearance; caved-in stomach, hollow cheeks: the life flow has little power; grey edging lead of around the gums as a typical sign: the bed of aggression, the home of basic trust is dull and colourless.

Handling: Careful detoxification, going about life more slowly; taking back one's expectations of efficiency; in the case of heart symptoms, taking care of matters of the heart.

Resolution: Living at a slower pace and more consciously, letting oneself be carried along by the flow of life; enjoying one's dwindling life energy with increasing calm and composure; reflecting on the essential, on the more profound meanings of life.

Archetypal principle: Saturn-Neptune.

Learning disorders

Symptom level: Not wanting to take in and take on anything; rejecting exchange with the surrounding world; in combination with →depression, →hyperactivity, →concentration disorders.

Handling: Staying oneself, developing one's own uniqueness; finding one's own attitude to life; getting what one really wants out of it; sensing one's own calling.

Resolution: Finding the way to oneself and reaching one's own centre; finding one's own vision, hearing the call and transforming it into a career preference.

Archetypal principle: Mercury-Saturn.

Leg fracture

(see also Bone fracture)

Physical level: Legs (mobility, progress, stability).

Symptom level: Serious situation, which prevents all movement and any progress in life, radically " putting the brakes on" and forcing those affected to sit tight; difficult situations are described as "a tough break"; Thigh: Break with the family tradition (the strength that one has brought along on the development path); Lower legs: Break with one's own ideas on the development path.

Handling: Consciously questioning and making a break with the continuity of life, one's own progress and the process of getting ahead.

Resolution: Pausing to be content in order to tap into new content; re-considering one's future path.

Archetypal principle: Saturn-Uranus.

Leg oedema

Physical level: Legs (mobility, progress, stability).

Symptom level: Build-up of spiritual water that has sunk down into the leg area: being heavy-footed and ungainly ("a clumsy clot"), the opposite of the ideal of elegant slimness;

frequently during pregnancy when the focal point (central weighting) of life has to be pushed downwards into the feminine pole; being bogged down: movement and progress are hindered or sluggish; the spiritual (water) element gathers in the lower area and directs attention to one's own roots.

Handling: Moving one's focal point (central weighting) down into the lower feminine pole: finding connection with the Earth; safeguarding one's standpoint: acquiring a sure footing, e.g. in discussions, not "losing the ground under one's feet"; "lowering oneself" emotionally, tackling down-to-earth problems; allowing spiritual stirrings to sink in deeply; giving in spiritually (since there is a compulsion to lie down); putting one's feet up in the concrete and figurative sense.

Resolution: Contemplation and calm; discovering one's true spiritual field of activity in down-to-earth areas; finding one's deepest basis, dropping anchor: arriving in the harbour (of marriage?).

Archetypal principle: Moon-Pluto.

Legasthenia

(reading and writing deficiency)

Symptom level: Problem of keeping order and the (right) order of things; having skipped over certain development stages or not completed them in the right order.

Handling: e.g. catching up on the crawling phase as part of a course of therapy; consciously giving chaos its own space; ritual exercises of ordering and sorting (e.g. mandala painting).

Resolution: Lending more expression to the feminine-intuitive level (particularly in the case of originally left-handed people forced to use their right hand); breaking through order and regulation on other levels; allopathically: attentively taking one step

after the other, without skipping over any stages on the path (of learning); slotting oneself into the existing life pattern (mandala).
Archetypal principle: Mercury-Uranus.

Leprosy

Physical level: Skin (boundary, contact, tenderness), nervous system (news service).

Symptom level: Biblical disease pattern which resulted in isolation and discrimination: the lepers were those banished and outcast by the community; today widespread "only" in Asia, Central Africa and Latin America since its treatment is a question of money and organisation; insidious conflict extending over decades (chronic infection): following an incubation period (preparatory dormant stage) of years to decades, there are fever reactions (general mobilisation of the body) and ulcerations (unresolved conflicts eating deep into one's own flesh); numbness of the extremities due to failure of the sensory nerves leads to unintentional self-mutilation; if untreated, ulcerations develop into mutilations (rotting away of the limbs and extremities and consequent surrender of the corresponding functions and subjects); disfigurement, e.g. lion-face (Facies leontina): being marked; the disease pattern leads (untreated) to lingering illness and death: having been given up by all others, finally giving oneself up as well.

Handling: Acute and long-term (allopathic) approach: antibiotic therapy to destroy the mycobacteria (leprae); long-term spiritual (homeopathic) approach: making oneself aware of the insidious conflict and addressing it down to one's deepest depths; general mobilisation for the conflict in the mental-spiritual respect; voluntarily giving up certain thematic groupings

marked by the disease pattern and sacrificing outer development areas in favour of inner ones.

Resolution: Accepting being an outsider, voluntary retreat (e.g. cloister); taking on the challenges thrust on one by Fate as a mark of distinction and facing up to the struggle for one's own life.

Archetypal principle: Neptune-Pluto.

Lesion

(chronic →Inflammation)

Physical level: The organism can be affected at almost any point.

Symptom level: Often still smouldering conflict which has now become chronic; (warlike) bound energies; unclarified situation, prolonged conflict; no real war, no real peace: rotten, lukewarm compromise; permanent frustration; only half-hearted resistance; struggle in which one no longer really believes; lack of energy prevents a genuine solution; fear of the consequences of acting and of responsibility; fear, respectively lack of courage/lack of strength to make a decision: stagnation, static warfare; fear of the sacrifices associated with a decision; refusal to learn the long-overdue lesson.

Handling: Locating and identifying the area and subject of the conflict; directing the energy of awareness to this area/subject; homeopathic, long-term solution: living under fire, holding out, sitting things out, taking one's time: Za-Zen; seeking one's centre, doing justice to both sides; bearing the restrictiveness of the situation until, having reached its climax, it expands again; allopathic, short-term solution: making decisions (freeing the sword from the scabbard; Latin: dēcīsiō = 'a cutting off'); transforming bogged down (potential) energy into living (kinetic) energy and vice versa (bringing a deadlocked situation back into movement; calming a hectic situation): playing with energies; having the courage to overstep one's own boundaries or to withdraw oneself completely; standing up honestly to the conflict and making firm decisions.

Resolution: homeopathic method: accepting response-ability: finding answers; developing empathy since the other side is also right (from its point of view); finding one's centre: harmony as a successful compromise between war and peace (the goddess Harmonia as the child of Venus – the goddess of love – and Mars – the god of war); consistent, tenacious search for the middle ground; acting by not acting: acting but being prepared to relinquish the fruits of one's actions in order to end the stagnation, but without tipping the balance to the other pole; recognition that great victories lead to great wars and that remaining still helps towards achieving inner peace; integration first of the one pole, then of the other; becoming whole/healed; becoming aware; readiness for reconciliation, genuine willingness for compromise ("If someone strikes you on the right cheek, turn to him the other also"); allopathic method: lively discussions and arguments ("Be hot or cold, the lukewarm I will spit out of My mouth").

Archetypal principle: Saturn-Mars.

Leucorrhoea

see Efflux

Leukaemia

(blood cancer; see also Cancer)
Physical level: Blood (life force), immune defence system (defence).
Symptom level: Degeneration in the immune defence system: usually an abnormal increase in immature defensive cells (white blood corpuscles) similar to defensive combat against an overpowering opponent, in which troops that are too young, untrained

and therefore ineffectual are thrown against the enemy, and in effect, then do more harm than good; desperate (re)actions; not being able to defend one's own skin (any longer) – having felt oneself to be defenceless, at the mercy of others and a victim one's whole life – often a sign of unacknowledged weariness towards life; hardly having taken oneself for real and definitely not having taken oneself seriously enough; swellings of the lymph nodes: intense activity in this area of defence as well; later often collapse of the immune defence system: inability to defend oneself after the preceding defensive battle, which has used up all of one's resources; having strayed so far off track from one's inherent development path with regard to resistance and defence that the body has to help the (forgotten/repressed) issue to express itself; the mental-spiritual growth in the area of resistance has been blocked for so long that it now runs riot in the body in an aggressive and random way, striking out in an uncontrolled way on the level of immunity; the cancer realises physically – in this case, in the domain of immune resistance – that (turnaround) which would be necessary in the same domain spiritually; great weakness as though badly knocked about by the defensive battle; bone and joint pains: the foundational structures (of life) and articulation (of one's own needs) cause pain; loss of appetite and listlessness: the hunger for life fades away; swelling of the liver and spleen: rush of life energy in the organ related to one's philosophy of life and questions of meaning and in the blood filter; bleeding under the skin: the life force flows away; anaemia: breakdown of the life energy.

Handling: Radically questioning the nature and working method of one's own system of defence, and if necessary, radically overhauling it, even if this involves the danger of being temporarily unprotected, i.e. entirely without defence; opening oneself up in the area of defence and attack to one's own outlandish ideas and bold fantasies, and courageously allowing them to flourish and expand; thinking back to early dreams of one's own forms of attack and defence; bringing these (back) to life and putting them into practice with wild decisiveness; in the certainty of having nothing more to lose, mustering courage for self-realisation/one's own method of defence (in life); taking advantage of the weakness as an occasion for thorough rest and inwardly gathering together one's own strengths; largely doing without external stability, outer mobility and stimuli, even if this causes pain: the strength that is now needed must come, above all, from within; following the path of the life energy and turning one's attention to the issues related to the liver (meaning of life, re-ligio[n] - reconnection); filtering everything superfluous and unnecessary out of the life flow; allowing all of the life energy to flow into the decisive battle, which must get under one's skin and go down to the very core of one's bones (one's foundations); at the same time, giving up resistance on the deepest level against one's own destiny; acceptance of the/(one's own) meaning of life and one's inherent tasks; taking up the fight for survival in an open(ly offensive) and aggressive way on the level of inner imagery; considering all the measures mentioned under →cancer: since cancer affects the complete organism, it must also be met across-the-board.

Resolution: Breaking with the old defensive structures that are foreign to one's own being; fighting in an aggressive and open(ly offensive) way for one's own (life) forms; recognising the necessity to switch from the physical and thus (life-)threatening level

to the challenging, but life-saving mental-spiritual level, and relying in this realm on the defensive struggling that is vital to life; discovering love that transcends all boundaries; setting oneself above external rule and standards laid down by oneself or others, and living and expressing oneself solely in accordance with the obligations of one's own highest law.
Archetypal principle: Mars-Pluto.

Leukocytosis
see Blood count, disturbed

Leukodermia
see Albinism, Vitiligo

Leukoplakia
see Psoriasis

Libido, loss of
see Listlessness

Lichen
(eczema, see also Dermatomycoses)
Physical level: Skin (border, contact, tenderness).
Symptom level: Lichen ruber planus: flat, nodular eczema; Lichen nitidus: bright, yellow-brown nodular eczema, particularly on the penis and in the crook of the arm; Lichen pilaris: nodules on the hair follicles particularly in young women around the age of 20, on the upper arms, upper thighs and buttocks; Lichen simplex chronicus (also Neurodermitis circumscripta): pigment-free lesions that can be up to palm-size and that are extremely itchy, particularly on the extensor surfaces of the extremities and the genitals; →Lichen sclerosus et atrophicus: on the genitals; problems with contact and/or distancing oneself: nodes as symbols of a problem, many small nodes = many small, subordinate

problems, which as a mass, can nevertheless become a substantial problem and then really compound the problem of contact in the form of a vicious circle; making oneself so unattractive that nobody comes to close to one in the sensitive areas of the genital region and the unprotected inner sides of the extremities (inward protection); on the outer or extensor sides; the aspect of shielding and defending oneself against the outside carry more weight.

Handling: Learning to defend one's skin in a more open way and thereby preventing unwanted contact in advance; making oneself aware of what is going on underneath one's own skin: allowing oneself to burst with rage if one feels like it; opening one's borders in the figurative sense if one feels like it and is itching so much (to do so); recognising the tendency to make oneself ugly in order to sidestep problems and tasks.

Resolution: Being at ease in one's own skin; accepting one's own body and reconciling oneself to it: sensing desire at its border areas and courageously satisfying its needs for contact.

Archetypal principle: Saturn-Venus.

Lichen sclerosus et atrophicus

(skin disease of the vulva; see also Pruritus vulvae, Vulval carcinoma)
Physical level: External genitalia (vulva [protective wall]), mucous membranes (inner boundary, barrier).
Symptom level: Affects women over the age of 60; the skin as the border to the outside loses its suppleness; the area of sexuality is lifeless, but (still) carries within it a great deal of explosive material for conflicts.
Handling: Opening the borders to the outside in the sexual area; presenting oneself as vulnerable and less "shameful"; seeking sensual

satisfaction, not only in excessive eating; bringing together the polar contrasts in one's own being.
Resolution: (Re-)discovering openness and the capability to be receptive; consciously approaching unity.
Archetypal principle: Venus-Pluto-Saturn.

Lid inflammation

(blepharitis)
Physical level: Eyelids (curtains of the soul).
Symptom level: On the basis of →inflammation, →allergy and →eczema, conflict arises over closing, respectively opening, one's eyes; in the mornings, problems opening one's eyes, which have become glued shut overnight: not wanting to face the day; instead, one would like nothing better than to just keep one's eyes shut; not wanting to confront day-to-day life; leaving the curtains closed: no performance takes place - no vision(s) can come to light.
Handling: Consciously owning up to one's current problems with the confrontation of life; taking a time-out (a breather), making room for introspection: sometimes consciously leaving one's eyes shut in order to not have to look at things more closely; no longer taking care of everything; fighting for one's peace and quiet, being committed to retreat in an open(ly offensive) way.
Resolution: Making good use of one's hard-won opportunities for retreat: instead of looking outwards, looking inwards and practising introspection in the sense of searching for one's overall vision. Archetypal principle: Sun/Moon-Mars.

Light dermatoses

see Photodermatoses

327

Limping

(see also Claudicatio intermittens)
Physical level: Legs (mobility, prog-ress, stability), feet (steadfastness, deep-rootedness).
Symptom level: Dragging one leg behind oneself: dragging oneself through life; running rough: unusual movement process; being hindered in moving forward (making progress) = being different: being an outsider.
Handling: Learning to stand up to being an outsider and being out of the ordinary; bringing original ("flipped out") elements into life; elevating the banal eccentricity of the limping movement process to a more sophisticated level: stepping out of line; ensuring creative surprises; bringing variety into monotonous life processes; getting ahead more slowly and more patiently.
Resolution: Emulating Hephaestus, the inspired god of metal-working and blacksmiths of the Greek Pantheon, who after being thrown from Heaven, was lame in both legs: he created wonderful works of art through his inspired spirit.
Archetypal principle:
Uranus-Saturn.

Lipid storage diseases

(e.g. Gaucher's disease)
Physical level: Liver (life, evaluation, reconnection), spleen (filter of the life force), more rarely, the bone marrow (defence, vitality, uniqueness), skin (border, contact, tenderness), lymph nodes (police stations).
Symptom level: Enlargement of the affected organs due to lipid (kerasin) deposits: fats are stored instead of burnt off; dropping out of neurological functions: disturbances in the passing on of information.
Handling: (instructions for parents, since those affected are children):

preserving the valuable aspects of life; but also retaining superfluous aspects for enjoyment; giving more room to the subjects of the meaning of life and enjoyment, but also to the regulation of one's own vitality; dis-covering central values and learning to put them to good use.
Resolution: Reconciling oneself with the meaning of life and learn-ing to accept and hold on to the over-abundance.
Archetypal principle: Jupiter-Saturn.

Lipoma

see Adipose tumour

Lipomatosis cordis

see Heart, fatty degeneration

Lipophilia

(literally: love of fat; fatty deposits at certain points of the body, with central weighting on the lower part of the body)
Physical level: Pelvis (sexuality, basis of life, resonance base), legs (mobility, progress, stability), feet (steadfastness, deep-rootedness).
Symptom level: e.g. 'saddlebags' phenomenon (in women) = fatty de-posits below the belt-line reminiscent of riding jodhpurs: emphasis of the lower feminine half of the body with simultaneous unconscious rejection of the feminine; this fat is not loved by the women affected, as the name 'liphophilia' would suggest, but is instead hated, since it draws attention to the relevant domain that has been avoided and given a back seat in consciousness.
Handling: Consciously directing one's central weighting to the tasks (left outstanding) in the feminine area: sexual desire, progress, deep-rootedness (finding one's place in life); emphasis of the feminine in consciousness.

Resolution: Reconciliation with one's own feminine fate; conscious acceptance of the lower pole of life which has come up too short, i.e. the lower body (in the macrocosm: the poor southern hemisphere of the world).
Archetypal principle: Venus/Moon-Jupiter.

Liposarcoma

(cancer of the fatty tissue; see also Cancer)
Physical level: Fatty tissue (overflow, excess reserves).
Symptom level: Aggressive destruction of the tissue for excess reserves and storage; degeneration in the area of over-abundance: wild and ruthlessly rampant growth; having strayed so far off track from one's inherent development path with regard to the formation of reserves and enjoyment of over-abundance that the body has to help the (forgotten/repressed) issue to express itself; the mental-spiritual growth in this thematic area has been blocked for so long that it now forges a path in the body in an aggressive and random way; the cancer realises physically in the structural area that (turnaround) which would be spiritually necessary in the corresponding area of consciousness.
Handling: Radically questioning the policies regarding reserves and savings that have been passed down to one, and if necessary, giving these up without a further thought; opening oneself up in the area of over-abundance and luxury to one's own outlandish ideas and bold fantasies; courageously pressing ahead with them and allowing them to expand; thinking back to early dreams of one's own forms of expression with regard to luxury, over-abundance and excess reserves; bringing these (back) to life and putting them into practice with wild decisiveness; in

the certainty of having nothing more to lose, mustering courage for one's own self-realisation/one's own path; providing expression for oneself in the area of over-abundance and luxury instead of allowing the body to speak up for itself: preferring to have a cluttered-up house than overloading one's body with clutter, although admittedly this also cannot be the intended endpoint of one's development; struggle over spiritual values instead of material ones; considering all the measures mentioned under →cancer: since cancer affects the complete organism, it must also be met across-the-board.
Resolution: Breaking with the old life that is foreign to one's own being and its handling of over-abundance and luxury; fighting in an aggressive and open(ly offensive) way for one's own forms (of life); wrestling for security in the figurative sense, which can ultimately only be found on the spiritual level: there is no security other than "in God's hands"; recognising the necessity to switch from the physical and thus (life-) threatening level to the challenging, but life-saving mental-spiritual level, and relying in this realm on expansive growth in the affected Archetypal area; discovering love that transcends all boundaries; setting oneself above external rule and standards laid down by oneself or others, and living and expressing oneself solely in accordance with the obligations of one's own highest law; taking the search for immortality and omnipotence (of the soul) into one's own hands.
Archetypal principle: Jupiter-Pluto.

Lips, cracked/chapped

Physical level: Mouth (absorption, expression, maturity – being able to speak for oneself), lips (sensuality).

Lisping

Symptom level: Fear of sensuality, which achieves its goal with lips that are repulsive; at the same time, cracked and chapped lips send a signal in the form of body fluid (soul) and blood (life energy) that something wants to come out of them: wanting to open up and give oneself up entirely to sensuality; tearing oneself to shreds in the area of sensuality or being torn over this point; "talking oneself ragged"; overly dry situation, too little soul (water) in the game of life.

Handling: Opening oneself up to sensuality, and thereby finding the right level that promises enjoyment; preferring to open one's mouth (lips) for kissing.

Resolution: Experiencing and enjoying sensuality and voluptuousness; spreading enjoyment with one's lips.

Archetypal principle: Venus-Saturn.

Lisping

Physical level: Tongue (expression, speech, weapon), mouth (absorption, expression, maturity – being able to speak for oneself).

Symptom level: Touching the front teeth with the tongue when pronouncing sibilants: an unfortunate "slip of the tongue" (manner of speaking); unclear, wishy-washy means of expression: not being (wanting to be) understood.

Handling: (for jointly-affected parents, whose problems are often reflected by the children): learning to direct the attention to dangerous sounds (hissing of the snake); emphasising sibilants; showing understanding and conveying to the child the feeling of being understood.

Resolution: Feeling oneself understood; finding understanding; finding the correct turn of phrase (manner of speaking); wanting to share one's views.

Archetypal principle: Mercury.

Listlessness

(lack of interest in sexuality; see also Frigidity, Impotence, Orgasm problems, Depression)

Physical level: Consciousness problem; starting from the genital region (sexuality, polarity, procreation), the whole organism is affected.

Symptom level: Boycott of life; stress due to work, children, lack of money, other problems; other things are more important; too much tension caused by one's career; expenditure at other points; loss of erotic tension after many long years of marriage, lack of imagination; no interest in intercourse and exchange; fear of one's own shadow: religious →feelings of guilt, fear of pregnancy, fear of infection; partnership problems: power struggles, lack of cleanliness, hate; difficulties with one's sexual role, self-assured women have a castrating effect on some men; certain medications (e.g. beta-blockers, sedatives) can make one chemically impotent; result of sexual abuse; dependency of desire on the female hormonal cycle.

Handling: Allowing the libido to flow into creative projects; concerning oneself with oneself and one's own issues; arranging one's life to be more enjoyable and sensual; not only valuing performance and action highly, but also simply being; valuing eroticism more highly; ensuring reliable contraception and clean relationships in the sexual area.

Resolution: Giving love a central place in life; learning the art of love (Tantra).

Archetypal principle: Venus-Saturn.

Liver abscess

Physical level: Liver (life, evaluation, reconnection).

Symptom level: Localised, relatively clear conflict in the area of one's philosophy of life, re-ligio(n) (from

Latin religāre 'to bind, tie again') or evaluation.

Handling: Aggressive, combative confrontation with the relevant subject that is causing the stir; struggling offensively over questions about the meaning of life; addressing the meaningfulness, respectively meaninglessness, of one's own life.

Resolution: Doing justice to the new elements that are causing the stir and struggling to reach a solution to the conflict; forging pathways towards one's own philosophy of life, respectively towards achieving intellectual autonomy.

Archetypal principle: Jupiter-Mars.

Liver cancer

(see also Cancer)

Physical level: Liver (life, evaluation, reconnection).

Symptom level: Degeneration in the domains of one's philosophy of life, re-ligio(n) (reconnection), questions about the meaning of life or in the domain of value judgements: wild and ruthlessly rampant growth on the physical level; profound conflict related to the meaning of life, which the person affected is unaware of or which appears un(re)solvable; having strayed so far off track from one's inherent line of development with regard to one's philosophy of life, spirituality and overall sense and meaning of life that the body has to help the (forgotten/repressed) issues to express themselves; the mental-spiritual growth in these areas has been blocked for so long that it now forges a path in the body in an aggressive and random way; the cancer realises physically in the thematically-related domains that (turnaround) which would be spiritually necessary in the corresponding domains of consciousness; aggressive destruction of functioning liver cells with the danger of a

collapse of the liver functions (similar prognosis to →cirrhosis of the liver).

Handling: Radically questioning the old customs and traditions that have been passed down to one concerning religion, philosophy of life and questions of values as far as they relate to one's own life, and if need be, ruthlessly destroying them, even if this involves the danger of having to obliterate much of the old in order to achieve spiritual autonomy; opening oneself up in the areas of life philosophy and religion to one's own outlandish ideas and bold fantasies; courageously and freely allowing them to flourish and expand; thinking back to early dreams of one's own religious goals, wishes and ideas about the meaning of (one's own) life, bringing these (back) to life and putting them into practice with wild decisiveness; in the certainty of having nothing more to lose, mustering courage for one's own self-realisation/one's own path; taking the growth impulse away from the body and directing it to more resolved (redeeming) levels; providing expression for oneself in the spiritual area instead of allowing the body to speak up for itself; considering all the measures mentioned under →cancer: since cancer affects the complete organism, it must also be met across-the-board.

Resolution: Pushing ahead with one's search for the actual meaning of life; recognising the necessity to switch from the physical and thus (life) threatening level to the challenging, but life-saving mental-spiritual level, and relying in this realm on expansive growth in the archetypal domain concerned; discovering love that transcends all boundaries; setting oneself above external rule and standards laid down by oneself or others and living and expressing oneself solely in accordance with the obligations of one's own highest law.

Archetypal principle: Jupiter-Pluto.

Liver, cirrhosis

Physical level: Liver (life, evaluation, reconnection).

Symptom level: Hardened standpoints with regard to one's value judgements and questions about the meaning of life: hardened liver due to conversion of functioning liver tissue into non-functioning scarred connective tissue (underlying diseases: →alcoholism, unhealed →jaundice, →poisoning): the liver is no longer up to its task; its issues come up too short; clinging stubbornly to the concept of the meaninglessness of life; often eventual shrinkage as the opposite pole to the initial expansion and growth (possible preliminary stage of a fatty liver); self-poisoning: the liver's laboratory operations collapse; reduction in performance increases in parallel with the progression of the cirrhosis; lust for life declines and disappears on all levels: loss of appetite (for life) to the point of apathy; flowing away of the lifeblood (bleeding tendency due to insufficient coagulation factors); □oesophageal varicose veins (varices) and stomach varicose veins (the so-called caput medusae, Latin: 'head of Medusa') due to blockage, respectively the backing-up of the flow of life energy in or in front of, the liver; process of feminisation in men, similar in effect to a castration, since female hormones can no longer be broken down: development of breasts, female pubic hair, regression of the testicles; abdominal dropsy (□ascites formation): the spiritual element builds up in the centre and cannot be kept in flow; liver stars (spider angiomas): instead of directing one's gaze at the stars in the heavens as an expression of the Great Order in which everyone has his/her place, stars are produced on the skin (bursting of minor blood vessels).

Handling: Making oneself aware of one's own hardening in questions about the meaning of life and one's value judgements, and making re-adjustments inwardly rather than re-modelling the liver; allowing over-indulgence that is beyond measure to shrink back; beginning to critically confront the toxicity of one's own lifestyle; giving up performance demands; turning one's attention to essential inner questions; distancing oneself from excessively greedy consumption of the world and learning to be modest; consciously giving oneself to and expending one's life energy on essential matters; confronting the blockage in one's own energy world which is leaving its mark on one's stomach; doing justice to the feminine pole of one's own life, breaking loose from the masculine (macho madness of many alcoholics); taking the soul (feminine water element in the stomach) seriously and collecting it (in one's centre); fasting as a healthy process of contraction and as a method for regaining the right measure.

Resolution: Allowing oneself to shrink back to a healthy measure in good time and finding one's way to what is essential (the meaning of one's own life) by means of good differentiation and evaluation; recognising in the disease pattern of cirrhosis of the liver (the fourth most common cause of death in Germany) the price of growth at any price.

Archetypal principle: Jupiter-Saturn.

Liver, congested

(see also Portal vein blockage)

Physical level: Liver (life, evaluation, reconnection).

Symptom level: Enlargement and blue/red discoloration of the liver: the life energy accumulates in the liver; the significance of the liver-related themes builds up; the increase in pressure of the tissue in the liver leads to a shrinking of the cells and an accumulation of fat: the liver tries to do justice to the increased weightiness (importance) with sham solutions (puffing up of the liver's dimensions due to fatty deposits); replacement of the declining liver tissue with connective tissue on the path to →cirrhosis of the liver: hardening of the matter.

Handling: Directing one's complete energy to the liver and the essential questions related to the themes of the liver: "What is the meaning of my life? Where do I come from? Where am I going? What are my values? What is the right measure for me?"; awareness of sham solutions which boil down to nothing more than boastful stirring and create much ado about nothing; concentration on the essential instead of becoming hardened.

Resolution: Concerning oneself with life and the prospects it has to offer; becoming clear in oneself about how to apply one's remaining life energy.

Archetypal principle: Jupiter-Saturn.

Liver diseases

(interpreted here using the example of hepatitis; see also Jaundice, Fatty liver, Liver, cirrhosis)

Physical level: Liver (life, evaluation, reconnection).

Symptom level: Frustrating remodelling attempts by the liver, which in the search for a solution just keeps on growing and growing, but without any plan or objective; eventually, it exhausts itself in this process until, in the end, there are hardly any functioning liver cells left, and instead only connective tissue remains: the overall sense of the liver and one's life structure is destroyed in the chaos of these seemingly desperate attempts at rescue and remodelling; unconscious chronic conflict with regard to matters of one's philosophy of life, religion and evaluation: actual neglect of these matters; aggressive,

strength-sapping struggle for the right measure; problems in estimating what is useful or harmful/poisonous; lack of moderation in taking things on board; overblown desires for expansion, overly high ideals, delusions of grandeur; loss of energy and potency as a corrective measure for taking on too much; melancholy and →depression (feeling "liverish").

Handling: Setting out on the search for meaning instead of leaving the liver to search for physical solutions; learning to appreciate and preserve the original order of life; consciously confronting issues of philosophy, spirituality and questions of meaning in an open(ly offensive) way; critical re-examination of what one considers to be the right measure; more conscious identification of what agrees with one, and what is harmful; recognising that it is the dose that makes the poison (Paracelsus); expansion in the areas of philosophy and religion instead of in the liver; confronting aspects of one's life philosophy in spirit (intellectually) instead of with spirits (alcoholic drinks) ("In vino veritas" is not enough); trusting oneself to take on more on the mental-spiritual level, and thereby taking the load off the stomach and liver; restricting oneself in the expenditure of (sexual and general) energy; learning sensible limitations and constraints; calming down and finding calm within oneself; giving life the correct (right) direction, an objective, orientation (to the core elements) and order; remodelling one's life, instead of the liver; committing oneself offensively to ensuring fair measures – both for oneself and others.

Resolution: Keeping one's life (liver) in the right measure(ment); gaining confidence; finding the one's own sense of meaning and putting it into practice in one's own life.

Archetypal principle: Jupiter-Mars.

Liver inflammation

see Liver diseases/Hepatitis

Liver spot

(Lentigo; see also Pigment flecks [chloasma, melasma], Birthmark [naevus], Freckles [Ephelides], Age-related symptoms [age marks])

Physical level: Skin (border, contact, tenderness).

Symptom level: (Insignificant) spots on one's "hide", being slightly marked; most probably only an aesthetic phenomenon, which should, however, be kept under observation due to a minimal tendency towards degeneration: as soon as the spots begin to grow, bleed or change noticeably in any other way, dermatological clarification is indicated; potential problem zones of uncontrollable growth.

Handling: If necessary, interpret the localisation and understand it as a call to attention to keep one's growth within sensible channels.

Resolution: Growth in the mental-spiritual and social domains so that the body remains relieved of the burden.

Archetypal principle: Jupiter-Pluto.

Lockjaw (tetanus)

Physical level: The complete organism is affected.

Symptom level: The pathogens that are at home in faeces and the ground penetrate through wounds, and by means of the central nervous system, cause lockjaw, which 40% of those afflicted fall victim to: energies from the lower shadow kingdom (excrement and earth, which naturally consist of the products of decomposition) break through the border to the upper world, penetrating into central areas and poisoning them; severe pains at the point of the injury and cramps which spread out: lockjaw (the so-called risus sardonicus

– 'sardonic grin' due to cramping), swallowing disorders, cramps of the facial muscles, exaggerated irritability, rock-hard cramps of the entire back, stomach and neck; the patient is responsive right to the point of death and thus fully experiences the torment; death eventually occurs from causes such as respiratory paralysis.

Handling: (in the sense of prevention; vaccination provides relatively reliable protection): coming to terms with the dark forces of the underworld in good time in order to protect oneself against surprise attacks; not shying away from conflicts and confrontations; letting out one's laughter before it ends up frozen on one's face as a cramped sardonic grin; allowing oneself to be stimulated by life in good time while one can still react to it; battling to not swallow and accept everything without objection; being straight with and strengthening oneself (from behind); showing backbone and not letting one's neck be bowed down.

Resolution: Consciously encountering the god Pan in all of nature; reconciliation with the primordial forces of the underworld; experiencing the enormous forces of one's own inner world before they put one in a vice; consciously experiencing what feats the muscles are capable of and delighting in these.

Archetypal principle: Mars-Saturn/Pluto.

Lockjaw (trismus)

(see also Teeth, grinding overnight)

Physical level: Lower jaw (weapons store), chin (strong will, forceful assertion).

Symptom level: Cramped power impulse and impulse of will of the upper and lower level, often corresponding to family/generation problems, in which the upper jaw usually stands for the family of origin and the lower

jaw for the individual; often unconscious conflicts in this respect between tradition and individuation.
Handling: Consciously facing up to the diverging interests within the family and biting one's way through in the figurative sense; developing bite instead of being like a dog with a bone.
Resolution: Applying one's power consciously and responsibly; standing behind the forceful pushing through of one's demands and one's enjoyment of the fruits that they bear.
Archetypal principle: Mars/ Saturn/ Uranus.

Long-sightedness

(see also Senile hypermetropia)
Physical level: Eyes (insight, perspective, mirrors and windows of the soul).
Symptom level: Disorder occurring mainly with increasing age; the point of sharpest vision recedes into the distance; the expansiveness and thus the possibility of maintaining an overview remain intact (parallel development that points in the same direction: forgetfulness for events that are temporally close, while those that are temporally distant are remembered): not perceiving and not wanting to believe what is close at hand and obvious, overlooking it; looking beyond and ignoring the day-to-day trivialities; removing the millstone of these day-to-day trivialities in one's immediate surroundings from one's neck; perhaps already considering oneself as something better; distancing oneself from adverse or angry feelings with regard to one's immediate life circumstances and wishes; need to get away and to get ahead, to flee into the future.
Handling: Gaining an overview, letting one's gaze wander in the distance, discovering perspectives in life; giving a lower priority to what is close at hand and concerning oneself with the wider context of life; giving the greater whole priority over the minor details of life; directing one's concentration/one's gaze to the horizon of life (extending one's horizon); developing distance to one's own life; aligning the important events in the overall design, and from this, developing (life) wisdom.
Resolution: Developing clear far-sightedness and an overview of the essential stations along the path of life; recognising the (great) arc of life; finding the guiding red thread in the labyrinth of one's own life; older (far-sighted) people should distance themselves to a certain degree from their own lives, in the same way that young (short-sighted) people are called on to allow events closer to them; finding and further developing the vision of one's own life.
Archetypal principle: Sun/ Moon-Jupiter/Uranus.

Low blood pressure

(hypotension; see also Connective tissue weakness)
Physical level: Blood (life force) finds no resistance at the walls of the blood vessels (transport routes of the life force), which give way and do not stand up to the pressure.
Symptom level: The limits (of the vessel walls) are not challenged; avoiding resistances and challenges; not going to the limit, drawing back in the face of conflicts and generally withdrawing oneself from life; apparent relinquishment of power, surrender of responsibility; retreat into the unconscious; taking flight into powerlessness (by blacking out), "playing dead" reflex; demoralisation with regard to one's own life; lack of steadfastness and uprightness:"feign"(t)ing spells (i.e. dizziness due to self-deception); the life energy current cannot find its way back to the centre

and remains blocked somewhere on the periphery; fear; cold feet: lack of grounding; having no vital connection with Mother Earth, with the feminine principle; not yet having found one's place in life; cold hands: not being inwardly prepared to make contact, to tackle life and get a grip on it; victim stance: frequently being reduced to the size of a snail and withdrawing into one's shell; being forced to the ground; being helpless, downtrodden, powerless (blacking out); passive resistance (not being able to get out of bed in the morning), tendency toward regression; boring life without tension, but long, because this is very kind on the heart; rejection of life (childish attitude): "Daddy (the husband) will sort it out"; frequent tendency toward →depression and defeatism and later in the course of life, transition to the opposite pole of high blood pressure. Handling: True relaxation instead of slackness; seeing one's own smallness and weakness against the wonder of Creation; yielding (to the greater law) and giving way without resentment; conscious abandonment instead of battling; letting oneself be caught and carried by Mother Earth; striving for connection with the Earth, deep-rootedness; handing over responsibility and power into higher hands ("Thy will be done"): exercises in subsequent development of basic trust (exercises which enable experiences of unity); lifting "It is more blessed to give than to receive" from the blood to the level of consciousness; owning up to one's lack of deep-rootedness and contact and accepting the boundless flow of events; consciously sacrificing oneself, instead of physically taking refuge in the victim role; regression in the sense of re-ligio(n) (Latin: 'to bind, tie again') = reconnection to the origin of life. Resolution: Humility; adaptability, elasticity, flexibility; sympathy

(misericordia); finding one's place in life and putting down roots: yielding to life.
Archetypal principle: Moon-Saturn.

Lower leg fracture

see Leg fracture

Lues

see Syphilis

Lumbago

(Lower back pain, see also Sciatica)
Physical level: Spinal column (dynamics and hold, uprightness).
Symptom level: Conflict between "lower" drives and "upper" demands: having been torn this way and that between superego and animalistic instinct, one is suddenly ripped apart and (painfully) pulls oneself together; overloading as compensation for a lack of self-assurance and feelings of smallness and inferiority; being torn this way and that in an uncontrolled manner that one cannot stand behind; tearing oneself apart, putting oneself out, bending over backwards; not standing up to things properly, and instead over-stretching the spinal column (in terms of mobility/flexibility); projection: feeling like others are using one as a voodoo doll and that it is their fault that one is putting one's neck and oneself out since they are making one's head spin with no involvement from oneself (German word for lumbago = Hexenschuss 'witches' jab').
Handling: Consciously demanding more of oneself and taking on greater loads; growing as a result of these challenging demands and gaining (self-)assurance; allowing oneself to be carried away more often and more courageously and learning to say 'yes' to one's own impulses and needs; consciously exerting oneself beyond the normal measure and

making the effort to do justice to one's own expectations; taking back projections and also recognising one's own involvement, even in so-called bad moves (twisting things the wrong way, contorted convolutions, a fling on the side and other problematic moves), which one cannot/does not want to own up to.

Resolution: Standing behind one's own needs and wishes in a positive way, adopting the right stance to life.

Archetypal principle:
Saturn- Mars-Uranus.

Lung abscess

Physical level: Lungs (contact, communication, freedom).

Symptom level: Localised conflict in the area of exchange, contact and communication; sitting on a volcano in the communications area which wants to erupt.

Handling: Aggressive, combative confrontation with the relevant subjects which have broken into and stirred up this problem area.

Resolution: Doing justice to the new elements that are causing the stir and struggling to reach a solution to the conflict.

Archetypal principle: Mercury-Mars.

Lung cancer

(bronchial carcinoma [above all in connection with →smoking] and adenocarcinoma [minor connection with smoking]; see also Cancer)

Physical level: Lungs (contact, communication, freedom).

Symptom level: Degeneration in the contact and communications area, e.g. exchange and contacts which do not correspond to the innermost core of one's being, but still consume a great deal of energy (bronchial tissue that has broken with its kind strikes out on its own); wild and ruthlessly rampant growth in this subject area; aggressive disturbance/total destruction of communication (primarily due to smoking; see also the underlying communications problem which is expressed in →smoking, secondarily due to cancerous proliferation); growth that infiltrates into foreign areas; intrusion into taboo areas; penetration through iron-clad borders (basal membranes): unlived, binding (loving) communication that transcends all boundaries sinks down into the body; contact and exchange processes that are capable of breaking down all boundaries occur in an aggressive and infiltrating way on the physical level of the body; struggling for air, not being able to breathe freely anymore: tight constraints and anxiety with respect to one's own enclave in life; having strayed so far off track from one's inherent development path in the contact and communications area that the body helps the (forgotten/repressed) issues to express themselves; the mental-spiritual growth in this area has been blocked for so long that it now forges a path in the body in an aggressive and random way; the cancer realises physically that (turnaround) which would be spiritually necessary in the corresponding area of consciousness; the search for immortality and omnipotence (of the soul) lives itself out in the cancer cells instead of in consciousness: Breakthrough to immortality (on the cellular level); the re-connection to the origin, the source of religion (from Latin religāre 'to bind, tie again') has sunk down into the regressive tendencies of physical cancer cells: regression on primitive (metabolic) levels.

Handling: Bearing in mind and looking closely at one's tendency in earlier stages (of the disease) to slowly drag oneself along in crab-like fashion (Latin: cancer = 'crab') (not going one's own way in the communicative respect).; opening oneself up in the area of contact and exchange

to one's own outlandish ideas and bold fantasies; courageously allowing them to grow and develop uncontrolled (by others); giving one's all for one's own path in life in an offensive and penetrating way: thinking back to early dreams and one's own forms of expression with respect to communication; bringing these (back) to life and putting them into practice with wild decisiveness; seeking and winning conflicts in the communications area; in the certainty of having nothing more to lose, mustering courage for one's own self-realisation/ one's own path: making boundless exchange and loving contacts a reality; courageously penetrating (intellectually) into foreign areas which do not "officially" concern one: forcing intellectual breakthroughs; return to a simpler, more modest way of life; returning to contemplation of one's own origins ("Where do I come from?"); reconciliation with the mortality of the body; looking forward to the actual goal: immortality (of the soul); considering all the measures mentioned under →cancer: since cancer affects the complete organism, it must also be met across-the-board; being receptive to binding, loving communication that transcends all boundaries; courageously enforcing it while destroying old communications structures using open(ly offensive) means; taking questions about the origin of everything and the sense of the whole into one's own hands, thereby taking the load off the cells of the body.
Resolution: Free expression; individual communication; recognising the necessity to switch from the physical and therefore (life-) threatening level to the challenging, but life-saving mental-spiritual level, and relying in this realm on expansive growth; discovering love that transcends all boundaries; setting oneself above external rule and standards laid down by oneself or others and living and developing oneself solely in accordance with the obligations of one's own highest law; establishing community on a higher human level; seeking communication with God (e.g. prayer, meditation); taking the search for immortality and omnipotence (of the soul) into one's own hands.
Archetypal principle: Mercury-Pluto.

Lungs, congested

see Lung oedema

Lung embolism

(most dangerous complication of leg vein thrombosis; see also Embolism, Thrombosis, Blood coagulation)
Physical level: Lungs (contact, communication, freedom).
Symptom level: Vitality which has become sluggish somewhere in the landscape of the body congeals to form blockage material in the communications area (lungs): solidified, sluggish life energy threatens the communication and exchange system; instead of reflecting flowing joy (for life), life has degenerated into (fulfilment of) obligations; circulation and breathing disorders in the dependent area of the lungs (lung infarction): no energy flow, no further spiritual exchange – both are sacrificed; threat to life due to blockage of the most important system which anchors us in the polar world of contrasts.
Handling: Acute (allopathic) approach: getting the energy flow moving again, clearing up blockages, ensuring (gas) exchange; long-term (homeopathic) approach: slowing down the flow of life energy and reducing the exchange volume; consciously and voluntarily sacrificing parts of one's communication and exchange; realising the threat to life if the body is forced to stage the issue; making a break in one's traditional way of supplying the communications

and exchange area with energy: finding more conscious forms of exchange; consciously sacrificing communications levels and contacts which have become superfluous; taking care of the contact area in a new way and with more attentiveness.
Resolution: Taking more time for oneself; slowing down the tempo of life, granting oneself rest; finding new forms of exchange.
Archetypal principle: Mercury-Saturn.

Lung fibrosis

Physical level: Lungs (contact, communication, freedom).
Symptom level: The fibrous tissue in the lung alveoli and in the connective tissue between them get out of hand, resulting in a loss of elasticity and gas exchange disorders; the communication with life is constrained by too much peripheral tissue, which hinders the specific lung tissue; too much peripheral communication, which causes the essential matters to come up too short.
Handling: Strengthening communicative bonds and coming to mutual agreements that are more strongly binding; replacing the rampant growth of the binding connective tissue on more sensible levels e.g. connections with others that grow to be more binding.
Resolution: Promoting bonding ability and binding commitment in the contact and communications area.
Archetypal principle: Mercury.

Lung inflammation

(pneumonia)
Physical level: Lungs (contact, communication, freedom).
Symptom level: Conflict ignites itself from germ-inating elements (pathogens), which stir things up in the communications area; combative conflict between contact (openness) and

distancing oneself; aggressive conflict in the area of exchange; war over one's contact with the world; pathogens such as pneumococci, which over half the population have in their lungs at all times, do not represent the actual problem, although they always play a role; it is more a question of the milieu and the (spiritual) breeding ground; pathogens such as SARS, on the other hand, are no real problem for us, but instead serve more as a distraction from the approx. 30,000 deaths per year (in Germany alone) caused by completely normal lung inflammation pathogens due to increasingly less effective antibiotics, respectively increasingly more resistant bacteria.
Handling: Allowing oneself to be stirred up in the communications area instead of throwing open the doors to being stirred up by pathogens; open(ly offensive) conflicts in the exchange area to the point of aggressive battles; committing oneself to waging wars in this respect; learning to distance oneself at the right point.
Resolution: Openness towards stirring suggestions and stimuli that are foreign to one; breaking down one's own communications barriers; getting to know the lobes of the lungs as wings of freedom and openness which enable us the freedom of exchange with all beings: with other people through the communication of language, which is based on the flow of breath; with animals and people through the same air we breathe and with plants through the circle of life, in which we take the oxygen which they produce and give them the carbon dioxide they need.
Archetypal principle: Mercury-Mars.

Lung oedema

(see also Oedema)
Physical level: Lungs (contact, communication, freedom).

Lung pressure, increased

Symptom level: Leakage of (spiritual) water from the vascular system into the exchange and communications area of the lung alveoli; the air (thought) element is forced out by the water (soul) element: the lightness of one's thoughts is drowned in the build-up of emotional backwater; drowning in and from one's own spiritual water.

Handling: Releasing the spiritual element from its narrow, prescribed paths and sending it into the communications channels; allowing emotions to penetrate into the worlds of one's thoughts; opening the exchange area to spiritual aspects; consciously immersing oneself in one's own spiritual worlds. Resolution: Bringing the watery spiritual worlds and airy worlds of thoughts into contact with each other and enabling exchange.

Archetypal principle: Mercury-Moon/Neptune.

Lung pressure, increased

see Cor pulmonale

Lupus erythematodes

(see also Auto-aggressive/Auto-immune diseases)

Physical level: Skin (border, contact, tenderness), particularly of the face, but also the upper chest and back, extensor surfaces of the hands and fingers; involvement of inner organs (→endocarditis [heart], →glomerulo-nephritis [kidneys]).

Symptom level: Being marked (by life) in the face: red with unlived aggression (flush of anger?); one's own border fortifications and contact surfaces are violently attacked from the inside out; instead of being directed outwards against outside enemies, the defensive strength is specifically directed against one's own border and contact structures: becoming one's own worst enemy; eating oneself up with unlived aggression that forces its way to the outside; spreading of the attack of unbridled aggressions to the kidneys (balance, partnership) and endocardium (feeling, emotion): the inflammation of the endocardium from the inside out due to the same conflicts shows how much one's heart is being turned into a skeleton closet: instead of being lived outwardly, the vital defensive forces attack one's own heart from the inside; the kidneys as organs of the (acid-base) balance also become the theatre for staging a civil war.

Handling: Showing one's (true) face in all honesty; allowing the energy to come to the surface: turning red with fiery enthusiasm and heated ardour instead of with (unconscious) anger; blossoming in the sense of flourishing; voluntarily bringing one's own borders into question; allowing oneself to be stirred up more often and more intensively in the figurative sense; directing the struggle to a higher level: combatively concerning oneself with oneself, and thereby taking the load off the immune defence system; offensively calling one's own borders and communications structures into question on the level of consciousness, even to the point of self-sacrifice; including the thematic areas of partnership, balance and feelings, and matters of the heart in the conflict as well; exercises which get under one's skin and scratch at the (external) glossy surface; fasting as a means of finding one's way back to what is essential.

Resolution: Courageously calling into question one's own appearance, one's partnership behaviour and one's handling of matters of the heart and offensive restructuring in these areas.

Archetypal principle: Pluto-Mars.

Lymph node inflammation

see Adenitis

Lymph node swelling, inflammatory

see Lymphadenitis

Lymphadenitis

(inflammatory lymph node swelling)
Physical level: Everywhere where lymph nodes (police stations) are found.
Symptom level: Expression of a delimited local conflict or within the framework of a more general conflict; war over a police station.
Handling: Making oneself aware of the subject of the conflict and having it out on the mental-spiritual level.
Resolution: Facing up combatively to the conflicts and having them out to the point of (re)solution.
Archetypal principle: Mars.

Lymphogran-ulomatosis

see Hodgkin's disease

Lymphostasis

see Elephantiasis

Lyssa

see Rabies

M

Macromastia

see Hypermastia

Macular degeneration

see Retinopathy

Mad cow disease

(Bovine Spongiform Encephalopa-thy – BSE; see Creutzfeldt-Jakob disease)

Malaise

(see also Vomiting/Nausea, Balance disorders, Jetlag)
Physical level: Balance organ in the inner ear (balance sensor), stomach (feeling, receptiveness), hormone system (control, information).
Symptom level: Not feeling at home in one's own body, not being oneself, not having it (all) together, not being in one's centre; being unable to digest something; inner tensions come dis-harmoniously to the surface.
Handling: Deeply sensing the spir-itual imbalance, tracing the source of the disturbance, paying attention to one's bodily sensations, listening closely inwardly.
Resolution: Accepting oneself as one is; not being of this world.
Archetypal principle: Sun-Moon-Venus-Neptune.

Malaria

(tertian or swamp fever; the disease pattern which overall costs the most human life on Earth)
Physical level: Blood (life force).
Symptom level: Periodically-recur-ring fits of fever with shivering attacks due to the breakdown of blood cor-puscles that are filled with plasmodia (single-cell parasites); the plasmodia then immediately search for new blood corpuscles and their breakdown after 48 and 72 hours (depending on the type of malaria) leads to the next fit of fever: periodic general mobilisation of the body as a reaction

to its energy carriers that have been infected and occupied by the enemy; these battle attacks are often accompanied by vomiting: feeling sick to one's stomach and wanting to once again be rid of what doesn't agree with one; Mars-driven (mosquito bite pierces the skin) intrusion of chthonic powers (the fever attacks often flush wild fantasies from dark shadow areas to the surface).

Handling: Courageously, offensively and feverishly searching for one's own rhythm and living in accordance with it with dedication and energetic commitment; opening oneself up to life with all of its tension and provocative elements instead of opening oneself up to provocative elements in the form of pathogens; working from the opposite pole: learning to defend oneself offensively and aggressively; taking on and defeating outer and inner enemies; going into battle time and again for one's own vital life interests; prevention: voluntarily penetrating into the dark realms of fantasy (inner journeys instead of the outer journeys during which tourists are most likely to become infected).

Resolution: Ability to put up a fight: taking on and conquering the inner opponents; correctly assessing one's own combat strength and courage before travelling to countries where malaria is prevalent (in earlier times, these were adventure trips; today these are luxury trips and the adventure often comes through the back door, namely in the evening with the mosquitoes); living according to one's own rhythm in a courageous and challenging way.

Archetypal principle: Pluto-Neptune.

Mammary carcinoma

see Breast cancer

Mammary gland inflammation

(mastitis; usually in the first weeks following delivery when nursing)

Physical level: The female breast (motherliness, nourishment, safety and security, sensuality, desire).

Symptom level: Conflict over nursing, nourishing, giving milk, mothering (war over the "milk bar"); wanting to mother too much; stirring elements (pathogens - from Greek. pathos "suffering, feeling, emotion") penetrate (into the tissue) via the maltreated milk sources (cracks around the nipple); danger of a deepening of the conflict (→abscess); other causes: insect bites which become infected, a partner who sucks or bites too much during loveplay; there is too much weighing on her chest and dragging her down: the child, the man, sexuality, the issue of supply (money issues); possibly also unconscious aggression because now she is supposed to give and has received too little in return; feeling oneself left alone in the partnership with the task of providing on all levels.

Handling: Owning up to the conflict over nursing and fighting it out internally: who has what rights to the mam(m)a/ry – the newborn because of the milk bar, papa as his source of desire, mama (and papa) and her figure?; allowing stirring subjects related to nursing (e.g. anxiety about the beauty of the breast); fighting out the conflict down to the very depths of the relationship (with the child, partner and one's own body) (e.g.: "What can I/do I not want to give with the mother's milk?"); learning to deal with the total dependency of the child, but also learning to see through its first ambitions to power; scaling back one's expectations with regard to motherhood; mothering oneself; reducing stress; allowing oneself to be helped.

Resolution: Inner willingness to nourish; accepting and enjoying womanhood without reservation; reorganisation of the hierarchy of relationships in favour of the new life: for a certain time, putting the child first (nursing) and the partner in second place.
Archetypal principle: Moon/ Venus-Mars.

Mandibular joint pains

Physical level: Jaw (weapons store), joints (mobility, articulation).
Symptom level: The collision of the claims to power of the upper level (= family of origin, the past) and the lower level (= the individual, the present) leads to cries of pain and cries for help from the joint, which can no longer deal completely with the tension; the unconscious conflict between tradition and individuation is typical of modern-day society.
Handling: Consciously facing up to the tensions of life; developing bite instead of snappishness; gritting one's teeth and biting one's way through life in a healthy way instead of being like a dog with a bone.
Resolution: Seeking a sustainable compromise between the higher and lower interest positions; finding an acceptable balance in the direction of balanced composure (in the Buddhist sense of Uppekha).
Archetypal principle: Mars/ Saturn.

Manic-depressive disease

(bipolar disorder; see also Depression)
Symptom level: Mood fluctuations from being over the moon one minute to the deepest depths of deathly despair the next; wandering through Heaven and Hell; motoric fluctuations from enormously enhanced to abnormally slowed down; 1. Mania:

Insomnia, exaggerated alertness, overflooding, enormous spiritual liveliness; cheerfulness for no apparent reason (for outsiders); →flight of ideas and compulsion to speak almost to the point of missioneering; over-exaggerated opinion of oneself beyond all measure: regarding oneself as the greatest and the best; 2. Depression: Inability to react to external stimuli, emotions at a low ebb; longing for death, feelings of inferiority.
Handling: Acknowledging the right to existence of both extremes, respectively polarity in general, and starting from the basis of one's experience of both extremes, setting out on the search for the middle ground; transforming the loud high spirits of forced cheerfulness into the serene high of the spirit; obtaining from the flight of ideas and one's compulsion to speak the courage for one's own, perhaps even also high-flying ideas and the ability to make inspiring speeches; by using one's boundless self-overestimation (or more accurately, Ego-overestimation) as a starting point, sensing one's own possibilities of reaching unity, one's centre and one's self; joyfully cheering to high heaven, making Heaven (the heavenly kingdom of God) a reality in oneself; from the experience of depression, picking up the ability to let oneself get involved with death and to come to terms with it long before it comes to take one with it; grounding exercises during the manic phase (learning to come back down to earth): simple manual work, garden work, daily sweating as a result of one's own efforts, etc.; spiritual exercises aimed at finding the centre: mandala painting and meditation, Tai Chi, Qi Gong, making pottery on the rotating potter's wheel, Hatha yoga, Uppekha meditation.
Resolution: Homeopathically: being tolerant of the great amplitude of

one's mood swings, e.g. finding a (more intense) life rhythm which enables the connection of both (extreme) poles; reconciling oneself with both extremes of mood, integration of the two souls in one('s own) breast, with each coming into its own; working allopathically from the opposite pole: finding one's centre: being at rest in oneself, with one's feet firmly rooted in Mother Earth and one's head uplifted to the Father in Heaven (Indian rule of life); moving away from the extremes ("Be hot or cold, the lukewarm I will spit out of My mouth") and making steps forward to the balanced centre ("If someone strikes you on the right cheek, turn to him the other also"): developing from the first biblical quote to the second: this requires a person to be so at rest in their centre that not even external attacks should be able to shake them from it.
Archetypal principle: Pluto (the extremes).

Mastitis

see Mammary gland inflammation

Mastodynia

(pains in the female breast)
Physical level: The female breast (motherliness, nourishment, safety and security, sensuality, desire).
Symptom level: Call for help of the breast without any discernible physical reason: call for loving attention and recognition; more "psychosomatic" than →mastopathy; fending off all contact; the breast does not want to be "used" physically any more.
Handling: Looking after the breasts and their related issues; directing attention to the areas of maternal nourishment and erotic desire; keeping unwelcome contact and shocks at arm's length; protecting oneself against unwanted advances and abuse.

Resolution: Reconciling oneself with one's own breasts and enjoyment of the themes related to them, such as nourishing and being nourished, sensuality and tenderness.
Archetypal principle: Moon/ Venus-Mars.

Mastopathia fibrosa cystica

see Breast cysts

Mastopathy

(most frequent disease of the breasts, benign tissue proliferation with the tendency to formation of →breast cysts; see also Breast nodes, benign)
Physical level: The female breast (motherliness, nourishment, safety and security, sensuality, desire).
Symptom level: Rampant growth of nodes (cysts) in the mammary ducts: the knotty nodes represent unresolved knotty problems/conflicts: having a lot of conflicts on one's chest; swelling of the breast as though nursing a baby: problems with providing nourishment, giving milk, being a mam(m)a/ry; fear of cancer: in the case of mastopathy, however, the nodes, although frequently painful, are less solid and not as firmly-attached (nevertheless, the danger of degeneration cannot be excluded): the pains are a cry for help, loving attention and tender care.
Handling: Owning up to one's unresolved problems in the breast area (nourishment, arousal) and adequately addressing these; owning up to one's conflict over nourishing, nursing and being a mother; asking oneself the questions that are important in the case of →cancer and responding to these: nipping problems in the bud in the sense of genuine prevention that goes far beyond normal early detection; giving the gift of

tender care and loving attention to the breast or letting it be given.
Resolution: Inner willingness to nourish (on whatever level); accepting and coming to love one's own breasts.
Archetypal principle: Moon-Jupiter/ Saturn.

Maxillary sinus inflammation

see Sinus inflammation

Measles

(see also Skin rash, Childhood diseases)
Physical level: Skin (border, contact, tenderness), eyes (insight, perspective, mirrors and windows of the soul).
Symptom level: heavy congestion; puffy, tear-stained eyes; blocked nose: sick to the eyeballs of everything; the eyes swollen shut; not wanting to hear or see anything more; internally an all-out war (high fever); externally/at the borders, the blooming of the typical skin eruptions (→efflorescences [Latin: 'beginning to flower']): not putting up with anything any longer; offensive struggle at one's own borders; the borders are painfully re-drawn and revised; flu-like accompanying symptoms: being in a huff, etc. (□influenza); over-sensitivity to light: wanting to spend the preparatory time prior to breakthrough of the new elements in the dark.
Handling: Opening oneself up voluntarily for the next step; opening and redefining one's borders – even if this is painful; having had enough (being sick to the eyeballs) of the old.
Resolution: Allowing something new to break through from the inside; making a development step that is due and redefining one's own limits.
Archetypal principle: Venus/ Saturn (skin) and Sun/Moon (eyes)-Mars (breakthrough into the new).

Median nerve paralysis

("Benedictine hand", monkey paw; see also Hand problems)
Physical level: Nerves (news service), hands (grasping, gripping, ability to act, expression).
Symptom level: The dropping out of the median nerve results in restriction of the ability to bend the wrist joint and the first three fingers ("Benedictine hand"), and the gradual degeneration of the ball of the thumb leads to monkey paw; the inability to close the hand prevents one from coming to grips with life, and obtaining one's fair share of it: a caricature of swearing an oath of confession; issue of honesty: the hands are always held in the open, i.e. harmless position, as when giving a harmless greeting; the oath-taking gesture reinforces the impression of putting on an unnatural display.
Handling: Accepting the compulsion to let go; releasing one's strong grip (in the area of possession).
Resolution: Taking an oath of commitment to a harmless stance towards life; being radically honest.
Archetypal principle: Mercury-Neptune.

Medication abuse

see Abuse, Drug addiction, Pharmacomania

Medication rash

(see also Allergy)
Physical level: Skin (border, contact, tenderness).
Symptom level: Offensive, unconscious rejection of the medication concerned.
Handling: "Breaking out", consciously defending oneself against this form of treatment.

Resolution: Offensive, courageous defensive reactions in the verbal area instead of in the physical (e.g. saying 'no' even if something comes from an authority such as a doctor).
Archetypal principle: Saturn-Mars.

Megalomania

(occurs with obsession, schizophrenia, alcohol abuse; frequently also as a more benign form without these underlying illnesses [narcissistic life theme])
Symptom level: Self-overestimation springing from deep feelings of inferiority and nothingness; overvaluing one's own spiritual and physical abilities beyond all measure; thinking oneself to be the greatest; hubris: mistaking oneself for God.
Handling: (In the case of →mental illness, first interpret and address the condition within the framework of the basic problem): becoming honest and recognising the feeling of being "high up on top" as simply a fear of the deep downfall; preserving the right quintessence of the feeling of greatness, but measuring it in accordance with the reality of others; recognising that, although admittedly one is very special in oneself, everyone else is also very special in their own way; seeing through the delusion and keeping one's eyes on one's overall objective: compare the myth of Icarus, who wanted to fly to the physical sun rather than becoming one with his inner sun; re-examining one's own attitude to greatness against the measure of reality, e.g. by means of Zen meditation.
Resolution: Becoming one with oneself: developing self-awareness; uniting oneself with the Greatest Being; entering into unity.
Archetypal principle: Jupiter-Sun.

Melancholy

see Depression

Melanoma

(see also Skin cancer, Cancer)
Physical level: Skin (border, contact, tenderness).
Symptom level: Disfigurement of the contact surface with the world, disgusting, black growth on one's own surface: dark, unlived shadow issues thrust themselves forward into the light of consciousness and threaten the life that one has led so far; rampant growth – without structure or order – in the area of one's own borders and norms and the area of direct contact; repulsive (unconscious) matters destroy one's (structural) integrity from the inside out and tear open the borders in a frighteningly ruthless way; disfigurement of one's own image: being compelled to honesty; typically triggered by conflicts relating to tainting and disfigurement (melanoma from Latin < Ancient Greek melas = 'black, dark' and -oma = 'disease, morbidity') or injury to one's (structural) integrity; having strayed so far off track from one's inherent development path with regard to the border and contact areas that the body must now take over the subject on its own initiative in order to help it to be let out (expressed) at all; the mental-spiritual growth in this area has been blocked for so long that it now forges a path in the body and strikes out in an aggressive and ruthless way; the cancer realises physically in the border and contact area that (turnaround) which would be spiritually necessary in the corresponding area of consciousness; the darkest shadow breaks forth out of the depths and threatens the existence that one has led until now.
Handling: Learning to define one's own limits, and on the basis of this capability, also trusting oneself to open oneself up: consciously and courageously opening up one's own borders with the world; opening

oneself up in the border and contact area to one's own outlandish ideas and bold fantasies; courageously allowing them to flourish and run wild; thinking back to early dreams of life and boundless visions and bringing these back to life with wild decisiveness; opening oneself up to the blackest shadow realm; considering all the measures mentioned under →cancer: since cancer affects the complete organism, it must also be met across-the-board.

Resolution: Discovering love for oneself and for the world that transcends all boundaries; setting oneself above standards laid down by oneself or others and living in an open and outgoing way solely in accordance with the obligations of one's own highest law; recognising the necessity to switch from the physical and thus (life-)threatening level to the challenging, but life-saving mental-spiritual level, and relying in this realm on expansive growth.

Archetypal principle: Saturn/ Venus (Haut)-Pluto/Jupiter (Krebs).

Melasma

see Pigment flecks

Memory loss

see Amnesia

Memory weakness

see Forgetfulness

Menière's disease

(see also Balance disorders, Hearing, hardness of, Deafness)
Physical level: Ears (hearing and obeying commands).
Symptom level: Build-up of the fluid in the inner ear (endolymphs); having stumbled onto unsteady ground: insecurity with regard to one's foundations in life; no longer being sure of one's

life; deceiving oneself about something with regard to the foundations of one's life; the ground is pulled away from beneath one's feet; one's steadfastness is brought into question; having climbed to dizzying heights.
Handling: Trusting oneself to the ever-changing interplay of life; voluntarily calling one's own standpoints into question; seeing through the so-called securities in life as a pretence; voluntarily giving up (material) stability; standing on one's own two feet in life and truly feeling its unceasing movements.
Resolution: Being honest in relation to oneself and one's life; bringing together one's life dream and reality; dancing along with the dance of life: elevating "everything flows" (Panta rhei) to a maxim in life.
Archetypal principle: Venus/Saturn (ears)-Neptune (dizziness).

Meningitis

Physical level: Brain (communication, logistics), cerebral membrane (protection).
Symptom level: extreme headaches: cry for help of the embattled central control headquarters; neck stiffness (opisthotonus): caricature of self-righteous rectitude, over-the-top hard-headedness; (in newborns): war against protective feminine forces; battle against the forces of the primordial mother; Ego problem ("thick skull"), resistance to the new incarnation, decision between this world and returning to the (Great) Mother; (in adults): repressed aggression; lack of willingness to contribute consciously to the struggle for life/to detach oneself from the primordial mother; sleeping one's life away, having lost the appetite for life; too little willingness to conquer one's own living environment; rigid bearing in the central control headquarters (stiff neck); battle of the polarities, imbalance between the

feminine-watery and masculine-fiery elements, respectively between dark maternal and light spiritual forces.
Handling: Fighting for one's own life; finding one's centre; connection of sensory thought with intellect; coming to grips with what is pressing down on one; risking war on the highest level; developing self-awareness and pride; leaving the mother's womb and re-solving its demands on a higher level.
Resolution: Re-birth, confrontation between protective feminine and for-ward-striving masculine forces.
Archetypal principle: Mercury/ Moon-Mars.

Meningoencephalitis

see Meningitis, Cerebral inflammation

Meniscus injury

(see also Sport accident, Accident)
Physical level: Joints (mobility, artic-ulation), knee (humility).
Symptom level: Squashing the Moon-shaped, cartilaginous disc in the knee: the buffer between the thigh (family tradition) and lower leg (one's own way) is ground down, torn or "flattened" by being overloaded; the shock-absorber (cf. the intervertebral discs of the spinal column) is used up; hubris: forcing a movement which demands too much of the knee, for which it is not designed; not having a grip on a situation in one's conscious-ness; stretching the buffer in one's knee to the limit; often sport injuries, in which one hasn't got a good mental grasp of the situation and thus forces the body into some inappropriate form of action; compensation for inner inflexibility through excessive external movements; Meniscus tear: the knee joint is incorrectly strained and over-stretched in its function as a hinge joint; Pinched/trapped meniscus: the knee joint is overloaded and the buff-ering disc is first pressed upon and then eventually squashed flat.

Handling: Risking more on the level of verbal articulation and performing more offensive moves intellectu-ally; pursuing new, unconventional paths on the level of consciousness; recognising and accepting one's own physical limits; making more courageous leaps in consciousness instead of doing (performance) sport; challenging and putting the connec-tion between tradition and one's own aspirations in life to the test without putting oneself too much out of joint; courageously and offensively com-mitting oneself to impending trials between the past and present which stretch one to the limit, all the while accepting the risk that the pressure might increase enormously; con-sciously putting oneself under pres-sure in the area of humility, and thus sparing the knee; learning about the issues related to the knee joint: humil-ity and submission; being upstanding and straightforwardly admitting which aspects of performance are really necessary.
Resolution: Courageously and offen-sively setting foot in new spiritual ter-ritory; testing the connection between old and young in one's own family for its ability to bear heavy loads and resolving the subject of humility with-out losing sight of one's own path of individuation.
Archetypal principle: Mercury/ Saturn (meniscus, knee joint); Mars (injury).

Menopause, male

(Climacterium virile; see also Depression)
Physical level: Genitalia (sexuality, polarity, reproduction), glands/hor-mones (control, information).
Symptom level: Out-of-the-ordinary aspects in outward behaviour that attract attention: suddenly dressing in the fashions of the young, driving an open-top sports cabriolet, having a

young girlfriend; the misunderstanding: instead of becoming like a child again on the mental-spiritual level, the attempt is made to do so on the social level; the result: childish behaviour. Turning into a "softie"/becoming effeminate: facial features soften/become more feminine, development of breasts; the misunderstanding: instead of realising the opposite feminine pole - the anima - in consciousness, the attempt is made to do so on the physical level; the result: external softening/effeminacy; prostate swelling; problems with passing water: the proud jet stream – the attribute that streams out the masculine charisma – becomes a pathetic trickle, and its owner is forced to remain on the toilet in the continual attempt to let go; a kink in performance: marks the kink in the path of life, the time of change, where turning around and turning back (inside oneself) should be on the agenda; depression to the point of suicidal tendencies; the misunderstanding: the now forthcoming task of concerning oneself with (dis)solution (letting go) and resolution (salvation), with dying as the goal of living, is transferred from the mental-spiritual level to the banal physical level.

Handling: Making oneself aware of the archetypal task of "becoming as a child" on the mental-spiritual level; bringing the anima - the feminine spiritual pole in every man - to life; practising letting go (e.g. in one's profession, sport, family); recognising the moment of the turnaround and using it to turn back (within); maturing from the role of father into that of the Grand Father; coming to terms with death.

Resolution: Making the re-connection in the sense of re-ligio(n) (from Latin religāre 'to bind, tie again') and consciously slotting oneself into the life pattern of the mandala.

Archetypal principle: Sun/ Mars-Uranus/Saturn.

Menopause, premature

(Climax praecox, undergoing the change as early as the third or early fourth decade of life)

Physical level: Genitalia (sexuality, polarity, reproduction), glands/hormones (control, information).

Symptom level: Regulatory disorders between the hypophysis and hypothalamus; being burnt-out, having had enough; usually affects intelligent, totally exhausted superwomen, who are so drained that "nothing works any more"; living in overdrive, too much activity, no rhythm; too much life energy is used up in too short a time; coming too quickly to the point of (the) change and turnaround, without wanting to believe this is true; overburdened women who often experienced periods that were far too heavy; premature physical maturity due to a lack of spiritual maturity; inwardly remaining the young girl; direct transition from young girl to old woman.

Handling: Adjusting oneself to the turnaround; celebrating the homecoming, the internalisation; learning that intensity flows not from quantity, but from quality (not lots of different adventures, but instead deep experience).

Resolution: Maturing internally for the change.

Archetypal principle: Moon-Uranus.

Menstruation, absent

(amenorrhea)

Physical level: Ovaries (fertility), womb (fertility, safety and security).

Symptom level: Rejection of womanhood through menstruation not setting in (primary amenorrhea), e.g. in the case of →anorexia or missing menstruation (secondary amenorrhea) as a result of contraceptive pills, stress, sorrow, incorrect diet or sensory overload; regression to the pre-sexual time, in which everything was less polar and therefore less (wo)/menacing and sex-based; not living in rhythm with one's own (sexual) determination; retaining one's life blood for oneself (e.g. in a nutritional crisis); thinking only of oneself, giving up one's openness to foreign (fertilising) influences; lack of willingness for self-sacrifice and giving of oneself; missing out on the chance for monthly cleansing and regeneration.

Handling: Conscious regression to the phases that go before becoming a woman (childhood, youth); exercises and rituals in order to resolve the tasks of the earlier phases: basic trust in the intrauterine period, childishness in childhood, learning in primary school, playing adolescent games, ecstasy exercises (sexuality, music, sport, dancing).

Resolution: Resolving being a child in order to be able to break loose from it; preparation for the first period and being a woman; corresponding (collective) rituals of transformation.

Archetypal principle: Moon-Saturn.

Menstruation, irregular

Physical level: Genitalia (sexuality, polarity, reproduction).

Symptom level: Not yet having arrived at a stable life rhythm as a woman: the little girl continues in her search (late puberty) or the mature woman cannot yet detach herself completely (early menopause); irregular cycle due to fear of fertility and sexuality.

Handling: Accepting polarity, consciously coming to terms with one's own rhythm and the great rhythm of "death and rebirth", life and death; learning to accept "regulations" that are essential to life. Resolution: Finding one's own rhythm as a woman.

Archetypal principle: Moon-Uranus.

Menstruation, painful

(dysmenorrhoea)

Physical level: Womb (fertility, safety and security).

Symptom level: Painful experience of being a woman; not being reconciled with one's own femininity; frequently transfer of the problem from the mother to the daughter: the subject is acted out in the child (spiritual inheritance); sexual problems: lack of ability to give oneself completely; painful registration of the period in the case of the unfulfilled desire to have a child; opportunity to flee; instrument of power; experience of being torn between external demands and inner needs.

Handling: Accepting one's own femininity; accepting the opportunities associated with being a woman; making a conscious (blood) sacrifice for one's own feminine task; learning to understand menstruation as a rest and recovery period and a cleansing ritual; giving loving care to one's body.

Resolution: Reconciliation with one's own sexual role and its corresponding life rhythms; accepting one's task in life; letting go and giving in completely to one's own feminine strength.

Archetypal principle: Moon-Mars.

Menstruation, too heavy

(hypermenorrhoea)

Physical level: Genitalia (sexuality, polarity, reproduction).

Symptom level: Heavy menstrual bleeding on the basis of a →hormonal imbalance or in the case of a →myoma which lasts up to seven days and results in →anaemia; the build-up and breakdown of an inadequate endometrium costs a great deal of life force (blood): expenditure with simultaneous saving of feminine energy and the "love hormone" oestrogen; bleeding oneself dry; not being in the female rhythm; being hard on oneself; the helper in need of help.

Handling: Putting one's energy into one's own inherent feminine interests; allowing one's passion and lifeblood to flow into one's own feminine task; doing away with things and creating order in order to shed what is outlived and old.

Resolution: Allowing strength and energy to flow abundantly; giving oneself up to one's own life energy and entrusting oneself to it; swimming along in the flow of life.

Archetypal principle: Moon-Pluto/ Jupiter.

Menstruation, too light

(hypomenorrhoea)

Physical level: Genitalia (sexuality, polarity, reproduction).

Symptom level: The feminine fertility pole demands little energy; becomes significant as an illness only in the case of an unfulfilled desire to have a child; sign of infertility, the fertilised egg is not provided with an adequate nest.

Handling: Becoming clear in oneself what form of fertility should be placed in the foreground; questioning one's desire for a child, creating a relationship and professional situation in which the hormones are able to come into flow and physical fertility makes sense.

Resolution: Following the mature female rhythm of life; taking time for the Archetypal Moon aspect in life.

Archetypal principle: Moon-Saturn.

Mental illness

(obsolete designation for a "pathological disorder of the psychic function";

see also Psychosis, Schizophrenia, Depression, Spiritual crisis)

Symptom level: Resistance to the dark side; collective fear of the shadow, heightened to the point of paranoia and manic delusions; subjects originally belonging to life are split off and the corresponding energies banished.

Handling: Taking the shadow aspects and forms for real and granting them importance, taking one's own dark sides seriously and paying them respect; acknowledging them instead of shoving them away.

Resolution: Shadow integration, individuation.

Archetypal principle: Pluto/ Neptune.

Mercury poisoning

see Amalgam poisoning, Heavy metal poisoning

Messies syndrome

(see also Addictions)

Physical level: Consciousness.

Symptom level: The home as a hoard of collected things, even as the name of the disorder suggests – of rubbish and mess; restriction of one's own living space; piling up rubbish in the outer world as an expression of the inner situation; danger of being suffocated by unprocessed things; not being able to deal completely with the outer world, its tasks and what it has to offer.

Handling: Making and preserving many inner experiences, then retaining what is important; learning to consciously take what one needs; learning to distinguish between what is important and unimportant; making something out of one's possibilities; contributing to creating a world of abundance; building up reserves (spiritual, intellectual, and as far as material reserves are concerned, building these up more with regard to

one's bank account), creating one's own world out of what is safe, secure and familiar.
Resolution: Retaining the essential; living with an attitude of (inner) plenty; learning to enjoy abundance.
Archetypal principle: Mercury/ Jupiter.

Meteorism

see Flatulence

Metrorrhagia

see Intermenstrual bleeding

Middle ear inflammation

(otitis media)
Physical level: Ears (hearing and obeying commands).
Symptom level: Aggressive conflict at the mucous membrane of the middle ear; suddenly-occurring ear pains: cry for help from the hearing organ; attacks of the shivers, fever: general mobilisation of the immune defence system; hardness of hearing: not wanting to hear/obey commands (the main period for middle ear inflammations is that phase of childhood in which it is a matter of exactly this issue); perforation of the eardrum with outflow of pus: discharge of the excess pressure from the middle ear cavity.
Handling: (for jointly-affected parents, whose problems are often reflected by the children): aggressive, offensive conflicts regarding the issue of hearing-listening carefully-obeying commands; opening up and tapping into the issue in all its possibilities: lending someone one's ear or turning a deaf ear; learning to hear outwardly and to listen carefully inwardly; learning to pay attention to others and one's own inner voice; allowing oneself to be shaken up thoroughly,

and throwing all of one's energies into the struggle over obedience; learning to sensibly define one's limits (e.g. distinct from parents and educators); supporting the outer shutting of one's ears in favour of turning inwards; promoting breakthroughs into new niches of consciousness.
Resolution: Listening closely to hear inner and outer voices and obeying their commands.
Archetypal principle: Saturn-Mars.

Midlife crisis

see Climacteric complaints, Menopause, male

Migraine

(hemicrania [headaches on one side of the head]; see also Headaches)
Physical level: Head (capital city of the body).
Symptom level: Headaches on one side of the head: one side of reality is hurting and is crying out painfully for help; one-sidedness in thinking and feeling; having fallen into a vicious circle through fixation on one-sided positions: one's distress (from Latin 'to pull in opposing directions') shows the dividedness in one's head and consciousness; (from a psychoanalytical perspective), reaction to narcissistic mortification (Freud: narzisstische Kränkung) (of the woman), i.e. the wounding of feminine self-esteem; forcing others to make allowance for one; getting what one would otherwise not receive; cold hands (as a sign of being communicatively withdrawn and shut off), which when warmed frequently trigger the migraine attack: migraine as the comeuppance for having shut oneself off for too long and as a method for discharging pent-up tension; conflict between instinctual drives and rational thought, thought tries to take the place of action; blocking erotic impulses in one's

head; often the unconscious attempt to live out sexuality in one's head, the migraine attack is similar in sequence to an orgasm: the head acts the part of the lower body; orgasm in one's head; the light apparitions preceding it can, according to Oliver Sacks, only be recognised as a higher, spiritual light if the lower light of sexuality is resolved (compare the migraine visions of Hildegard von Bingen).

Handling: Reconciling oneself with sexuality in one's head and then returning it to its place below; getting to know and love one's own depths; conquering the sexual underworld; bringing together instinctual and rational thought functions: combining thought and action; putting what has gone to one's head back in its place; learning to say 'no' honestly and foregoing using a migraine as an excuse; learning to set one's limits with people close to one; recognising one's own needs and forcefully asserting one's demands on oneself and others before the migraine takes over this task; creating a harmonious balance between commitment to service and the needs of the Ego.

Resolution: Bringing together the right (feeling) and the left (thought) hemispheres of the brain; transforming the one-sidedness (feeling of only being half a person) into a unified whole (two halves form an orb, a well-rounded affair): accepting the two sides of one's human existence (light and shadow); finding the light in the dark (Hildegard von Bingen); reconciliation with one's own sexuality and its place in the body on the lower level.

Archetypal principle: Mars-Venus-Uranus.

Milk accumulation

(galactostasis)

Physical level: The female breast (motherliness, nourishment, safety and security, sensuality, desire).

Symptom level: Stoppage of the milk flow due to inadequate emptying or obstruction of the flow: the breast swells up dangerously, the child no longer receives nourishment; unconscious inhibition against allowing the stream of nourishment to flow; not being able to give from one's heart; wanting (to give) too much, and with the cramping, not being able to give or unconsciously not even wanting to give (for example, because one has too little oneself – in the figurative sense).

Handling: Going within oneself in order to reflect on one's own motivation towards nursing and nourishing; sensing whether I myself even actually have enough in order to be able to give freely; taking hot showers can allow the milk to flow again.

Resolution: perhaps consciously standing behind one's inability to nurse or providing for oneself to a sufficient extent that giving becomes possible again and comes from the heart.

Archetypal principle: Moon-Saturn.

Milk, intolerance

(a distinction should be made between the intolerance of 1. Milk sugar (lactose intolerance), 2. Milk protein, 3. Breast milk; see also Digestive complaints, Allergy)

Physical level: Small intestine (analysis, assimilation).

Symptom level: Cow's milk is actually not a suitable drink for humans; in terms of composition, it has little in common with human breast milk; children should ideally be nursed until they can switch to other forms of nourishment, and no longer need the breast milk substitute (Comparative composition: Carbohydrates: human milk 7 %, cow milk 4.8%; Fat: human milk 4%, cow milk 3.5-4%; Protein: human milk 1.5%, cow milk 3.5 %; Trace elements: human milk 0.3 %, cow milk 0.7 %). 1. Half of the adult population (2. billion people) and 900 million children and young people cannot produce any lactase for the metabolism of lactose since dairy farming has only been practised for the last 12,000 years (within the overall framework of evolution, the organism needs a great deal of time to adapt to new conditions). 2. Denial of life: Rejection of the basic building blocks of life = proteins (Greek protos = 'first, most important'), especially casein and whey protein (albumins and globulins), in the milk. 3. Rejection of the mother/the maternal principle and its gifts.

Handling/Resolution: 1. Making oneself aware of the situation and avoiding milk; 2. Treating the →allergy; 3. (For jointly-affected mothers, whose problems are often reflected by the child): reconciliation with one's own mother (role); becoming aware of other levels where one's own gifts are rejected; dealing with the issue of rejection.

Archetypal principle: Moon-Saturn.

Mineral loss

see Demineralisation

Miscarriage

(spontaneous abortion/abortion, premature termination of pregnancy, weight of the foetus below 500g; see also Stillbirth [weight of the foetus at least 500 g])

Physical level: Womb (fertility, safety and security).

Symptom level: Flight of the fruit (the unborn): genetic defect as an expression of an inherited affliction; the task appears unresolvable or too difficult; termination of a short development; flight of the mother from a physical, spiritual or social situation that is demanding too much of her: pushing away an uninvited guest; unconscious abortion; rising inflammations as an expression of conflicts rising up from below; stress, overwork as a sign of a lack of involvement.

Handling: (For the mother): learning, once decisions (conceived at higher levels) have been made, to stick to them, be receptive to them and to uphold them; examining one's desire for a child with regard to unacknowledged rejection at a deeper level; nest-building exercises in the physical and spiritual respect.

Resolution: Giving reconciliation with the theme of life as a gift and receiving it as a gift as well; accepting the will superior to one's own wishes and will.

Archetypal principle: Moon-Uranus, Pluto.

Mitral insufficiency

(see also Heart valve insufficiency, Heart defect)

Physical level: Heart (seat of the soul, love, feelings, energy centre), heart valves (valves of the life and energy flow).

Symptom level: Both constriction and leakage at the same time; Sisyphus task in the engine of the life flow: the forward surging of the life flow is bought at the cost of significant steps backwards; tendency towards regression; problems with retreating; lack of supportive backing in life; not being able to keep one's trap shut, finding it difficult to say 'no'.

Handling: Intentionally going forward but also slipping back in life: reacting to every step forward with appropriate retrospection; consciously taking back one's life energy; learning to withdraw into one's shell; conscious regression; developing openness for one's own regressive steps.

Resolution: Consciously taking on the Sisyphus situation as a task in life; reconciling oneself to the fact that life is taken back again and again.

Archetypal principle: Sun-Saturn.

Mitral stenosis

Physical level: Heart (seat of the soul, love, feelings, energy centre).
Symptom level: Resistance in one's heart; central obstacle in the centre of one's own life which devours a large part of one's vitality; major unacknowledged anxiety experience; being without additional reserves; life has become pale and colourless; slinging one's passion and lifeblood at one's environment; not receiving enough mental-spiritual energy (nourishment).
Handling: Learning to take on restrictions; accepting doing without as a necessity; acknowledging narrow limits; accepting spiritual powerlessness (blacking out); seeing through demonstrations of power and recognising them as just "feign"ting spells (bouts of deception).
Resolution: Humility in the face of obstacles that one can do nothing about; working from the opposite pole: integrating expansiveness and the free flow of energies into life.
Archetypal principle: Sun-Saturn.

Mola hydatiformis

see Hydatiform mole

Monkey paw

see Hand problems

Monocular vision

see Squinting

Mononucleosis

(Pfeiffer's glandular fever)
Physical level: Lymph nodes (police stations), liver (life, evaluation, reconnection), spleen (filter of the life force, vitality store).
Symptom level: Generalised conflict (usually in the period following the onset of sexual maturity) which can spread to all possible areas of the immune defence system; period in which individuation begins, accompanied its associated conflicts; swellings in the domain of the entire lymph system, and especially the lymph nodes, liver and spleen (particularly affects young people and older children): emphasis of the local police stations, as well as the issues related to the liver, such as philosophy and meaning of life, evaluation and finding one's own correct measure, as well as the issues related to the spleen, such as filtering, storage and production of the life energy; fever; general mobilisation of the complete immune defence system against the enemies (mononucleosis viruses); frequently associated with the fear of binding oneself emotionally (is also often called the "kissing disease").
Handling: Taking on the struggle and the confrontation with external challenges (for example, with the opposite sex): conflict at the local level and comprehensive mobilisation of the complete system; grappling with questions related to the meaning of life, value judgements and the problem of finding the right measure; practising confrontation and struggle; learning to control the flow of the life energy; struggling to achieve independence; letting out one's aggression in the form of fever.
Resolution: Waging inner struggles with complete commitment; coming to terms with central subjects of life such as relationships; courageously tackling individuation.
Archetypal principle: Mars-Jupiter.

Morbus Basedow

see Basedow's disease

Morbus Bechterew

see Bechterew's disease

Morbus Boeck

see Sarcoidosis

Morbus Cushing

see Cushing's syndrome

Morbus Menière

see Menière's disease

Morbus Scheuermann

see Scheuermann's disease

Mouches volantes

see Eye floaters

Mouth, bad taste in

Physical level: Mouth (absorption, expression, maturity - being able to speak for oneself), tongue (expression, speech, weapon).

Symptom level: "Having swallowed a bitter pill", "something is not to one's taste", something has left a sour taste in one's mouth; always feigning good taste, continually bowing to foreign tastes.

Handling: Recognising for oneself the true flavour of the things which one has to swallow; learning to live with one's own "bad" taste and undertaking to do something in the direction of developing better taste; learning to stand up for one's own taste even if this is judged by others as bad.

Resolution: Certainty in one's tastes.

Archetypal principle: Venus/Jupiter-Saturn.

Mouth, cracking at the corners

see Cracked skin

Mouth, dryness of

Physical level: Mouth (absorption, expression, maturity - being able to speak for oneself).

Symptom level: Lack of the feminine-spiritual element: no oil in the works; an excess of the archetypally masculine aspects: talking too much (running off at the mouth); preparation for battle instead of commitment to a subject; fear (e.g. before giving a speech); keeping one's lips sealed; reluctance, readiness to flee ("flight or fight?"); longing for the opposite feminine pole; thirst, desire to moisten one's lips.

Handling: Recognising the predominance of the masculine-combative quality and re-examining one's own motivation; making oneself aware of one's own situation of reluctance or danger: What is endangered?; recognising the restrictiveness and venturing into it completely until it is transformed into expansiveness.

Resolution: Integrating more of the feminine-spiritual element: approaching matters with feeling; tuning into the situation and being in synch with it.

Archetypal principle: Moon-Saturn.

Mouth of the uterus cancer

(see also Carcinoma in situ as a preliminary stage of this form of cancer, and Cancer)

Physical level: Mouth of the uterus (lower mouth), mucous membranes (inner boundary, barrier), womb (fertility, safety and security).

Symptom level: Border combat; too many assaults have been allowed; inability to protect oneself adequately against attacks and assaults.

Handling: Offensively dealing with issues related to sexual self-determination; recognising one's own injury and chronic over-stimulation in

this area; learning to protect oneself against assaults and attacks from foreign interests on one's own femininity; considering all the measures mentioned under →cancer: since cancer is a disease pattern affecting the whole organism, it must also be met across-the-board; seeing through what traditionally-accepted medicine proposes as "prevention", i.e. using better prophylaxis measures than vaccination and smears: obliging the partner to take appropriate hygiene measures; the best and only genuine prophylaxis: addressing the conflict issues in a mental-spiritual way.
Resolution: safeguarding one's own interests with regard to conflicts in the intimate area; recognising the necessity to switch from the physical and thus (life-) threatening level to the challenging, but life-saving mental-spiritual level, and relying in this realm on expansive growth; discovering love that transcends all boundaries, setting oneself above external rule and standards laid down by oneself or others, and living and expressing oneself solely in accordance with the obligations of one's own highest law.
Archetypal principle: **Moon-Pluto.**

Mucoviscidosis

(congenital metabolic disease with thickening of the secretion of the mucous-producing glands of the lungs, pancreas and intestines)
Physical level: Metabolism (dynamic equilibrium), lungs (contact, communication, freedom), intestines (processing of material impressions), pancreas (aggressive analysis, sweet enjoyment).
Symptom level: Blockages (slimy mucous congestion and constipation); changes in organ structure (fibroses) due to the thick and sticky secretions: learning to adjust oneself to conditions that challenge one to have it out;

obstructive "stick-to-it-iveness" in the area of the slimy, feminine mucous element; slimy mucous congestion of the lungs: overinflation and disturbance of the gas exchange (→pulmonary emphysema): communications problem; the lung problem results in secondary strain on the heart (→cor pulmonale); strain on the liver (→cirrhosis of the liver): problems with finding a sense of meaning; frequent infections (and allergies) due to the blocked glandular outlets.
Handling: Concerning oneself intensively with the exchange in the lungs, making use of physiotherapy and psychotherapy; in physical terms: percussion, aspiration and breathing exercises, in spiritual terms: communications and contact exercises; actively supporting the digestion and processing (of the intestines); allowing oneself an enormous amount of time in the feminine realm of slimy mucous and orientating life towards it on all levels; actively and consciously striving to find a sense of meaning in life; becoming aware of one's inner phlegmaticness; recognising and processing slow-moving and sticky elements in one's own being.
Resolution: Coming into contact and exchange with the surrounding world despite the conditions which make things heavier going and continually pushing one's absorption and processing of the world further forward.
Archetypal principle:
Mercury-Moon/Saturn.

Multiple sclerosis

(see also Paralysis, Balance disorders, Seeing double, Urinary bladder inflammation, Auto-aggressive/Auto-immune diseases)
Physical level: Myelin sheaths of the nerves (news service).
Symptom level: Literally translated: multiple areas of hardening (in the communications area); withdrawing

oneself with the greatest possible harshness, enormous self-discipline with regard to control and suppression; turning away from one's own strengths and capabilities; putting the brakes on (slowing oneself down) and finally coming to a complete stop (paralysis); aggression directed against oneself: "Me against myself"; rigid stance towards oneself, but also towards others and the surrounding world; lack of consideration of one's own needs: being hard on oneself as judge and jury; with the further progression of the disease pattern, also eventually becoming inconsiderate towards one's environment; great fear of loss of control, that things could run off the rails and that one may not be able to keep the reigns in one's hands; tendency to exertion of control and influence: desire to plan everything in advance, with the simultaneous lack of adequate challenges; iron principles and moral attitudes, rigid standpoints; perfectionism; tendency to put the blame on oneself; tendency to hubris (being overbearing); wanting to force the world into shape (and into submission) according to one's own, often rigid notions; taking a path which is usually not one's own and is therefore heavygoing; fulfilling the needs of others before they even express them and overlooking one's own; subordinating one's own dream of life to that of the often authoritarian father; in the case of paralysis of the legs: being bound by compulsions; no longer knowing whether one is coming or going; no longer being able to move forwards or get away, but also no longer being able to keep up; in the case of paralysis of the arms: no longer being able to fight back, not being able to get a grip on things; blockage of the activity on the nerve level; vision problems: smouldering conflict over sight and insight; no longer being able /willing to look closely at things; double vision: measuring with double standards; →balance disorders, "feign"ting spells (dizziness): standing on unsteady ground; →fatigue: wanting to switch off, refusal to take part in life; →urinary bladder inflammations: conflicts with letting go, holding back of one's own spiritual flood; no longer being able / willing to feel; rejection of the female pole; the disease pattern forces regression into childish spheres of experience: those affected do not need to do anything more, but are simply pushed (in a wheelchair); everything has to be taken off them; they learn what they least wanted and were least able to bear: being dependent and at the mercy of others; in the end, everything has to be taken off them, which is almost the equivalent of a regression to the situation of being fully cared for in the womb.

Handling: Recognising one's hardness towards oneself and others and transforming it into consistency; searching for traces of hardness, obstinacy, rigidity, doggedness in one's own life; seeing through the firmness of moral standpoints as rigidified stiffness; recognising perfection as belonging to God: developing openness to one's own faults; recognising one's own way as the most heavygoing, but also the only rewarding way; struggling to achieve one's own line, one's own uprightness (towards oneself); turning one's gaze from outside to inside: introspection and insight; recognising and acknowledging both sides of polarity as having equal rights; learning to experience and live with the flowing movement of reality: "Panta rhei" ('everything flows'); granting oneself rest: outer and inner; shaking off the harness altogether and letting loose once and for all instead of continually building up and letting go of tension by hitching and unhitching it; learning to let go in an open(ly offensive) way; reconciling oneself with the feminine aspect of the soul and its feelings and sensibilities; giving way and letting things happen, emphasising the feminine pole; accepting one's own painful weakness, allowing the river (of tears) to flow.

Resolution: Giving up perfectionism; surrendering oneself in the positive sense (to one's fate): accepting rhythmic processes in one's own up and down (swings) and one's own swimming (in the sea of life); subordinating oneself to the law (Saturn) of life: "Thy will be done" instead of exerting control over everything and everybody; return to contemplation of the inherent mental-spiritual homeland of mankind, re-ligio[n] (from Latin religāre 'to bind, tie again').

Archetypal principle: Mercury/Moon-Neptune-Saturn.

Mumps

(parotitis epidemica; see also Childhood diseases)

Physical level: Parotid gland (ears = hearing and obeying commands).

Symptom level: Inflammatory conflicts and swellings of the parotid glands (hamster cheeks): conflicts over the production of the archetypally feminine lubricating fluid (saliva); spreading to other fluid-producing glands is also possible, e.g. also to the pancreatic gland (the problems spread to one's digestion); in adult males, the testicles are also affected in 25% of cases (spreading of the conflict to the issues of masculinity, fertility), in 30% of cases the cerebral membranes are affected (extension of the conflict to the central control headquarters); as in other childhood diseases, this is an infection, in other words, a conflict through which the child is prompted to leaps in maturity and development (the tension/uncertainty before the next step); in the specific case of mumps, it is – conspicuously - a matter of portraying

something; puffing up one's cheeks or being overblown and cheeky: an attempt to develop one's own, more imposing personality, which has slid down into the body.

Handling: (for parents and children): openly staring a growth step in the (child's) personality in the face; for the child, it is a matter of becoming more imposing; for the parents, of accepting the new position of the child with good will, although it initially makes a somewhat overblown impression; concerning oneself with the oil in the gearbox; conflict over the production of the feminine lubricating and digestive fluids; accepting the extension of the conflict to the issues of processing and digestion of material impressions (intestines) and also immaterial impressions (brain); if necessary, also including the field of masculinity and fertility in the critical conflict; generally being open in the face of new developments; developing willingness to deal with conflicts and consciously making allowance for them since conflicts are indispensable for growth.

Resolution: Offensively and combatively breaking with a piece of one's own experience of being a child; adjusting oneself to conflicts with the feminine pole, which will persist until a further element of breaking loose (free) from the motherly world is achieved; undertaking courageous and conscious steps (also through conflicts and pains) into new territory; taking an open(ly offensive) stance with regard to one's own inner steps forward.

Archetypal principle: Moon-Mars.

Muscle ache

Physical level: Musculature (motor, strength) of the motoric system.

Symptom level: Painful symptoms of fatigue, and in extreme cases, even small muscle fibre tears in the motoric domain, caused by the accumulation of metabolic waste residues: painful signs of demanding too much of a motoric area which was under-trained for the given task; pushing things too far; limits established by habit have been overstepped (too recklessly and at the expense of the body).

Handling: Paying attention to the gap between one's expectations and one's own (cap)abilities; remaining active in order to stimulate the circulation and promote the removal of the waste residues: gentle(!) further training; taking a positive approach to answering the help calls that the muscle tissue is sending for more attention: attention for muscles means movement: passive through massages, hot baths and hot-water bottles; active through new challenges such as sport.

Resolution: Remaining active on the mental-spiritual-muscular level.

Archetypal principle: ars.

Muscle hardening

see Myogelosis

Muscle/joint tension

(see also Cramps)

Physical level: Musculature (motor, strength), joints (mobility, articulation).

Symptom level: Over-stretching of the muscles and joints = tension over and beyond normal limits (dystonia): pushing rigorous effort too far: being too rigorous with oneself; rigidity shows the spiritual corset that one is living within.

Handling/Resolution: Expending one's efforts at the right place and the right time; understanding the interplay of polarity in the build-up and release of tension and recognising the inter-connection of both poles.

Archetypal principle: Mars-Saturn/ Uranus.

Muscle pains

see Fibromyalgia, Muscle rheumatism, Amalgam poisoning

Muscle rheumatism

(soft tissue rheumatism; see also Rheumatism)

Physical level: Musculature (motor, strength).

Symptom level: Blockage of the activities in the motoric domain: e.g. feeling "rusted up" in the morning; inhibition of the expression of aggression towards the world; being forced to rest in order to put an end to compensating for inner rigidity and obstinacy with over-activity; auto-aggression gets stuck in the muscles as inflammation: not owning up to one's own aggressions; →feelings of guilt if hostile impulses cannot be compensated for by sacrifice and service; build-up of the residues from undigested problems.

Handling: Voluntarily restricting oneself in the motoric area; learning to draw back more outwardly and become more courageous inwardly; encouraging the confrontation with oneself (auto-aggression) and with one's own flexibility; questioning altruism and submissiveness; fasting: getting back to the essence; re-digesting and resolving undigested problems (breaking down waste residues).

Resolution: Giving things (oneself) a rest; reflecting on one's own inner life; bringing egoism, inflexibility, inability to adapt, bossiness, and aggression out of the shadow area.

Archetypal principle: Mars-Saturn.

Muscle slackening

see Atonia

Muscle tear

(muscle rupture; see also Accident, Work accident/Domestic accident, Sport accident, Traffic accident)
Physical level: Musculature (motor, strength) of the motoric system.
Symptom level: Over-stretching of the muscle leads to it tearing: interruption of one's mobility; over-the-top demands on one's mobility burst the limits of one's actual abilities in a painful way; tearing oneself to pieces for one's ambition, for a matter/situation or also for a person.
Handling: Voluntarily stretching oneself more in consciousness; taking the load off the body; grasping things in consciousness; stretching inwardly and winding up as much momentum for one's own actions as one's own capacity to bounce back will allow; straining hard beyond all measure in order to make the impossible possible after all, but doing this in consciousness instead; preferring to pause and reflect before one reaches the end of one's tether.
Resolution: Extending and stirring oneself up intellectually; facing up to things in the right way; consciously guiding and directing the body; resolving trials that stretch things to the limits on the mental-spiritual level.
Archetypal principle: Mars-Uranus.

Muscle twitching

(Tics; see also Tourette's syndrome, Twitching of the limbs, Restless legs)
Physical level: The area of the skeletal musculature (motor, sources of strength).
Symptom level: Uncontrolled discharges of pent-up, held back energies, which each have meaning in their own way: Making faces and grimaces: impulses of mocking and ridiculing; Winking: giving signs, seeking allies; Adjusting one's glasses: wrestling to find the right view; Scratching oneself: expressing one's own consternation, something has gotten "under one's skin" and one is "itching" to do something about it; Clearing one's throat: finally also wanting to say something (→compulsive coughing).
Handling: using one's sources of power in passing; allowing the available energy to flow unnoticed into life; freeing oneself, overcoming stagnation and standstill with energy.
Resolution: Allowing a fireworks display of motion to spark throughout the body, e.g. by means of ecstatic free dancing.
Archetypal principle: Mars-Uranus.

Muscular atrophy

(see also Atrophy)
Physical level: Possible everywhere in the area of the musculature (motor, strength).
Symptom level: Unused muscles begin to waste away (atrophy due to inactivity after being in plaster or as a result of a largely sedentary lifestyle); degenerative muscular atrophy due to disorders of the stimulating motoric nerves; no longer being in full possession of one's powers, dependency due to lack of strength; momentum for motion dwindles, is given up (not uncommonly in order to "put the squeeze" on others for the purpose of getting help from them); depending on the localisation and function of the muscle concerned, different underlying problems are involved.
Handling: Taking the load off the affected area in the figurative sense; ensuring the support of others in a conscious way.
Resolution: Letting oneself and one's own demands shrink back more.
Archetypal principle: Mars-Neptune.

Muscular strain

(see also Accident, Work accident/
Domestic accident, Sport accident,
Traffic accident)
Physical level: Joints (mobility,
articulation), musculature (motor,
strength).
Symptom level: Overdoing something, going too far, over-stretching
something; wanting to force something beyond its physical limits;
tensing the nerves to breaking point:
"fraying one's nerves".
Handling/Resolution: Broadening
and stretching oneself in the mental-spiritual sense in order not to
overload the body; not over-stretching
one's overall span; voluntarily putting
spiritual flexibility to good use based
on one's own initiative.
Archetypal principle:
Mars-Jupiter-Uranus.

Mutism

see Autism

Myasthenia

(fatigue paralysis)
Physical level: Transverse musculature (motor, strength) of the motoric
system.
Symptom level: Rapid fatigue of the
broad muscle strength to the point of
complete fatigue paralysis: no longer
being able/willing to do anything;
speech paralysis: no longer being
able to let anything out (express oneself); swallowing paralysis: no longer
being able to get anything down and
even to the point of fatal respiratory
paralysis: shutting down of contact
with polarity.
Handling: Allowing oneself peace
and serenity in the mental-spiritual
area; consciously entering into
silence (cf. various orders such as
the Carmelites); foregoing all assimilation, renouncing material possessions; adapting oneself to overcoming

the polarity which is manifested in the
inhaling and exhaling of breathing.
Resolution: Consciously attuning
oneself to life in the world beyond,
where communication takes place
without words, nothing more has
to be assimilated, movements take
place without muscle power and the
laws of polarity have been revoked.
Archetypal principle: Mars-Neptune.

Myasthenia gravis

(see also Muscular atrophy)
Physical level: Musculature (motor,
strength), eyelids (curtains of the
soul).
Symptom level: Connection with the
thymus gland, which has normally
receded in adults, but in this case,
remains active longer or starts to
grow again: being stuck in the childhood phase, desire for mothering;
not wanting to mature and become
independent; loss of independence
in the concrete sense, often accompanied by attempts at compensation:
particularly emphasising being grown
up although without corresponding
maturing of the emotional character
traits (e.g. the man always looks
for his mother in his wife or marries
child-like women who are rejected as
soon as they become independent);
inclined to be easily offended like a
child, snapping suddenly and going
off in a huff if one is not the focus of
attention; tendency to move oneself
into the focus of attention out of
weakness; propensity for stomach
problems: one's centre causes one
pain; drooping eyelids (→ptosis) as
a typical symptom: withdrawal from
the world, leaving the curtains drawn,
hiding behind them.
Handling: Consciously allowing oneself to be weak, seeking help like a
child; going back and reliving puberty/
adolescence in order to be able to put
it behind one; conscious withdrawal,
regeneration and introspection;

intentionally leaving the curtains drawn and concerning oneself with oneself alone.

Resolution: Finding the inner child in oneself instead of outwardly regressing to a child; engaging in the deep immersion and introspection (of Buddha)

Archetypal principle: Mars-Neptune.

Mycoses

see Dermatomycoses, Candidamycosis

Myelitis

see Spinal cord inflammation

Myeloma

(plasmocytoma) see Bone cancer

Myocardial rupture

(rupture of the myocardium (heart wall)) see Cardiac infarction

Myocarditis

(heart muscle inflammation; see also Inflammation)

Physical level: Heart (seat of the soul, love, feelings, energy centre).

Symptom level: Unresolved heart conflict which could unhinge the life that one has led so far; war that has flared up around the energy centre of life (the heart): heart-rending conflict, struggle for one's own life, everything is at stake; conflict-charged relationship; inner weeping of the heart; often unconscious longing for death; danger of giving up one's own centre.

Handling: Crying in a heart-melting way; waging an open(ly and offensive) struggle over one's centre in life, over matters of the heart (muscle); courageously having out central life-and-death conflicts; getting set inwardly for the (all-decisive) battle;

allowing The Old Adam (i.e. one's previous life) to die.

Resolution: Recognising and accepting life as a perpetual struggle for one's own centre; venturing the struggle for the whole.

Archetypal principle: Sun-Mars.

Myodegeneratio cordis

see Heart degeneration

Myogelosis

(muscle hardening)

Physical level: Musculature (motor, strength) of the motoric system.

Symptom level: Localised, pressing, painful muscle hardening due to over-exertion or on the basis of an inflammation.

Handling: Developing willingness to face conflict with respect to inner flexibility; restricting oneself outwardly to essential movements and undertaking inner steps.

Resolution: Maintaining one's relationships with the outside world through concentrated application of one's motoric flexibility.

Archetypal principle: Mars-Saturn.

Myoma

(myoma uteri)

Physical level: Womb (fertility, safety and security).

Symptom level: Unfulfilled or unconscious desire for offspring: the child's-head-sized myoma develops in the location for having children; outgrowths bloom on the level of fertility ("it's blooming crazy!"); the unconscious desire for fertility exceeds the actual number of one's children; frequently occur as a result of the discrepancy between modern social compulsions and the old tradition of having a lot of children; also sometimes occur if the old-age provision of the woman threatens to fall through, since in evolutionary terms, children were the traditional answer to this problem: giving old, outmoded answers to the challenges of modern-day life; misdirected, but benign growth: having slipped back down to a regressive physical level since it has usually been long since overtaken by one's current period of life.

Handling: Elevating fertility and growth to the mental-spiritual level; having brainchildren (i.e. mental-spiritual conception); creating more resolved (redeeming) outlets for one's own fertility, e.g. mental, artistic creativity and wildly proliferating ideas; taking care to ensure a reliable old age provision in good time.

Resolution: Making the archetype of the Grand Mother a reality: becoming a mother to new life – on the appropriate level depending on one's age.

Archetypal principle: Moon-Jupiter.

Myopia

see Shortsightedness

Myositis

see Dermatomyositis

Myxoedema

(see also Thyroid gland hypofunction)

Physical level: Thyroid gland (development, maturity), subcutaneous connective tissue (protection, insulation).

Symptom level: Mucous substances are deposited in the subcutaneous fatty tissue: development of a thick skin; bloated, yellowish cold skin: lifeless expression; thin, fragile hair: the issues of freedom and power are in a bad state; retention of salt and water: the feminine spiritual element is retained on the physical instead of on the spiritual level and causes the body to swell up; the basal metabolism declines drastically: the life

processes come to a standstill; the cholesterol level rises: expression of the regressive basic attitude directed at withdrawal and sealing oneself off; biding one's time until death without any drive in a sluggish, semi-conscious way that is characterised by disinterest in the outside world: shutting oneself off from the outside world; being left cold by everything, playing dead; lack of interest in life; almost all cases of apparent death and "being buried alive" come from this realm.

Handling: Growing a thick skin against the outside world in the figurative sense and developing inner liveliness behind these thick walls; withdrawing oneself from outside life and winding down the number of activities: voluntarily foregoing outer freedom and power; letting things happen; taking oneself to heart spiritually; letting everything old die; conscious coming to terms with dying and death; concerning oneself with subjects beyond one's (material) boundaries (transcendence).

Resolution: Inner withdrawal; becoming a conscious wanderer between the worlds: experiences of transcendence.

Archetypal principle: Mercury-Saturn/Neptune.

N

Nail biting / chewing

Physical level: Fingernails (claws, aggression).

Symptom level: Fear of (one's own) aggression; blunting one's own weapons (claws), biting down one's own aggression, amputating one's claws; in children: fear/→feelings of guilt about outwardly putting one's aggression into action; reflection of the fear of the parents towards aggressions; not trusting oneself to get a grip on one's life; too little outlet for the life force; hunger for aggression; defiance of restrictive parents.

Handling: (also for jointly-affected parents, whose problems are often reflected by the children): Developing respect for one's own vital powers; taking back the outwardly-directed physical aggressions; owning up to one's tendency to back away from life; creating outlets for the inner vitality: from external outlets (sport, hearty nourishment requiring good chewing) to internal outlets (living courageously); sensing and satisfying one's own powers and one's own hunger for life.

Resolution: Being outwardly more defensive and inwardly more courageous: facing up to life, showing one's inner claws.

Archetypal principle: Mars-Mars.

Nail fungus

(see also Athlete's foot, Dermatomycoses, Candidamycosis)

Physical level: Finger- and toenails (claws, aggression).

Symptom level: Being too weak to show one's claws and defend one's own skin (weak defensive situation); one's own weapons (claws) are taken over by foreign invasion troops; being deprived of the use of one's own claws; in particular, it is non-living tissue which falls victim to fungal infections (fungi are saprophytes, which live on dead organic matter).

Handling: Becoming more willing to compromise; taking one's mental-spiritual defence system back a notch, as this takes a load off the body, thus allowing it to improve its own defence system; fostering the involvement with foreign impulses; letting in foreign elements; making room for foreign elements and making

them one's own instead of letting oneself be taken over by what is foreign; opening up those areas which are no longer used and consequently no longer needed, i.e. lifeless areas that have died off, to foreign life impulses; taking in vital (living) nourishment, which yields nothing to the fungus; consciously making the daily choice: either nourish the fungus with dead nourishment that has no nutritional value or oneself with vital (living) nourishment.

Resolution: Allowing foreign impulses and life forms to get close to one's borders; getting to know them, accepting them, and integrating them into one's own life; in the long term, bringing life into one's own living terrain (in consciousness); bringing dead areas back to life.

Archetypal principle: Mars-Pluto.

Narcolepsy

(sleepy state [somnolence], daytime sleepiness [hypersomnia], uncontrollable compulsion to fall asleep [narcolepsy])

Physical level: Usually a consciousness problem.

Symptom level: First clarify and interpret the basic situation (frequently also related to organic brain processes); exhaustion; fear of the (performance) requirements of the day/ general activity; turning the day into night; taking flight into dream worlds/ into the consciousness of earliest childhood, copping out of responsibility; approaching everything slowly ("sleepyhead"); fear of being born.

Handling: Allowing oneself to enter the narrow realm of fear until it opens up into expansiveness; consciously exploring the dream worlds of the other side (dream yoga, conscious lucid dreams, etc.); re-living the state of childhood unawareness (therapeutically) in order to be able to let go of it once and for all; reconciling

oneself with one's own birth trauma (reincarnation therapy); once again returning to the Paradise of the womb, and then with the event of the birth, consciously taking one's leave from it; seeing the day as a symbol of life, and approaching it as if it were a ritual.
Resolution: Discovering the essence of responsibility (i.e. the ability to respond) in finding answers to life; seeking answers – even in sleep ("The Lord grants sleep to those he loves"; sleeping on a matter once again before deciding).
Archetypal principle: Neptune.

Narcomania

see Drug addiction

Nasal bone fracture

Physical level: Nose (power, pride, sexuality).
Symptom level: Having stuck one's neck out too far (just follow your nose), warning shot: "getting one's nose put out of joint"; as a result of this shot across the bows - the blow to the nose and its subsequent fracture - the personality is challenged and rattled; good therapy for excessive curiosity ("Little Master/Miss Nosey) and the need to stick one's nose (John Thomas) in everywhere (the size/shape of a man's nose has long been believed to indicate the size/shape of his penis); braking of the push to move forward; finding oneself on the wrong (training) ground.
Handling: Paying attention to warnings; keeping one's nose more in one's own business; practising restraint.
Resolution: Correcting one's course in response to warnings about the path in life that one has taken so far.
Archetypal principle: Mars-Saturn/ Uranus.

Nausea (dizziness)

see Kinetoses, Balance disorders

Nausea (upset stomach)

see Vomiting/Nausea, Pregnancy complaints, Malaise

Neck cysts

(see also Cysts)
Physical level: Neck (assimilation, connection, communication).
Symptom level: Remains of early embryonic development stages, which are normally completely outgrown and then disappear, e.g. remains of gill pouches, flaps and passages from the early aquatic origins of life: having been arrested in development; being stuck in an early development stage; something has remained open and unfinished; the unfinished state of humankind becomes a personal task; the human legacy demands special attention from those concerned.
Handling: Examining life for open developments, open ends, open spots; making oneself aware of these and paying them special attention; discovering any catches that one has become hooked on; keeping in mind the unfinished sides of one's own personality.
Resolution: Reconciliation with one's own history; consciously pushing development ahead and bringing it to a conclusion.
Archetypal principle: Venus/ Saturn-Moon.

Neck fracture

(see also Paraplegia)
Physical level: Back of the neck (strength, vulnerability), cervical vertebra (column) (being easily swayed, flexibility of the head).

Symptom level: "Breaking one's neck" = (almost) killing oneself; (unconsciously) (wanting) to bring this life to an end: many suicides and executions deliberately aim at the neck; no longer being able to feel the connection between the life one is leading and the actual sense of life.

Handling: Making oneself aware that one (unconsciously) did not want to continue living this life in this way, and that it is now time to turn to something completely different.

Resolution: Accepting the extreme twists and turns of Fate and resolving the new assignments resulting from them (→paraplegia).

Archetypal principle: Saturn-Uranus.

Neck pains

Physical level: Back of the neck (strength, vulnerability), neck (assimilation, connection, communication).

Symptom level: Cry for help from the overloaded neck, the weak point of the spinal column ("Who is breathing down one's neck?"); fear of new hard knocks to the neck and other bad experiences which have already been incurred at this sensitive point; obstinacy and stubbornesss can lead to hard-headedness, which is painful and makes the central control headquarters inflexible, →neck stiffness.

Handling: Paying attention to the cries for help and recognising their message (What does the neck have to be relieved of? Which old patterns from bad experiences or which unresolved conflicts are hanging around one's neck like a millstone? What expectations of further hard knocks are causing concern and already hurting in advance?); admitting to, acknowledging and getting over old hard knocks.

Resolution: Directing attention to the neck – the most sensitive point of the spinal column; reconciling oneself

to the blows from behind and hard knocks of the past so that the neck does not have to cry out in fear nor remind one of the pain.

Archetypal principle: Venus-Mars.

Neck stiffness

Physical level: Back of the neck (strength, vulnerability), neck (assimilation, connection, communication).

Symptom level: Obstinacy, stubbornness and hard-headedness: inflexibility of the central control headquarters; going through life wearing blinkers; unconscious refusal to acknowledge all sides and facets of the world.

Handling: Following one's own way in a straightforward way without being sidetracked; heading for the essential with concentration and consistency; making oneself aware when one is being shown something that is right under one's nose; recognising and avoiding distractions.

Resolution: A single viewpoint which contains everything (recognising the whole in the part).

Archetypal principle: Venus-Saturn.

Necrosis

(decay of cells leads to the dying off of delimited areas of tissue)

Physical level: All areas of the body can be affected.

Symptom level: Areas of the body which have died off correspond to deserted or completely dead subject areas: abandoned battlefields.

Handling: Admitting to oneself that the domains of consciousness belonging to the dead areas are also in agony; sensing subjects in one's own life which have died off or been abandoned and can no longer be brought to life; where possible, revitalising lifeless, but important subjects; taking leave of what has died off and making adjustments to compensate for their functions in some other way.

Necrospermia

Necrospermia

Resolution: Letting old, hand-ed-down patterns and habits that get in the way of life, etc. die off on the mental-spiritual level.
Archetypal principle: Saturn-Pluto.

Necrospermia

(immobility of the male sperm with resulting inability of fertilisation; see also Akinospermia, Infertility)
Physical level: Testicles (fertility, creativity), epididymis (fertility, maturity).
Symptom level: Disease pattern which is becoming more frequent; the fertility of men in industrialised countries is declining drastically (fewer and less mobile sperm); our performance-driven society produces many pollutants which ruin the sperm, thus allowing it to correct itself in this unresolved way; in the case of the unfulfilled desire to have a child/infertility, it is nowadays almost always the man who is the "primary cause".
Handling: Owning up to the lack of fertility: becoming less fertile (performing less) on figurative levels, but all the more so in the body: taking the action-man trip down a notch; simplest therapy: a real holiday (without "doing" anything) and instead letting simply things happen; reigning in the performance trip and giving free rein to (new) life; coming to (oneself); also doing things which produce nothing and from which nothing results.
Resolution: Being calmer outwardly, but inwardly livelier and (spiritually) more fertile.
Archetypal principle: Mars-Pluto/Saturn.

Nephritis

see Glomerulonephritis

Nephrolithiasis

see Kidney stones

Nephroma

see Kidney cancer

Nephrosclerosis

see Kidney, contracted

Nephrosis

(kidney degeneration)
Physical level: Kidneys (balance, partnership).
Symptom level: Degeneration of the kidney ducts (as a result of feverish infections, poisoning, fat metabolism disorders) leads to loss of protein in the urine (→albuminuria) and →oedema in the body; materials essential for life are lost due to the damage to the kidney filter; a back-up of the spiritual water develops in the body; vital life elements are allowed to pass through unused.
Handling: Allowing oneself to let more pass; letting things just flow through one.
Resolution: Becoming more generous (e.g. in the partnership), also passing on and letting go of essential things.
Archetypal principle: Venus-Saturn.

Nerve inflammation

(Neuritis, see also Trigeminal neuralgia)
Physical level: Almost all regions of the body can be affected, nerves (news service).
Symptom level: Constant pain in contrast to the recurring aches of neuralgia: cry for help; sensibility and motoric breakdowns in the functional area of this nerve: conflict in the area of a nerve or the subject connected with it; breaksdowns in the domains of feeling and activity.
Handling: Aggressively addressing the subject related to this nerve; persistent confrontation with the subject without slacking off; freshly

reactivating one's news service system and staying on the trail of hot communications topics.

Resolution: Committing oneself to the struggle and fighting it out in an open(ly offensive) way to the point of resolution.

Archetypal principle: Mercury/Uranus-Mars/Saturn.

Nerve pains

(neuralgia, neuropathy, polyneuropathy; see also Nerve inflammation (above))

Physical level: Nerves (news service).

Symptom level: Intermittant pains (cries for help) from the supply area of a nerve; unresolved, smouldering conflicts in the subject area of the part of the body connected with this nerve.

Handling: Learning to call for help and also to accept help; letting out one's aggressions and finding courageous ways to live them out constructively.

Resolution: Understanding the call for help; courageously and offensively ensuring relief.

Archetypal principle: Mercury/Uranus-Mars.

Nervous breakdown

Physical level: Nerves (news service).

Symptom level: Blowing of the fuses in the central control headquarters, emergency br(e)aking, pulling the rip cord, before it becomes really dangerous; disrupted communication due to overloading: total breakdown of traffic in the nervous system, traffic jams, obstructions; seeing oneself too much as the central point of focus and simply diving under and staying submerged in the middle of all the overloading ; too much input, hardly any or even no output at all: chasing after life and allowing oneself to be hounded; lack of confidence in one's

ability to convince oneself and one's environment of one's worth; being torn this way and that, living highly charged under various tensions; ignoring the rules of communication and mediation; frequently striving too hard to please everybody, and thereby forgetting oneself; overloading oneself in order to look good for others; being driven ("You are going to drive me crazy!").

Handling: Admitting to oneself the total state of overload of the central control headquarters: being glad that the fuses blew, thereby preventing any more serious damage; voluntarily closing down communication for a temporary period until a reorganisation and reorientation has taken place: developing "nerves of steel"; temporarily reducing the input and increasing the output; screening oneself off, temporarily letting nothing more in and allowing as much as possible to flow out and away; learning to first let go before something further is accepted and added to the information store; granting oneself rest, giving up the e(x)ternal struggle; instead of allowing oneself to be over-stimulated by the huge number of impressions and demands, learning to distance oneself consciously and in good time; making efforts to achieve an overview early on, taking a bird's-eye view and learning to be selective; working from the opposite pole (allopathically) in the case of objective overloading of robust types (which is much rarer than the breakdowns of over-sensitive types): taking the load off the head as the only centre of command and control and all decision-making, and additionally enlisting the aid of the heart (feeling, intuition) and the gut (instinct, gut feeling).

Resolution: Making an alliance with the heart: communication from heart to heart; acting on one's gut feelings.

Mercury-Uranus.

Nervousness

(see also Nervous breakdown)
Physical level: Nerves (news service).
Symptom level: One's own demands with regard to the speed of life, variety and performance cannot be fulfilled by the body; wanting to realise too much too quickly, sensory overload; the lines are too weak for the high level of input; overloading disrupts the connections; impending breakdown of the networks.
Handling: Admitting to oneself the state of overload of the communications channels; temporarily reducing the input; voluntarily closing down communication for a temporary period until a reorganisation and reorientation has taken place; granting oneself rest, temporarily giving up the e(x)ternal struggle.
Resolution: Taking the load off the head, and instead bringing the heart (feeling, intuition) and the gut (instinct, gut feeling) more strongly into the game of life; listening carefully with the heart; learning to act on one's gut feelings; living vibrant life energy; allowing oneself to be stimulated and exposed to situations that make one tingle with vitality instead of trembling with inner unrest.
Archetypal principle:
Uranus-Mercury.

Neuralgia

see Nerve pains, Trigeminal neuralgia, Intercostal neuralgia

Neuritis

see Nerve inflammation

Neurodermitis

(see also Allergy)
Physical level: Skin (border, contact, tenderness).

Symptom level: Being challenged by allergic skin reactions: "something is itching and grating one"; aggressive form of obtaining loving attention, which is demanded by affected children at the top of their voices; reaction to an allergen (often milk, suggestive of a mother conflict) which provokes and arouses and is experienced either as pleasantly exciting or irritating; passion/ inner fire/ fury thrusting its way to the surface: "bristling with excitement"; struggle down to one's very lifeblood against symbolic concepts of an enemy as represented by the allergens (for interpretations, see: →allergy); over-reaction, overblown concept of the enemy; strong unconscious aggressiveness; the burning aggression is written all over one's face; it disfigures the fac(ad)e; using the need to avoid the allergens as a method for tyrannising one's environment and thereby living out aggressions: unconscious power games; build-up of aggression, suppressed vitality; insatiable need to scratch open one's skin, to break down one's own borders; bristling with excitement (on the wrong level); wanting to burst with anger; feeling oneself to be outcast like a leper (shutting oneself off from the community), secreting oneself. away
Handling: Making oneself aware of one's own needs, which are getting under one's skin; voluntarily allowing oneself to be challenged: life with all its many stimuli is allowed to stir one up; consciously letting the many stimuli come in and letting oneself be lured to come out; courageously opening the borders; consciously letting in the symbols classified as hostile and recognising and accepting them in their whole meaning; becoming more responsive; allowing oneself to bristle with excitement more often; letting the borders (skin) be easier to pass through in order to

be able to foster more contact and exchange; relieving the body again of the exercise of aggression and becoming more aggressive and offensive oneself: daring to live; becoming more adept at rapid-fire responses; learning to defend one's own skin and to open its floodgates as required; consciously taking on demanding challenges and allowing them to demand a lot of one in order to grow more as a result of the demands; acting offensively; (learning) enjoyment of eroticism; seeking conscious confrontations with the areas that one is avoiding and resisting.

Resolution: Scratching around in one's consciousness for long enough until one knows what is itching and irritating one, what is getting under one's skin and what is firing up one's soul; grasping the red-hot irons (Mars) in life; putting up a bold front to life (Latin frons, -tis 'forehead').

Archetypal principle: Venus/ Saturn (skin)-Mars (inflammation).

Neuropathy

see Nerve pains

Neurosis

(see also Heart neurosis, Stomach neurosis, Anxiety, Phobia)

Symptom level: In general: ways of reacting that deviate from the "norm", often on the basis of aberrations with respect to time (the patients do not behave in a manner that is appropriate to the given situation; instead, their behaviour belongs to a completely different time), which causes suffering to those affected; in particular:

1. Anxiety neurosis: Restrictiveness problem, which is frequently connected with the unprocessed initial experience of restriction during birth;
2. Depressive neurosis: Lack of reconciliation with one's own mortality;
3. Compulsive neurosis: Failed rituals that have sunk down into the unconscious;
4. Hysterical neurosis (an formerly frequently-occurring special form: conversion neurosis): In their form of expression, the hysterical symptoms already plainly show the problematic issue; they present it in the form of stageworthy theatrics, so to speak – over-the-top self-promotion;
5. →Perversions in the sense of a sexual neurosis: Combining sexual gratification with unusual ideas;
6. Character neurosis: Character deviations from the "norm";
7. Compensating neurosis: Attempts to obtain benefits or compensation which one would not normally be judged as being entitled to.

Handling: (on the basis of experiences with reincarnation therapy):

1. Making oneself aware of one's birth trauma and clarifying it;
2. Reconciling oneself with the subject of dying – death – (re)solution;
3. Uncovering sunken rituals and reconciling oneself to the tasks that have remained open;
4. Making oneself aware that the vying for attention is a front for the search for real love;
5. Digging up and laying bare the roots of unusual imprintings;
6. Recognising and resolving the aspect of one's own character that one is suffering under;
7. Digging up and laying bare the roots of what– on the surface – seem to be misguided expectations.

Resolution: (in general for neuroses): Making oneself aware of the basic aberration with respect to time and finally arriving at a life in the current moment instead of making the attempt to master new situations with old programmes; acknowledging and letting go of the past (as happens, for example, in reincarnation therapy).

Archetypal principle (in general for neuroses): Pluto in combination with practically all other principles, in particular Moon (soul); especially: 1., 2. and 3. Pluto/Moon-Saturn; 4. Pluto/ Moon-Uranus-Sun; 5. Pluto/ Moon-Mars/Uranus; 6. Uranus; 7. Pluto/ Moon-Saturn.

Nicotine poisoning

(see also Smoking, Poisoning)
Physical level: The whole organism is affected, but above all, the blood vessels (transport routes of the life force).
Symptom level: If one is not used to it, even small doses of nicotine lead to →balance disorders, →headaches, →(increased) saliva production, outbreaks of sweating, vision disorders, →heart failure, →cramps, and ultimately, →delirium; the nicotine content of just 10 g of tobacco is fatal for an adult; chronic nicotine poisoning as a result of regular smoking leads to sensory disorders →circulatory disorders of all vessels – beginning from the feet, via the genitalia (there is a high impotence and infertility rate amongst smokers) to the heart and brain; poor vision, gastric disorders, decline of the reaction capability, chronic infections in the area of the respiratory tract, dramatic increase in the probability of →cancer, above all in the area of the lungs (→lung cancer), although the rate of →stomach cancer is also 10 times higher than amongst non-smokers.
Handling: Acknowledging one's dependency and seeing through the relevant individual spiritual pattern underlying one's urge to smoke: a spectrum which leads from the sensual-oral vicarious satisfaction substitute via the relief of stress (letting off steam) to social aspects, such as brandishing a glowing baton.
Resolution: Identifying one's own smoker archetype and selecting an alternative, more constructive and

less dangerous level of resolution for the smoking problem.
Archetypal principle: Neptune.

Night blindness

(hemeralopia)
Physical level: Eyes (insight, perspective, mirror and window of the soul), rods of the retina (photographic plate of the eye).
Symptom level: No longer being able to orientate oneself in the dark, but also wanting to remain in the dark; fear that the light (of recognition) could blind one or reveal one's own shadow; already beginning to lose track of things at twilight; endangerment in the evening time, when things become eventful; helplessness in the shadow kingdom; lack of adjustment to the female half of the day; not being aware of one's blindness to the female half of reality.
Handling: Voluntarily giving things a rest and staying home (within oneself); looking inwards and intensifying one's inner vision with regard to one's own feminine reality; owning up to the difficulties with the dark side of the day (the female half of reality); turning towards the bright sides (the light) and living and enjoying them intensively; allowing the night to be night again and giving things a rest externally (activities in the dark, when one cannot see anything, are dangerous), and instead looking inward; shadow therapy: learning to see in the dark; illuminating the shadow kingdom.
Resolution: Courage to take (one's own) dark sides for real and to take them seriously, making the dark side of the day the homeland of the soul; finding one's actual home in the worlds of spiritual imagery.
Archetypal principle: Moon/ Sun-Saturn/Pluto.

Nightmares

(see also Sleep problems, Anxiety)
Physical level: Usually a consciousness problem.
Symptom level: Meeting with one's
own misdirected strength; attempt at
conflict resolution which was rejected
in the light of day; night-time shadow
therapy; fear of not being able to
meet the demands of one's life task.
Handling: Bringing pressing and suppressed conflicts into one's daytime
consciousness and confronting them
courageously; continuing unfinished
dreams as guided visualisations,
since solutions to symbolic happenings can be found in the dreams
themselves; learning to dream lucidly;
exercises in letting go.
Resolution: dealing conclusively with
existential anxieties and one's material existence; willingness to follow
one's own unique path; cultivating a
well-developed conflict culture; openness to spiritual truths.
Archetypal principle: Saturn-Pluto.

Nipple, chapped

Physical level: The female breast
(motherliness, nourishment, safety
and security, sensuality, desire).
Symptom level: Conflict over nursing, nourishing, mothering (war over
the "milk bar"): too much unconscious
mothering?, worn docking point?,
already being completely frayed?;
tearing open one's breast (or allowing
it); suppressing the cries of pain due
to the sore, chapped milk source
when nursing; being torn between the
child and the partner, being torn in
different directions, being torn within
oneself, tearing open one's breast for
others (see also the Christian symbol
of the Pelican, which tears open its
own breast in order to nourish its
young with its blood); she has so
much on her chest that is dragging
her down (child, man, the issue of
supply, responsibility) that she and
her breasts cannot hold it out, but instead sustain visible damage; danger
of escalation towards → mammary
gland inflammation.
Handling: Owning up to one's conflict over nursing and fighting it out
internally: who has what rights to the
mam(m)a/ry – the newborn because
of the milk bar, papa as his source of
desire, or mama (and papa) because
of her figure?; fighting out the conflict
down to the very depths of the relationship (with the child, partner and
one's own body) (e.g.: "What can I/
do I not want to give with the mother's
milk?"); learning to deal with the total
dependency of the child on the one
hand, but also learning to deal with its
first ambitions to power on the other;
scaling back one's expectations with
regard to motherhood; mothering
oneself; reducing stress; allowing
oneself to be helped.
Resolution: Total devotion to life: to
the new one (the child), but also to
one's own in relation to the mother
and lover role; developing inner
willingness to nourish; accepting and
enjoying womanhood without reservation; reorganisation of the hierarchy
of relationships in favour of the new
life: for a certain time, putting the child
first (nursing) and the partner in second place, and then later vice versa
(with regard to the breast).
Archetypal principle: Moon/
Venus-Mars.

Nipple, inverted

(nipple drawn in below the level of the
areola)
Physical level: The female breast
(motherliness, nourishment, safety
and security, sensuality, desire), nipple (nourishment, desire).
Symptom level: Introverted instead
of extroverted willingness to nourish;
neediness of one's own instead of
the need to satisfy (nourish) others;
active giving is rejected both in the

area of nursing (Archetypal principle - Moon) and seducing (Archetypal principle - Venus); retreat to a large degree in two essential points of feminine being, usually on the basis of earlier disappointments.

Handling: Homeopathically: first and foremost taking care of the satisfaction of one's own needs; turning oneself inwards more and looking after oneself: getting one's own fill (satisfaction); developing a tendency towards letting oneself be conquered in the relationship with one's partner; making oneself aware that the partner should make an effort, and that the woman (like her breast) is not to be had so easily; allopathically: turning out (exposing) the nipple to the powerful sucking of the baby/man, and as a result of the tugging of the baby/man, becoming capable of nursing; in other words, becoming an extroverted woman in terms of nourishing ability and thereby in addition to the Moon archetype (nursing, nourishing) developing the seductive archetype of Venus, because the nipples of the breast, in addition to their feeding function, are also alluring and oriented towards the partner (Venus principle).

Resolution: Reconciliation with the polarity of giving and taking: nourishing and being nourished; satisfying and being satisfied.

Archetypal principle: Moon-Venus.

Nosebleed

(epistaxis)
Physical level: Nose (power, pride, sexuality).
Symptom level: (for jointly-affected parents, whose problems are often reflected by the children): life energy and joy for life run off in a demonstrative way via the nose (harmless, but creates an impression for the parents and child); children symbolically and unconsciously show their intimidation and endangerment by sacrificing their own lifeblood; by means of this dramatic blood sacrifice, which is clear for all to see, those affected indicate how badly things are going with them; momentary increases in pressure when the blood rushes to one's head: letting off (excess) pressure.

Handling: Acute therapy: remaining calm and laying the head back; placing a cold, wet cloth on the neck; ensuring that the blood does not rush to the child's head too often (which also frequently happens in their sleep); letting out the life force at the body's safety release valves (its openings) in the figurative sense: emphasising the body (e.g. through sport and games) instead of relying only on the intellectual level; all physical activities which toughen one up are primarily suitable for directing the lifeblood into the body musculature, and secondly, beneficial for the mostly delicate constitution of those affected; taking care that children do not waste their life energy: sensitive small beings of the homeopathic Phosphorous Type tend to nosebleeds and to demand too much of themselves (mentally).

Resolution: Reconciling oneself with the endangerment of the life (entrusted to one).

Archetypal principle: Mars-Mars.

Nose-picking, chronic

Physical level: Nose (power, pride, sexuality).
Symptom level: Symptom classified as improper because of its sexual connection but which also has the character of a popular plague: stimulation of the genital regions via the corresponding reflex zones through stimulation of the erogenous zones on the inside of the nose; (unconscious) attempt to stimulate one's own vitality.

374

Handling: Making oneself aware of the symbolic and reflexological connections; seeking erotic satisfaction by direct means.

Resolution: Realising and enjoying fulfilling eroticism and genital sexuality.

Archetypal principle: Mars-Venus.

Nursing problems

(see also Milk accumulation, Breast-milk production, deficient)

Physical level: The female breast (motherliness, nourishment, safety and security, sensuality, desire).

Symptom level: (In the case of the mother): lack of willingness to nourish the child; not wanting to give any more of oneself, or in the situation of a seemingly never-ending nursing period: not allowing the child to continue along its development path; wanting to keep it as a babe in arms; (in the case of the child): spurning the mother through her milk, or in the situation of a seemingly never-ending nursing period: the only method of the child to keep the mother for itself.

Handling: Reconciliation with the (nourishing) mother role, one's own child(hood), as well as the father of the child and his demands; coming to terms with one's own awareness of deficits; in the case of rejection of the milk by the child: children who were originally rejected themselves can express rejection on their part in this way; sometimes the rejection which the mother experiences in this way from her child can only be recognised and accepted when viewed within the chain of lives.

Resolution: Developing oneself towards the state of understanding and life situation in which there is enough for all.

Archetypal principle: Moon-Saturn/Pluto.

Nutrition-related damage

(amongst adults in industrialised countries)

Physical level: Metabolism (dynamic equilibrium), joints (mobility, articulation), blood vessels (transport routes of the life force), ultimately all types of tissue and organs are affected.

Symptom level: From →arteriosclerosis to →rheumatism, from →obesity and →being underweight to →high blood pressure; in Germany, such diseases cause losses to the economy of over €70 billion per year; ultimately a problem of a lack of awareness: as a rule, too much of the wrong foods are eaten, above all far too much animal protein and too much refined, processed food robbed of its essential nutrients (ready-made meals, fast food, etc.).

Handling: "You are what you eat": eating and living in a fast, fleeting and rushed way or in a consciously-balanced and nourishing manner; seeing through the mechanisms of one's own incorrect diet and the compensation for basic needs, such as that for sensuality by over-eating and eating the wrong foods; developing an understanding of the "species-appropriate" (i.e. suitable for homo sapiens) diet that is fit for human beings; finding out what one really needs (to live).

Resolution: Enjoying a species-appropriate, sensually-fulfilling, balanced and nourishing diet that is suitable for one's type; placing quality above quantity at all levels of assimilation.

Archetypal principle: Moon/Venus-Saturn/Jupiter.

Nyctophobia

(pavor nocturnus, fear of the dark; see also Anxiety, Phobia)

Symptom level: Fear, even of the twilight, which heralds the (dark) night, and symbolises the downfall of the light; (unconsciously) recognising the night symbolically as the feminine side, the shadow of the bright day, and fearing it as such; feeling oneself to be completely at the mercy of the shadow kingdom when in the dark; helplessness vis-à-vis one's own shadow, which being associated with the night, now threatens to rise up. Handling: Owning up to one's difficulties with the dark side of the day (and reality) and recognising that the night should be assigned to the shadow kingdom; one's own shadow therapy: learning to see and accept one's own dark night sides. Resolution: Having the courage to ensure that the dark sides (of oneself) are taken on, taken for real and taken seriously. Archetypal principle: Moon-Saturn-Pluto.

Nymphomania

(see also Addiction: Sex addiction) Symptom level: Pathologically-increased desire for sex and sexual intercourse in women; almost uncontrollable longing for the sexual opposite pole - the man. Handling: Intensive processing of the issue of polarity; conscious sexuality in the sense of a ritual; tantric attempts to discover love in the depths of sexuality. Resolution: Recognising sexuality as simply the physical aspect, whose spiritual component is love. Archetypal principle: Pluto.

Nystagmus

(rapid eye movement, involuntary eye movement) Physical level: Eyes (insight, perspective, mirrors and windows of the soul). Symptom level: Unsteady, wandering gaze; hunted, driven, unbalanced impression, restless dissatisfaction

searching for a target; being nervous and making others nervous; finding no stability (in life?); avoiding (eye) contact. Handling: Consciously allowing one's gaze to wander; inner movement in the sense of seeking and finding; consciously wandering and travelling; viewing the world in order to develop a worldview; consciously making contact. Resolution: Acknowledging one's own shadow world; fulfilling the longing to wander, allowing the searching gaze to set off on the search for happiness and healing in the sense of becoming whole. Archetypal principle: Uranus.

O

Obesity

Physical level: Fatty tissue (overflow, excess reserves), stomach (feeling, receptiveness). Symptom level: Outer fullness instead of inner fulfilment; being at war with the pleasure principle; battling with one's own weight (weightiness); search for caring attention, love and security; a need for love and enjoyment that is lived out through eating: vicarious satisfaction substitute ; excess weight gained due to "comfort eating"; eating as a reward; eating as a substitute for the feeling of unity and an overflowing heart; protective layer against a loveless environment: insulation/isolation in one's own (protective) fortress (nothing in the body insulates as well as fat: hardly any warmth can be lost to the outside, but none can get in either); desire to be left in peace in one's own fortress of fat; playing hide-and-seek behind yellow walls: dodging reality; fleeing from

376

one's own sex appeal; not wanting to live out one's own sexual role; problems with polarity: allowing one's own sexuality to be submerged in baby-fat (regression); creating one's own buffer zone, a crumple zone to protect against getting "knocked up"; putting on more; feigning pregnancy with a round figure, and in this way, simulating fulfilment; not being well-disposed towards oneself: weighing oneself daily and hating oneself for the result; being fed up with oneself; carrying the unlived load of other levels; feelings of weightiness (importance), authority and power.

Handling: Learning to recognise and accept one's own weight as fitting for the moment; ensuring loving attention and reward through other means of enjoyment than eating, e.g. sensual sexuality, erotic rituals, gentle massages, artistic pleasures; with regard to eating: consciously nibbling temptations with enjoyment; eating rituals; seeking substitutes for the substitute of "eating"; recognising and acknowledging excess weight gained due to comfort eating as a temporary life-preserver in order to then let go of it again when love starts to flow again; learning to protect oneself in other ways than the insulation/isolation of fat: striking back verbally with a sharp tongue and pointed remarks, arming oneself with arguments instead of with pounds and becoming adept in rapid-fire comebacks; learning to accept one's own sexual role and show it outwardly; learning to accept knockbacks as a result of flirting; becoming weightier on more developed levels; fighting for and earning the rewards that one believes one is entitled to; learning to grit one's teeth and bite one's way through life, learning to take on and digest life; working to develop new lifestyles (which are more personally valid for one), as well as a new inner form that the outer form can orientate itself

towards: fasting for healing purposes as a conscious ritual for the transition to new patterns; exercise/sport within the optimal aerobic range.

Resolution: Love which embraces the body, soul and spirit; feeling well-rounded, gaining spiritual weight: carrying weight (importance) instead of being overweight; taking up room; extending one's area of influence; inner fulfilment.

Archetypal principle: Jupiter-Venus.

Obstipation

see Constipation

Occupational illness(es)

(see also Poisoning)

Physical level: All areas of the body can be affected.

Symptom level: Various symptoms, depending on the occupation.

Handling: Asking oneself what one's occupation gives one,and what it takes, what one is missing in "this job", why and how it is making one ill.

Resolution: Inwardly listening to (heeding) the call which is heralding one's true calling, and making this into a profession.

Archetypal principle: All possible, depending on the area of the body concerned.

Oedema

(hydropsy; see also Ascites formation in the case of cirrhosis of the liver; Foot oedema, Leg oedema, Cerebral oedema, Lung oedema, Quincke's oedema)

Physical level: Connective tissue (connection, stability, binding commitment).

Symptom level: Accumulation of water in the tissue of the legs and feet in particular: blockage and build-up of the spiritual element in the lower area; emphasis of the feminine lower pole of the body due to its weightiness (importance); making things nice and cushy for oneself, building a moat to protect oneself.

Handling: Holding (getting) back the spiritual element and directing it into the lower, feminine areas; paying attention to which regions most need to be watered, respectively infused, with spirituality; taking the lower half of the body for real and taking it seriously; allowing room for one's own problem zones; not allowing oneself to be boxed in; taking what one needs spiritually (spiritual water); ensuring better grounding; stepping out in grander style.

Resolution: Occupying and reconciling oneself with the feminine, spiritual aspects in the figurative sense; safeguarding the body against being overflooded with spiritual water; standing up for one's greater needs.

Archetypal principle: Moon-Neptune.

Oesophagal inflammation

see Reflux oesophagitis

Oesophageal varices

(varicose veins of the oesophagus; see also Liver, cirrhosis)

Physical level: Oesophagus (food pipe - nutrition supply).

Symptom level: In cases of portal vein hypertension due to liver problems (first clarify and interpret the basic problem [typically cirrhosis of the liver]), the life energy backs up as far as the area of the food pipe: danger of a life-threatening loss of life energy (potentially-fatal haemorrhaging).

Handling/Resolution: Clarifying the underlying problem of the meaning of life; bringing the pent-up life energy back into flow again.

Archetypal principle: Mercury-Jupiter/Pluto.

Oesophagitis

see Reflux oesophagitis

Oligophrenia

see Debility

Open leg ulcers

(ulcus cruris; see also Varicose veins, Connective tissue weakness)

Physical level: Skin (border, contact, tenderness), connective tissue (connection, stability, binding commitment).

Symptom level: A creeping, crawling process that drags on endlessly as a result of being physically "thin-skinned"; attempt at openness on the level of an open leg wound; means of detoxification; smouldering wounds from deep injuries which one has sustained in life and which do not want to heal; lack of forgiveness and willingness to close off the wounds; clinging tightly to misery and suffering.

Handling: Opening one's borders and floodgates in the mental-spiritual respect and letting out what wants to be let out, even if one is reluctant to see what then rises up out of the depths; opening up the inner windows again, opening oneself up, letting in a breath of fresh air (oxygen and ozone therapy often lead to an improvement – but they can also become dangerous if they close the only window and no other window [higher up] is opened; looking after the border of one's skin, taking care of the (only) open point; getting rid of the poison via other channels ("spitting poison and bile"); bringing other possibilities of detoxification to light; danger of nursing the wound shut using naturopathic means without paying attention to the spiritual dimension, which then often results in self-poisoning because the poisons can no longer be eliminated.

Resolution: Opening up spiritually and thereby giving the body the chance to close up the border of the skin again; forgiving in order to be able to forget; reconciling oneself and making peace.

Archetypal principle: Venus/ Saturn-Pluto.

Orchitis

see Testicles, inflammation

Orgasm problems

(difficulties in coming to an experience of unity during sexual intercourse; above all, a complaint of women, but in fact, more frequent in men, although the latter usually hide behind the misconception that ejaculation is an orgasm; see also Frigidity)

Physical level: Starting from the genital region (sexuality, polarity, procreation), the whole organism is affected; ultimately a consciousness problem.

Symptom level: sign of a degenerate art of lovemaking which, in relying only on mechanical, physiological processes, has hit rock bottom; inhibition against letting (oneself) go and letting oneself fall (often originating very early on in life on the level of a lack of basic trust); fear of, respectively inability, to die (the orgasm as the "little brother" of Death, death of the Ego as the lifting of the Me-You boundary); not being able to surrender oneself completely; wanting to uphold the final control.

Handling: Learning the art of love (Tantra, Kama Sutra); exercises in letting go: exercises in letting oneself fall into water; breaking loose in unbridled dance exercises, ecstatic music or sports experiences, Samadhi tank or floating exercises in water; spiritual exercises culminating in experiences of unity (connected breathing);

making oneself aware of one's dominating need for control; learning to see through the lack of trust in the situation/one's partner; play-acting as a form of "behavioural therapy" until it finally happens to one; exercises which lead to the surrender of intellectual control and bypass the archetypally masculine "doer"/ "go-getter" pole, such as "inner journeys" (guided visualisations).

Resolution: By giving up one's Ego, finding the way to one's self; recognising and experiencing the unity of all life: experiences of pure being; trusting oneself to the flow of life in the sense of "Thy will be done".

Archetypal principle: Venus-Saturn (inhibition)/Uranus (exclusion)/Neptune (lack of devotion)/Pluto (fear of loss of control).

Ornithosis

see Psittacosis

Ossification

Physical level: Above all, cartilage tissue (elasticity, binding commitment) that has ossified in the course of life.

Symptom level: Causing what is soft to harden; being hard on oneself; sacrificing one's flexibility in favour of exaggerated stability.

Handling: Preferring to be consciously stricter and more disciplined with oneself; applying stricter standards to the flow of one's own life, rather than walling in the wings (lobes) of the lungs in an ossified, inflexible rib cage and allowing the blood vessels, as the channels of the life energy, to petrify.

Resolution: Becoming a student (disciple) of life, learning to value (self-) discipline; accepting and fulfilling existing structures in the sense of the life mandala.

Archetypal principle: Saturn.

Osteochondropathia juvenilis deformans

see Scheuermann's disease

Osteodystrophia fibrosa generalisata

(Recklinghausen's disease)
Physical level: Parathyroid glands (balance between ossification and instability), bone system (stability, strength).
Symptom level: Hyperfunction of the parathyroid glands has the effect that an excess of parathyroid hormone interferes with bone development and the metabolism of minerals: disintegration of the overall structure due to bone cysts and deformations, distension and spontaneous breaks (→bone fracture): breaching of norms and structures; break with norms and rules, chaos in the structural domain; the rise in the calcium level of the blood leads to hardening (calcification) in the kidneys (balance, partnership); increased density of the bone (osteosclerosis) of the base of the skull: cranial nerve failures (e.g. →facial paresis); pigment anomalies: being marked (with distinction) (in a mild form).
Handling: Taking the load off the body by taking the task away from it: more lax approach to norms and prescribed structures, remodelling them to suit one's own purposes; bending and fitting of the norms to one's own ideas; conscious break with structures which are no longer useful; allowing creative chaos to move into the structural domain; learning to see through rigidifications in the partnership domain of balancing contrasts.
Resolution: Creative handling of structures and norms; adapting them to one's current needs; playing with them.
Archetypal principle: Mercury-Saturn/Neptune.

Osteomyelitis

see Bone marrow inflammation

Osteonecrosis

(dying off of the bone)
Physical level: Bones (stability, strength).
Symptom level: Dying off of the old structures on the physical level, which goes down to the bone; giving up stability and structure on the bone level; the previously-valid norms and laws break away and disintegrate: a process which affects one down to the marrow.
Handling: Letting go of security, stability and structure instead of clinging on to them; allowing one's accustomed stability and familiar structures to disintegrate; letting the old norms and laws break down or even actively throwing them overboard; preferring instead to encourage the signs of disintegration of one's own old structures; consciously questioning one's own strength and staying powers (ability to hold out); recognising that the stabilising structures themselves must become softer at the innermost core, for instance, as is the case for men in the second half of life when it becomes a matter of realisation of the anima (the inner woman).
Resolution: Allowing the old structures which have supported life for so long to die off; bringing everything about oneself into question right to the very depths; courage for transformations which extend to the very bones and even down into their marrow.
Archetypal principle: Saturn-Pluto.

Osteoporosis

Physical level: Bones (stability, strength).
Symptom level: One's own structure becomes brittle; there is a lack of inner stability and security; one can

no longer rely on one's own inner structure; one's inner strength and dependability are brought into question; 1. Functional reasons for the increasing loss of calcium from the bones in men and women: Due to the lack of movement and exercise, the muscles, tendons and bones are not put under enough pressure (everything that is under-used starts to be broken down by the organism, e.g. arm or leg muscles after being immobilised in a plaster cast; "use it or lose it"); incorrect nutrition; 2. Content reasons: Behind the declining physical agility lies the corresponding decreasing mental-spiritual agility of modern people; loss of calcium from the bones in order to get rid of ballast; everything which those affected do not voluntarily throw overboard in terms of ballast at the midpoint of their life is given away by the body in the substitute form of calcium loss from the bones; in order to lighten one's load on one's way back to the origin in the circle of life (mandala), whatever has become superfluous is simply cast off ; for the way home – the return of the soul – extremely sturdy bones are no longer so necessary; attempts at deception through the use of hormones only succeed to the extent that the body is led to believe that it is not yet time for the change (of life direction in the mandala): it then stops jettisoning ballast, but this also has the effect that life stays blocked at the midpoint, and thus necessarily remains only half-complete.

Handling: Consciously calling into question the structures which have carried one through life thus far; no longer depending on anything as being secure or taking anything as a given; giving life a new supporting framework; redefining the inner structure; jettisoning ballast: both concretely in the form of excess weight as well as in the figurative sense: letting go of things which can make no

useful contribution to the homeward journey of the soul; adjusting oneself inwardly to new life tasks following the change: activities requiring such sturdy bones as in one's youth are not fitting for this time of life; facing up to the new pattern of life instead of trying to squeeze past it and remaining nailed stuck to the midpoint through the use of hormones; finding a secure hold in one's own spiritual structure; leading a life which is satisfying and fulfilling to the feminine or masculine pole.

Resolution: Making the change from outer to inner activity: lightening one's load externally in order to prepare oneself inwardly for the essential demands of time.

Archetypal principle: Saturn.

Osteosarcoma

see Bone cancer

Ostitis deformans

(Paget's disease)

Physical level: Bones (stability, strength).

Symptom level: One or more bones thickens and become distorted; this is accompanied by bone loss, with the result that even minor causes can lead to spontaneous fractures; primarily affects men of advanced age: the life structures become outwardly impressive, but are capable of bearing little inwardly, and in the end, even break away spontaneously.

Handling: Letting old structures break apart; making oneself aware of the hardening and deformation of one's own personality; allowing the old, outlived framework of life to die off.

Resolution: Coming to rest and allowing new, dependable structures to grow – smaller, but more reliable ones; developing the wisdom of age and becoming gentler and more flexible; spending time with one's

grandchildren and one's own inner child.
Archetypal principle: Saturn-Uranus.

Otitis externa

see Auditory canal inflammation

Otitis media

see Middle ear inflammation

Otosclerosis

(ossification of the miniature bones of the ear [auditory ossicles])
Physical level: EMars/hearing (hearing and obeying commands).
Symptom level: Ossification of the miniature bones of the ear, with the result that they can no longer articulate together in a flexible way: one's adaptive flexibility in terms of listening carefully and obeying is lost; becoming inwardly more rigid as far as the issues of paying attention and hearing/obeying commands are concerned; becoming set in one's ways with regard to outer vibes/vibrations, retreating into one's snail shell (Latin: cochlea) and becoming hardened, even fossilising; rigid obedience.
Handling: Concentrating oneself inwardly (on one's inner voice) and being rigorous and strict with oneself; distancing oneself more strongly from the outside world and listening more to one's own inner self; with the loss of one's ability to adapt to the outside world, conquering the inner world instead, and learning to trust in one's own inner voice.
Resolution: Early retreat; carefully listening inwardly, hearing the commands of one's inner voice; only listening to what is truly interesting and important for oneself.
Archetypal principle: Saturn-Saturn.

Ovarian cancer

(ovarian carcinoma, see also Cancer)
Physical level: Ovaries (fertility).
Symptom level: Usually affects women between the ages of 65 and 70; the tumour often only produces symptoms when metastases have already colonised the entire stomach cavity and fluid from the tissues floods the stomach (→ascites formation); wounding at the source of life, primordial female trauma; always coming up too short; often as a precursor to the disease, there have been problems with one's children or family projects, which one cannot detach and dissociate oneself from; the fruits of one's labour become a threat; also not uncommon, sticking it out for too long in a relationship which has been deeply dissatisfying simply to satisfy external expectations (tradition, care); sacrificing oneself and one's own possibilities: this sacrifice sometimes reaches its ultimate climax in death from cancer.
Handling: Learning to protect oneself against attacks and assaults from outside interests on one's own creativity; releasing one's own children, and above all one's daughters, on the internal level as well; critically questioning one's own tendencies towards self-sacrifice; considering all the measures mentioned under →cancer: since cancer affects the complete organism, it must also be met across-the-board.
Resolution: Consistently going one's own feminine, creative way; recognising the need to switch from the physical and therefore (life-) threatening level to the challenging, but life-saving mental-spiritual level, and relying on expansive growth in this realm; discovering love that transcends all boundaries, setting oneself above external rule and standards laid down by oneself or others, and living and developing oneself solely

382

in accordance with the obligations of one's own creativity and highest law,
Archetypal principle: Moon-Pluto.

Ovarian carcinoma

see Ovarian cancer (above)

Ovarian cysts

Physical level: Ovaries (fertility).
Symptom level: Accumulations of fluid in the cavities of the ovaries, which only become dangerous in the rare case of them bursting open, or if extremely large, through them taking up too much space (nowadays can be examined at the early stage by ultrasound although they do not usually need to be operated on): spiritual water accumulates in the ovaries; stress-related hormonal disorders form the basis for misdirected growth, which in turn can cause bleeding: loss of life energy; disturbance of the cyclical follicle formation: falling out of (female) balance; simulated ovulation and great activity in the area of fertility without letting oneself get truly involved with the subject; swallowed down (encapsulated) tears, problems with the motherly principle (with one's own motherly aspects or one's own mother); feeling oneself to have been stunted in one's own creative potentials and unconsciously being angry about this; the unexpressed discontent shuts itself away in the form of a cyst.
Handling: Tackling the subject of fertility using the powers of the soul; becoming aware of one's true intentions in the domain of one's own fertility: admitting to oneself what one as a woman really wants to have growing here and what allows one to grow as a woman.
Resolution: Reconciliation with the role of fertility in one's own life.
Archetypal principle: Moon-Saturn.

Ovarian insufficiency

(inadequate performance of the ovaries)
Physical level: Ovaries (fertility).
Symptom level: Underdevelopment of the genitals: lack of fully-fledged sexuality; deficient formation of secondary sexual characteristics, such as breasts: being maladjusted in one's outward appearance as a woman; not being willing/able to stand behind one's outward appearance as an adult woman; disruptions of the menstrual cycle due to deficient follicle maturity: hampered/hindered fertility.
Handling: (in addition to allopathic replacement of what is lacking hormonally): owning up to one's refusal to become a fully-fledged woman with all its sexual consequences; learning to accept one's own sexual role and accepting and loving the outward appearance of a woman; owning up to the problems with one's own fertility and learning to face up to them (on all levels).
Resolution: Homeopathic approach: developing the animus (masculine spiritual qualities); allopathic approach: appreciating and accepting oneself as a woman: reconciling oneself with womanhood.
Archetypal principle: Moon-Saturn

Ovaries, inflammation

Physical level: Ovaries (fertility).
Symptom level: Cry for help of the feminine (lower) pole; conflict over the conception of children (procreation); combative conflict over fertility, creativity; danger of infertility due to chronification, adhesions, scars; very common in our anti-children, post-modern era: hidden behind the conflict is often a decision not to have children for pragmatic reasons that contradicts the wishes of one's

own soul, and which then – due to being unacknowledged – becomes physically manifested; unconscious rage against oneself because of this decision.

Handling: Turning one's attention to the issue of femininity and giving it recognition and respect; wrestling with oneself and the situation regarding one's own fertility/one's own offspring (also in the figurative sense) in an open(ly offensive) way; finding the courage to also fight for old models (many children, a large family) if these are one's own ideals; combatively confronting one's own creativity/one's brainchildren; finding a dynamic balance between the extreme positions.

Resolution: Bringing one's own children/own works into the world; allowing all one's courage and strength to flow into creative processes and dealing with conflicts consciously and courageously, developing an effective conflict culture.

Archetypal principle: Moon-Mars.

Ovaries, suppuration

(pyoovarium; see also Ovaries, inflammation, Fallopian tubes, suppuration, Adnexitis)

Physical level: Ovaries (fertility).

Symptom level: Usually occurs in combination with suppuration of the Fallopian tubes; severe acute or chronic conflict in the area of sexuality and fertility; the debris of war (pus) blocks creative expression.

Handling: Fighting to push through one's own ideas of fertility.

Resolution: Offensive confrontation with one's own creativity on all specifically-feminine levels.

Archetypal principle: Moon-Mars.

Over-sensitivity to pain

(hyperalgesia)

Physical level: Skin (border, contact, tenderness).

Symptom level: The skin's over-sensitivity to pain attracts attention; high sensitivity, tendency to be easily irritated.

Handling: treating the relevant zone of oversensitivity with respect to the corresponding organ domain (reflex zone phenomena); transforming physical sensitivity into emotional sensibility.

Resolution: Alertness for the signs from within: listening carefully to one's inner voice and bringing its message to the surface.

Archetypal principle: Venus/Saturn-Moon/Uranus/Neptune.

Ovulation, absent

(anovulatory cycle; see also Ovarian insufficiency, Hormone disorders, female)

Physical level: Ovaries (fertility).

Symptom level: The most natural form of contraception at an early age, during menopause or in times of great stress; protective mechanism in order not to conceive a child during times of extreme stress and/or spiritual overburdening; the woman cannot warm herself to the idea of conceiving children; fear of binding commitment; resistance towards an unsuitable partner; too much concentration on one's brainchildren (i.e. mental-spiritual conception).

Handling: Withdrawing the energy from external projects; reconsidering life and career plans; coming to rest; not dashing around so much outwardly (for oneself and others).

Resolution: Being in balance; creating security and a restful nest for oneself; tapping into and living out one's creative potential.

Archetypal principle: Moon/
Uranus-Saturn.

Ovulation pain

Physical level: Ovaries (fertility).
Symptom level: Ovulation (the bursting forth of the egg) becomes painful;
one's own feminine fertility becomes
a painful problem and cries out for
attention; sensibility has swung in the
opposite direction to over-sensitivity;
rejection of the "death and re-birth"
process.
Handling: Directing great sensitivity
into sensible channels; attentively
following and adapting oneself to the
cyclic process.
Resolution: Willingness to come
to terms with bursting forth into the
unknown and the daring venture of
motherhood; battling courageously for
one's own fertility.
Archetypal principle: Moon-Mars/
Uranus.

Oxyuriasis

see Threadworm infestation

Ozaena

(atrophic rhinitis, stinky nose)
Physical level: Nose (power, pride,
sexuality).
Symptom level: Evil stench from the
nose due to chronic contraction of the
nasal mucous membrane; purulent
secretions and dry crusts, which
stink as they break down (women
are much more frequently affected;
frequently of syphilitic origin, but
also as a consequence of incorrect,
long-term overuse of chemical nasal
sprays, which dry out the mucous
membrane): being a stinker, instead
of having a good nose for things;
being cut off from one's own intuition
and ability to get wind of things; unwilling (unable) to rely on one's own
hunches ("I can smell it in the air",
"scenting danger"); repelling others

by means of one's own effusions (the
nose as a weapon [of deterrence]):
isolating oneself from the world;
possibility of deterring erotic partners
up-front if one is someone that others
turn their noses up at; form of (unconscious) forward defence (like the
skunk); effectively establishing one's
limits and marking one's territory in a
lasting way; unresolved (unredeeming) possiblity for attracting attention
to oneself.
Handling: Making oneself aware of
one's own situation and recognising
the consequences; securing one's
territory against intruders in a more
pleasant way; tracking down the
deeper spiritual reason why one does
not want any close contact; making
an impression in a more developed
way and building up one's own personal (resonance) field.
Resolution: Reflecting back on
oneself and ensuring order in this
respect: keeping one's nose in one's
own business instead of poking it into
everyone else's
Archetypal principle: Mars-Pluto.

P

Paget's disease

see Ostitis deformans

Pain

(see also Phantom pain)
Physical level: Wherever sensitive
nerves (news service) are found, pain
is also possible.
Symptom level: Being compelled
to register sensation and feeling;
warning system of the body; call for
help by the tissue for better circulation or relief; inflammatory pain
related to aggressive conflicts; pain
from the wounds inflicted by physical

injuries; nerve pain stemming from oppressed, constricted pathways; the spiritual pains of a tormented soul: unlived, suppressed rage or even an act of self-punishment in the case of feelings of guilt; extreme (social or relationship-based) constriction can cause fear to the point of pain.
Handling/Resolution: Reacting to warnings as early as possible; responding to calls for help; using aggressive conflicts in the tissue as an occasion for more courageous confrontations on the mental-spiritual level; admittedly, this means that the pain is initially simply transferred; however, there is then a better chance of getting completely over and done with the subject on the spiritual level; using pains stemming from physical wounds as prompts to explore the parallel wounds which have arisen in the soul; using nerve-related pains to come to the aid of quashed impulses and suppressed information; coming to terms with spiritual pains on their own level, e.g. by turning one's attention to aspects of the soul that are lacking adequate care, relieving oppressed and over-loaded aspects of the soul of this burden, turning one's loving attention to wounded aspects of the soul and providing support for struggling areas of the soul; passion instead of passionate suffering.
Archetypal principle: Mars-Moon.

Panaritium

see Whitlow

Panarteritis

(arterial wall inflammation)
Physical level: Blood vessels (transport routes of the life force), arteries (energy pathways).
Symptom level: Conflict over the energy flow: the energy pathways have been overrun with war and are being fiercely fought over.
Handling: Critically addressing the issue of one's distribution of energy.
Resolution: Wrestling offensively and aggressively with the issue of one's distribution of energy.
Archetypal principle: Mars-Mercury.

Pancarditis

(all-out war over the heart) = endocarditis + myocarditis + pericarditis; (see relevant entries)

Pancreas, inflammation

(pancreatitis)
Physical level: Pancreas (aggressive breakdown [analysis], sweet enjoyment).
Symptom level: War in the explosives factory (doubly dangerous); common prior history: seeking refuge in alcohol and eating binges = ruinous sparing of consciousness while over-taxing the stomach; conflict avoidance or avoidance of confrontation and analysis.
Handling: Thinking and analysing more offensively, courageously and aggressively; trusting oneself to address highly-charged issues and to break them down into their individual details; turning (self-) destructive forces into creative work; relentlessly and courageously drawing out the best from one's own depths.
Resolution: Addressing the three basic forces of life: the creative, the conservative and the destructive principle (Sun, Saturn, Pluto).
Archetypal principle: Mars, Mercury.

Pancreatic cancer

(Pancreatic carcinoma; see also Cancer)

Physical level: Pancreas (aggressive breakdown [analysis], sweet enjoyment).

Symptom level: Aggressive destruction of pancreas cells with the danger of causing the digestive functions to collapse; degeneration in the area of aggressive breakdown of foods; wild and relentlessly proliferating growth of the degenerate gland cells; almost always starting from the head of the pancreas, three times more common in men than in women; having strayed so far off track from one's inherent line of development with regard to the breakdown and digestion of life that the body must help the (forgotten/suppressed) subjects to break through again; often a conflict over nourishment: not getting what one believes one is entitled to, or what one had already secretly regarded as one's assured possession; mental-spiritual growth in relation to this subject has been blocked for so long that it now forges a path in the body in an aggressive, uncontrolled way; in the area related to the subject concerned, the cancer realises in physical form that (turnaround) which would be spiritually necessary in the corresponding area of consciousness; early spreading of the malignant growth to subjects such as partnership and balancing of opposites (kidneys), exchange and communication (lungs) and meaning of life (liver).

Handling: Radically questioning the old, customs and traditions with regard to the breakdown and digestion of life that have been passed down to one and relentlessly destroying these if necessary; opening oneself up in the area of breakdown and digestion for one's own outlandish ideas and bold fantasies, and allowing them to flourish and expand courageously and freely; thinking back to early dreams, wishes and ideas about the processing of life, and bringing these (back) to life with wild decisiveness;

in the certainty of having nothing more to lose, drawing courage for self-realisation/one's own path; taking the growth impulse away from the body and directing it to more clarified (redeeming) levels; considering all the measures mentioned under →cancer: since cancer affects the complete organism, it must also be met across-the-board.

Resolution: Breaking with old ideas for processing things, digestion possibilities, analysis methods, assessments and judgements that are actually foreign to one's own being, and struggling aggressively in an open(ly offensive) manner for one's own way (in life) and meaning of life; finding expression in the spiritual area, in the world of meaning, instead of letting the body speak for itself; recognising the necessity to switch from the physical and thus (life-)threatening level to the challenging, but life-saving mental-spiritual level, and relying in this realm on expansive growth in the affected (Archetypal) area; discovering love that transcends all boundaries, setting oneself above external rule and standards laid down by oneself or others, and living and expressing oneself solely in accordance with the obligations of one's own highest law.

Archetypal principle: Mercury-Pluto.

Pancreatic carcinoma

see Pancreatic cancer (above)

Pancreatic insufficiency

Physical level: Pancreas (aggressive breakdown [analysis], sweet enjoyment), small intestine (breakdown (analysis), assimilation).

Symptom level: Lessening of one's ability to be critical; inner abandonment of the ability to get to the bottom of things; lack of understanding for details.

Handling: Consciously limiting self-criticism and criticism from outside; occasionally letting things just slide and not being too critical; learning to enjoy superficialities; emphasising the broad outline.

Resolution: Meeting life confidently.

Archetypal principle: Saturn-Mercury/Mars.

Pancreatitis

see Pancreas, inflammation

Panic (attacks)

(see also Anxiety)

Symptom level: Stifling restrictiveness, lack of openness towards life; misunderstanding with regard to the "end of life".

Handling: Confronting the god Pan and learning to stand one's ground; reconciling oneself with one's own mortality: fear of death is the restrictive narrowing of oneself before dying.

Resolution: Dying before dying; see information about Angelus Silesius and many other Christian mystics.

Archetypal principle: Saturn-Uranus-Pluto.

Papilloedema

see Cerebral compression syndrome

Papilloma

(benign growth of the skin or mucous membrane) see Ureteral papilloma

Paralysis

(paresis; see also Respiratory paralysis, Intestinal paralysis, Facial nerve paralysis, Median nerve paralysis, Myasthenia, Paraplegia)

Physical level: Musculature (motor, strength).

Symptom level: 1. Slack paralysis: absolute adynamia (lack of strength), having no power to push through one's will; 2. Spastic paralysis: great strength, but tense and uncontrollable, so therefore senseless; one's own desires and ideas have to remain unfulfilled; being locked up in the prison of one's own body in a gentle (slack paralysis) or violent way (→spasticity); not being able to get a grip on the outside world; paralysing fear, fleeing into helplessness.

Handling: 1. Learning to let go on the figurative level represented by the limb in question; 2. Also putting one's own strength to use without purpose or concrete objective; detaching oneself from the outcomes of one's own actions; letting go of one's ambition of being able to control the world; recognising the aspect of fleeing (e.g. from responsibility) in the paralysis; seeing through the paralysis as the most perfect "excuse" of all.

Resolution: Giving oneself completely, letting go of one's ambitions of controlling and being a "doer" and "go-getter".

Archetypal principle: ars (musculature)-Neptune (paralysis)/Uranus (spasticity).

Paranoia

(see also Spiritual crisis, Mental illness)

Symptom level: Mental disorder with systematised delusions, but in which the remaining powers of thought are often unaffected and remain quite intact; psychotherapy frequently fails due to the reluctance of the person affected to perceive any illness; within the field of psychiatry, it is claimed that it is not possible to determine the origin of the system of delusions; within the framework of esoteric philosophy or Jungian psychology, however, the origin is very evident: the people affected are inundated with shadow aspects which become part of their normal consciousness, while at the same time, the normality of our world recedes into the background behind these aspects, slipping into the shadow realm so to speak; inflationary overflooding with dark spiritual aspects which become overpowering, eventually taking over command of the central control headquarters of the brain and determining consciousness; the normality which has sunk down into the shadow realm only pops up on rare occasions in the form of so-called "islands of clarity" (Podvoll); persecution mania (belief that everyone is out to get one): shadow aspects that have been projected outwardly finally catch up with one; →megalomania: expectations for one's own life that have been separated off for too long suddenly flood one's consciousness; delusions of love and jealousy: those affected are flooded with unrealistic notions of love.

Handling/Resolution: Grounding on all levels: establishing as much contact as possible with the "normal" world (the family, social group, etc.) (→spiritual crisis); rebuilding the ability to distinguish between inner and outer reality, strengthening once again the lost boundary membrane between the upper world and the underworld, but without setting it in stone; taking seriously the deep spiritual longing which suddenly surfaces in many patients, although without encouraging spiritual exercises; prevention: making friends with the contents of one's shadow aspects (as soon as possible) and recognising these as one's own (as yet) unlived spiritual elements; accepting these and integrating their energies back into life instead of separating them off completely.

Archetypal principle: Saturn Neptune-Pluto.

Paraplegia

(see also Accident, Work accident/ Domestic accident, Sport accident, Traffic accident)

Physical level: Spinal canal (data highway) in the spinal column (dynamics and hold, uprightness).

Symptom level: Getting one's backbone/ back broken: getting one's will broken, being incapacitated/placed under disability, with the result that one can no longer be straight with oneself; breaking one's neck / one's back: losing one's life; lack of a lively relationship between the head and the lower body; complete blockage: powerlessness in relation to one's own lower pole; the feminine side appears to one as a foreign body; no feeling for the right time for material and spiritual giving; fall back into earliest childhood.

Handling: Learning to respect the will of others ("Thy will be done"); consciously processing one's close scrape with death; learning the significance of polarity by means of the example of the interplay between the upper and lower body; learning to give and give away freely and unconditionally; perceiving the regression to the learning level of a child as an opportunity to become like a child again in the figurative sense; taking (on) the staying (behind), respectively staying down (at school), not as a punishment, but as an opportunity to catch up on something that one had previously missed out on; directing one's central weighting in life inwards/downwards and getting to know and appreciate one's feminine side; discovering tenderness in place of sex; coming back down to Earth (from possible periods of high-flying); learning to forcefully assert oneself and to act from the calm of the sitting position; consciously letting go of standing, withstanding and standing up for oneself, and discovering other ways of facing up to life.

Resolution: Recognising the value of life in itself (irrespective of its terms and conditions); humility: looking up at the world from below; giving of oneself completey: having the world at one's feet.

Archetypal principle: Uranus (accident)-Saturn (handicap)/ Neptune (paralysis).

Parasomnia

see Sleep problems

Paratyphus

see Typhus abdominalis

Paresis

see Paralysis

Parkinson's disease

(paralysis agitans)
Physical level: Brain (communication, logistics), nerves (news service).
Symptom level: Intention tremor: whenever a movement impulse arises, it is hindered by tremors; in other cases →paralysis: on the basis of general (spiritual) inflexibility, the overexaggerated willpower becomes clear (disease pattern of Tito, Mao Tse-tung, Pope John Paul II.); wide gulf between one's expectations for achieving something in the world and inner paralysis/rigidity; being gripped by the fear of death or filled with great rage (trembling); wanting to shake off one's dread/experience of reality; rigidity of expression and movement; keeping a straight face, zombie existence; fear of failure, showing a well-oiled front; communication disorder; inability to adjust oneself to changes that are essential to life: changes in the weather and phases of the Moon can exacerbate the situation, as can other changes; the paralysis

can also cripple the vocal cords as organs of communication; cold hands and feet as an expression of contact problems; the frequently-observed wringing of the hands and wrestling for words shows the unbroken will; discrepancy between wants and abilities: people possessing great willpower, who must learn that not everything is doable by far; having blocked out a lot in terms of emotions and feeling in difficult relationships (family, social, political); having given one's all and worn oneself down; but still not having managed to convince others intellectually or shape one's environment according to one's own ideas; the resulting anxiety or rage is shown by the trembling; the mask-like poker face documents the rigidification which has arisen; exhaustion of the masculine pole due to overexaggerated expenditure of energy; threat to life due to respiratory paralysis: the break with communication and exchange becomes clear.

Handling: Digesting a life full of over-activity: establishing outer calm for the benefit of inner mobility; voluntarily "eating humble pie" and "putting less on one's plate"; paying attention to quality; concerning oneself with death and (re)solution; staring reality straight in the eye until it loses its power to terrorify (fixed, impenetrable gaze); venturing all the way into the narrow realm of one's own fear until it is transformed into expansiveness; learning to show one's true face; coming back down to Earth; exercises which revolve around inner balance and serve to help one find one's way (back) to one's own centre.

Resolution: Recognising the unity of humankind and the world; changing from being a monument (for others) into an inwardly lively and outwardly calm person (following one's own path).

Archetypal principle: Saturn/ Uranus.

Parodontitis

Physical level: Gums, periodontium (basic trust).

Symptom level: Preliminary stage of loss of the root; the conflict over deep basic trust flares up at the tip of the root and in the surrounding periodontium (parodontitis apicalis); loosening of the teeth with advanced age (parodontitis marginalis = preliminary stage of →parodontosis) on the basis of chronic conflicts centred around basic trust that has been exhausted; the build-up of dental calculus (tartar) deposits around the neck of the tooth provides favourable conditions for the formation of periodontal pockets in which chronically suppurating →inflammations occur.

Handling: Open(ly offensive) confrontations with the issue of basic trust and committed struggle for basic trust; seeing through the ineffectual attempts to bolster and prop up one's own weapons (i.e. by encircling them with walls of plaque) and providing genuine protection and corresponding care of one's weapons; recognising the conflict-ridden undermining of the basis of one's own vitality and courageously counteracting it; creating a dependable place of regeneration for one's weapons: just as we regenerate ourselves every night in bed, the teeth must also be able to regenerate themselves in the tooth bed (periodontium) in order to stay in good shape; exercises in gaining basic trust.

Resolution: Leading an offensive and courageous life and putting one's weapons into use for the red hot issues of life; getting a grip on life.

Archetypal principle: Moon/Mars (periodontium)-Mars (inflammation).

Parodontosis

(contraction of the gums)

Physical level: Gums, periodontium (basic trust), teeth (aggression, vitality).

Symptom level: The contraction of the complete periodontium (gums, periodontal membrane and alveolar bones), frequently as a late after-effect of chronic and deep-set →inflammations of the gums, i.e. of conflicts in the area of basic trust; the contraction of the gum tissue and degeneration of the root of the tooth lead to loosening of the teeth or even to them falling out: the bed, respectively the basis, of vitality shrinks away, resulting in badly- anchored weapons; uprooted, unhealthy aggression; shows the deficits in basic trust and courage to face life; exposed neck of the teeth: exposure of the roots of aggression, until laid bare and naked, they can no longer give the tooth enough hold; the wobbly weapons correspond to the exhaustion of one's own vitality - one's vital powers begin to waver; hate that has sunk into the shadows, aggression set adrift; aggression that has died off, decaying vitality, resignation.

Handling: Laying bare the roots of the aggression problem right down to its very depths; admitting to oneself that one's aggression and vital strength have no sound basis; concerning oneself with the issue of basic trust and sinking one's efforts into ensuring that the teeth can continue to perform their aggressive work (of shooting off at the mouth); admitting to oneself how naked, exposed and forsaken one's own weapons already are and becoming active in standing by them: creating a dependable place of regeneration for one's weapons: just as we regenerate ourselves every night in bed, the teeth must also be able to regenerate themselves in the tooth bed (periodontium) in order to stay in good shape; exercises in belated establishment of basic trust.

Resolution: Building a nest for the weapons of the mouth and not only tending to (looking after) and being tender to (caring for) them, but also to their basis; establishing basic trust, and building on this foundation, leading an offensive, courageous life; getting a grip on life; apart from in the first months of pregnancy, basic trust arises from experiences of unity (peak experiences), as is the objective of almost all meditation practices. Archetypal principle: Moon/Mars-Neptune (contraction).

Parotitis epidemica

see Mumps

Paunch

see Fat belly, Obesity

Pavor nocturnus

see Nyctophobia

PCP

see Rheumatism

Pediculosis

see Crablouse infestation, Headlouse infestation

Pelvic vein thrombosis

(see also Thrombosis, Leg oedema)
Physical level: Pelvis (basis of life, resonance base), legs (mobility, progress, stability).
Symptom level: Congealment and clumping of the life energy: the life flow is (painfully) hindered; danger of →lung embolism (stopping of vital communication); the return path of the life energy to the centre (the fountain of youth) is blocked; something lays itself at cross purposes to the return energy transport: not getting anything, or not getting enough in return for what one has given out – in the left (feminine) or the right (masculine) area; disturbed life flow in the pelvis and leg area (often in connection with long periods of immobility and hormone pills); blockage in the leg: emphasis of the lower extremities and the lower (feminine) pole of the body; painful, heavy and therefore clumsy and swollen leg due to the build-up of spiritual water that has sunk to the bottom; cry for help from the affected leg for the disposal of the built-up residues; hindering of movement and progress: being forced to rest.
Handling: Concentrating on one's own vitality; voluntarily slowing down the life flow and steering the ship of life into calmer waters; voluntarily putting emphasis on giving over taking; giving the lower, female area more loving attention and awareness (more weight); finding one's point of focus (i.e. central weighting) (in rest), approaching things with inner calm; letting oneself fall emotionally and thus allowing oneself to arrive at one's true self.
Resolution: Reconciliation and harmonisation of the two poles of giving and taking; contemplation in the form of a calmer flow of the life energy in order to discover the true central focus of one's spiritual tasks; enjoying giving of oneself to the point of being totally spent (without ulterior motives); working from the opposite pole: considering returning to the origin.
Archetypal principle: Moon-Saturn.

Penis cancer

(see also Cancer)
Physical level: Penis (desire, power).
Symptom level: Aggressive destruction (usually) of the lance (penis) tip: destruction to the point of total loss of the instrument of power; almost always the result of prolonged, chronic conflicts (→inflammations) of the inner foreskin, in which the smegma (foreskin lubrication) also comes into play (issue of cleanliness):

degeneration in the area of one's aggressive thrusting forward (self-assertion) of masculine-phallic strength; wild and ruthlessly rampant growth of the degenerated skin cells, almost always starting from the head of the penis; having strayed so far off track from one's inherent line of development with regard to masculine thrusting forward (self-assertion) and procreation that the body helps the (forgotten/repressed) issues to break through again; mental-spiritual growth in relation to these subjects has been blocked for so long that they now manifest themselves in an aggressive and random way; the cancer realises physically in the phallic area that (turnaround) which would be spiritually necessary in the corresponding area of consciousness.

Handling: Radically calling into question the old, handed-down customs and traditions with regard to masculine thrusting forward (assertion), sexual-phallic behaviour and sexuality in general, and if necessary, ruthlessly destroying these; opening oneself up in the area of masculinity and procreation to one's own outlandish ideas and bold fantasies and courageously and freely allowing them to flourish and expand; thinking back to early dreams and one's own objectives, wishes and ideas in relation to sexuality, masculinity and procreation, bringing these (back) to life and putting them into practice with wild decisiveness; beginning on the mental-spiritual level and fighting on the outermost front; in the certainty of having nothing more to lose, mustering courage for one's own self-realisation/one's own path; taking the growth impulse away from the body and directing it to more resolved (redeeming) levels; considering all the measures mentioned under →cancer: since cancer affects the complete organism, it must also be met across-the-board.

Resolution: Providing expression for oneself in the mental-spiritual area instead of allowing the body to speak up for itself; recognising the necessity to switch from the physical and thus (life-)threatening level to the challenging, but life-saving mental-spiritual level, and relying in this realm on expansive growth in the domain of creativity; discovering love that transcends all boundaries; setting oneself above external rule and standards laid down by oneself or others and living and expressing oneself solely in accordance with the obligations of one's own highest law.
Archetypal principle: Mars-Pluto.

Penis, inflammation of the cavernous body

Physical level: Penis (desire, power).
Symptom level: Unconscious conflict over the firm standing of the "little man"; civil war in the dwelling of one's own body instead of the battle of the sexes.
Handling: Courageously and offensively making oneself aware of one's problems dealing with the phallic forces and making use of them in one's relationship instead of directing them against oneself.
Resolution: Bringing hot sex and burning desire into the game of life.
Archetypal principle: Pluto-Jupiter-Mars.

Pericardial sac inflammation

(pericarditis, armoured heart)
Physical level: Heart (seat of the soul, love, feelings, energy centre).
Symptom level: Unresolved conflict in the area around the heart; stockpiled spiritual conflicts of the heart; besiegement of the heart by

aggressive spiritual energies; danger of strangulation of the heart due to spiritual backwater that has been discharged by the conflict and stored up (pericardial sac tamponade); a matter of heated conflict that is close to one's heart (muscle); vain attempts to pack one's heart in cotton wool (weakening, softening of the heart) or to wall it in (armoured heart); stone-walling the centre of one's heart (with calcium).

Handling: Learning to fight for one's own centre and matters of the heart; applying oneself with burning passion to the protection of one's own centre; bringing to light more firmness and determination in matters of the heart, loving in a heart-melting (heart soften-ing) or strong (armoured heart) way, fighting for all-embracing, caring love.

Resolution: Protecting one's own innermost self, standing up and fight-ing for the protection of one's own centre; placing caring for the capital of the body's landscape in the centre of one's life.

Archetypal principle: Sun-Mars.

Pericarditis

see Pericardial sac inflammation

Perineal tear

see Birth complications

Period pains

see Menstruation

Periosteum inflammation

see Periostitis (below)

Periostitis

(shin splints, see also Bone marrow inflammation, although the conflicts here only extend as far as the perios-teum and not into the marrow)

Physical level: Bone surface (stabil-ity, strength).

Symptom level: Conflicts (→inflam-mation) that go right to (the skin of) one's bones/to the outskirts of one's own internal structure; profound con-flict which can lead to cracks in one's feeling of self-esteem; war over sta-bility and the structures in one's life, struggle over the protective sheaths of the framework; offensive conflicts over norms and laws.

Handling: Dealing with conflicts that go down to the bone; allowing one's accustomed stability and familiar structures to be called into question; conducting an open(ly offensive) struggle in the area of norms and laws.

Resolution: Calling everything about oneself into question right down to the bone.

Archetypal principle: Saturn-Mars.

Peritonitis

(see also Stomach perforation)

Physical level: Abdominal cavity, starting primarily from the stomach (feeling, receptiveness) and intestines (processing of material impressions).

Symptom level: War, struggle for survival; dispute over the body's cen-tre – the abdominal cavity; everything revolves around the stomach, around one's own navel: contemplating one's navel; "playing dead" reflex.

Handling: Addressing the matters of one's own centre; contemplating one's own (spiritual) naval in (good) time; giving the stomach phases of absolute rest (e.g. by fasting; fasting every night for at least 12 hours, and every year for at least one week).

Resolution: Acting courageously and offensively from one's own centre; trusting one's gut feeling: perceiving and taking seriously the navel (hub) of one's (own) world.

Archetypal principle: Mercury/ Moon-Mars.

Permanent erection

(priapism; e.g. as a result of prostate and urinary bladder illnesses)
Physical level: Penis (desire, power).
Symptom level: Energy (blood) blockage in the organ of (pro)creation (first interpret the basic illness); high pressure in the "magic wand", but no release valve; permanent arousal with pain, and without sexual stimulation and ejaculation: unconscious permanent readiness for copulation and fertilisation; danger of ending up at the opposite pole of →impotence.
Handling: Clarifying the relationship to phallic energy; becoming aware of the basic problem; dispatching energy and attentiveness to the sexual domain; creating outlets for the pressure to be creative; developing permanent readiness to address the issue of polarity.
Resolution: Thrusting life energy into creational processes; standing up for one's own masculine sexuality.
Archetypal principle: Mars-Pluto.

Pernicious anaemia

(Biermer's disease)
Physical level: Large intestine (unconscious, underworld).
Symptom level: Lack of Vitamin B12 due to stomach mucosa problems leads to disorders in the maturation of the red blood corpuscles – the carriers of the life force; loss of performance: no longer wanting or being able to do things; dizzy "feign"ting spells (→balance disorders) and blackouts: deceiving oneself and fleeing from responsibility; difficulties with walking: no longer managing to move forwards; jaundice (icterus): backup in the breakdown of the blood; →burning tongue, atrophy of the tongue musculature: despite the burning desire ("a fiery tongue"), having nothing more to say.

Handling: (after administration of Vitamin B12): withdrawing oneself from the performance-based, go-getter domain; being honest and giving up responsibility, laying functions aside; putting the brakes on outwardly in favour of inner development; letting out what one is burning to say for as long as this is possible.
Resolution: Shifting down a gear in one's activities instead of throttling the flow of the life force.
Archetypal principle: Pluto-Mars-Saturn/Neptune.

Perniones

see Chilblains

Pertussis

see Whooping cough

Perversions, sexual

(see also Fetishism, Neurosis)
Physical level: Starting from the genital region (sexuality, polarity, procreation), the whole organism is affected; ultimately a consciousness problem.
Symptom level: (examples):
1. Paedaphelia (love of young boys, well-accepted in ancient times): sign of immaturity; polarity problem; not involving oneself with the sexual opposite pole;
2. Games with urine ("drinking nature's champagne"; "foreign urine therapy") and faeces: confronting suppressed shadow subjects on the concrete level;
3. Sex with animals (bestiality): regression in evolution; vain attempt to reconcile oneself with one's animalistic sides;
4. Sex with corpses: vain attempt to learn to love death;
5. Sadomasochism, piercing: attempt on the concrete level to bring together aggression (Mars) and love (Venus);

6. Domination: subjugating oneself sexually to the opposite pole instead of honouring it on the figurative level and serving the feminine principle;
7. Group sex: attempt to compensate for the lack of quality (content: love) with quantity (form).
Handling: Bringing awareness into one's concrete actions; deviating from the norm in more sophisticated domains.
Resolution: Elevating the level; some examples: from bestiality to Francis of Assisi, from eating faeces to shadow therapy; bringing so-called abnormal perversion into resolved form: becoming an extraordinary person.
Archetypal principle: Pluto-Uranus.

Pes varus

see Club foot

Petit mal

see Epilepsy

Pfeiffer's glandular fever

see Mononucleosis

Phantom pain

Symptom level: Lost limbs, but also teeth, continue to cause pain although they have long since ceased to be physically present; the structures continue to exist in consciousness as long as their image has not been deleted in the astral domain: cries of help from an unprocessed shock/loss situation.
Handling/Resolution: Consciously re-enacting the experience of the loss once again (even operations under full anaesthetic can be brought to one's awareness using the techniques of reincarnation therapy) in order to be able to really let go of the lost limb.
Archetypal principle: Neptune/Mars.

Pharmacomania

(compulsive desire to conjure up pleasant states by means of suitable medications, flowing transition to →drug addiction)
Symptom level: Drugs used include, above all, psychotropic medications, such as Lexotanil, but also pain-killers and sedatives, and even all the way up to narcotics in order to get "high"; increasing medication abuse, in particular, also in connection with the new "designer drugs".
Handling: Owning up to one's lack of freedom; acknowledging one's dependency as a precondition for being able to free oneself of it; ensuring the desired consciousness states on more resolved (redeeming) levels: calmness, balance, ecstasy, happiness, etc.
Resolution: Finding the way to freedom by acknowledging one's own bondage and allowing oneself to be helped in the process: "Only you alone can do it, but you cannot do it alone" (realisation from the field of AA groups).
Archetypal principle: Neptune.

Pharyngitis

see Sore throat, Inflammation

Pheochromocytoma

(adrenal gland medulla tumour; see also High blood pressure)
Physical level: Adrenal glands (centre for stress regulation, water balance and sex life).
Symptom level: The production of noradrenalin and adrenalin from the tumour results in suddenly-attacking hypertensive crises with extreme blood pressure peak levels: initially coming under extreme pressure in phases; later transition to permanent high blood pressure: no longer being able to get out of the pressure situation.

Handling: Voluntarily placing oneself under great pressure in the struggle over the main decisive (life-and-death) issue; sorting out which problem that repeatedly places one under great pressure without really being resolved the tumour symbolically corresponds to.

Resolution: Vigorously facing up to the great struggle and clarifying the underlying problem.

Archetypal principle: Mars-Jupiter/ Pluto.

Phimosis

(narrowing of the foreskin on the penis)

Physical level: Foreskin (curtain in front of the spearhead).

Symptom level: Constriction of the foreskin which is usually congenital, but also sometimes arises from chronic inflammations, and which has the result that the foreskin can no longer be drawn back over the glans: not wanting to leave the protective shield of childhood; not being able/willing to show the spearhead/ pinnacle of masculinity: not facing up to one's own masculinity; being ashamed of one's sexuality and desire; not wanting to expose oneself out of fear of being revealed; difficulties in "making a stand like a man" and unveiling the "glistening jewel of masculine potency": difficulties in withdrawing one's sword from the scabbard and making decisions (Latin: dēcīsiō = 'a cutting off'); if the problem is not cleared up surgically, this often leads to the avoidance of women and fear of them, and thus impairs life as a whole.

Handling: Circumcision as takes place in some cultures as a puberty ritual: the glans as a symbol of the now unfolded male potency is freed for all time; in our society, physical enlargement, or if necessary, operation (circumcision significantly before puberty and without the surrounding ritual framework is not enough for becoming a man, although it does still enable a step in this direction); making oneself aware of one's constriction in the sexual-masculine area and doing away with it on all levels before it becomes even more troublesome than keeping the member clean already is; developing the courage to show and demonstrate one's masculinity; becoming a good lover (with staying power), since the glans, due to being laid bare by the circumcision and the resulting continual stimulation, becomes less sensitive (an advantage for the female partner, although sometimes a disadvantage for the man); if not corrected, there is also the danger of later penis cancer based on the potential for inadequate hygiene (penis cancer in circumcised men is just as unknown as cancer of the uterus is in the corresponding cultures).

Resolution: Making oneself aware of the pre-determined constriction, or the constriction which has arisen in the course of various conflicts in the area of one's own masculinity; opening oneself up to this area and staking out the space one needs in order to become a grown man (allowing one's member to grow to masculine size and uprightness).

Archetypal principle: Mars/ Moon-Saturn.

Phlebitis

see Vein inflammation

Phlegmon

(suppurating inflammation of the connective tissue)

Physical level: Connective tissue (connection, stability, binding commitment).

Symptom level: Usually spreads out through gaps in the tissue and thus also brings with it the danger of an overall general sepsis: deep-seated conflict tending to chronification on the level of inner connections and binding commitment; this becomes widespread by eating its way into out-lying gaps of the body and brings with it the danger of the situation bursting its banks and turning into a life-threat-ening poisoning.

Handling: Fighting out wars down to the deepest levels and committing oneself to great battles which fling a great deal of conflict matter to the surface and smash a lot of delicate porcelain to pieces (war debris in the form of pus); intervening and putting a stop to the threat before it is too late.

Resolution: Not shying away from even the deepest conflicts in order to protect one's life.

Archetypal principle: Mars.

Phobia

(see also Anxiety, Agoraphobia, Claustrophobia, Heart neurosis, Can-cer, fear of, Nyctophobia)

Symptom level: Experiences that frequently stem from completely different times and the correspond-ing behaviour accompanying these threaten the present time: aberrations with respect to time, as in the case of neurosis and chronic anxiety con-ditions which, as those affected are often fully aware, have no basis in reality, but which they cannot come to grips with due to not having seen through the symbolic components involved, such as:

1. Carcinophobia (see Cancer, fear of; fear of the all-engulfing, destruc-tive aspect of cancer illnesses): getting to know and accept the all-en-gulfing, destructive aspect of one's own being; getting to know the dark goddesses Hekate and Kali.

2. Fear of heights/acrophobia (fear of falling, →vertigo): finding the arche-typal fear of the Fall from Paradise in oneself and accepting it.

3. Recognising animal phobias and the learning tasks inherent in them: recognising in the snake one's own snake-like aspects (seduction into polarity, temptation); in the spider, one's own spider-like aspects (laying devious traps, shying away from open conflict, sucking others dry, (ab)using the masculine principle only for pro-creation purposes); in the dog (wolf), one's own unconscious aggression (aggressive barking, baring one's teeth); in rats, (symbol of filth and dirt) impure tendencies (transmitters of the Plague); in mice, the aspects of being lightning-fast, uncontrollable and erotically-cuddly, but at the same time, getting in everywhere and being a thieving freeloader (living off the table and supplies of others).

4. Erythrophobia (fear of →blushing): accepting one's own shame, on the one hand, and sexual desire on the other; recognising one's own feelings of inferiority and dependency on the opinions of other people.

Handling: (general): finding and accepting the nature of what is feared in one's own unconscious; correcting the time aberration by making clear to oneself which other time period the relevant adverse experience belongs to; reincarnation therapy.

Resolution: Reconciling oneself with this part of the soul and liberating the energy that is tied up here for use in other areas.

Archetypal principle: Saturn (the restriction of fear in general)-Pluto.

Photodermatoses

(light dermatoses; see also Allergy [light as an allergen])

Physical level: Skin (border, contact, tenderness).

Symptom level: Reacting to bright sunlight or tanning lamps with irrita-tion and blister formation: (uncon-sciously) sensing the brightness, the light side of reality, the masculine pole as dangerous, and fighting against it on one's own border and contact area (opposite pole: archetypally feminine Moon); fever and general feeling of malaise: general mobilisation against the light and its symbolism; shunning one's own inner light: people who tend to assume the worst of themselves (light shadow); one's own shadow resists the symbolism of the light.

Handling: Critically confronting one's own light side; facing up to one's own apparently glowing reflection in an open(ly offensive) way and determining whether everything that is glittering truly is light; reconciling oneself with both sides of one's own soul: the acceptance of the shadow also leads to one being better able to bear the light.

Resolution: Developing awareness of one's own light sides and thus taking on the dark aspects of the soul more lightly.

Archetypal principle: Saturn/ Venus (skin)-Sun/Pluto.

Pickwick syndrome

(being extremely overweight with heart-lung syndrome; see also Obesity)

Physical level: Heart (seat of the soul, love, feelings, energy centre), lungs (contact, communication, freedom), stomach (feeling, receptiveness).

Symptom level: The lungs are so blocked by too much fat and the raised diaphragm (also due to fat) that this results in insufficient gas exchange; consequences include arterial oxygen deficiency, increase in the red blood corpuscles and pronounced desire to sleep (somnolence): consciousness disorders due to too many waste residues (CO_2) in the flow of the life energy; symptoms associated with extreme →obesity: search for security and safety behind one's own walls (nothing insulates/isolates better than fat); protective layer against a loveless environment; desire to be left in peace in one's own fortress of fat; not wanting to live out one's own sexual role; feeling of importance and power; weight(iness); vicarious satisfaction substitute; search for caring attention/love: "putting on weight due to comfort eating"; outer fullness instead of inner fulfilment; reward through eating; avoidance of reality (somnolence); not being favourably disposed towards oneself.

Handling: Reducing communication to the outside world: getting in contact and communicating with oneself instead; recognising on the basis of the deficient supply of energy that one could get by with much less; climbing to another level of consciousness; realising security in other ways: rapid-fire responses, well-padded financial cushions at the bank, etc.; realising weightiness (importance) on the social level; finding more resolved (redeeming) access to the Venusian realm of enjoyment; seeking inner fulfilment; striving for a well-rounded attitude towards life; rewarding oneself by other ways and means than eating: consciously nibbling with delight, sensual eating rituals; gentle massages; working out new patterns for life, a new inner form; gritting one's teeth and biting one's way through in the concrete sense; conscious fasting for healing purposes.

Resolution: Love which embraces the body, soul and spirit; feeling well-rounded, gaining spiritual weight.

Archetypal principle: Mercury-Jupiter-Venus.

Pigeon chest

Physical level: Rib cage (sense of self/Ego, personality)

Symptom level: Narrow rib cage with keel-like projecting breastbone and trough-shaped indented sides of the chest; on the basis of vitamin D deficiency and lack of sunlight, or congenital: deprived children (in the shadow realms of life) who lack vitamins (the stuff of life) and sun (life energy); in some cases, constriction of the heart and the lobes (wings) of the lungs: the areas of feeling and communication are constrained; high flying is greatly hampered with wings that have been clipped in this way.

Handling: Resigning oneself to one's own restricted space, then slowly filling it with life and expanding it; restricting communication, controlling feelings; getting to know and appreciate one's own darkness, the basis.

Resolution: Filling out the space that Fate has allocated one and making the best out of it.

Archetypal principle: Saturn (rib cage)/Sun (heart)/Mercury (lungs)-Saturn (restriction).

Pigment deficiency

see Albinism (congenital form which affects the whole body); Vitiligo (acquired form on localised areas of the skin)

Pigment flecks

(chloasma, melasma; see also Liver spot [lentigo], Birthmark [naevus], Freckles [Ephelides], Age-related symptoms [age marks])

Physical level: Skin (border, contact, tenderness).

Symptom level: Dark skin flecks arise during pregnancy or as a result of hormone therapies, respectively taking contraceptive pills; mark (of distinction), feminine stigmatisation; not feeling comfortable in one's female role; protective darkening, covering up; being blackened (denigrated) or marked.

Handling: Accepting the dark flecks of one's own being; acknowledging and accepting the mark of distinction instead of feeling oneself to be

marked; recognising pregnancy or fertility and even just womanhood in general as a mark of distinction; owning up to one's darker sides; developing a thicker, darker hide that is therefore less sensitive and consequently safer; defending one's own skin.

Resolution: Marking oneself with distinction; living up to one's own distinctiveness; standing by one's own shadow; ensuring protection.

Archetypal principle: Moon/Venus-Pluto.

Pimples

see Folliculitis

Pituitary adenoma

Physical level: Hypophysis (pituitary gland; harmony and adaptation at the highest level)

Symptom level: Benign tumour that often produces hormones, more commonly affecting women; 1. Eye symptoms because the tumours press on the path of the optic nerves; 2. Other symptoms depending on the hormones produced: prolactin results in galactorrhoea (milky discharge; 30 % of cases); 3. Growth hormone (HGH): →acromelagia (all possible extremities of the body, such as the chin, tip of the nose, etc. begin to grow again, 20% of cases); 4. ACTH production (excess production of cortisol): →Cushing's syndrome (10% of cases).

Handling: 1. In the case of eyesight coming under pressure: call to look less to the outside and more to the inside, insight instead of outlook; 2. Involving one's own maternal-feminine side in the life flow; becoming more generous with one's archetypally feminine gifts; 3. Venturing further into the world, taking up more room, coming out of oneself more courageously; enabling one's own courageous and space-taking growth on mental and spiritual levels; 4. Concentrating on one's own inner centre.

Resolution: 1. Acquiring inner ability to see through things; becoming insightful, all-seeing; 2. Freely making a gift to the surrounding world of one's own anima (one's feminine gifts); 3. Growing beyond oneself on the mental-spiritual level; 4. Strengthening one's own centre and recognising it as what is essential.

Archetypal principle: Mercury-Jupiter.

Pityriasis versicolor

("sun fungus"; see also Dermatomycoses)

Physical level: Skin (border, contact, tenderness).

Symptom level: Yellow-brown to black, pea-sized flecks which flow together to form patterns and lend the skin a dirty appearance: tainted impression; peeling of the skin in branflake-shaped form after scratching: being too weak to defend one's own skin, which becomes a hotbed for fungal eczema to play around in; "bristling with energy"; despite the protective acid layer, one's own border fortifications are occupied by the fungus; all non-living material can fall victim particularly easily to occupation by fungi (fungi are saprophytes, which feed on dead organic matter).

Handling: Clearing up what lies behind the dirty impression that one's own border and contact areas are making to the outside world; opening one's borders in the mental-spiritual respect in order to be able to remain unscathed; opening oneself up to new and foreign impressions and making them one's own instead of allowing oneself (the body) to be taken over by foreign intruders; developing willingness to give: being clear about the essence of every symbiosis: mutual dependence on one another, mutual reliance on one another, mutual using

of one another; living and letting live, an interplay of You and Me; confronting the issues of freeloading and sponging off others: "Where do I allow others to freeload off me, and where do I myself freeload off others?"; opening up one's own areas that are no longer used and consequently no longer needed, i.e. lifeless areas, to new and foreign life impulses; making one's own unused abilities available to others; taking in vital (living) nourishment, which fungi do not like.

Resolution: Confronting stimulating elements at the contact areas with the outside world in a courageous and open(ly offensive) way and allowing them get in(volved with oneself) ; opening oneself up to life, even also including its aspect of death; bringing life into one's own living terrain (in consciousness); bringing the dead areas back to life.

Archetypal principle: Venus/ Saturn-Pluto.

Placenta previa

(displacement of the placenta close to or over the cervix; see also Birth complications)

Physical level: Womb (fertility, safety and security).

Symptom level: (In the case of the mother): inability to give up the child; (in the case of the child): hopeless perspective on life; (for both): being reliant on outside aid.

Handling: Meditating on the mother role in the sense of Khalil Gibran: "Your children are not your children. They are the sons and daughters of Life's longing for itself..."; (for the mother and the later adult): obtaining outside aid in the case of blockages and obstructions along one's path (in life); learning to willingly accept assistance.

Resolution: Learning to deal with obstacles; doing away with them; not

allowing oneself to be discouraged, even in hopeless situations.
Archetypal principle: Moon-Saturn.

Placental insufficiency

(see also Birth complications)
Physical level: Womb (fertility, safety and security).
Symptom level: (In the case of the mother): inability to nourish the child adequately until the end; (in the case of the child): lack of nourishment due to sclerosis of the placenta villi, circulatory disorders of the placenta (e.g. in the case of nicotine, alcohol and drug consumption, incorrect diet, an overload of pollutants, after prolonged use of the pill), or in the case of children carried over term.
Handling: (On the part of the mother): making oneself aware of one's deficient ability to nourish or one's attacks against the unborn (e.g. through smoking) and exploring the (underlying) reason; admitting to oneself to what degree this situation endangers the life of the child (e.g. impairing the development of intelligence).
Resolution: Reconciling oneself with the pregnancy and the mother role at an early stage; finding support for oneself; instilling trust in the child; nourishing and serving it.
Archetypal principle: Moon-Saturn.

Placental separation, premature

(see also Birth complications)
Physical level: Womb (fertility, safety and security).
Symptom level: Occurs almost only in combination with other existing threats such as →gestosis, →eclampsia, →high blood pressure, bleeding disorders, accident or an umbilical cord that is too short. (In the case of the mother): wanting to get rid of the

child prematurely and thereby putting the child's and one's own life at risk; over-reaction in the case of panic and shock; wanting to push the problem away; (in the case of the child): life-threatening, premature ejection; (for both): being reliant on outside (operative) help.
Handling: Making friends with the mother role in order to hold it out to the end; scrutinising one's willling-ness to give a child the gift of life for unconscious, ambivalent or contrary tendencies; (for the mother and the later adult): willingly accepting help from outside and admitting to oneself how necessary it is.
Resolution: Patiently and humbly waiting for the right moment; doing what must be done voluntarily and in the correct sequence (i.e. responsibility = ability to respond to the demanding challenges of Fate).
Archetypal principle: Moon-Uranus.

Plantar warts

(see also Foot-sole warts)
Physical level: Sole of the foot (deep-rootedness, grounding).
Symptom level: "The thorn in one's flesh"; painful contact with the ground, painful standing and understanding, painful deep-rootedness; tense relationship with Mother Earth.
Handling: Treading more gently/taking a softer stance; learning to deal more carefully with the Earth and with one's own roots; learning to stand up for oneself even in painful and difficult situations; asking oneself where the shoe (of life) is pinching; also letting in painful impressions, voluntarily allowing oneself to be impressed.
Resolution: Allowing understanding (for painful situations) to grow.
Archetypal principle: Mars-Neptune.

Plasmocytoma

see Bone cancer

Pleural inflammation

(pleuritis)
Physical level: Pleura (tensioning framework and envelope of the lungs).
Symptom level: Conflict in the area of communication (take into account basic diseases such as → pericardial sac inflammation, lung infection, and above all, →pulmonary consumption);
1. Dry inflammation with discharge of aggression (irritable coughing, "coughing up" what one really thinks), painful, accelerated, shallow communication (breathing);
2. Damp inflammation with communication blockages (respiratory distress); general mobilisation (fever); leakage of spiritual fluid (pleural effusions).
Handling: Dealing with conflicts relating to the communication area (the scene that one mixes in); stating one's opinion to others openly and offensively ("Who could be a good source of friction?"); communicating in a quicker, easier and more unconstrained way; behaving with more care towards one's own communications organs ("What is rubbing me up the wrong way?"); engaging in general conflicts; letting out the spiritual; sharing oneself /one's ideas.
Resolution: Courageously stamping out a path for one's own opinions in the high-tension field of communication; letting out (expressing) spiritual subjects, taking them seriously and giving them importance; realising oneself in life and in communication with others; working from the opposite pole: once again becoming flexible and fluent (able to glide smoothly).
Archetypal principle: Mars-Mercury.

Pleuritis

see Pleural inflammation

PMS

see Pre-menstrual syndrome

Pneumonia

see Lung inflammation

Pneumothorax

Physical level: Lungs (contact, communication, freedom), pleura (outer lining of the lungs; tensioning frame, which expands the lungs), pleural space (low-pressure system for elastic expansion of the lungs).
Symptom level: Usually occurs due to the breakthrough of tubercular cavities into the pleural space or due to external injuries (first clarify and interpret the basic situation); air, which pushes its way into the pleural space, reduces the low pressure which is necessary here, causing the corresponding lobe of the lung to collapse: this leads to the dropping out of the exchange (of breathing) on this side; air on the wrong level stops the airing process; the inner wings (lobes of the lungs) are clipped.
Handling: Consciously reviewing one's own willingness for exchange and communication; coming to terms with the air element and learning to integrate it correctly; clarifying which of one's own behavioural patterns could make the rib cage, as a symbol of personal power, the victim of a violent attack on its (structural) integrity; recognising the situation of "being a lame duck" and opening oneself inwardly to again unfolding and spreading one's own wings.
Resolution: Reconciling oneself with the process of exchange – which the lobes (wings) of the lungs ensure – in order to fly through life on them.
Archetypal principle: Mercury-Uranus.

Podagra

see Gout

Poisoning

(intoxication; intentional poisoning, see Suicide; otherwise see also Self-poisoning, Botulism, Accident, Work accident/Domestic accident, Heavy-metal poisoning)

Physical level: Primarily the stomach (feeling, receptiveness), then the complete organism.

Symptom level: Accidental assimilation of dangerous materials through misjudgement of the danger and/or carelessness: pushing the digestion of the world too far; carelessly and unconsciously overestimating one's own capabilities with regard to handling the various elements and dangers of life.

Handling: Carelessness in dealing with spiritual poison (such as gossip, malicious rumours, holding grudges, being easily offended, etc.); recognising the poisoning of one's own life basis; identifying slipshod handling of the (processing of the) world; developing a better nose for dangers; consciously believing oneself capable of more and relieving the body of the substitute role.

Resolution: Awareness and attentiveness in dealing with the world and its dangers.

Archetypal principle: Neptune/ Pluto (depending on the poison).

Poliomyelitis

see Infantile paralysis, spinal

Pollacisuria

(frequent urge to pass water)
Physical level: Urinary bladder (withstanding and relieving pressure).
Symptom level: Persistent urge to urinate, which nevertheless leads to the emptying of only small quantities of urine, e.g. in case of an →enlarged prostate, →urinary bladder inflammations and →urinary bladder stones: persistent call to let go.

Handling: Adjusting oneself to letting go and practising it on figurative levels in order to take the burden off the urinary bladder; spiritual exercises in letting go: meditations, group dynamic exercises.

Resolution: Making friends with the necessity of letting go of everything one has ever received; accepting the necessary constraints that are enforced by the polarity of giving and taking.

Archetypal principle: Moon-Pluto.

Polyarthritis

see Rheumatism

Polyglobulia

see Blood, thickening of; Blood count (haemogram), disturbed

Polyneuropathy

see Nerve pains

Polyposis intestinalis

see Intestinal polyps

Polyps

see Adenoids, Intestinal polyps, Cervical polyps, Uterine polyps

Portal vein blockage

(see also Liver, cirrhosis; Oesophageal varices)

Physical level: Portal vein: blood supply (life force) to the liver (life, evaluation, reconnection).

Symptom level: In the case of liver problems (first clarify and interpret the basic problem), in particular, cirrhosis of the liver, the life energy from the liver backs up into the body: formation of →oesophageal varices, bleeding

→haemorrhoids, caput medusae-Latin: 'head of Medusa'- varicose veins on the belly - as a result of the vitality backup.

Handling: Making oneself aware of the backup of the life energy, which then puts the region concerned with the meaning of life, evaluations and finding the right measure under pressure; directing vitality into other areas and letting it become visible in those areas: finding more suitable forms of expression.

Resolution: Letting out (expressing) the thematic area of the physically over-taxed liver more in the spiritual respect in order to take the load off the physical level; clarifying for oneself the question of the meaning of life.

Archetypal principle: Mars/Jupiter-Pluto.

Portiocarcinoma

see Cervical cancer

Post-natal depression

Physical level: Metabolism (dynamic equilibrium); abrupt change in hormone levels after giving birth.

Symptom level: Being overwhelmed by reality; having to let go of the pregnancy in one fell swoop; turning away from the (day-to-day) life that is looming on the horizon; tendency to flee; asking too much of oneself due to the modern-day role model of the successful working mother; if the child is nursed on demand, the sleep rhythm may end up being interrupted every one to two hours, with the result that there is never enough time for dream phases: the inner images and voices which consequently can no longer be processed become increasingly powerful and force their way into waking consciousness: visual and auditory →hallucinations.

Handling: Creating niches (of consciousness) for oneself in order to be able to withdraw to them when necessary; reconciling oneself with the mother role and the responsibility that goes along with it; consciously accepting the death of tried-and-trusted customs; letting go of the newborn, releasing it into life; consciously becoming more open to border areas between other realities; ensuring longer phases of unbroken sleep (→three-month colic) or consciously committing oneself to the increased state of alertness; taking it as a form of spiritual exercise.

Resolution: Reconciliation with the new life period and task: commitment to the new life situation; readiness for inner growth: growing from being a woman into being a mother.

Archetypal principle: Moon-Neptune/Pluto.

Post-partal psychosis

see Post-natal depression (above)

Posture defects

(see also Round back, Hollow back)

Physical level: Spinal column (dynamics and hold, uprightness).

Symptom level: The existing, but unlived inner stance is let out (expressed); the shadow area becomes visible.

Handling: Taking the message in the (incorrect) stance for real and taking it seriously; helping the previously-unlived inner stance to come to life, relieving the body of the burden; possible exercises on the physical level Hatha yoga, Tai Chi; on the mental-spiritual level: mandala painting and meditation.

Resolution: Assuming a centred stance, in which the inner and the outer aspects correspond to each other.

Archetypal principle: Saturn.

Precancerosis

(tissue change; vague term, which is frequently misused to scare people: given that this is a society in which half of the population is suffering from cancer of one sort or another, and in view of the frequently long development time of the disease pattern, preliminary stages of cancer are naturally widespread, and are often no indication of a real threat [a dormant cancer "pet" as proposed by Hackethal = a slowly-growing prostate cancer which has little or no influence on life expectancy and only becomes a threat due to unnecessary operations]; see also →Cancer)

Physical level: Indications are possible in many types of tissue.

Symptom level: Traditionally-accepted medicine: tissue changes which frequently develop into cancer, and should therefore arouse suspicion; Alternative medicine: various indications from tissue acidity to changes in capillary-dynamolysis (German: Steigbilder [L.Kolisko] - diagnosis procedure originating from anthroposophic medicine), blood composition, etc.

Handling: Addressing the applicable problem of the affected area of the body; confronting oneself preventatively with the cancer pattern of normopathy (→cancer), recognising it and making it superfluous.

Resolution: Going one's own way.

Archetypal principle: Pluto-Jupiter.

Preclampsia

see Eclampsia

Pregnancy complaints

Physical level: Stomach (feeling, receptiveness), glands/hormones (control, information).

Symptom level: Feelings of dizziness ("feign"ting spells):

(unconsciously) not bringing two conflicting things into alignment (→kinetoses, balance disorders), pregnancy and one's life plan contradict each other; one's own, perhaps unacknowledged, intentions are thwarted; →vomiting/nausea (emesis = vomiting 5 to 6 times per day, hyperemesis = unstoppable vomiting, with the danger that the organism may dry out and the metabolism will then go haywire): typical - in fact nowadays regarded as more or less normal - reaction to the unaccustomed over-abundance of female hormone in the initial acclimatisation phase: refusal to accept the new (hormone) situation, the new social role; rejection of one's own female role/ motherhood; low identification with femininity prior to this point; unconscious resistance towards the child, respectively the man who fathered it, whom the woman sometimes can no longer stand (the smell of); "not wanting to bear what he has saddled her with"; lack of desire to make oneself available as a nesting and breeding ground and to put one's own interests on the back burner for so long; she finds it sickening, it makes her want to be sick and so she does; she urgently and continually wants to get rid of something which she rejects or is disgusted by; the attempt to suppress the new situation comes to nothing; often the only possibility for getting social or professional pressure off her back.

Handling: Taking account of the situation in which one finds oneself in all honesty; reconciling oneself with one's own womanhood in this new dimension: meditations on the mother role, processing of one's own mother relationship; addressing the issue of the father of the child and his role in one's life (body); reconsidering one's own life planning and becoming aware of the natural hierarchy, according to which the

child displaces the partner and career from first place; facing up to the new situation and making decisions; detaching oneself from old attitudes and issues which are no longer fitting and only lead to nausea and reluctance; possibly cancelling the amniocentesis appointment, or at least getting it over with as quickly as possible, and committing oneself unconditionally to the unborn child.
Resolution: Truly throwing up (one's arms and surrendering to the situation); giving in completely.
Archetypal principle: Moon-Uranus.

Pregnancy, false

(pseudogravidity; has become quite rare nowadays due to early ultrasound examinations and pregnancy tests; see also Hydatiform mole)
Physical level: Womb (fertility, safety and security), stomach (feeling, instinct, enjoyment, centre), genitalia (sexuality, polarity, reproduction).
Symptom level: Conflict between extremely strong desire for a child and unconscious fear of responsibility or between sexuality and motherhood; puffing oneself up with no content behind it; adopting the bearing of pregnancy without having to bear the consequences; pregnancy as a possibility for exercising power; keeping up appearances (of a pregnancy): conflict between appearance and reality.
Handling: Learning to be responsive to womanhood, sensing one's responsibility for one's own sexual role; clearing up one's own birth trauma in case it is the fear of birth which is preventing genuine pregnancies; reconciliation with sexual aspects as the natural basis of pregnancy; to the extent that there is a discrepancy in judgement between dirty sex and motherhood as the will of God, working on the issue in order to arrive at a natural re-alignment; reconsidering in

the direction of more developed forms of exercising feminine power.
Resolution: Reconciliation with the full depths of one's own womanhood.
Archetypal principle: Moon-Neptune.

Pregnancy psychosis

see Post-natal depression

Pregnancy toxicosis

see Eclampsia

Premature birth

(see also Birth complications)
Physical level: Womb (fertility, safety and security).
Symptom level: 1. For the mother: →vaginal inflammation due to a localised immune deficiency, which rises up and triggers labour pains: inability to adequately defend the entrance into one's own underworld; conflict over the exit, which pushes forward into the physical centre of the abdominal cavity and contests with the child for the nest; (unconsciously) wanting to be rid of the child as soon as possible; prematurely wanting delivery from the obligation of having to carry it any more (to full term); wanting to give the child life as soon as possible; cutting the umbilical cord, separating from the child too quickly; due to anguish and suffering, being unable to build a spiritual nest for the child. 2. For the child: Fleeing by rushing headlong to the outside (→birth complications: breaking of the waters): "Just get me out here already!"; premature escape from the oppressing restrictiveness; courage to forge ahead; curiosity.
Handling: 1. On the part of the mother: consciously addressing premature separation tendencies, rash decisions, the handling of obligations that have been undertaken, overhasty gifts; opening oneself up

to the feminine Moon archetype. 2.
On the part of the later adult: Taking
care to choose the right moment;
noti(ci)ng one's own tendencies to
flee by rushing headlong into things;
in various situations, keeping an eye
on one's tendency to come too soon;
cultivating conscious handling of
one's own curiosity; questioning one's
own courage: Is it simply due to a
lack of imagination?; learning to allow
one's own fruits to ripen until they fall
(almost) by themselves.
Resolution: Mastering the art of
choosing the right time: "There is a
time for everything."
Archetypal principle: Mars-Moon/
Uranus.

Pre-menstrual syndrome

(PMS; see also Menstruation, painful)
Physical level: Ovaries (polarity,
procreation).
Symptom level: The effect of the
hormone progesterone is aimed at
breaking down the endometrium if no
fertilised egg has "nested" in it; not
being able to adjust oneself physically and spiritually to the process of
breaking down and letting go; tension
in the lower body: tense life situation
in the area of femininity; headaches:
conflict extends to the central control
headquarters; breast tenderness:
pain at (once again) not being able
to do justice to the motherly Moon
aspect; rage at not having any fruitful
(fertile) relationship; "Don't touch me!"
Handling: Monthly retreat; taking
menstruation as a time-out; paying
more attention to one's own (bio)
rhythm.
Resolution: Giving oneself completely to the female cycle of "death
and rebirth"; letting the monthly dying
process happen; recognising and experiencing menstruation as a taboo in
the positive sense (instead of working

and holding things out: conscious
letting go).
Archetypal principle: Moon-Pluto.

Presbyacusis

see Senile deafness

Presbyopia

see Senile hypermetropia

Priapism

see Permanent erection

Proctitis

(rectal inflammation)
Physical level: Rectum (underworld).
Symptom level: Inflammatory conflict
over the rectum = the hoarding and
giving up of material treasures; often
exacerbated by an overly-stimulating
lifestyle which includes alcohol and
the overuse of strong spices.
Handling: Critically and combatively
confronting the issue of hoarding and
letting go of material wealth; committing oneself to the struggle over the
final station on the journey of material
nourishment and deciding it in one's
favour; living a highly-stimulating life
on more sophisticated levels: finding
pungency and spice in life in the figurative sense.
Resolution: Clear, clean, circumstances with regard to letting go
(taking leave).
Archetypal principle: Pluto-Mars.

Progenia

(the lower set of teeth projects beyond the upper set, reversed overbite;
as the opposite pole, see Prognathia)
Physical level: Upper and lower jaw
(weapons store), mouth (absorption,
expression, maturity – ability to speak
for oneself).
Symptom level: predominance of the
animalistic forces over the spiritual;

energetic power to forcefully assert one's will: the more distinctly the lower jaw projects forward, the less compromising one's will is in forcefully asserting itself; not making a friendly face.

Handling: Developing more subtle (more human) forms of forceful assertion, forcefully asserting oneself through using one's brains; learning to articulate oneself; learning to retreat, respectively to give in.

Resolution: Standing up for one's own animalistic needs, but also transforming and developing them further as far as possible.

Archetypal principle: Mars-Pluto.

Progeria

(premature ageing in children)

Physical level: The whole organism is affected.

Symptom level: Ageing sets in during childhood or at the age of around 20 years with →stroke, →hair loss, →arteriosclerosis, →rheumatism among other symptoms; age becomes the dominating life theme, suppressing everything else; in the form of a caricature, these young people force those around them to keep their unlived ageing in mind.

Handling: Seeking out and living structure, discipline, maturity – the qualities of age; ageing consciously.

Resolution: Reconciling oneself with ageing as a priority – diametrically opposite situation to the case of children with →Down's syndrome, who have to reconcile themselves with childhood.

Archetypal principle: Moon-Saturn.

Prognathia

(unusually-pronounced projection of the upper jaw in front of the lower jaw; as the opposite pole, see Progenia)

Physical level: Upper and lower jaw (weapons store), mouth (absorption,

expression, maturity – ability to speak for oneself).

Symptom level: Less pronounced power to push one's will and oneself forward, power interests that have been taken back: backing off from life, fleeing into the spiritual; seemingly not wanting to hurt a fly, harmlessness.

Handling: Mustering courage to make oneself aware of one's own defensive structures in order to back off in a well-targeted way, and if necessary, to be able to hold oneself back; consciously giving up self-restraint and taking what one needs or what one is due.

Resolution: Directing one's will to inner goals.

Archetypal principle: Mars-Mars/Neptune.

Prolapsus uteri

see Uterine prolapse

Prolapsus vaginae

see Vaginal prolapse

Prostate cancer

(see also Cancer)

Physical level: Prostate (guardian at the threshold to the second half of life, sperm supply), genitalia (sexuality, polarity, reproduction).

Symptom level: Similar in appearance to →prostate enlargement, which is why this subject should also be included here; aggressive destruction of the prostate gland from the inside out; degeneration in the area of the supply system for the male semen and the lubricating fluid for sexual intercourse; wild and ruthlessly rampant growth of the degenerative prostate cells under the influence of male hormones, often triggered by loathsome conflict in the sexual area that eats away at one; having prematurely finished with one's masculine sexuality;

409

having strayed so far off track from one's inherent line of development that the body helps the (forgotten/repressed) issue to break through again; mental-spiritual growth in relation to this subject has been blocked for so long that it now manifests itself in an aggressive and random way; the cancer realises physically in the prostate area that (turnaround) which would be spiritually necessary in the corresponding area of consciousness: offensively expanding growth above and beyond the rut of one's own accustomed role pattern.

Handling: Radically calling into question the old, handed-down customs and traditions with regard to the masculine share in procreation and sexuality in general, and if necessary, ruthlessly destroying these; opening oneself up in the area of masculinity and fertility to one's own outlandish ideas and bold fantasies, and courageously and freely allowing them to flourish and expand; allowing one's own creative growth impulses to sprout and ensuring that things run in a well-oiled fashion; helping to restore the prostate to its usual secondary role as the producer of lubricant for sexual intercourse; fostering a more developed notion of sensuality and sexuality, which leads to long, wonderful love-making feasts; thinking back to early dreams and one's own goals, wishes and notions of eroticism and love and bringing these (back) to life and putting them into practice with (wild) decisiveness; in the certainty of having nothing more to lose, mustering courage for self-realisation/one's own path; taking the growth impulse away from the body and directing it to more resolved (redeeming) levels; considering all the measures mentioned under →cancer: since cancer affects the complete organism, it must also be met across-the-board.

Resolution: Breaking with old ideas that are actually foreign to one's own

being in the affected area of procreation and sexuality and struggling aggressively in an open(ly offensive) manner for one's own way (in life) and one's own meaning of life; providing expression for oneself in the mental-spiritual domain instead of letting the body speak up for itself; recognising the necessity to switch from the physical and thus (life-) threatening level to the challenging, but life-saving mental-spiritual level, and relying in this realm on expansive growth in the affected area; discovering love that transcends all boundaries; setting oneself above external rule and standards laid down by oneself or others and living and expressing oneself solely in accordance with the obligations of one's own highest law; recognising ecstasy as a goal.

Archetypal principle: Moon/Mars-Saturn/Pluto.

Prostate enlargement

(prostate hypertrophy)

Physical level: Prostate (guardian at the threshold to the second half of life, sperm supply), genitalia (sexuality, polarity, reproduction).

Symptom level: Mid-life crisis which gives one a warning reminder of the impending turnaround and the need to let go: the proud jet stream - the attribute that streams out the masculine charisma - becomes a pathetic trickle; not being able to let go: through the persistent urge to go, being forced to practise accordingly (on the toilet) and thereby being hindered in life; suffering from a build-up of waste water: no longer being able to get rid of everything (urine residues) and thereby being put under strain; fear of becoming older, letting go and giving up (things to others); putting oneself under pressure (particularly spiritually, sexually, etc.); hindering the flow of the spiritual energy; not being able to let go appropriately of what is old and outlived; "growing protest" of the prostate against having been largely ignored over the course of a long life; the actual task of the prostate – the production of lubricating fluid so that everything runs smoothly during sexual intercourse – is hardly called upon by the men affected; the sexual activities frequently do not last long enough for the lubricant production of the prostate to even spring into action; further background: frequently occurs in men who are dissatisfied with their position, who no longer enjoy any regard, and who in consequence, do not possess any self-esteem because they have never found the way to their unconsciously-sensed greatness; not having lived up to one's own unconscious expectations of oneself as one was never able to grow beyond oneself, and therefore also couldn't develop a positive attitude towards sexuality (anyone who does not consider themselves lovable naturally remains a poor lover); the prostate then outgrows its limits instead.

Handling: Approaching one's own feminine pole; turnaround in the life mandala; taking back of masculine delusions of grandeur; voluntarily concerning oneself with letting go and integrating corresponding exercises into one's life; consciously and committedly living out what has remained open in the sexual domain; learning to love and live eroticism in a form which includes contact with one's own feminine side; enabling the physical side of love to run in a well-oiled way; taking stock at the turnaround point leading into the years of one's change of life: Have the demands of the way there, and the preparations for the way back been fulfilled?; integrating a new form of conscious masculinity (trusting in the youthful, vital masculinity of the way there is no longer sufficient).

Resolution: Acknowledgement and processing of the issue of polarity; letting go of what is superfluous for the homeward journey of the soul; enjoying age and experience and outgrowing one's limits on the mental-spiritual level.

Archetypal principle: Moon/Mars/Saturn-Jupiter/Pluto.

Prostate inflammation

(prostatitis)

Physical level: Prostate (guardian at the threshold to the second half of life, sperm supply), genitalia (sexuality, polarity, reproduction).

Symptom level: Triggered by coli-bacteria or cocci via the urinary tract: stirring aspects which spread from the anal or urethral area; aggressive struggle for the supply gland of the semen, which often spreads to other genital organs, such as the seminal vesicles (→adnexitis in men); conflict between "feminine" and male-orientated sexual behaviour, between the weakling (softie) and the He-man (macho).

Handling: Consciously having out conflicts over one's own sexuality; helping to restore the prostate to its usual secondary role as the producer of lubricant for sexual intercourse; accepting the confrontation and being ready for the forthcoming fight: preferring to open oneself up on the mental-spiritual level to new stimulations rather than opening up the prostate gland to the stimulation of pathogens; watching out for attacks which spill over from the waste matter and waste water area; practising cleanliness in the figurative sense and careful separation of the different areas; letting oneself get more involved in one's own sexuality, i.e. giving up stereotypical gender roles, such as the macho and softie.

Resolution: Facing up to the challenges in the area of the prostate gland in a courageous and open(ly offensive) way = nourishment of the sperm (organisms) and preparation of the gliding/guiding substance.
Archetypal principle: Moon/Mars/Saturn-Mars.

Protrusion, dental

(horsey teeth)
Physical level: Teeth (aggression, vitality).
Symptom level: Leaning towards forward-directed, unbridled aggression.
Handling: "Baring one's teeth", openly expressing vitality and aggression, going on the offensive.
Resolution: Finding the right measure when dealing with defensive aggression.
Archetypal principle: Mars-Jupiter.

Pruritus

see Itching

Pruritus vulvae

(itching in the area of the outer female genitalia; see also Itching, Lichen sclerosus et atrophicus)
Physical level: Vulva (protective wall), mucous membranes (inner boundary, barrier).
Symptom level: Love, eroticism and the sweetness of life attract and stimulate one (though unacknowledged) so strongly that outer boundaries are often aggressively torn open (by scratching); resistance to the partner, resistance to one's own and foreign sexual practices, self-punishment; unfulfilled sexual fantasies or traumatic experiences in the sexual domain, which bring themselves to mind in this way.
Handling: Letting oneself get involved with both the light and dark sides of one's own personality; granting oneself one's own feminine desire

and showing it; allowing the issues of "polarity" and "sexuality" to once again come close to one and come inside.
Resolution: Discovering, acknowledging and living out one's own sexual desire.
Archetypal principle: Venus-Mars.

Pseudarthrosis

(false joint)
Physical level: Long bones of the skeleton (bones = stability, strength).
Symptom level: Following a fracture (first clarify and interpret the basic situation [bone fracture, accident]), the ends of the fracture do not grow together again, but instead form a new joint at a point not intended for this purpose; the ends of the fracture become covered with cartilage, and a joint capsule forms, which can then even become filled with synovial fluid: abnormal mobility in the affected section of the limb.
Handling: Making clear to oneself the excessive demands on the body which led to the break; distancing oneself from a repeat of similar excessive demands, thereby giving the body the confidence that this will not happen again and that therefore no joint is necessary at this point, except in the case of an accident; instead of forcing the body to create a joint at an unsuitable point, preferably becoming more double-jointed and agile in consciousness: learning to articulate oneself and to better adjust oneself to the challenges on the level of consciousness.
Resolution: Preferring to demand more of oneself in consciousness rather than demanding too much of the bones; (creatively) heightening one's mental-spiritual agility.
Archetypal principle:
Uranus-Saturn.

Pseudocroup

see Croup

Pseudogravidity

(pseudocyesis) see Pregnancy, false

Psittacosis

(ornithosis; see also Avian influenza)
Physical level: Affects the complete organism.
Symptom level: Infectious ideas from the realm of the air (birds) challenge one to battle; fever: general mobilisation against the invading enemies (viruses); coughing: expression of aggression ("coughing up" what one really thinks); lung inflammation: war over exchange and communication; nosebleeds: loss of life energy; overall poor general condition: being run down in terms of life energy.
Handling: Defending oneself with all one's might in order to safeguard the (structural) integrity of the landscape of the body; expressing one's opinions clearly, distinctly and in an open(ly offensive) way; daring to engage in combative confrontations over the issues of communication and exchange; sacrificing life energy and pitching it into the struggle.
Resolution: Courageously facing up to the challenge and opening oneself up to new, offensive impulses while still defending and preserving one's own sphere of life and interests.
Archetypal principle: Uranus/Mercury-Mars.

Psoriasis

(see also Skin rash)
Physical level: Skin (border, contact, tenderness).
Symptom level: Forming a hard shell, arm(our)ing the borders; character armour (Wilhelm Reich); often an exaggerated need for security; often comprehensive attempts at adaptation and currying favour out of fear or because one is seeking protection; fear of getting hurt: "the soft core hidden behind a rough exterior"; clearly marking one's limits in all directions: not letting anything more in or out; going to extremes in setting limits leads to isolation; considerable losses of the important building blocks for life (in the form of protein) due to the formation of flaky skin: sacrificing oneself for one's border fortifications; the breakdown of these armoured borders leads to severe losses (the former GDR can be seen as a good analogy for the pattern of psoriasis in the form of a country).
Handling: Learning to protect oneself in a different way in order to relieve the body of the burden of this task; creating a protected area for oneself, in which one can oversee and determine what gets in and what gets out; discovering and learning to enjoy one's own sensitively-soft core in this inner protected area; recognising the consequence of total armouring and total isolation; preferably learning to invest the basic building blocks of life in more sensible protective measures than in the formation of flaky skin to act as physical armour: e.g. learning to defend oneself verbally (developing a sharp tongue and the ability to make rapid-fire comebacks, arming oneself with penetrating arguments and building oneself up comprehensively with knowledge; making clear to oneself that even the strongest armour will develop chinks sooner or later, with the accompanying threat of loss of the life energy (blood) and the easy invasion of dangerous enemies (pathogens); psychotherapy.
Resolution: Setting one's limits, and through doing so, being able to open oneself up again: becoming vulnerable and capable of being wounded again in order to experience the wo(u)nd/erment of life; opening oneself up

again to the flow of lively vitality, love and caring attention.
Archetypal principle: Venus/ Saturn (skin)-Saturn (armour).

Psychosis

(see also Spiritual crisis, Manic-depressive disease)
Symptom level: Break (through) of the protective membrane between superficial consciousness and deeper layers even as far as the collective unconscious; overflooding of the (upper) consciousness with contents from the unconscious, which in such abundance can scarcely be processed, if at all; sudden breach of the dam wall holding back the shadow realms, which – long suppressed – now gain the upper hand; aberrations on the consciousness level; in the struggle between intellect and one's emotional being, the former draws the short straw and the latter takes over command; shadow aspects can appear on the scene on both levels (the ice-cold intellect and maniacal rage); taking flight from unbearable states of consciousness into supposedly-better illusory worlds, which are, however, experienced as completely real; endogenous psychoses (incomprehensible for classical, orthodox psychiatrists) and symptomatic psychoses (due to poisoning or drugs such as LSD) do not differ in principle, and simply have different triggers for the flight from reality; often arising at decisive points in life: instead of risking the great leap into adulthood, motherhood or one's profession,the leap is made to another consciousness level (cutting [oneself] loose from one level, latching onto another); giving away the responsibility for one's own life, allowing oneself and one's interests to be governed by others (such as in psychiatric care), regression to the dependent child level; paying a high price for denial.

Handling: Attempts at grounding – coming down or back to this Earth with both feet firmly on the ground: simple manual tasks which require little concentration (such as hoeing the garden); substantial, regular diet (not sensitive, vegetarian-style, but instead coarse and hearty); daily sweating through one's own (exertion of) power; no spiritual exercises with closed eyes, no meditations, except at the most Za-Zen (with open eyes), Hatha yoga or Tai Chi; usually, however, exercises involving movement (long walks) are accepted much better, since the patients want to get moving (inwardly), but cannot find the starting point; orientation exercises in the body: bodywork of the type advocated by Milton Trager, Feldenkrais or bioenergetics; careful psychotherapy to enable orientation and processing of the shadow contents that are forcing their way to the surface: attempt to make contact with that part of one's being which still retains perspective (the "islands of clarity" proposed by Podvoll, one's [spiritual] Self); containment of the flood of images for a short time is sometimes necessary, often by means of allopathic suppression (medications) in order to open up a starting point for the therapy.
Resolution: Finding the (stable) bridge which connects the two worlds, the outer and inner, respectively the left and right hemispheres of the brain, with each other; reconciliation with the dark parts of one's own spiritual life, which express themselves in the →hallucinations and other mental lapses associated with the psychoses.
Archetypal principle: Moon-Uranus/ Neptune/Pluto.

Ptosis

Physical level: Upper lids (eyelids = curtains of the soul).

Symptom level: Drooping of the upper lids due to paralysis of the lid muscle: (tired) bedroom eyes.

Handling: Examining one's own wearily-arrogant (facial) expression with regard to its broad symbolic meaning, in particular, whether one is letting oneself down (overall); recognising the effect of the continual invitation into the bedroom on oneself and others; remaining aware of the opposite pole with its call to keep one's eyes open.

Resolution: Taking things easy with respect to oneself and the world; repeatedly drawing one's gaze away from the outer world in favour of introspection.

Archetypal principle: Saturn-Neptune.

Puberty acne

(see also Folliculitis, Skin rash, Inflammation)

Physical level: Skin (border, contact, tenderness).

Symptom level: Inner struggle thrusts its way to the surface; breakthrough of pubertal sexuality across the border: attempt to force it back; the "hot" subject of sexuality and partnership inflames the (skin) border; stimulation and pressure of the new, and fear of the new; self-protection against encounters by means of pimples, not letting anyone close to oneself; lack of self-esteem; unconscious disfigurement of one's own appearance in order not to have to look the hot conflict issue in the eye; as a result: aggravation of the situation through continued unlived sexuality; being ashamed of one's own sexuality; attacking one's own boundaries and prescribed norms on the physical instead of on the consciousness level; scarred acne face: old battlefield of puberty conflicts; desire to squeeze the pimples and thereby give oneself scars.

Handling: Discovering and experiencing sexuality within the framework of puberty; obtaining loving attention for oneself (and for one's contact organ - the skin); seeking erotic skin contact by means of puberty games, going to the disco; opening the (skin) borders from inside to the outside; giving in to one's pressing sexual urges; sunlight brings improvement: ensuring warm, loving attention for the skin; examining, exploring and giving way to the pressure which one has come under; instead of pressing out the pimples, learning to ex-press one's sexual needs.

Resolution: Making the breakthrough to the other sex; enjoying the outbreak of sexuality.

Archetypal principle: Venus/Saturn (skin)-Mars (inflammation).

Puberty, premature

(acceleration)

Physical level: The whole organism is affected in terms of its growth and development.

Symptom level: Early onset of puberty, accelerated physical development, often with decelerated psychological maturity.

Handling: Promoting spiritual growth, but breaking down the performance-based mentality and over-the-top ambition.

Resolution: Speeding through mental-spiritual processes; ensuring balance between the body and soul; venturing earlier and more courageously onto the erotic-sexual playing field.

Archetypal principle: Venus-Uranus.

Puerperal fever

see Childbed fever

Pug nose

see Rhinophyma

Pulled muscle

see Muscular strain

Pulmonary consumption

(pulmonary tuberculosis, TBC)
Physical level: Lungs (contact, communication, freedom).
Symptom level: The airy lung tissue becomes caseated and transforms itself into the material; the airy lightness and freedom turns into a hard cheese-like substance: the lightness of being is lost; consumption (of the body): discontinuing communication and slipping away; taking flight from a hard, restrictive reality perceived as unbearable; creeping conflict, which without many symptoms (if untreated) often drags on until death: the patients fade away relatively unobtrusively ("the silent disease"); developing on the basis of immune deficiency (undernourishment, incorrect diet, addictions, other lung problems), the (tuberculosis) pathogens can usually only gain a foothold in the lungs after repeated attacks and then cause the conflicts to flare up; fatigue and lack of appetite reveal the tendency to shrink away from things; weight loss indicates the unconscious intention to make oneself scarce; not wanting to be part of this coarse world; the only slightly-raised (subfebrile) temperatures show that no violent struggle is going on here – the patients are too weak for that – but rather that a smouldering fire has been ignited in the depths of the communications and contact organ of the lungs; while nowadays TBC is more a disease of the poor and troubled mileus, it was in earlier times also the noble way out of a normal life that one considered oneself to be too fragile and weak for; prior to the introduction of penicillin, the depletion of the population due to consumption was enormously high: taking flight from an overly traditional, restrictive reality perceived as unbearable (first to the sanatorium, which was usually found in an attractive, high location, well above the profane world with its hardships, and then into the world beyond); preference for the illusionary dream world, rich in imagery, which was further encouraged by "air and light baths"; preferring not to be a part of this sorry world; sanatoria were in themselves already an artificial world, but the dreams and illusions of many affected patients went even further; open and closed TBC differ with regard to the danger of infection: in the first case, high danger, in the latter case, non-existent.
Handling: In addition to the (allopathic) warlike elimination of the mycobacteria by means of tried-and-tested antibiotic combinations, devoting oneself as soon as possible to the silent conflicts that get stuck into one in a barely noticeable way in the area of communication and exchange; reducing one's mental-spiritual defences in order to release the body's defences from their substitute role and strengthen these again; making oneself aware of one's tendency to steal away from heated contacts; recognising one's tendency to flee from the contact and communications area and giving in to these in the external domain, but also taking care to ensure that one comes into deeper contact with oneself; in addition to the airy-light confrontation on the level of thoughts, also "getting down to the nitty-gritty", "reaching out" and realising oneself communicatively; forging concrete plans instead of losing oneself in "castles in the air"; establishing firm facts and communicating projects with substance instead of producing cheesy rubbish in one's own lungs.
Resolution: Deepening the relationship with transcendence, the flirting with the world beyond, in a conscious

and effective way – without using the lungs as a means of flight for stealing away from polarity; realising oneself in life and in one's communication with others.

Archetypal principle: Mercury-Neptune (see Thomas Mann: "Der Zauberberg" (The Magic Mountain), in which the basic consumption pattern is portrayed very accurately).

Pulmonary emphysema

(hyperinflation of the lungs)

Physical level: Lungs (contact, communication, freedom), rib cage (sense of self/Ego, personality).

Symptom level: Puffing up of the communications area at the cost of genuine exchange (first clarify and interpret the basic problem, such as →asthma or →bronchitis): the breathing function begins declining, since the air can no longer be exhaled completely; the (right side of the) heart suffers damage; artificial powerfulness through the inflated rib cage (inflation of the Ego), which is expanded from the inside by the alveoli (air sacs) of the lungs: behind the claim to power, the powerlessness becomes apparent; overemphasis of taking in (air) as opposed to letting (it) go; rigidity (barrel chest), which allows neither flexibility nor openness to the life energy (breath); overinflated people use the controlling "deep, chesty tone of utter conviction" although they are not at all convinced of themselves, but are instead suffering from a lack of self-confidence; life degenerates into a struggle for survival.

Handling: Expanding one's communication and contact area from the inside out; extending one's sphere of power and influence through one's own efforts; ensuring more consistency and structure in the exchange; owning up to the caginess and communication constraints that

are concealed behind the illusions of grandeur; acknowledging one's own powerlessness and accepting it as a starting point and task; recognising the dangers for the area of the heart and the emotions that is posed by the constrained communication and the impaired exchange; learning to share parts of oneself instead of puffing oneself up; recognising communication as a bipolar affair, in which every taking involves the corresponding giving; taking on more spiritually in order to relieve the body of the problem of taking; giving less away spiritually and retaining more for oneself in order to make it easier for the lungs to solve the problem of letting go.

Resolution: Discovering the function of the lungs as wings; flying on the wings of expressed thoughts and the lightness of balanced communication; establishing the harmony of giving and taking.

Archetypal principle: Mercury-Jupiter.

Pulmonary stenosis

Physical level: Heart (seat of the soul, love, feelings, energy centre); lungs (contact, communication, freedom).

Symptom level: Lack of openness to the flow of life in the direction of energy exchange; restriction/hindrance of the life energy; undersupply of the lungs and therefore the body with fresh life force (Prana); back-up of the energy into the middle of the heart: right cardiac hypertrophy with the danger of right-side heart failure.

Handling: Reducing the energy exchange and consumption on other levels, e.g. in the financial and social domains in order to relieve the body of this task; letting the current of life energy flow in a more concentrated and conscious way; learning to get by with less, to be more modest;

417

concentration of one's life energy on matters of the heart (muscle).

Resolution: Living more consciously through better utilisation of one's life energy.

Archetypal principle: Sun/Mercury-Saturn.

Pulmonary tuberculosis

see Pulmonary consumption

Pyelitis

see Renal pelvis inflammation

Pyelonephritis

see Glomerulonephritis

Pyoovarium

see Ovaries, suppuration

Pyosalpinx

see Fallopian tubes, suppuration

Pyromania

Symptom level: Inclination to start fires (particularly amongst firemen!).

Handling: Igniting a fire in oneself until the flames of enthusiasm rage out of control; confrontation with one's shadow which, if ignored, tends to blaze a path in unresolved (unredeeming) and dangerous ways.

Resolution: Getting to know and appreciate one's inner fire.

Archetypal principle: Mars.

Q

Quincke's oedema

(see also Allergy, Urticaria, Oedema)

Physical level: Skin (border, contact, tenderness), particularly of the face (visiting card, individuality, perception).

Symptom level: Blushing (out of anger or shame) rises up into one's face and stays there: the face in flames (branded), burning like fire; monstrous face (puffed up): one's shadow looks out at one from the mirror (cf. Oscar Wilde: "The Picture of Dorian Gray"); loss of face; Medusa head: being scary and scaring off, devouring; suppressed aggression (→allergy): one's face is burning (because of dishonesty, a symbolic slap across the face, malicious pleasure = German: Schadenfreude); swelling up instead of piping up in protest; something (evil) is written all over one's face (although one refuses to believe this is true).

Handling/Resolution: Making friends with and reconciling oneself with one's other (dark) side; making oneself aware of one's shadow instead of forcing the body to live it out; grimacing when bearing it instead of grinning and putting on a brave front; voicing unpleasant truths.

Archetypal principle: Venus/Saturn-Pluto/Mars.

R

Rabies

Physical level: The whole organism is affected.

Symptom level: The smallest wounds which come into contact with the saliva of animals infected with the rabies virus become the entry point for this disease pattern, which is still always fatal if left untreated; increasing states of agitation alternating with periods of lethargy; spastic muscle cramps, in particular of the larynx, which lead to vehement refusal to drink and which produce large quantities of thick, sticky saliva – reminiscent of animals foaming at the mouth; without treatment, death occurs due to →respiratory paralysis or →heart failure.

Handling: (assuming, of course, that there is immediate immunisation following infection) - Preventive measures in the concrete sense: being careful of normally-timid wild animals, which behave conspicuously tamely or at the other extreme very aggressively; since the incubation period is quite long as a rule (3 to 7 weeks), animals suspected of carrying the virus can be observed long enough to begin immunisation treatment in good time; doing without masculine rituals practised in the past by hunters, such as cutting off the tail of any dead foxes found: such ill-gained "trophies" can occasionally prove to be life-threatening. Preventive measures in the extended sense: getting to know one's own rabid rage and stark raving madness in good time before having to encounter these in the concrete sense; being sufficiently reconciled with states of agitation and the animal in oneself so that one can be safe from unexpected attacks.

Resolution: Exercising the necessary care in handling the animalistic aspects of nature; acknowledging their wildness; coupling one's animal(istic) love with understanding and preventing it where necessary, both in the concrete and in the wider sense.

Archetypal principle: Pluto.

Rachitis

(rickets – the "English disease")

Physical level: Above all the bone system (stability, strength).

Symptom level: Disease pattern triggered by lack of Vitamin D and sunlight, which due to inadequate calcification in the bones leads to their softness and deformation: a deficiency of light and love in the life of the child prevents the development of firm structures (bones); soft bones suggest inadequate structuring of life; the deformation of the bones shows how deformable all structures still are at the beginning of life, especially the spirit and soul, but also the hardest material itself: the bone.

Handling: (for jointly-affected parents, whose problems are often reflected by the children): Vitamin-D prophylaxis in the first months of life and exposure to natural daylight nowadays reliably prevent the disease pattern; bringing light into life on all levels; giving loving attention and tenderness and conveying security and safety.

Resolution: Becoming aware of the softness and deformability of the soul, spirit and even the skeletal framework of the child and being appropriately responsible in dealing with them; guaranteeing love and dependable security as the basis of the developing life.

Archetypal principle: Saturn-Moon.

Radiation accident

see Irradiation

Rage, fits of

(see also Aggressiveness)

Symptom level: Built-up aggression breaks through in the area of the least resistance or in the area of a weak spot and discharges itself tempestuously (in terms of the macrocosm, compare volcanic eruptions or earthquakes); lack of courage to express one's own aggressions at the point where they arise; loss of control with regard to one's own energies: the (spiritual) fuses blow all of a sudden.

Handling: Getting to know aggression and learning to appreciate it; creating outlets for it in constructive areas; consciously allowing the fuses to blow where it makes sense, e.g. in the experience of orgasm, but also on all other occasions involving ecstatic letting go (dancing, sport, music); only then later switching to the opposite pole and learning control (the tantric control of sexual energy also only makes sense if this force has already been experienced in its primitiveness).

Resolution: Becoming aware of one's own energies and consciously playing with them (Heraclitus: "Everything flows", "War is the father of all things"); having the courage for one's own expressive powers.

Archetypal principle: Mars-Uranus.

Rash

see Skin rash

Raynaud's syndrome

(see also Low blood pressure, Circulatory disorders)

Physical level: Blood (life force), fingers (getting a grip on the world; see also in Part 1 the specific sign-ificance if only individual fingers are affected), hands (grasping, gripping, ability to act, expression).

Symptom level: Cold, dead fingers and hands: no real desire for lively, warm interpersonal contact; at the very least, conventional contact does not come from the heart; laying down of all ability to act: not being able to get a grip on life: "my hands are tied"; not being able to defend one's own skin; unconscious hate.

Handling: Owning up to the under-cooled contact situation and creating space for oneself: ducking under into one's own inner self; taking time out to be alone; taking back the expectation of handling things successfully in the outer world; ceasing to strive for protection; learning to surrender and trust (oneself).

Resolution: Getting to know one's own impulses that are hostile to life and being able to handle them.

Archetypal principle: Mercury-Saturn.

Recklinghausen's disease

see Osteodystrophia fibrosa generalisata

Rectal cancer

(most frequent intestinal cancer; see also Cancer, Anus praeter, Constipation)

Physical level: Rectum (under-world), large intestine (unconscious, underworld).

Symptom level: Frequently develops on the basis of constipation (stinginess): chronic stimulation (irritation) of the borders of the shadow kingdom (mucous membranes of the large intestine); unresolved shadow subjects: terrible, unappetising, nasty conflicts; degeneration in the area of excretion and letting go: holding things back hinders the process of growth – the process of "death and rebirth" is interrupted if one remains sitting on the dead (typical problem of the masculine materialistic "collect-and-keep" society, and for this reason, a very widespread type of cancer); unconscious and ruthlessly proliferating growth in the underworld; having strayed so far off track from one's inherent development path in the area of letting go and excretion that the body helps the (forgotten/

repressed) issue to express itself; the mental-spiritual growth in this area has been blocked for so long that it now forges a path in the body in an aggressive and random way; the cancer realises physically that (turn-around) which would be spiritually necessary in the corresponding area of consciousness; hindering the de-scent (of waste) when crossing from one world into the next; basic fear of being drowned by the flood of one's own inner chaos; thrift to the point of outright stinginess, which stands in the way of one's actual task; hostility towards development: "not doing one's business"; having deviated from one's own life concept: fear of living for oneself; "degenerate" (i.e. not corresponding to one's own nature) connection to the shadow kingdom of the unconscious; unlived offensive force strikes out; aggression forges a path in the underworld; regressive orientation; regression on the physical level of the body.

Handling: Learning to muck out one's inner spiritual waste (Heracles, who had to muck out the Augean stables, can serve as a model ex-ample from mythology); learning to preserve essential elements (on the mental-spiritual level); consciously problematising the issue of letting go and recognising it as a task on the journey of life; extending the borders of the shadow kingdom; delving deeper into the fear of one's own inner feminine flood until it clears up by itself; rejecting certain types of business (which are only related to material aspects); opening oneself up in the area of letting go to one's own outlandish ideas and bold fantasies; considering the measures mentioned under →cancer: since cancer affects the complete organism, it must also be met across-the-board; admitting to oneself the deviation from one's in-herent task in life; re-contemplation of one's essence, of what is one's own;

exploring the feeling of fear towards what is inherently one's own; looking for unusual (unprescribed) ways of shadow confrontation; bearing down on the unconscious with courage and offensive force.

Resolution: Courageous and open(ly offensive) integration of one's own shadow world in an individual/ (one's own) way; recognising the necessity to switch from the physical and thus (life-)threatening level to the challeng-ing, but life-saving mental-spiritual level, and relying in this realm on expansive growth; discovering love that transcends all boundaries; setting oneself above external rule and stan-dards laid down by oneself or others, and living and expressing oneself solely in accordance with the obliga-tions of one's own highest law.

Archetypal principle: Pluto-Pluto.

Rectal inflammation

see Proctitis

Rectal prolapse

see Anal prolapse

Reflux oesophagitis

(see also Rupture)

Physical level: Oesophagus (food pipe, nutrition supply), stomach (feel-ing, receptiveness).

Symptom level: Conflict over swal-lowed nourishment which, now mixed with acidic gastric juices, presses back up from the stomach into the food pipe: something leaves a sour taste in one's mouth and ignites a burning conflict; the closure at the lower end of the oesophagus is de-fective because of a so-called hiatus hernia (the most frequent form of dia-phragm hernia): parts of the stomach press upwards into the upper world located above the diaphragm; reflux without inflammation: unprocessed matters come back up again, wanting to be re-processed.

Handling: Aggressive conflict over what has been assimilated; sensing one's own sourpuss elements (acerbity) and asking oneself what is making one so angry; making oneself aware of the attacks spilling over from the nest area into the upper world; reducing the pressure in the digestive area: eating a sensible diet; ensuring natural (dis)order in the underworld: if a bubbling witches' cauldron has been created, cleaning it up.

Resolution: Consciously and slowly assimilating only what is digestible and ensuring adequate processing. Archetypal principle: Moon-Mars/Uranus.

Regression

see Depression

Rejection reaction

(following organ transplants)

Physical level: Immune system (defence); all parts of the body where transplants are performed.

Symptom level: Natural attempt by the organism to preserve its (structural) integrity and protect itself from the foreign (tissue); self-defence by the immune system; rejection of an (organ) donation = not being able to accept the organ as an undeserved gift (imbalance between giving and taking).

Handling: Making oneself aware of the rejection and the deeper layer at which the original disease pattern is continuing to claim its rights, thus preventing the acceptance of the simple solution of the donation; integrating the subject initially symbolised by the failed organ, and now again by the replacement organ.

Resolution: Becoming friends with the donated organ at the level of inner imagery; applying the defensive stance to other areas: for the preservation of one's own integrity; self-defence in the mental-spiritual respect with simultaneous openness for new momentum and suggestions/ideas; gratitude; accepting the gift of (new) life; adopting the foreign as one's own consciously and with humility. Archetypal principle: Mars-Saturn.

Renal pelvis inflammation

(pyelitis)

Physical level: Renal pelvis (catchment funnel), kidneys (balance, partnership).

Symptom level: Spiritual conflicts on the basis of →kidney stones or germ-inating elements which have risen up from the the bladder (→urinary bladder inflammation): shadows coming to light (waste water of the bladder), chronic hardening and solidification of unresolved partnership problems as the trigger.

Handling: Confronting the underlying partnership problems; addressing the still provocative issues which one wanted to get rid of spiritually (bladder); learning to fight for harmony and inner balance.

Resolution: Committed willingness to fight for the sake of spiritual harmony; fostering a constructive conflict culture in the partnership area. Archetypal principle: Venus-Mars.

Respiratory arrest

see Apnoea, Sleep apnoea

Respiratory distress

(e.g. with bronchitis, lung inflammation)

Physical level: Respiratory tract (exchange), lungs (contact, communication, freedom).

Symptom level: Being cut off from polarity; "gasping for air", not being

able to catch one's breath, shortness of breath; problems with the lightness of the air element and the free-flight into the world of thoughts and imagery; refusal to communicate with life; inhalation problems: rejecting life, not allowing it in or close to oneself; exhalation problems: not being able to give (any longer), lacking belief in receiving anything in return; having already given one's all (being spent).
Handling: Recognising what is taking one's breath away, and taking the wind (for breathing) out of one's sails; asking oneself where the overload lies; breathing exercises: practising taking while also letting giving happen; exercises with connected breathing; practising exchange on the mental-spiritual level; spiritual exercises related to polarity: consciously moving within the scope of one's own possibilities.
Resolution: Getting by with less exchange and communication; restriction to the essential with respect to energy, becoming sparing with (one's own) energy, making better use of it; when one's breathing stops, feeling the closeness to transcendence.
Archetypal principle: Mercury-Saturn.

Respiratory paralysis

Physical level: Lungs (contact, communication, freedom), respiratory centre (control of exchange).
Symptom level: Being cut off not only from oxygen, but also the Prana flow: paralysed communication; paralysis of the energy supply; the giving up of taking and (consequently also of) giving; while in the state of being cut off from polarity, approaching the transcendental experience of unity.
Handling: Breathing exercises; exercises related to polarity; clarifying the question of whether there is still something essential to take in;

reducing external communication in favour of inner communication.
Resolution: Consciously adjusting oneself to the transition into the transcendental world (in the state of deep meditation, one's breathing also often stops when one transcends the borders of polarity).
Archetypal principle: Mercury-Neptune.

Respiratory tract diseases

(see also Bronchial asthma, Cold diseases, Influenza)
Physical level: Nose (power, pride, sexuality), gullet/throat (assimilation, defence), larynx (distribution), windpipe (exchange), lungs (contact, communication, freedom).
Symptom level: Shutting oneself off from the outside (nose blocked, throat congested, voice hoarse, ears blocked, eyes reddened, bronchia tending to be closed off); outward expressions of aggression (coughing, snorting, sneezing); disturbance of vitality, rhythm, build up and release of tension, exchange.
Handling: Learning to shut oneself off from the outside; creating one's own space, keeping one's environment at a distance ("Don't get too close to me!"); offensively defending one's living space ("coughing up" what one really thinks, "snorting").
Resolution: Standing up for one's own needs; drawing one's borders in good time; ensuring one's living space with all one's might.
Archetypal principle: Mercury-Saturn, Mars (coughing), Uranus (sneezing).

Restless legs

Physical level: Legs (mobility, progress, stability).
Symptom level: Restless condition of the legs; continual, compulsive

movement, above all when one is trying to rest; one is forcibly run off one's feet; unrest in getting ahead.

Handling: Getting moving again; stirring oneself from the spot and getting ahead; taking the legs into one's hands.

Resolution: Inner, spiritual progress.

Archetypal principle: Jupiter-Uranus.

Retained testis

(cryptorchism; retention of a testicle in the abdominal cavity or the inguinal canal)

Physical level: Testicles (fertility, creativity), genital region (sexuality, polarity, procreation).

Symptom level: Historical-evolutionary-based retention of the testicles, which fail to take part in the descent into the sexual region: the body manifests spiritual immaturity; testicles (gonads) which remain on the upper, higher (and less suspicious) level lose their function (become infertile): rejection of the descent into the lower, fertile domains (reaches) of sexual matters (e.g. overly clean fantasies); the symptom is often similarly embarrassing to the person affected as the related subject which is thereby being prevented: holding back one's own masculine creative possibilities, and in consequence, often feeling oneself of less worth and inferior to "normal" men, but in particular with respect to women.

Handling: (for jointly affected parents, whose problems are often reflected by the children): allowing sexuality to live in the (sexual) underworld from the very beginning; recognising the danger of infertility (on all levels) and the budding feelings of inferiority in good time and preventing them by the (enforced) descent into the underworld; if necessary, forcible correction of the position (of the testicle): 1. The descent can

be effected by means of hormone therapy or 2. operation = 1. Allowing more of the masculine aspect to flow in and 2. Forceful displacement of the attributes of masculinity into the underworld (scrotal) sacks provided for this purpose.

Resolution: Understanding that the creation of new life is only possible in the underworld (of the sexual), just as the metamorphosis of dead matter into new life (or vitamins) can only take place in the kingdom of the dead of the intestines; making friends with one's own masculinity, reconciling oneself with it and enjoying it.

Archetypal principle: Moon-Pluto.

Retching

(see also Vomiting)

Physical level: Neck (assimilation, connection, communication), gullet (assimilation, defence).

Symptom level: "Something gets stuck in one's throat", "not wanting to swallow something"; closure of the throat against something that is pushing its way to the surface; preferring to choke rather than integrate something; something wrongly taken on board is flung out again.

Handling/Resolution: Learning to shut oneself off forcibly from outside influences and to correct faults through one's own efforts.

Archetypal principle: Venus-Pluto.

Retinal detachment

(ablatio retinae; see also Blindness)

Physical level: Eyes (insight, perspective, mirrors and windows of the soul), retina (photographic plate of the eye).

Symptom level: 60% of cases with →shortsightedness, 35% due to old age, 5% in cases of absence of the crystalline lens of the eye; flashes, haziness, seeing shadows as the foreshadowers of partial blindness: having seen something so terrible that it shatters one's picture of things and perhaps even tears the canvas (screen); warnings overlooked in the spiritual become physically so apparent that they can no longer be overlooked; they indicate that something is wrong with one's perception of the world; losses in one's field of vision: no longer being able to perceive the whole reality; becoming blind to parts of the outer world; tendency towards total loss of sight (complete →blindness.

Handling: Learning to take for real (perceive) what has been overlooked in the figurative sense; becoming insightful; directing one's gaze specifically to the essential; focussing oneself and one's gaze; consciously honing it and homing it in; learning to look inwards.

Resolution: Placing inner images on a par with/above external images; inner orientation, insight.

Archetypal principle: Sun/Moon-Uranus.

Retinal diseases

see Retinopathy

Retinal inflammation

(retinitis)

Physical level: Eyes (insight, perspective, mirrors and windows of the soul), retina (photographic plate of the eye).

Symptom level: Triggered by too much light (snow blindness, autogenous welding); a flash burn on the light-sensitive photographic plate of the eye occurs: such burns are comparable to those caused by sunburn; conflict in the background of one's vision; conflict over the transport vessels of the life energy in the eye.

Handling: Ensuring more light in the mental-spiritual sense; encouraging flashes of inspiration and sudden brainwaves instead of physical energy flashes; letting things dawn on

one and being enlightened more often in the figurative sense.

Resolution: Exposing oneself to the spiritual light.

Archetypal principle: Sun/Moon-Mars.

Retinitis

see Retinal inflammation

Retinopathia pigmentosa

Physical level: Eyes (insight, perspective, mirrors and windows of the soul), retina (photographic plate of the eye).

Symptom level: Congenital problem, usually emerging in early childhood, which causes the vision cells responsible for light sensitivity to degenerate and can lead via increasing restriction of the field of vision to the point of →blindness; inability to adjust oneself adequately to darkness: problems in dealing with one's shadow, the dark part of one's own existence; conflict fought out against the background of vision; conflict-laden confrontation with the images of life; wanting to blend something out and not see it; giving priority to thinking over feeling.

Handling: Withdrawing oneself inwards and concentrating on the essential; owning up to one's own difficulties with the dark sides of life and accepting them; orientating oneself to the inner light at an early stage in life.

Resolution: Acknowledging and honouring one's own deepest feelings; adjusting oneself to the inner divine light; allowing a light to dawn on one in the figurative sense.

Archetypal principle: Sun/Moon-Mars-Saturn.

Retinopathy

(retinal diseases; see also Retinal inflammation)
Physical level: Eyes (insight, perspective, mirrors and windows of the soul), retina (photographic plate of the eye).
Symptom level: Non-inflammatory degeneration of the retina due to minor haemorrhaging with →diabetes mellitus, →high blood pressure (first clarify and interpret the basic situation): danger of →blindness.
Handling: Voluntarily complying with the call to look less to the outside and to look more to the inside; making inner instead of outer journeys; developing one's intuitive perception, emphasising the sixth sense instead of the first sense.
Resolution: Insight instead of outlook; arriving at one's own centre.
Archetypal principle: Sun/ Moon-Saturn.

Retracted testicles

see Retained testis

Rheumatic pains

see Twitching of the limbs

Rheumatic pericarditis

see Pericarditis

Rheumatism

(polyarthritis)
Physical level: Joints (mobility, articulation), musculature (motor, strength).
Symptom level: Rusted-up, blocked joints (the joint lubrication, which corresponds to the oil in a machine, is used up): deadlocked situation, comparable to the seizing of a piston in an engine (anyone who does not get enough exercise rusts up: in

actual fact, the joints need physical movement in order to remain well lubricated, in the same way that inner flexibility is necessary so that everything in life runs in a well-oiled way); old, outlived subjects (waste residues, rheumatism nodes) block any further steps forward and the possibility of getting a grip on one's (inner) life; grit in the works: one's articulation capability silts up due to the lack of inner movement; stiffness in the morning, which forces one to rest outwardly, shows the rigidity with which those affected face the day and life; inhibition of aggression in consciousness and instead aggressive attacks against one's own joints; auto-aggression/ pain remains stuck as inflammation in the joints: not being able to face up to one's own aggressions; often unlived, suppressed criticism of oneself and others; not getting along with one's connections (usually in the family, but also in the professional field): the disappointed dream of harmonious, peaceful relationships now has to be enforced through suffering ("dictatorship for the good of all"); instead of battling to establish a position, it is now to be achieved through suffering ("whoever suffers (endures) so much must be rewarded after all"); blockage of the activity in the muscular area: being forced to rest in order to put an end to compensation of one's inner rigidity/obstinacy through over-activity; →feelings of guilt with simultaneous "benevolent tyranny" or illness if hostile impulses cannot be compensated for by sacrifice and service; build-up of undigested problems; in particular: Finger joint: Conflict over getting a grip on life; Wrist joint: Conflict over the ability to handle things; Elbow: Conflict over elbowing one's way through (forceful assertion); Hip joint: Conflict over forward progress in life and the meaning of life; Knee joint: Conflict over humiliation and humility;

Ankle joint: Conflict over getting one's chance to make the leap.

Handling: Living in a more open(ly offensive) way; fighting for one's own agility and articulation in the world; recognising the vital energies that one has directed against oneself and re-directing them into the mental-spiritual area; accepting the enforced rest and using it for inner struggles; transferring one's central weighting from outer to inner activity; recognising and observing one's combative assaults on the life of others (the rheumatism itself is sometimes also misused for such purposes), and also learning to see through cramped (forced) sacrifice as an attempt of this type; honest questioning of altruism; retraction of projections; starting to work on the undigested problems which are manifesting themselves in the (rheumatism) nodes; conscious fasting for clearing up the nodes and cleansing the connective tissue of corresponding deposits.

Resolution: Bringing egoism, inflexibility, inability to adapt, bossiness and aggression out from the shadow area; developing mental-spiritual agility.

Archetypal principle: Mercury (joints)/Mars (muscles)-Pluto (auto-aggression)-Saturn (inhibition).

Rhinitis

see Cold diseases

Rhinitis atrophicans

see Ozaena

Rhinophyma

(pug nose, rummy nose; see also Rosacea)

Physical level: Nose (power, pride, sexuality).

Symptom level: Grotesque, bulbous swelling of the nose ("hooter"), which dominates and disfigures the whole face and blazes like a red traffic light; exacerbated by alcohol abuse: the red, rummy nose of the heavy drinker; unconscious desires for power bear unsightly fruits; lack of sexual and aggressive stimulation manifests itself physically; undeveloped genital/phallic sexuality: suppressed wishes for unrestrained excesses and degeneracy in the domains of sexuality or power; growth impulses that have come up too short; red clown's nose: meddlesome, sticking one's nose in everywhere, nosy.

Handling: Fostering spiritual interests instead of consuming spirits; in order to take the burden off the nose, directing one's sexual fantasies into one's waking consciousness and to the applicable places in the body; making oneself aware of one's desires for unrestrained excesses and expansion instead of pushing these away into the body; acknowledgement of one's own desires for power, unlived pride and libido-driven sexuality; becoming more brazen and meddlesome; also taking oddball paths if these are one's own; looking after one's "sniffer" and getting wind of things.

Resolution: Letting one's nose show one the way: "always following one's nose"; growing and unfolding (developing further); radiating vitality and drawing attention to oneself; transforming being marked into being marked with distinction.

Archetypal principle: Mars-Mars.

Rib fracture

Physical level: Rib cage (sense of self/Ego, personality), ribs (safety, protection, adaptation).

Symptom level: Reaction to particularly constrictive/binding situation: attempt to force the denied openness with violence; attempt to open the heart area from outside with violence and to help the wings (lobes) of the lungs to freedom; break-in of outside

forces into the well-protected cage for the most central organs.
Handling: Voluntarily opening the chest area from inside rather than having it broken open from the outside; giving the heart and the wings (lobes) of the lungs all the inner freedom they can use; also opening oneself inwardly for extreme impacts and impulses.
Resolution: Risking flexibility and exchange from the heart; taking off on flights of fantasy; developing greater emotional agility.
Archetypal principle: Saturn-Uranus.

Rings under the eyes

see Eyes, rings under

Roemheld's syndrome

Physical level: Stomach (feeling, receptiveness), intestines (processing of material impressions), heart (seat of the soul, love, feelings, energy centre).
Symptom level: The overwhelmed underworld (distended intestinal loops) creates pressure on the centre of the emotions and feelings (of love) (the heart); the intestines put the heart under pressure; the shadow kingdom pushes its way upwards and puts the squeeze on the heart, causing it to feel ill; something which stinks touches one's heart; not really (being capable of) digesting what one has taken to heart; something is weighing on one's heart which is creating pressure; the desire to relieve the pressure leads to one raising a stink; being wedged in, standing with one's back to the wall.
Handling: Perceiving the underworld more consciously and learning to see through to its effects on other levels; making oneself aware that everything which cannot be processed in the

kingdom of the dead pushes its way upwards again and (in addition to headaches) can also cause heart problems; sounding out (tapping) and listening (with a stethoscope) to the oppressed, stressed heart for effects from the shadow realm; placing value on the digestibility of (spiritual and physical) nourishment and bringing oneself to create the necessary preliminary conditions, such as good chewing (understanding); not turning one's heart into a skeleton closet, but instead voluntarily opening it up in order to let out the emotions (Latin e-movere = 'to move out'); letting off steam even to the point of making a stink, or better yet: letting things out (expressing them) openly; seeking confrontation instead of raising a stink about something via the back door; setting off on the search for the deeper sources of the pressure.
Resolution: Digesting/processing things appropriately; taking the load off the heart by solving the problems of the underworld; shadow therapy.
Archetypal principle: Sun/Moon-Pluto.

Rosacea

(see also Rhinophyma, Puberty acne)
Physical level: Skin (border, contact, tenderness).
Symptom level: Reddening of the skin based on a foundation of unnaturally-increased sebaceous secretions (seborrhoea), which can extend from minor vascular distensions to the formation of pustules and papules, as well as to the proliferation of sebaceous glands, and thus eventually to disfigurement: the face blooms red like a rose and attracts attention; conflict-laden (inflammatory) basic setting, upon which a warlike battlefield can develop; last desperate attempt at puberty and growing up.
Handling: Identifying shame as the source underlying the redness/

reddening; tackling the subject of puberty/growing up and helping the corresponding aspect of sexuality to break through; allowing a new stage in life to blossom with the same glow as the rosacea; finding other, more resolved (redeeming) ways of attracting attention to oneself.

Resolution: Making oneself aware of the tasks connected with the characteristic qualities of the prevailing period of life and giving them the chance to blossom; allowing oneself to bloom.

Archetypal principle: Venus/Saturn-Mars.

Rotary vertigo

(see also Balance disorders, Menière's disease)

Physical level: Balance organ in the inner ear (balance sensor).

Symptom level: Losing control: standing on unsteady ground; not yet having found the "right way to go about things"; instead of making the wheels turn and setting things in motion, things turn and move around one in an uncontrolled way.

Handling: Conscious (spiritual) exercises, giving up control (learning to let go); rediscovering child-like play (various spinning and twirling games); dancing waltzes without "feign"(t)ing spells (dizziness due to self-deception); ensuring that, in the extended sense, everything or at least a great deal revolves around oneself; consciously getting things moving in life, twisting and turning oneself instead of falling victim to physical illusions of movement.

Resolution: Finding the right way to go about things in life; discovering the pleasant aspects of letting oneself go (Dervish dancing: whirling to the point of trance-like ecstasy).

Archetypal principle: Neptune.

Round back

Physical level: Spinal column (dynamics and hold, uprightness), back (strenuous effort, uprightness).

Symptom level: Over-stretched back musculature as a protection for the more vulnerable front side, which is kept hidden; unlived humility; bowed down/broken child/adult; bowing to superiors but treading inferiors underfoot ("suck-up" and "arse-crawler" mentality); "doubling up with effort", lack of straightforwardness; strength that has been surpressed; lack of strength in letting out (expressing) oneself; no firm hold; bending oneself out of shape to avoid rubbing anyone the wrong way; bowed down and humiliated; lack of stable backing.

Handling: Making a stand against things before one's back is broken; consciously sensing opportunistic, conformist adaptations and recognising their incompatibility with inner, and in the long term, also outer uprightness; finding stable support in one's own life axis; being one's own backing; opening the heart and communications area (lungs); learning to walk tall; becoming upright and honest.

Resolution: Through awareness, allowing genuine humility to grow out of humiliations.

Archetypal principle: Saturn.

Rubella

(see also Skin rash, Childhood diseases)

Physical level: Skin (border, contact, tenderness).

Symptom level: Something new aggressively blazes a path into the life of the child or young person, bursting open the border of the skin from the inside; a necessary development step in the direction of self-realisation is imminent and must be fought for; the body becomes a drilling ground.

Handling/Resolution: (also for jointly-affected parents, whose problems are often reflected by the children): preparing oneself for new steps in life in an open(ly offensive) way; making oneself aware of the importance of this development step, which in the case of women, indirectly provides protection against later problems in pregnancies; adolescents must learn to pay attention to their own inner voice, and live self-confidently, i.e. but also to detach themselves from prescribed parental patterns and compulsions.

Archetypal principle: Mars/ Uranus.

Rummy nose

see Rhinophyma

S

Sacroiliac pains

see Back pains, Sciatica, Lumbago

Saddlebags

see Lipophilia, Obesity

Salivation, increased

Physical level: Salivary gland (appetite, desire, closeness).

Symptom level: Unsatisfied hunger for life: something is making one's mouth water; drooling expectantly over one's expectations in life in a lustful and lascivious way.

Handling: Obtaining and assimilating what one is lusting after; learning to stand up for one's own desires.

Resolution: Switching to the spiritual level and satisfying one's hunger for life and experiences in this domain.

Archetypal principle: Moon-Venus/ Jupiter.

Salmonella enteritis (salmonellosis)

see Intestinal inflammation

Salpingitis

see Fallopian tubes, inflammation

Sarcoidosis

(Boeck's disease, connective tissue tumours)

Physical level: Connective tissue (connection, stability, binding commitment); all organ structures can be affected, but above all, the lymph nodes of the lungs and the subcutaneous tissue.

Symptom level: Painless, usually lentil-sized or smaller tumours, appearing on the trunk and on the face, but also on the arms and legs, which as a rule, are harmless, and usually disappear spontaneously (connections with →pulmonary consumption are probable): harmless blemishes of one's outer appearance; in the rare third and final stage, resulting in fibrous (connective tissue), there are structural changes in the organs – the lymph nodes of the mediastinum (the space between the lobes of the lungs) – which can then lead to displacement problems: impairment of communication and exchange.

Handling: Intensifying binding commitment and growth at the cost of superficial communication; feeling oneself to be marked and marking oneself with distinction.

Resolution: Growing in matters related to connections and binding commitment and relieving the body of what it is doing for one in terms of being binding; fostering the growth and proliferation of ones talents.

Archetypal principle: Jupiter/Moon.

Sarcoma

see Bone cancer, Liposarcoma, Cancer

SARS

see Lung inflammation

Satyriasis

(see also Addiction: Sex addiction)

Symptom level: Pathologically-increased sex drive in men; seemingly unconquerable longing for sex and sexual intercourse and therefore also for the opposite sexual pole, i.e. women, which is intensified by social taboos on the subject.

Handling: Intensive consideration of the issue of polarity; conscious sexuality in the sense of approaching it as a ritual; tantric attempts to discover love in the depths of sexuality.

Resolution: Recognising sexuality as simply a physical aspect, whose spiritual component is love; quality instead of quantity.

Archetypal principle: Pluto.

Scabies

Physical level: Skin (border, contact, tenderness)

Symptom level: Something lively gets under one's skin and irritates (itches) one, particularly at night: the scabies mites eat out their characteristic winding burrows directly under the skin and darken it with their excrement; at the end of the burrow, they leave behind small blisters, which itch severely particularly at night; aspect and feeling of uncleanliness: being marked by the ("shitty") trails of the parasites; nowadays often the trigger for panicky obsession with cleanliness, feelings of shame with regard to one's tainted impression; "being eaten up by something" (feeling insulted, bad-tempered); feeling of being undermined/infiltrated, of no

longer "being home alone" (which we never are anyway).

Handling: Also allowing oneself to be stimulated by seemingly unclean aspects (particularly at night); taking on stimuli as challenges; letting lively elements get close to one and allowing them to get under one's skin, thereby leaving behind clear tracks in the spiritual domain; letting oneself get involved with the "parasites", tolerating them, "living and letting live"; learning to share (oneself/one's views); critically re-examining one's own feeling of cleanliness with respect to life (lively elements); allowing oneself to get involved with contacts which get under one's skin.

Resolution: Meeting lively elements with openness, even down to their smallest, humblest and seemingly most inferior forms; living and letting live.

Archetypal principle: Venus/ Saturn (Haut)-Pluto (parasites, freeloaders).

Scar hernia

(see also Rupture, Umbilical hernia)

Physical level: Anywhere where scars have been left behind following injuries.

Symptom level: (recent) Opening up of an old wound; improper closure of a wound promotes the giving way of the scar; there is still pressure behind the scar which it cannot withstand; having come under pressure due to old problems which were first acute at the time of the injury.

Handling: Making clear to oneself how little one is completely over and done with the wound (bearing a grudge?); reconsidering the old wound and taking new approaches to promoting its healing; consciously going back to the relevant old experience in order to process what has remained open; making oneself aware of the (spiritual) pressure behind the scar and giving way to it; becoming aware of old wounds which have not healed sufficiently; becoming aware of inner wounds which have never healed completely.

Resolution: Taking new approaches in order to finally resolve (clear up) old issues once and for all.
Archetypal principle: Saturn-Uranus.

Scar proliferation

(scar keloid)
Physical level: Scars on the body surface, skin (border, contact, tenderness).
Symptom level: Scar proliferations following operations and severe burns as a sign that the event has not passed one by without leaving a mark and has not been completely processed; the connective tissue of the scar begins to proliferate and form unsightly scar beads, as if the event which led to the scar does not want to be forgotten; strikingly frequent occurrence if it is particularly important to the person affected that no scars or only tiny scars should remain (bikini-appendix scar): having learnt little or nothing from the traumatic events and therefore continually being reminded of this opportunity; scar keloids practically always occur following burns caused by atomic explosions, which shows that we generally cannot be completely over and done with the effects of this power on our organism.
Handling: Calling back into consciousness the event which led to the scar and coming to terms with it spiritually; recognising the meaning of the scar/the old injury, and again rolling out the story of how the scar came to be; relieving the organism of the task of keeping the memory alive by voluntarily keeping it alive oneself.
Resolution: Reconciliation with the original event; preserving it in consciousness without suffering from it any further.
Archetypal principle: Saturn (scar)-Jupiter (proliferation).

Scarlet fever

(see also Skin rash, Childhood diseases)
Physical level: Skin (border, contact, tenderness).
Symptom level: Angry red, inflamed throat with swollen tonsils and neck lymph nodes: serious conflict flares up at the point of entry into the inner world of the body; pain in the neck and pain when swallowing: having swallowed enough, further swallowing hurts too much; vomiting: the situation makes one "want to be sick", wanting to let out (express) something and be rid of it; raspberry-like tongue and breaking out in a scarlet-red rash (innumerable dark red spots) on the body: a vital, angry red energy breaks through to the outside; aggressions discharge themselves physically; danger of the inflammatory conflicts spilling over into the sinuses ("being sick to the eyeballs of something"), joints (articulation problems), kidneys (relationship, harmony problems), cerebral membranes (central regulation problems); rheumatic fever as a further possible complication: general defensive battle whose progression drags the joints and heart valve defects in its wake ("scarlet fever licks the joints and bites the heart").
Handling: Affected children have the task of fighting their way onto their own feet, thereby breaking out of the victim role which has been prescribed by the family or tradition, and also actively and combatively escaping from their martyr situation (a feeling similar to being wounded by thousands of needles); many attempts may be necessary for this purpose (scarlet fever can be contracted several times); tasks of the jointly-affected parents,

whose problems are often reflected by the children: supporting the aggressive struggle over letting in new impulses; providing loving attention, which makes tough chunks easier to swallow and helps to get rid of old patterns and ways of life; conscious changeover to and changing in line with the new era: allowing the new, unfamiliar energies to break through and break out with great force; instilling courage to prevail in the battle that is raging outwardly on the skin and inwardly in the soul; paying attention to secondary theatres of war: allowing frustration tolerance to develop; encouraging articulation and allowing oneself to develop; keeping relationship and harmony needs in mind; working on central questions related to the regulation of life; working to encourage the development of aggression in the sense of being fired up to lead a courageous life which values challenges and allows aggressive thinking.

Resolution: Meeting the new stage of life with openness; allowing what is as yet still unfamiliar to break through; tackling the impending development step with courage and rejoicing over the result.

Archetypal principle: Mars-Uranus.

Scheuermann's disease

(Osteochondropathia juvenilis deformans; see also Back pains)

Physical level: Spinal column (dynamism and stability), back (strenuous effort, uprightness).

Symptom level: Intervertebral disc tissue intrudes into the end plates of the vertebral bodies, thereby deforming them, and eventually leading to a rigid, →round back; bowed position without flexibility: having become fixed in a humiliating position; one's poor inner stance is clearly shown outwardly (hanging one's head in the

direction of hard-headedness); problems with uprightness: such problems emerge above all in adolescence at a time when instinctual drives are most strongly trying to push to the surface, often without the possibility of any release.

Handling: Supporting the interpenetration of feminine and masculine elements as forming the backbone and stability of life: allowing feminine energies to penetrate into masculine domains and fertilise them; concentrating on a humble stance as a matter of basic principle: allowing strength to flow into one's humble stance as a means for loosening up (resolving) strong rigidity.

Resolution: Humility.

Archetypal principle: Saturn.

Schizophrenia

(split personality; see also Hebephrenia, Mental illness)

Symptom level: Disturbed interpersonal and social connections, with at the same time, often outstanding intelligence; →hallucinations, absent-mindedness, illogicality, distorted perceptions from the perspective of the so-called normal people; splitting up and fragmentation of thought, feeling and action, when measured against what is considered usual and normal; often delusions of persecution, which from the point of view of those affected, nevertheless make sense, because they are, in fact, pursued and confined by "normal people", either in the form of physical confinement in corresponding institutions or through inner chemical captivity by means of psycho-pharmaceuticals; the disorders described suggest a flight from our normal world into a shadow world which appears unreal to us, but which is experienced as depressingly real by those affected; according to Joseph Campbell, schizophrenic breakdown is "a journey leading inwards and backwards in order to catch up on something that has been missed or to regain something that has been lost, and thereby bring life back into alignment".

Handling: (also for jointly-affected family members): creating points of access to the world of experience of the person affected; recognising the splitting of reality into two sides that we are all subject to due to polarity as the basis of every development; getting to know and accept the shadow kingdom with appropriate tour guides.

Resolution: Being able to distinguish between the shadow world and reality and learning to keep them apart.

Archetypal principle: Uranus-Neptune-Pluto.

Sciatica

(see also Intervertebral disc prolapse)

Physical level: Spinal column (dynamics and hold, uprightness), intervertebral discs (female pole of the spinal column), nerves (news service).

Symptom level: Aggravation of the sciatic nerve or usually the nerves emerging from the spinal cord channel with considerable pain due to pressure (often displaced intervertebral disc); dislocation of the life axis or conflicts (→inflammations); intervertebral disc problem: (excessive) existential pressure; the soft, feminine element is caught in the stranglehold between two hard masculine elements and pinched/squeezed (has the squeeze put on it?); overloading (e.g. as compensation for lack of self-assurance and feelings of inferiority): taking too much on (to one's shoulders) / saddling oneself with a burden (allowing oneself to be saddled), overloading/ overburdening/ overstretching oneself in order to make an impression and blot out the correct impression; often existential

pressure to ensure the livelihood for oneself and above all for the family; tearing oneself to pieces because one does not consciously "have a firm grasp" of something; search for recognition; pressure which gets on one's nerves; inner pressure blazes a path to the outside; side-stepping inner pressure: painful ways out; in the case of dislocation: one's life (world) axis has slipped out of alignment; in the case of spinal column displacements: getting caught/ deadlocked; humiliation in the case of a lack of uprightness: "crooked as a dog's hind leg"; uprightness pushed too far in the form of righteousness: "stick in the mud".

Handling: Allowing oneself to be challenged (provoked) in the central command area (sciatica) (for all steps forward and upward); making oneself aware of existential pressure and the role of the female pole; shifting the soft, feminine elements of one's own existence more into focus; consciously carrying (bearing) the burden of one's own existence; recognising and giving up overload situations as compensation for insecurity: subjecting the burdens on one's own shoulders to critical examination; experimenting with the life axis and the focal point of life; finding a more fitting orientation; putting back into line what has slipped out of alignment; straightening out deadlocked matters; putting things back to rights (even if it is painful); using the enforced rest for reflection.

Resolution: Restriction to the essential; transforming humiliations into humility; humbling oneself; being honest with oneself, and building on that basis, also with the world; moving and giving way inwardly.

Archetypal principle: Jupiter/ Mars-Saturn.

Scleroderma

(skin hardening)

Physical level: Skin (border, contact, tenderness), mucous membranes (inner boundary, barrier).

Symptom level: Hardening of the skin and the subcutaneous tissue: hardening of the borders; shutting oneself off inwardly and outwardly; contraction and atrophy of the skin and subcutaneous tissue: one's feels trapped in one's skin ("it's enough to make one want to burst"); the body shows one the narrowing and limiting of one's living space in the figurative sense, which those affected are not aware of.

Handling: Conscious setting of limits towards the outer world; strengthening of one's shielding against outside influences: reduction of direct external contacts; building up a thick skin; retracting one's feelers, reducing the borders and surfaces for exchange; opening oneself up inwardly and discovering one's own inner world; consciously owning up to one's own narrowness and restrictiveness and accepting these.

Resolution: Retreat inwards and conquering the opposite pole from within one's own inner world: from this safe platform, extending the borders and opening oneself up to the world; becoming one with oneself in order to be able to open up again from this starting point.

Archetypal principle: Venus/Saturn-Saturn.

Sclerosis

(hardening)

Physical level: Various areas of the organism can be affected.

Symptom level: Hardening, e.g. of the arteries (→arteriosclerosis), the skin (→scleroderma), the neuroglial tissue in the central nervous system (→multiple sclerosis).

Handling/Resolution: Ensuring concentration, well-defined limits, structure formation and clarity.

Archetypal principle: Saturn.

Scoliosis

see Spinal column, curvature

Screaming children

(often identical to children with distended bellies; see also Three-month colic)

Physical level: Pains (physical/spiritual), usually of unknown origin.

Symptom level: Despair expressed by the children at the top of their voice which can bring the parents to the limits of their own despair; outbreaks of aggression, which, in those who are testimony to it, can easily mobilise their own unprocessed aggression problems.

Handling: (For parents, whose problems are often reflected by the children): often improved by going for a drive in the car: something happens in the sense of vibration (swinging motion); gentle massages which convey loving attention and a feeling of safety and security; owning up to one's own mood swings and letting them out (expressing them); accepting the ups and downs of emotions in oneself and the children; making oneself aware of one's own unexpressed pain and suffering; finding ways to let out one's own suppressed screams; recognising and acknowledging aggression as a vital basic force; doing without what is difficult to digest (in concrete terms: overly frequent and incorrect nourishment, in the figurative sense: panic whenever the child cries); learning to have patience and to serve others; learning to be a mother/father to the limits of what is bearable; giving one's best and then learning to preserve inner calm despite the outer storms.

Resolution: Making peace with the mother/father role; building a nest and also conveying the corresponding nest feeling.
Archetypal principle: Mercury (communication)-Mars (aggression)-Moon (child).

Scurvy

(Vitamin C deficiency disease)
Physical level: Blood (life force), gums (basic trust), skin (boundary, contact, tenderness), mucous membranes (inner border, barrier), bones (stability, strength), joints (mobility, articulation).
Symptom level: Haemorrhaging (life force flows away and escapes), which usually begins in the gums (basic trust) before spreading into the mucous membranes (inner borders), skin (outer border), and joints (articulation), and eventually leading to painful structural changes of the bones (stability, strength); nowadays only occurs in mild forms in the case of an unbalanced diet (lack of fresh fruit and vegetables).
Handling: (assuming, of course, that sufficient Vitamin C is first administered): ensuring that one takes in enough fresh life energy in the form of fruit and vegetables; allowing one's own life energy to flow into the inner and outer border areas, into mobility, articulation and the structural domain; changing one's supporting structures – even if this causes pain.
Resolution: Bringing life into the Saturnine domain (= borders and structures) in one's own life.
Archetypal principle: Saturn.

Seasickness

see Kinetoses, Balance disorders

Seborrhoea

Physical level: Skin (border, contact, tenderness).

Symptom level: Excessive sebaceous secretions result in a face which looks as though well-oiled (seborrhoea oleosa) or which, due to peeling of the skin (seborrhoea sicca = dry) in greasy, branflake form, catches the eye; forms the basis for various skin problems, such as →rosacea, →puberty acne or also →rhinophyma.
Handling: Bringing more lubricating fluid into play; oiling the machine so that everything runs in a well-oiled way again (like "greased lightning"); trying to move through things glibly like an eel instead of rubbing oneself raw against everything; smoothly overcoming resistance; increasing physical secretions (e.g. sweating due to sport), expressing more with one's face.
Resolution: Finding and showing one's true face.
Archetypal principle: Venus/ Saturn (skin)-Jupiter (oil).

Seeing double

Physical level: Eyes (insight, perspective, mirrors and windows of the soul), retina (photographic plate of the eye); e.g. in the case of multiple sclerosis: brain (communication, logistics).
Symptom level: Having a double take on the world/reality; no longer bringing together the two sides of polarity; the polar division of the world into two contrasting aspects is forced upon one optically; being torn between these two sides of reality.
Handling: Making clear to oneself that everything has two sides and that this always includes the opposite pole; learning to see the opposites/ contradictions in one's own life and to acknowledge their existence.
Resolution: Always taking both sides of a matter for real; always keeping the polarity

of all Creation in view and knowing there is unity behind it.
Archetypal principle: Sun/Moon-Mercury.

Self-poisoning

(Auto-intoxication, see also Poisoning)
Physical level: The whole metabolism (dynamic equilibrium) is affected.
Symptom level: Unprocessed issues begin to poison and block one's own organism; no longer managing to get certain tasks completely over and done with.
Handling: Becoming outwardly more venomous instead of poisoning oneself inwardly; granting and taking more time for oneself for certain cleaning up and cleaning out measures; making oneself aware of which spiritual subject areas one has not managed to get over and done with and which of these threaten to block and poison one's life.
Resolution: Finding ways to eliminate the accumulated toxic elements from one's life; managing to deal conclusively with life and its waste products.
Archetypal principle: Neptune-Pluto.

Semi-consciousness

(e.g. in cases of →epilepsy, →alcoholism)
Symptom level: Clouding of one's consciousness with complete blackout of the conscious control mechanisms and reduced processing of external stimuli (for hours or days on end): allowing things to happen (to one) in an unresolved (unredeeming) way; taking leave from responsibility for oneself and others; being reliant on the support of others; turning away from the outside world and immersing oneself in the inner world; mood changes; behavioural changes to the point of completely uncharacteristic actions such as sexual and

criminal offences: shadow aspects force their way up from below into consciousness.
Handling: Voluntarily giving up one's powers of influence over the outer world for a time; shutting oneself off from the outer world and consciously turning inwards; consciously handing over responsibility to others; learning to consciously and gratefully accept support from outside; consciously allowing oneself to get involved with other, even dark moods; consciously getting to know one's own dark wishes and longings that are foreign to one's sense of self and instead attributable to the shadow kingdom; (psycho) therapy with regard to the basic problem.
Resolution: Contemplation; knowing and accepting oneself down to one's profoundest depths; allowing oneself to get involved with (existing) reality.
Archetypal principle: Neptune.

Senile deafness

(presbyacusis; see also Age-related symptoms)
Physical level: Ears (hearing and obeying commands).
Symptom level: The outer world gradually withdraws itself from one acoustically.
Handling: Recognising the demand to turn oneself away from the outer world, and towards the inner world.
Resolution: Listening carefully to one's own inner voice and obeying it.
Archetypal principle: Saturn.

Senile gangrene

see Gangrene

Senile heart

(see also Heart failure, Age-related symptoms)
Physical level: Heart (ability to love, emotion).

Symptom level: Enlargement of the heart, frequently occurring in old age due to cardiac insufficiency, which shows up on X-ray images as a shoe-shape; attempt, which is unsuccessful in the long term, to meet over-taxing challenges by expansion of the heart; one's centre of life expands at a substitute level; failure with regard to a central life theme; surrender is looming in central life areas; the end of life takes concrete form in the enlargement of the heart.

Handling: Return to one's own original heart themes and desires; expansion of one's own matters of the heart; opening up and stretching oneself to meet the flow of life and life energy; concrete spiritual exercises: fasting therapy in order to give the physical heart the chance to return to (its original) slim shape, and instead letting one's heart expand in the figurative sense.

Resolution: Taking care of one's own centre and the centre of one's own life; allowing the heart to expand beyond itself, and to broaden and open itself in the figurative sense; creating room in one's own heart for the whole world; opening up one's own heart to the world and all people, learning to love; finding (final) rest.

Archetypal principle: Sun-Saturn/ Neptune.

Senile hypermetropia

(Presbyopia; see also Age-related symptoms)
Physical level: Eyes (insight, perspective, mirrors and windows of the soul).
Symptom level: The aspects that are close at hand and one's death that is coming ever closer appear as increasingly out of focus and blurred; the aspects that are far off remain clearly in focus; life appears longer; perceptions of growing old and of ecstasy (Greek ékstasis = displacement,

trance): what is temporally close at hand become blurred.
Handling: Taking on the challenge of letting go of the day-to-day triviality that are close at hand in order to obtain an overview of the expansiveness of life: having a broad view of the greater connections of life.
Resolution: Reconciliation with what is distant and one's overview of the things of life; maintaining a retrospective view and finding the guiding golden thread in one's own life; recognising the (distant) objective; learning to appreciate the far-sightedness and wisdom of old age.
Archetypal principle: Jupiter-Sun/ Moon.

Sepsis

see Blood poisoning

Septum defects

(congenital heart defects with defects in the heart septum)
Physical level: Heart (seat of the soul, love, feelings, energy centre), heart septum (threshold in our centre between this side and what is beyond).
Symptom level: No real separation of the heart into a left and right side: half-hearted entry into polarity; remaining closely associated with unity (due to the ever-present threat of death); having a hole in one's heart: missing something in one's centre, defects of the heart (muscle).
Handling: Operative closure of the hole in the heart forces those affected into the world of polarity and thus into the confrontation with it; making openness of the heart a reality on the spiritual level; opening one's heart in the figurative sense so that the physical heart can remain closed in its centre.
Resolution: Striving for unity on the figurative level: being one with all; becoming one heart and one soul

with all sentient beings and the whole of Creation.
Archetypal principle: Sun-Saturn.

Sexual diseases

(venereal diseases that are sexually transmissible; see also Aids, Amincolpitis, Carcinoma in situ, Candidamycosis, Chlamydia infection, Crablouse infestation, Gonorrhoea, Herpes genitalis, Syphilis, Trichomoniasis, Dermatomycoses)
Physical level: All areas of the body can be dragged into their wake, the entrance gate for the problems is the sexual region (sexuality, polarity, procreation).
Symptom level: Particularly negatively-evaluated group of disease patterns, although such cases should never be a matter of value judgements, but instead always only of interpretations; after all, statistically speaking, all of life is a sexually-transmitted disease that in any case ends fatally; contrary to the actual biological purpose of sexual intercourse, which is the transfer of sperm organisms, in this case, other creatures end up being transmitted instead, which set totally different life forms in motion; riskiness of sexual intercourse with ever-changing partners: biology appears to take sides in rewarding faithfulness; (unconscious) conflicts over sexuality and gender identity: →feelings of guilt with regard to sexual impulses; sexually-related feelings of guilt with the unconscious tendency to punish oneself (of one's own accord) for having a fling on the side: (unconsciously) putting oneself and partners off the sexual area; suffering due to stimulating elements in the form of pathogens because one has been aroused without really granting it to oneself.
Handling: Acknowledging sexuality as an integral part of a fulfilled life; however, if it exists isolated from the mental-spiritual, it tends to integrate the lively vitality that is lacking by other means; allowing oneself to be ecstatically aroused, instead of opening oneself up to arousal in the form of pathogens; opening up one's own borders for one's partner and for erotic ecstasy; protecting oneself by maintaining cleanliness in sexual matters; making oneself aware that even the smallest of conflicts and uncleanliness in dealing with the sexual domain, which stands symbolically for the involvement with polarity; can be the breeding ground for all kinds of, and potentially also serious, complications; liberating the sexual domain from negative value judgements and learning to recognise and enjoy it as a guarantee for the survival of humankind and as a realm of desire; learning to be selective: the right choice of partner solves the problem that is created by screwing things up in the first place; using the flame of sexuality to also set the soul on fire; allowing one's whole being to be consumed by the fire of ecstasy.
Resolution: Leaving form and content together: sexual love in combination with mental-spiritual love leads to firm relationships and is the most effective form of prevention against the danger; overcoming the problem of dealing with polarity and putting the corresponding revelations into practice in one's everyday life; discovering in sexuality deep forces extending to all levels of existence (Tantra yoga).
Archetypal principle: Venus-Pluto.

Sexual intercourse, painful

see Dyspareunia

Sexually transmitted diseases

see Sexual diseases

Shingles

(Herpes zoster; see also Facial erysipelas)

Physical level: Stomach (feeling, instinct, enjoyment, centre), more rarely also the face (trademark, visiting card).

Symptom level: A long-held back border conflict discharges itself aggressively and painfully; the patient feels like screaming since the outbreak is so painful: screams that have been stifled for too long discharge themselves; something that already got under one's skin or on one's nerves much earlier now takes advantage of a period of weakness and breaks forth; active outbreak of resistance from within; rosy rash blossoming on the surface boundary to the outside: not having allowed one's own being to blossom sufficiently (be shown to the outside) in the past; long-suppressed impulses shoot up from below, planting strange blossoms on one's own skin: unlived (love) conflicts on the contact organ of the skin; burning emotions (love, jealousy, revenge) vent themselves via the skin (compare in mythology the burning robe of Medea, the burning river Lethe); the symptom forces honesty: the patient cannot bear contact of any sort and is over-sensitive; frequently also the theme of defilement and disfigurement (closeness between burning love and impure desires); frequently deeply-rooted insecurity due to the loss of a great love (which can be anything from a lover to a favourite task or projects of the heart).

Handling: Breaking forth; combative opening of one's own borders to offensive energies erupting from within; giving space to one's own long pent-up inner forces, even though this may be difficult and painful; blossoming, making space for oneself and expressing something unsaid; letting things out in a direct (unflowery) way; creating energy from openness.

Resolution: Setting unexpressed, underlying forces free; rejoicing in one's own creations; adorning oneself with one's own blossoms; enjoying the openness of one's own borders.

Archetypal principle: Venus-Mars.

Shivering attack

Physical level: The whole organism is affected.

Symptom level: Involuntary and uncontrollable cramps shake the body to the core: no longer being in control of oneself; lettting oneself be thoroughly shaken up; attempt by Fate to shake one into action for impending (typically combative) tasks; feeling ice-cold even while burning with high fever.

Handling: Allowing oneself to be shaken to the core and waking up to the demands of the moment; allowing oneself to be rattled and mixed up in order to arrive at new realisations (re-shuffling the cards, putting the pattern together in a new way using the same jigsaw pieces); no longer being in control of oneself, but instead allowing one's own vital forces to run their natural course; discovering Kundalini shaking meditation (Bhagwan-Osho) as a ritual in order to get the life flow back into motion again; being either hot or cold, but in any case, going to the extreme.

Resolution: Reflecting on the myth of Arjuna from the Bhagavad Gita, who was (mentally) shaken up by Lord Krishna until he was finally prepared to take up his struggle, and allowing this to have an effect on one.

Archetypal principle: Mars-Uranus.

Shock

see Collapse

Shop window disorder

see Claudicatio intermittens

Shortsightedness

(myopia)

Physical level: Eyes (insight, perspective, mirrors and windows of the soul).

Symptom level: Typical disorder in young people, who tend to see only their own immediate surroundings: lack of overview and far-sightedness; short field of vision with broad demands; "not being able to see the wood for the trees": not seeing something that is right under one's nose; cramped and tense eye muscles clearly show the corresponding view of the world, often an overall pinched, (strained) expression in order to bring some degree of focus into the images of the world by means of "squinting"(partly closing one's eyes); cumbersome view of the world; making things difficult to bear for oneself; wanting to bring everything up close in order to check it out; strong subjectivity, "seeing everything through one's own eye(glasse)s", "only seeing as far as the end of one's nose", strong egocentricity; one cannot trust one's own eyes; feelings of unease with regard to one's life circumstances; withdrawing, turning inwards; difficulties in dealing with the future; lack of self-awareness, which is why the point of vision that is in sharpest focus is brought ever closer by Fate; refusal to see the world as it really is: blurred view of the world; softening effect for everything that is more distant: illusionary misperceptions of reality; everything comes (too) close (for comfort); things up close become distorted out of the fear of missing something (the ambitious overachiever typically wears glasses); over-emphasis of thinking, neglect of

feeling: the body rectifies the situation by restricting one's vision (= thought, perception); fear of life, suppressed anxiety and rage, which results in burying one's nose in books instead of facing up to life; symptom of the intellectual; using eyeglasses to protect one's eyes (and oneself) from the world; placing a glass pane between oneself and the (dangerous) world.

Handling: Concentrating on what is close at hand and most obvious; developing respect and confidence with regard to one's own analytical capabilities; learning to rely on one's capability of concentration; what is far off is removed from one's field of view: instead of developing idealistic theories on how to save the world, (re)solving the pressing problems in one's own living environment; recognising and taking on one's own field of view as a task in itself: wise constraint; learning to be modest (with one's own area of responsibility); making oneself the centre of one's (own) world; learning to look outwards and to recognise and understand the world from the standpoint of this centre; making the world into what one would like to see in it; the hands-on idealism of youth, which can prove itself in the concrete task that is close at hand; asking oneself what one does not want to see; "taking the scales from one's eyes"; becoming softer and milder in one's judgement of the more remote environment (using the softening effect also in the figurative sense); critically placing one's own ambition under the microscope; working from the opposite pole: learning to look beyond the end of one's own nose; not relating everything to oneself, but developing a healthy distance to things.

Resolution: Maintaining the right distance from oneself and the world: seeing oneself honestly and realistically (in the world); allowing one's own subjects and problems to get

(close) to one; allowing oneself to feel emotions and allowing closeness; insight, clarity in self-awareness; mildness in judging the outer world; also living out one's emotional side.
Archetypal principle: Sun/Moon.

Shoulder-arm syndrome

Physical level: Shoulder (load-bearing capacity, stance), arm (power, strength).

Symptom level: No longer being able to raise one's arm due to →pain; no longer being able to put up the flagpole (to proudly fly the banner of life); having had one's wings clipped, no longer being able to spread one's wings and take flight, crash-landing; having tried for a long time to get a grip on things (life) using the affected side; now no longer being in a condition to do so; inability to seize hold of things and show who is the master in one's own house; painful shoulders cry for help and relief; one has overloaded oneself (above all with day-to-day trivial odds and ends) and is not aware of this burden; unconsciously bearing too much responsibility for others without receiving the anticipated thanks, which causes pain.

Handling: Giving it a rest, doing more things which one could do even with one arm tied behind one's back and giving the rest the cold shoulder; voluntarily granting the affected side the (recovery) break which has been forced upon one anyway and shifting one's weighting to the remaining side for what is most essential (right/masculine side: power/wielding the sword, bending the world to one's will; left/feminine side: requesting with humility, being receptive/ offering up the bowl, clinging on, holding tight; making use of the time of rest in order to ask oneself with regard to the affected side: What is causing such pain in my own life that this side is refusing to take part in it?; interpreting the pain as cries for help from the affected shoulder and identifying what is weighing down on this particular shoulder, what is blocking one's arm or who is tugging at it trying to seize control.

Resolution: :Looking after the left feminine side or checking that one's right(s) is/are observed; making peace with the attached problem or letting it go.

Archetypal principle: Mercury (Arm)-Saturn (inhibition).

Shoulder capsule weakness

see Arm dislocation

Shoulder pains

see Shoulder-arm syndrome

Shoulder tension

(to the point of stiffness and intractability; see also Shoulder-arm syndrome)

Physical level: Shoulder (load-bearing capacity, stance).

Symptom level: One of the most flexible joints is in danger of stiffening up very quickly, if forced to rest, and to thus show one's own stiffness and intractability; overloading due to tense straining and (muscle) tenseness: reluctantly dragging around what has been inwardly rejected; hardening due to excessive strenuous effort; fear (protecting/hiding one's head between one's shoulders).

Handling: Making oneself aware of one's burdens and obligations; identifying oppressive loads/burdens that one is bearing reluctantly; shaking off what is unbearable; recognising the true nature of things which one originally shouldered voluntarily, but which in the meantime have become burdens(ome): honestly clarifying how much one can take (on); whatever cannot be carried in a relaxed way, but instead only by means of tense straining, should preferably be dropped altogether.

Resolution: Freeing oneself from oppressive loads; developing the strong shoulders which others will want to lean on.

Archetypal principle: Mercury-Saturn.

Shyness

see Anxiety

Sight, loss of

see Blindness

Silicosis

Physical level: Lungs (contact, communication, freedom).

Symptom level: Connective tissue transformation of the lungs due to long-term irritation caused by inhaling dust containing silicic acid (mainly amongst miners working underground): the light-weight wings (lobes of the lungs), which are adapted to the air element, are converted into heavy tissue corresponding more closely to the earth element; shortness of breath and lack of air due to the continual decrease of the lung capacity, with accompanying disruption of the heart function: the capacity for exchange and communication is reduced as a result of long-term irritation, thereby laying the groundwork for →pulmonary consumption and →lung cancer: preparation for the end of communication.

Handling: (assuming, of course, that the "dusty" activity is discontinued): instead of taking things lightly, recognising the gravity of one's own communication situation; making clear to oneself that continuing to follow the beaten path that one has struck so far will bring one's vital, life-sustaining

exchange with the world to a complete standstill and thus lead to certain death; learning to recognise and respect limits; making oneself aware of the physically-imposed reduction of the exchange volume and freeing oneself of external distractions; returning to oneself and establishing communication with one's own inner being; coming to terms with one's own mortality and adjusting oneself to death.

Resolution: Transforming one's communication with the outside world into communion with oneself and with God.

Archetypal principle: Mercury-Saturn.

Singultus

see Hiccupping

Sinus inflammation

(Sinusitis)

Physical level: Nose (power, pride, sexuality), sinuses (lightness, airiness).

Symptom level: 1. General: Fear of conflicts: "being (chronically) sick to the eyeballs of something", "chronically in a huff"; tendency to deferential, exaggeratedly-friendly behaviour instead of forcefully asserting oneself and confronting the problems; preferring "slimy toadying", "sucking up to others", being "unctuous", reacting in a "slick, slippery and smarmy" way; 2. Frontal sinuses: being a "blockhead"; not having any intuition at one's disposal; 3. Maxillary sinus: Inhibition of aggression; bending down (submission) is often extremely painful and shows honestly that this is not what it is all about; 4. Nasal cavities/ethmoid bone cells: blocked "sniffer" shows that something is off key, which often also precipitates in a nasal twang.

Handling: 1. Seeing through one's own state of being chronically withdrawn and frustrated; consciously neglecting the air element (relying less on intellectual airing of the head in the form of being a "brainbox" and racking one's brains); recognising the restriction and blockage in one's own head on the figurative level; withdrawing oneself inwards into one's own space and creating space for oneself; working from the opposite pole: giving vent (Latin ventus = 'wind') (to one's resentment); fasting as a possibility of seeing through the inner blockage and allowing the outer blockage to flow away: cleansing; regaining the lightness that is one's due and swapping it for the hard-headedness;
2. Fronting up to a person or situation (Latin frons, -tis – 'forehead'), encouraging the confrontation; having the effrontery to stand up for oneself and struggle courageously;
3. Living out aggressions instead of bending over backwards: sinking one's teeth in, biting one's way through life, gritting one's teeth, biting off one's own chunk of (the cake of) life;
4. Conducting a confrontation with one's own personality, courageously calling oneself into question.
Resolution: Freeing up one's head again as old matters are cleared up and space for new elements arises; prevention: keeping one's head clear for what is important (for living).
Archetypal principle: Mars-Uranus.

Sinusitis

see Sinus inflammation (above)

Skin cancer

(see also Cancer)
Physical level: Skin (border, contact, tenderness).
Symptom level: Wildly proliferating growth in the domains of one's own limits and norms and direct contact; having strayed so far off track from one's inherent development path with regard to the domains of limits and contact that the body has now had to take over these issues on its own initiative in order to give expression to them; the mental-spiritual growth in these areas has been blocked for so long that it now forges a path in the body and strikes out in an aggressive and ruthless way; the cancer realises physically in the domains of limits and contact that (turnaround) which would be spiritually necessary in the corresponding area of consciousness.
Handling: Consciously, courageously and dedicatedly opening one's own borders to the world; opening oneself up to the surrounding world in love; opening oneself up in the domains of limits and contact to one's own wild ideas and bold fantasies, courageously and daringly allowing them to grow and flourish; remembering early dreams of life without limits and deeply-binding commitment and bringing these back to life with wild decisiveness; adopting all the measures mentioned under →cancer: since cancer affects the complete organism, it must also be met across-the-board.
Resolution: Discovering love for oneself and the world that transcends all boundaries, setting oneself above external rule and standards laid down by oneself or others; living openly and joyfully enjoying contact solely in accordance with the obligations of one's own highest law, but at the same time, still being able to rely all the while on one's own strength with regard to drawing borders against foreign assaults; recognising the necessity to switch from the physical and thus (life-) threatening level to the challenging, but life-saving mental-spiritual level, and relying on expansive growth in this realm.
Archetypal principle: Venus/Saturn-Pluto.

Skin cracks

see Cracked skin

Skin flecks

see Age-related symptoms, Liver spot (Lentigo), Pigment flecks (chloasma, melasma), Birthmark (naevus), Freckles

Skin hardening

see Scleroderma

Skin inflammation

see Dermatitis

Skin itching

see Itching

Skin rash

(see also Efflorescences, Puberty acne, Eczema, Itching)
Physical level: Skin (border, contact, tenderness); the exact localisation shows the level at which the problem is occurring.
Symptom level: Anxiously-aggressive (eruptive) defence against a conflict forcing its way through to the outside or something new breaking through the borders; the interior wants to get out into the light of awareness; something held back/ repressed wants to break through the border of suppression in order to come into sight (awareness); often very old, possibly even unresolved problems that have been brought along into this life are reflected outwardly (Caution: do not drive them back inside with allopathic therapies such as the administration of cortisone); (violently) flinging open one's own border from the inside; borders are called into question by hidden underlying energies; the subjects breaking through often betray impure, dark tendencies, i.e. shadow aspects;

scaring others away, keeping them at arm's length from one's body/skin while at the same time attracting them in the sense of making them curious.
Handling: Turning one's inside outside in the figurative sense; consciously addressing border conflicts: breaking out in the figurative sense; making one's own borders easier to pass through (from the inside out); courageously and consciously keeping unpleasant contemporaries at arm's length; allowing what has been long suppressed to rise up into consciousness and acknowledging it; voluntary questioning of one's own limits and norms or those adopted from others; taking the shadow for real and taking it seriously: what is forcing its way up and breaking out?
Resolution: Being aware of one's aggressions and creating release valves for them (erupting in the figurative sense and saving one's skin); voluntary border openings, liberation of the unconscious from the inside out; sensual contact.
Archetypal principle: Venus/ Saturn (skin)-Mars (rash).

Skull-brain trauma

see Brain concussion, Cerebral contusion

Skull fracture (basilar)

(see also Accident, Work accident/ Domestic accident, Sport accident, Traffic accident)
Physical level: Head (capital of the body).
Symptom level: Smashing of the bones of the skull due to the application of extreme force from outside: break-in into the capital of the body's terrain; threat to life due to the associated internal injuries and the frequently-occurring increase in intra-cranial pressure; the base of the skull is the

issuing point for many cranial nerves and vessels: threat to communication and supply.

Handling: Keeping oneself open at the highest (governing) level to all foreign, outside impulses; allowing the hardness of reality to get right up close to one; voluntarily allowing old structures of thinking and acting to go to pieces.

Resolution: Preferring instead to beat one's brains out in the search for solutions to dangerous problems.

Archetypal principle: Mars/ Saturn-Uranus.

Sleep apnoea

(see also Apnoea, Snoring)
Physical level: Lungs (contact, communication, freedom), respiration centre in the brain (communication, logistics).

Symptom level: Brief respiratory arrest during sleep (long breathing pause), which is ended by a deep intake of breath: shutting oneself off from the (night-time dream) world for a dangerously long time; once again managing to escape the jaws of death.

Handling: Consciously reconciling oneself with dying.

Resolution: Acknowledging the kingdom of the dead, the big brother of sleep.

Archetypal principle: Moon/ Neptune-Saturn.

Sleep disorders

see Insomnia

Sleep problems

(see also Narcolepsy, Insomnia, Somnambulism, Snoring, Sleep apnoea)
Physical level: Usually a consciousness problem.

Symptom level: 1. General: no longer managing to get one's daily life

completely over and done with; being off the mark; not being able to let go of the day; physical and spiritual constriction, coldness; fear of Ego-loss and loss of control;

2. Fitful sleep: nightly struggle over conflicts which were not cleared up during the day;

3. Disturbance of the waking-sleeping regulation (parasomnia): a life which has fallen out of its natural rhythm;

4. Talking in one's sleep: something which is putting the soul under pressure, but was not allowed to be said out loud during the day, makes itself heard;

5. Waking up tired: lack of regeneration during sleep due to worries weighing one down; "throbbing headache" often due to chronic sleep deficit or alcohol or drug abuse;

6. Waking up with a scream: fear, horror, being rudely awakened by problems;

7. Waking up too early, but not feeling refreshed;

8. Painful night-time erection: unresolved tension, unsatisfied masculinity.

Handling: 1. Getting rid of overstress; ensuring the optimum room for sleeping; trusting in oneself and allowing oneself to fall (asleep);

2. Recognising the night as the regulative and processing phase of the day and being happy that the conflicts avoided during the day can at least find room for themselves in this way;

3. Experimenting with one's sleeping and life rhythm until the ideal rhythm has been realised;

4. Bringing honesty to the light of day; clearing up secretiveness;

5. Falling asleep rituals; clearing up built-up problems, for example, by means of psychotherapy in trance;

6. Looking behind the terrible secret, daydreaming;

7. Identifying and removing the hindrance to regeneration,

8. Living out sexual needs in the partnership.

Resolution: 1. After a satisfying day's work, harvesting the fruits of the night; living openness and expansiveness;

2. During the night, solving those things which appeared insoluble during the day easily and in one's sleep; sleeping on things and waking up with solutions; in the case of concrete worldly problems, actively using the night for development, above all, in the sense of Indian yoga sleep or Tibetan dream yoga;

3. Realising one's life (rhythm) (all of life is rhythm); getting into (one's own) flow;

4. Voluntarily and courageously speaking one's mind about matters which are weighing one down in order to take the load off the soul;

5. Voluntarily and openly nudging subjects of the night into one's daily life focus;

6. Undertaking inner journeys and airing the secret of the shadow;

7. Achieving the ideal sleep situation;

8. Enjoying a fulfilled (love) life.

Archetypal principle: . and 2. Moon-Neptune; 3. Uranus-Moon; 4. Mercury-Neptune; 5. Neptune; 6. Neptune-Pluto-Mars; 7. Moon-Saturn; 8. Mars-Saturn..

Sleepwalking

see Somnambulism

Small intestine, inflammation

see Crohn's disease

Smallpox

(variola major)

Physical level: Skin (border, contact, tenderness).

Symptom level: Reddish-flecked nodes of inflammation on the skin, which within the space of 6 days transition via a blister stage into suppurating pustules, and then around the 12th day, finally scab over: numerous inflammatory conflicts which converge into a single major threat, thus challenging one to an open(ly offensive) and committed confrontation; if the mucous membranes are also afflicted from the beginning and bleeding occurs, the progression is fatal; vaccination (formerly compulsory) can prevent or at least weaken the disease, but carries the danger of fatal infections stemming from the vaccination itself; if the disease pattern is survived, the characteristic pockmarks usually remain behind as a reminder of the life-and-death struggle; general weakness with nausea, headaches, fever up to 41°C: general mobilisation for a war in which everything is at stake; vomiting: the patient wants to get rid of whatever has been picked up (through the air or through direct contact) that is now hurting the central control headquarters; the weakness betrays the potentially-fatal threat.

Handling: Committing oneself to a merciless and aggressive, life-and-death struggle; mobilising all forces for this all-out war; retaining the characteristic scars (in consciousness) as a reminder of the threat to life.

Resolution: Continually keeping in mind the threat to life in the world of polarity and reconciling oneself to it; acknowledging the aspect of struggle in life.

Archetypal principle: Mars-Pluto.

Smell, over-sensitivity

see Hyperosmia

Smoker's leg

(Endangitis obliterans; see also Circulatory disorders, Gangrene, Claudicatio intermittens, Smoking)

Physical level: Blood vessels (transport routes of the life force), legs (mobility, progress, stability), feet (steadfastness, deep-rootedness).

Symptom level: Allowing one's own legs to die off: no longer sending the life force all the way down into the legs/feet; having given up one's expectations of moving forward or upward or any further development; long since "having got cold feet"; no longer being able to approach anyone anymore; the feet cannot bear anymore: having no hope left.

Handling: Owning up to the strangulation of one's own future prospects in the outside world: directing all efforts inwards; owning up to one's great fear (of life); venturing into the narrow realm of one's own fear until one's own expansiveness opens up behind it; owning up to one's inner surrender of all hopes in the contact domain and for the future: asking oneself whether one has the courage to risk new development inwards.

Resolution: Being honest with oneself: "Do I want to just let my body rot alive and become numb and to let myself become mentally-spiritually sluggish and numb as well or will I give myself a push and find solutions inside which can no longer be expected on the outside?"

Archetypal principle: Saturn-Pluto.

Smoking

(see also Addictions, Nicotine poisoning, Lung cancer, Cancer)

Physical level: Lungs (contact, communication, freedom), blood vessels (transport routes of the life force); general increase in the risk of practically all types of cancer.

Symptom level: Substitute for genuine communication and freedom; longing for adventure and the big, wide world; the cigarette as a social balancing pole; search for stability, liveliness, activity; problems with the oral and Venusian aspects; contact and enjoyment disorder ("flirting" with the cigarette); hunger for enjoyment and ecstasy; taking flight from daunting contact situations: vanishing in a cloud of smoke, putting up a smokescreen; fear, insecurity, inhibitions; crawling away into one's innermost self; safety release valve for nervousness and inner pressure (role of cigarettes in war); a volcano which smokes, but does not erupt; aggression (letting off steam); auto-aggression, chronic state of war (→bronchitis); smoke as a substitute form of discharge of an unacknowledged claim to power: a stinker, "raising a stink about something"; accompanying symptom in times of great upheaval; in puberty: method for boosting one's ego; creation of an artificial adult image; false (feigned) maturity; the emancipatory claim "goes up in smoke"; "plenty of smoke, but no fire"; self-reward, self-gratification; dishonesty, self-overestimation: "blowing smoke", "fuming over nothing", "nothing but smoke and mirrors".

Handling: Owning up to the communications problem and working on it; discovering other possibilities for finding support; holding on dearly to people instead of cigarettes; truly committing oneself to life and courageously living out what the advertising of one's own cigarette brand projects; finding one's footing in the realm of Venus: discovering enjoyment beyond smoking; seeing through the cigarette as an instrument of flight and finding less dangerous ways of retreating; looking for other (more courageous) ways of letting off steam; owning up to aggressiveness and applying it to the necessary confrontation with the surrounding world; emancipating oneself in a more resolved (redeeming) way; creeping up behind impending transitions and getting ready to pounce; ensuring just rewards and satisfaction for oneself; using fasting as the way in to the way out; maintaining a clear view instead of clouding things and learning to see through the smokescreen; consciously giving oneself space for dreams and taking off into flights of fancy.

Resolution: Taking the needs experienced in smoking for real and taking them seriously in order to look for more exhilarating ways to satisfy them.

Archetypal principle: Venus-Mercury-Mars.

Snakes, fear of

see Phobia

Sniffles

see Cold diseases

Snoring

(see also Sleep apnoea)
Physical level: Breathing (exchange, law of polarity).
Symptom level: People who consciously concern themselves little with the unconscious tend to sink into a particularly deep sleep at night: too much slackening after too much tension; working against resistances every night; snorers sleep longer, because their sleep is less regenerating and close to stressful; not achieving a harmonious balance between giving and taking, between breathing in and breathing out: irregular interplay of the poles, being out of rhythm; disturbed contact to the surrounding world: wanting to be (alone) on one's own at night; keeping all others (including the partner) at arm's length each night; inability to ensure enough space and respect for oneself during the day/to set the tone; hard, coarse

communication comes out at night; expressing the unsaid in a rough way; lack of harmonious exchange with the world reduces one's overall feeling of wellbeing in life as well as general longevity (reduced life expectancy of heavy snorers); depriving others of their (night-time) peace and quiet: unconscious bid for dominance which disturbs everyone except oneself; making others aggressive with one's own unconscious aggression ("sleeping like a log while sawing logs").

Handling: Owning up to one's difficulties with the feminine side of the day (life); paying more attention to the shadow side - the dark feminine pole of the soul; also recognising the lack of harmony in one's communication during the day; finding other methods to ensure one's peace and quiet, at least during the night: noticing that one's greatest source of hindrance and disturbance is oneself; ensuring space and respect for oneself through the use of loud tones in the light half of the day; making oneself aware of one's own claims to dominance: finding more resolved (redeeming) levels and methods of exercising power.

Resolution: Awareness that harmony consists of both halves of reality and relies on a balancing of the poles.

Archetypal principle: Mercury-Saturn, Neptune-Mars.

Soft tissue rheumatism

see Muscle rheumatism

Somnambulism

(lunatism/sleepwalking)
Symptom level: In the mildest form: sleeping uneasily during the full moon and being haunted by wild dreams from the shadow kingdom; not being able to sleep due to the influence of the full moon: in this way, being forced to grant the moon

the honour of a night vigil; getting up while in the state of being carried away and directed by the world of inner images and without waking up to the world of intellectual day-to-day consciousness: doing odd things that are incomprehensible to one's waking consciousness, doing things that are problematic to the waking consciousness and often seemingly dangerous "with the certainty of a sleepwalker"; the suppression of vital impulses during the day leads to them being lived out at night; the irrational and unreasonable aspects are only allowed to come out and live at night; in English, there is a clear awareness of how closely "lunatics" (the insane) are in league with the "lunar" powers of the Moon; in French, the connection between the Moon and different moods is expressed in the phrase être bien/mal luné = to be in a good/ bad mood; these proverbial mood changes associated with the Moon, however, are more likely to be those of sensitive people reacting to the forces of the Moon.

Handling: With the help of the Moon, letting the night come into its own again: conscious processing of the day and one's life within the inner world of [dream] imagery by taking dreams seriously; consciously initiating these by means of a life that is more favourably inclined to the archetypally-feminine world of spiritual imagery; learning to pay attention to the Moon and her energies and to (ap)praise these appropriately; paying the Moon the respect due to every archetypal principle, and in particular, to this central feminine archetype; under the influence of the lunar forces, gaining access to nocturnal areas of consciousness as the shadow side of the day and consciously journeying around in these areas; learning to appreciate the qualities of this other side of our reality and learning to deal with them ever more consciously; in

time, also allowing the certainty of the sleepwalker to flow into the activities of one's day; taking the linguistic connections between the Moon and rhythm, as well as to moodiness and what appears (to the masculine-dominated waking consciousness) to be mental illness, as prompts for recognising one's own closeness to these areas, and even learning to appreciate them.

Resolution: Seeing the symptoms of sensitivity to the phases of the Moon, and in the wider sense, also of sleepwalking, as an opportunity to make contact with the other side (of one's own being); allowing oneself to be led and guided by other inner forces; increasingly recognising oneself as being guided; following up one's "wanderlust" between the worlds on the level of consciousness.

Archetypal principle: Moon (-Neptune).

Somnolence

see Narcolepsy

Soreness

see Intertrigo

Sore throat

(see also Cold diseases, Tonsillitis, Influenza)

Physical level: Neck (assimilation, connection, communication).

Symptom level: The passageway to the interior becomes a battlefield; uproar in the police stations (tonsils) which guard the narrow gateway; swallowing is painful and is rejected: no longer wanting to accept (swallow) everything; the poor sucker begins to fight back; having too much on one's plate; having swallowed down too many unsaid things; having simply swallowed for too long and conformed to the ideas of others; having lost (sight of) oneself.

Handling: Combatively defending the way into one's own inner being; boldly refusing to take certain things on board; feeling the pain of swallowing unpleasant things and truths and transforming it into combat strength; asking oneself self-critical questions about what one no longer wants to swallow; having the confidence to say even critical things out loud.

Resolution: Being on one's guard and no longer swallowing everything uncritically, knocking things back.

Archetypal principle: Venus-Mars.

Spasticism

Physical level: Skeletal musculature (motor, strength).

Symptom level: Increased tension in the motoric system (musculature); clumsy movements that are difficult to control: one is in a permanent state of tension; this wound-up, over-the-top state shows one's overstretched willpower: wanting too much, and in this way, achieving nothing, or even totally the opposite.

Handling/Resolution: Recognising one's straining and concentration on levels of consciousness in order to take this load off the body; making oneself aware of one's permanent readiness for action and struggle and putting this into practice in the figurative sense; transforming physical tension and strain into strenuous inner activity.

Archetypal principle: Mars-Pluto/Uranus.

Speech disorder

see Aphasia, Dysphasia

Spiders, fear of

see Phobia

Spider veins

(dilation of small veins under the skin surface)

Physical level: Blood vessels (transport routes of the life force), connective tissue (connection, stability, binding commitment).

Symptom level: Vulnerability, sensitivity, easily impressed or insulted; desire for flawlessness, stability, firmness of character is barred by "harmless little blemishes".

Handling: Increasing one's mental-spiritual impressionability: meditative attentiveness exercises; clarifying which structures one would most like one's own vitality to emerge from: allowing the life force to come to the surface more in the figurative sense; pursuing desires for flawlessness on the level of consciousness.

Resolution: Accepting small flaws as belonging to the polar world.

Archetypal principle: Mercury/Venus-Uranus.

Spinal column, curvature

(see also Back pains)

Physical level: Spinal column (stability and dynamism, uprightness).

Symptom level: Skewed situation, development has ended up on the wrong track; not being in alignment; swerving to avoid something; deviation from the centre in a central area: backing away from the feminine (left) or masculine (right) pole; growing away from one pole of reality; crooked ploys with regard to the life axis; wanting to worm one's way through life, dodging uprightness, wanting to steer round obstacles: "No matter how I twist and turn things, I still cannot manage it"; bending over backwards for something; growing towards one of the parents: to the domineering mother on the left or to the domineering father on the right; often a tradition of a lack of straightforwardness and honesty, which carries through one's line of ancestors.

Handling: Truly placing oneself on the preferred side and resolving (redeeming) it; understanding one's inclination to crooked ploys and keeping this in mind; consciously spinning crooked ploys (physically) and taking (appropriate) roundabout ways; learning to steer around obstacles: finding the smooth path to the centre; making oneself aware of one's general tendency to compensation; deviation to the left: turning one's attention more to one's own matters of the heart or of one's own anima (feminine part of the soul); deviation to the right: concerning oneself more with one's Archetypally masculine side, turning one's attention to the animus (masculine part of the soul).

Resolution: Smooth adaptation to the necessities of life; being at home on both straight and crooked paths; inner balance around one's own life axis.

Archetypal principle: Saturn-Uranus.

Spinal column fracture

Physical level: Spinal column (stability and dynamism, uprightness).

Symptom level: Sudden break in one's life axis (→accident) that nothing revolves around anymore; things are no longer in alignment, danger of →paraplegia; both the structural column function and the dynamic movement function are quashed; the outer corset points to the lack of inner hold; the life axis disintegrates in old age (senility) in a drastic and painful way (→osteoporosis).

Handling: Consciously breaking up the general continuity; considering new paths in essential areas; voluntarily laying oneself down to rest and admitting to oneself that essential

things are no longer in the correct relationship to each other; sorting out decisive problems and bringing them back into alignment; casting off ballast, exploring spiritual domains.

Resolution: Bringing the life axis that everything revolves around back into position and re-aligning it; allowing it to fuse together differently; learning to strengthen the weakest link in the column of life; trusting oneself to the homeward journey of the soul.

Archetypal principle: Saturn-Uranus.

Spinal cord inflammation

(myelitis)

Physical level: Central nervous system (news service), spinal cord (data connection from top to bottom).

Symptom level: Conflict, war (infection) over the data highway of the organism, resulting in blockages at the relevant local horizontal levels, but also in the central connection from top to bottom and vice versa; central and local regulation and control are being fiercely fought over, the logistics of life are at stake.

Handling: Courageous and combative struggle over the regulation of one's central tasks and life affairs.

Resolution: Directing all of one's energy into a re-structuring of one's control system for life.

Archetypal principle: Mercury/ Uranus-Mars.

Spiritual crisis

(Kundalini process; see also Psychosis)

Symptom level: Due to spiritual exercises being taken too far, the membrane between the shadow kingdom and daytime consciousness dissolves and the soul is exposed without protection to the shadow aspects; the highly sought after openness that one has pursued too quickly and often too ambitiously becomes a curse: those affected are no longer the master in their own house (body): inner visions inundate the patients and gain power over them; fear (e.g. of dissolving into thin air or losing oneself) becomes overpowering; the →panic of the Ego over its demise becomes the overriding life feeling.

Handling: Attempts at grounding in order to establish a secure body feeling as a basis for bearing one's ongoing experiences: e.g. garden work which leads to sweating; in fact, everything which promotes a connection to the body, including sex, provided that it leads to exhaustion, and is not carried out with tantric ideals in mind; hearty food, which by all means can be allowed to weigh the body down; nature walks which emphasise the contact with the ground; material connectedness in various forms, such as tidying up and cleaning (symbolically coming to terms with the lower world by putting it in order); all further sensitisation measures (such as meditation and other spiritual exercises aimed at transcendence) must be put on hold for the time being; no drugs of any sort, or only the classic drug for letting off steam – nicotine – if the person concerned has this particular addiction.

Resolution: After having involved oneself with the fire connection (Kundalini energy), the water element (going under in the sea of feelings and visions), the lightness of the worlds of thought (air), also letting oneself get involved with the earth element on a daily basis and letting it into oneself in a practical way; acknowledging the shadow kingdom without clinging tightly to it; only raising one's head to the Father in Heaven when the roots of one's feet are firmly planted in Mother Earth.

Archetypal principle: Neptune (resolution)-Saturn (border).

Spitting (while speaking)

Physical level: Mouth (absorption, expression, maturity – ability to speak for oneself).

Symptom level: Spitting when speaking, spitting on others when talking: unconsciously letting out (expressing) contempt and aggression; watery speech = language of the soul: the lack of inner spiritual participation is seen and felt outwardly; "talking oneself ragged"; the dry mouth leads to the expulsion of small particles of phlegm: unacknowledged fear situation; regression to the dribbling of the small child.

Handling: Making oneself aware of the levels that unconsciously resonate alongside one's speech; seeking more conscious ways of expressing aggressions and contempt; ensuring more resolved (redeeming) outlets for the spiritual element in one's own expression; owning up to one's fear when speaking; becoming like a child again in spiritual aspects.

Resolution: Making room for the things/contents which come up too short in one's own means of expression.

Archetypal principle: Mercury (speech)-Mars (aggression) Moon (soul, child).

Splayed feet

(see also Flat feet, Hallux valgus)

Physical level: Feet (steadfastness, deep-rootedness).

Symptom level: problems with one's stand(point); flaring apart of the tunnel-like arrangement of the bones of the middle of the foot; the transverse arch has been walked flat (e.g. due to wearing unsuitable footwear); collapse of the (typically human) transverse arch: the foot becomes broader; loss of elasticity; unnatural flair.

Handling/Resolution: Learning to swim more freely on the Earth's surface; spreading oneself less thinly and striving for a secure footing; stepping forward (progressing) in flow and with ease.

Archetypal principle: Neptune.

Splenic fever

(anthrax)

Physical level: Skin ([most frequent form of splenic fever] boundary, contact, tenderness), lungs (contact, communication, freedom), intestines (processing of material impressions).

Symptom level: A suppurating carbuncle develops from a pustule at the entrance point of the pathogens; if the disease pattern spreads beyond this point, it is almost always fatal; fever, lymph-node swelling: general mobilisation and localised defensive struggles; inflammation processes which break down the blood: struggles which consume one's life force; aggressive life-and-death struggle which ignites at one's external border.

Handling: Waging the struggle for one's own life with all one's strength; defending one's own (skin) border with all one's resources down to one's very lifeblood; if necessary, preparing oneself for crossing the threshold into the world beyond.

Resolution: Defending one's skin courageously and in an open(ly offensive) way; reconciliation with one's own mortality.

Archetypal principle: Mars-Saturn/Venus (skin), Mars-Mercury (lungs, intestines).

Splenic tumour

Physical level: Spleen (filter of the life force).

Symptom level: Swelling of the spleen in the course of many infectious diseases, but also in the case of diseases of the blood, liver blockage or heart defects (congested spleen):

the area responsible for blood cleansing swells up; the filtering activities of the life energy must be strengthened.

Handling: Consciously cleansing, filtering and monitoring the flow of the life energy in a better way; ensuring expansion in this area.

Resolution: Expansion of the field of influence of the dark goddesses Hekate and Kali: shifting the task of giving life and taking it away again into the foreground, and letting this subject help one to grow.

Archetypal principle: Saturn-Mars-Jupiter.

Spondylitis

(inflammation of the spinal column; see also Bechterew's disease, Back pains, Inflammation)

Physical level: Spinal column (dynamics and hold, uprightness), back (strenuous effort).

Symptom level: Inflammation of the vertebral bodies (first clarify and interpret the basic situation): aggressive struggle over uprightness and straightforwardness, and over the life axis, respectively its masculine aspect.

Handling: Waging an open(ly offensive) struggle over the foundations of one's own uprightness; standing up for oneself; remaining true to oneself.

Resolution: Being in alignment.

Archetypal principle: Saturn-Mars.

Sport accident/injury

(see also Accident)

Physical level: All areas of the body can be affected.

Symptom level: Pushing things too far physically and not "getting a firm grip on them" spiritually; this incorrect stance leads to problematic positions in the relevant sports activity; mental-spiritual inflexibility is compensated for by over-the-top demands on the body.

Handling: Becoming more courageous in the figurative sense, and in return, being more respectful of the body and its limits; re-deploying one's own ambition to more sensible levels.
Resolution: Gratefully accepting one's own physical parameters; allowing oneself to be challenged in the mental-spiritual respect and daring to follow new and even unusual paths.
Archetypal principle: Mars-Saturn-Uranus.

Sprain

(see also Foot sprain, Accident, Work accident/Domestic accident, Sport accident, Traffic accident)
Physical level: Joints (mobility, articulation), musculature (motor, strength).
Symptom level: Putting up too much resistance in an awkward way; being held responsible for a mistake and being called to account: being suddenly "wrenched into shape".
Handling/Resolution: Facing up to responsibility; recognising mis(s)-takes and integrating these into life as something that is miss-ing.
Archetypal principle: Mars-Saturn/Uranus.

Spring fever

(metabolic balance)
Symptom level: In former times, caused by diet and nutrition (exacerbated by Vitamin C deficiency occurring in the spring); with the changing of the seasons, rejecting change in a symbolic sense; shrinking back with fear from the rising of (one's own) juices (sap); fighting against one's own Mars-driven forces by struggling against offensive Mars activity in nature (trees catapulting seeds and erupting with blossoms, vegetables shooting out of the ground, spiky seedlings piercing through Mother Earth, buds bursting their seed cases); fear of breaking out into new pastures, of the energy which is expressed everywhere in the spring; having missed one's hibernation period; not having stored up enough energy.
Handling: Grasping and accepting change as the essence of Creation; facing up to one's own vital energy with openness; learning to take pleasure in it; learning to love the new as an opportunity for growth.
Resolution: Living in harmony with the characteristic qualities associated with the prevailing period of time: rest and activity each at the right time; aligning oneself with the natural course of the seasons.
Archetypal principle: Moon/Mars

Sprue

see Coeliac

Squinting

(strabismus, functional monocular vision: the images of the aberrant eye are suppressed)
Physical level: Eyes (insight, perspective, mirrors and windows of the soul).
Symptom level: Difficulty in giving life a clear direction; undirected gaze; shutting out one pole (the images of the squinting eye are filtered out by the brain, and therefore do not contribute to creating the overall picture in order to avoid seeing double), one-eyed view of reality; often occurs in periods of weakness in childhood (such as serious disease patterns): the children can no longer align the images and perceptions being experienced and withdraw to just one pole; also arises frequently when torn this way and that and unable to decide between the mother and father image, with the result that the eyes then do it on the physical level and each one goes its own separate way: if the right eye squints, then the father and his perspective is

excluded; in the case of a squinting left eye, the view of the mother is rejected; one-sided view: both sides of reality (of polarity) can no longer be held out, the contradictions have become unbearable; loss of half of one's field of view; not being willing/able to truly take things for real: the world becomes flat; two-dimensional worldview: insight in an unresolved form; inability to judge distances, to recognise the depth of things, to see different perspectives: flat world without any (mental-spiritual) depth; what is seen is always subject to doubt in the case of squinting, since one half of the view is missing. Inward squinting: the aberrant eye is directed inwards; tendency to remain at home with one's parents and to remain a child; need for security, introversion. Outward squinting: wanting to escape to the outside, wanting to break out of a difficult situation, not being able to find one's own centre; attempt to get around something; being evasive, not "coming to the point" (Hebraic hamartanein = 'missing the point, segregating oneself, sinning'), extroversion. Slight squint: considered attractive, reveals a certain weakness in one's perception of the world and thus also the need for help (which is often considered by men as attractive in women).

Handling: Making oneself aware of the diverging tendencies of one's own being; perceiving one's problems in finding one's direction; devoting oneself as intensively as possible to the one visible side (masculine or feminine) until there is a Resolution of the related theme(s); using the recognition of the restriction of one's own vision to just the one dimension as the starting point for developing an understanding of deeper dimensions in a figurative regard; compensating for the missing eye, the missing dimension through efforts of consciousness in order to learn to clearly recognise the depth of reality after all and to develop different perspectives; learning to face up to one's need for help; openly showing that one is (still) missing something for completeness; learning to restrict oneself (to one half of reality); aligning oneself with just the one side instead of observing the world from all sides; recognising life in its entirety in every individual aspect.

Resolution: Learning to see through Maya as the pale and flat reflection of true reality; learning to recognise the unity behind the world of polar duality; allowing genuine insight to grow out of the one-sided view; developing simple-mindedness with respect to unity.

Archetypal principle: Sun/Moon-Uranus.

St. Vitus's dance

(chorea)

Physical level: Higher areas of the basal ganglia (local communications nodes), nervous system (news service).

Symptom level: Inherited disorder of the neurotransmitter metabolism, which breaks out between the 30th and 50th year of life and ultimately leads to the breakdown of the central control headquarters (brain) (progressive →dementia); eccentric-looking, irregular flurries of movement, which burst forth suddenly and involuntarily; worm-like contortions, which the patients cannot control: creating a pitiful impression ("a wretched worm"); the hands and feet in particular perform movements reminiscent of mudras in temple dances (Greek chorea = dance): "performing a devilish dance"; outside of the flurries of movement, there is a slackening of the musculature: fleeing from one's own determination; hunger for life; unlived "Sturm und Drang" ('Storm and Stress') period.

Handling: Accepting the inescapability of one's own fate and using the time that one has been given as a gift; learning to recognise and accept the sword of Damocles hanging over one; concerning oneself with the issues of determination and freedom; coming to terms with one's family inheritance; putting the religious "Thy will be done" into practice; practising Uppekha (serenity); orientating oneself in line with one's centre of life; integrating ritualistic, ecstatic dances into life (patients are only free of complaints during ecstatic singing and dancing); translating the call to dance through life and to resonate in synch with everything – to celebrate the moment – into action.

Resolution: Consciously dancing the dance of life in line with the rules of the prevailing moment.

Archetypal principle: Uranus-Saturn.

Stabbing pains (in the chest)

see Heart problems

Steatorrhoea

see Fatty stool

Sterility

see Infertility

Stillbirth

(see also Miscarriage)
Physical level: Womb (fertility, safety and security).
Symptom level: Reaping death in life.
Handling: Taking one's leave of the dead child; grieving rituals; entering into an inner dialogue with the child and learning to accept its decision; occupying oneself with the teaching of reincarnation; addressing one's own mortality; pastoral care, self-help groups, psychotherapy, reading the Tibetan Book of the Dead.

Resolution: Knowing that our fate lies at every moment in God's hands or in the hands of a higher power; recognising that every gift that we receive from life must be given up again; seeing through the illusion of time.

Archetypal principle: Moon-Saturn.

Stomach cancer

(see also Stomach diseases, Cancer)
Physical level: Stomach (feeling, receptiveness).
Symptom level: In the usually long previous history of chronic irritation, aggressive (unconscious), sourpuss state (acidity), affectations of a spoilt child, resignation; something about one's own life lies heavy on one's stomach and cannot be digested: this then develops into an apparently-insoluble conflict; one's own nest is unconsciously brought into question and threatens to rupture from the inside out; the stomach wall as the symbol of the walls of the early nest of childhood is eaten away in a destructive-aggressive way, and the eroded remains begin to run wild and spread out; degeneration in the domains of feeling and receptiveness, e.g. absorption of things and feelings which do not correspond to the innermost core of one's being, but still consume a great deal of energy; (unconscious) wild and ruthlessly rampant growth in one's emotional world and the area of receptiveness; having strayed so far off track from one's inherent development path in the domains of feeling, nesting and receptiveness that the body helps the (forgotten/repressed) issues to express themselves; the mental-spiritual growth in these areas has been blocked for so long that it now forges a path in the body in an aggressive and random way; the cancer realises physically

that (turnaround) which would be spiritually necessary in the corresponding area of consciousness; unlived, binding loving feelings and comprehensive exchange that is capable of transcending all boundaries have sunk down into the body; the search for immortality and omnipotence (of the soul) lives itself out in the cancer cells instead of in consciousness; re-connection to the origin, the source of re-ligio[n] (from Latin religāre 'to bind, tie again'), has sunk down to the regressive tendencies of physical cancer cells.

Handling: Aggressively freeing oneself from the (golden) cage of childhood; becoming independent and learning to stand on one's own two feet; attacking the old nest of one's origin in an aggressive and open(ly offensive) way, and from the energies that are left over, creating something that is completely new and completely individual; opening oneself up in the domains of feelings and receptiveness to one's own outlandish ideas and bold fantasies; courageously allowing them to grow and develop without control (by others); thinking back to early dreams with respect to one's own comfortable nest, the realm of feelings and receptiveness towards the world; bringing these (back) to life and putting them into practice with wild decisiveness; in the certainty of having nothing more to lose, mustering courage for self-realisation, as well as for one's own path and nest; experiencing binding, loving feelings that are capable of transcending all boundaries; courageously living these out in open(ly offensive) ways, even if this involves destruction, for example, of old, childhood nest structures; taking questions about the origin of everything and the sense of the whole into one's own hands, thereby taking the load off the cells of the body; considering all the measures mentioned under

→cancer: since cancer affects the complete organism, it must also be met across-the-board.

Resolution: Providing expression for oneself rather than allowing the body to speak up for itself instead; recognising the need to switch from the physical and therefore (life-) threatening level to the challenging, but life-saving mental-spiritual level, and relying in this realm on expansive growth; discovering love that transcends all boundaries; setting oneself above external rule and standards laid down by oneself or others, and living and expressing oneself solely in accordance with the obligations of one's own highest law.

Archetypal principle: Moon-Pluto.

Stomach cramps

Physical level: Stomach (feeling, instinct, enjoyment, centre).

Symptom level: Hard-bitten way of digesting experiences, impressions and the world.

Handling: Consciously approaching the processing of the impressions more courageously, offensively, energetically, combatively; accepting the bits that are hard to digest as a challenge which could benefit one; recognising the stomach as a mediator between (pure?) feelings of the heart and instinctive (animalistic?) interests of the lower body.

Resolution: Digesting the world (Buddhism: Bhoga = "consuming and digesting the world"), i.e. digesting all the fruits of karma (=being consciously prepared to reap what one has sown); living on the basis of gut feelings.

Archetypal principle: Mercury-Pluto.

Stomach, descended

Physical level: Gut (feeling, instinct, security), stomach (feeling, receptiveness).

Symptom level: A slackening of the bands which hold the stomach in place causes it to slump lower: letting oneself sag in the area of nesting, security, and the home of the spirit; overstretched, large stomach due to chronic overstuffing, which sinks deep down into the stomach cavity: not getting enough.

Handling: Approaching things related to the area of one's own nest in a looser way; consciously relaxing and allowing things to slide; letting the soul "just hang loose" instead of the stomach; ensuring adequate provisions on the figurative level in order to be able to take the load off the stomach; getting one's fill without stretching the stomach to the point of feeling ready to burst.

Resolution: Looking after one's own safety and security, as well as family and home with relaxed and well-balanced poise.

Archetypal principle: Moon-Neptune.

Stomach diseases

(stomach ache, nausea and all preliminary stages of irritation and inflammation to the point of ulcers)

Physical level: Stomach (feeling, receptiveness).

Symptom level: Swallowing resentment: "bottling something up"; not living out aggressions: "being a sourpuss"; attempt to digest the feelings one has swallowed: aggression (acidity) goes no-where; lack of ability to consciously deal with aggressions and clear up conflicts/problems self-responsibly; excess stomach acid creates a feeling of pressure and prevents absorption of new impressions: loss of appetite; longing for the childhood paradise free of conflicts: appetite for baby-food/mashed food (diet that is light on the stomach), not wanting to swallow any hard lumps, refusal of raw food; refusal to leave

the nest, having become stuck in the basic attitude of the child, oral-aggressive fixation, demand to be cared for and spoilt without giving anything in return; living and eating should be free of challenges and aggravations.

Handling: Making oneself aware of one's feelings and the longing for maternal safety and security/the paradise of childhood, as well as one's desire to be loved and taken care of; consciously processing conflicts; consciously digesting impressions; abandoning one's façade of independence, ambition and forceful assertiveness; living out aggressive ambition; destroying one's own nest; receiving and giving love not only through the stomach, but above all through the heart and genitalia.

Resolution: Destroying the old nest in order to be able to build one's own.

Archetypal principle: Moon-Saturn-Mars.

Stomach mucosa, inflammation

(gastritis; see also Stomach diseases)

Physical level: Stomach (feeling, receptiveness), mucous membranes (inner boundary, barrier).

Symptom level: 1. Irritation: a soul rubbed raw, regressive desires for security; doing a great deal to please others and for the benefit of the community; happily fulfilling the hopes of others, and in the process, often forgetting one's own; being quickly piqued and insulted and acting the sourpuss, when one's own interests are overlooked by others; oral fixation: paradisiacal fantasies; becoming a "bellyacher" for others because one is so quick to take offence and due to one's clinging need for protection; grit (ill will) in the works;

2. Inflammation: battle and war to the bitter and bloody end in a region where security and harmony should reign; conflict between good-natured

willingness to take things on board and aggressive resistance (to something which is making one want to be sick); directing one's own aggressive forces (acid) against oneself: "being acerbic", "something leaves a sour taste in one's mouth"; swallowing emotions ("a poor sucker") instead of letting them out (Latin e-movere = 'to move out'); not being able to accurately estimate one's own weakness and demanding too much of oneself (overly spicy food, too much stress, etc.); continually tending toward self-criticism; being quick to take the blame for everything onto oneself and calling oneself and one's way of life into question; lack of self-confidence.
Handling: Letting out resentment at the right point; putting aggression to use more consciously; allowing emotions to rise up and letting them out (expressing them); reducing exaggerated efforts at achieving safety and security; taking back one's desires to be spoilt; becoming independent of the need for care; ripping into things on the appropriate level; on the one hand, learning to fight back against what has been swallowed and is making one want to be sick; on the other hand, finding safety, security and commitment in the right place (directing one's development away from the maternal nest into one's own nest); recognising one's tendency towards self-destruction; learning to handle and live with emotions.
Resolution: Steps forward on a more mature, adult level.
Archetypal principle: Moon-Mars.

Stomach neurosis

(nervous stomach)
Physical level: Stomach (feeling, receptiveness).
Symptom level: Pains (stomach ache, cramps, burning, stabbing pains): call for help; vomiting: one feels sick to one's stomach, spewing something (which one finds) indigestible back out again; having swallowed something heavy which is weighing one down; something is pinching and aggravating one, but is out of place in the stomach; one feels a burning sensation on one's tongue (or first of all, in one's stomach as well) to say something, but this should, in any case, be processed on the mental-spiritual level rather than the physical level; the stabbing pain in the pit of one's stomach indicates an injury on the figurative level.
Handling: Spouting out once again what one cannot use; uttering one's opinions instead of spluttering and getting rid of food in this way; assimilating in the figurative sense what is pinching and aggravating one; saying out loud what one's tongue or stomach is burning to express: burning needs and emotions want to be burned up through activity; old injuries want to be digested and often also responded to.
Resolution: Getting to know and appreciate the stomach as a display instrument for one's spiritual tone (mood); taking its messages for real and taking them seriously; yielding completely (to the flow of life).
Archetypal principle: Moon-Mercury.

Stomach perforation

(see also Stomach ulcer)
Physical level: Stomach (feeling, receptiveness).
Symptom level: First clarify and interpret the basic problem; danger of life-threatening bleeding (loss of life energy) and →peritonitis: breakout from the safe and secure cage, the nest of childhood; offensive breakthrough into the great, wide world of the stomach cavity; abdominal guarding (défense musculaire); eating a hole in one's own stomach.

Handling: Actively and combatively breaking out of the nest of childhood; creating free outlets to let out one's own feelings and emotions; learning to assert oneself aggressively instead of swallowing aggressions and bottling them up inside; creating release valves and outlets for offensive emotions; risking invasions.

Resolution: Gaining life-saving access to the big, wide world; taking on responsibility, exerting influence.

Archetypal principle: Moon-Mars/Uranus.

Stomach ulcer

(see also Stomach diseases, Ulceration)

Physical level: Stomach (feeling, receptiveness).

Symptom level: Undigested, unexpressed emotions and feelings are swallowed and digested on the physical level; the digestive enzymes that are secreted, and above all, the hydrochloric acid in the gastric juices eat through one's own stomach wall due to a lack of material alternatives: ripping oneself to shreds; pouring salt (acid) into open wounds; not having out conflicts, and instead reacting in an insulted and "acerbic (acidic)" manner; abdominal guarding (défense musculaire) in the stomach cavity; stay-at-home types unwilling to leave the nest (→stomach diseases), who – although the group is so important to them – nevertheless do not feel themselves to be accepted members of their community; in order to achieve this welcoming reception/acceptance, their own diverging interests are suppressed even more and emotions swallowed, although this rarely leads to success; associated symptom of gastric bleeding (much rarer and less dangerous than bleeding from the duodenum): life energy is lost and reappears in the form of tarry stools (pitch black); one's own vitality

is adapted and sacrificed to the kingdom of the dead.

Handling: Making oneself aware of and admitting one's feelings and the longing for maternal safety and security/the paradise of childhood and the desire to be loved and cared for; consciously processing conflicts: being strict and hard with oneself; consciously digesting impressions; abandoning the façade of independence and forceful assertiveness; rejecting what one as a poor sucker had previously just swallowed without resistance; becoming harder, more courageous; blowing apart the childhood nest that has now become a cage.

Resolution: Leaving the nest of childhood in order to free oneself and become grown-up and independent.

Archetypal principle: Moon-Mars.

Stomach upset

(see also Stomach neurosis)

Physical level: Stomach (feeling, receptiveness).

Symptom level: The stomach does not like what has been indulged in, or at least not in such abundance: it is upset; one cannot digest what one has asked of oneself or one's stomach: weighed down feeling after eating binges or drinking sprees; overload in the domain of further processing: biting off more than one can chew; wanting to integrate too much; asking too much of oneself; frequently amongst children who cannot yet determine their limits well enough and thus overestimate or even do not yet know their digestive and processing capabilities – when they have then recognised the problem, they react by becoming upset.

Handling: Paying attention to quality and quantity, before one upsets one's stomach; learning to truly enjoy: allowing the qualities of the goddess Venus (such as aesthetics, harmony, beauty) to reign at the dining table; shifting the emphasis from quantity to quality.

Resolution: Fulfilment instead of fullness or even just getting one's fill.

Archetypal principle: Moon-Jupiter.

Stomatitis

see Aphtosa, Stomatitis aphtosa (below)

Stomatitis aphtosa

(see also Aphtosa)

Physical level: Area of the tongue and oral mucous membrane (mucous membrane = inner border, barrier; mouth = absorption, expression, maturity - being able to speak for oneself).

Symptom level: Inflammatory, small ulcers, which lead to white →necroses (areas of dead tissue) and later suppurate; very painful conflicts in the area of taste; rotten compromises when it comes to the purity and suitability of meals; saliva flow: one's mouth is watering and reveals one's (unconscious) desire for the raging conflict; fever: shows the body's readiness for general mobilisation in the battle over the mouth and one's right to speak for oneself.

Handling: Conducting many small offensive and courageous confrontations with regard to the issues of taste and one's choice of food (e.g. after fasting); asking oneself what is good for one; offensively knocking back what does not agree with one; consciously fighting against rotten compromises in matters of quality, quantity and awareness; committing oneself to the critical confrontation with devotion and strong desire; mobilising all forces for this open(ly offensive) battle for one's own mouth (right to speak for oneself).

Resolution: Consciously and critically selecting which things are taken on board.

Archetypal principle: Moon-Mars.

Stomatitis epidemica

see Foot-and-mouth disease

Stony concretions

(lithiasis; see also Gall bladder, Urinary bladder, Kidney stones)

Physical level: Different areas can be affected; most frequently, the area of the kidneys (balance, partnership), bile duct (aggression, poison and bile), intestines (processing of material impressions) and urinary bladder (withstanding and relieving pressure).

Symptom level: Energies become set in stone; certain matters can no longer be kept in solution and thus precipitate; reacting in a hardened, stony way: becoming set in one's ways in the face of certain problems; turning into a rigid pillar of salt (like Lot's wife, who turned back): no longer flowing along in a forward-looking way in the stream of life; salts (the material that most stones are made of) represent a merging of the basic (feminine) and acidic (masculine) forces, and as such, are something completely new and neutral that is capable of combining these extremes; stones as the catalyst for →colics, which launch a field offensive against the obstacle in ever-recurring waves of attack, similar to the contractions associated with labour, in an attempt to give birth to it and accompanied by the corresponding labour pains.

Handling: Confronting the corresponding energies with consistency, clarity and hardness; trying to get rid of (expel) what can no longer be brought to the point of (re)solution; consciously trying to get over and done with certain matters that one is oversaturated with; it is precisely those matters in which one has reached saturation point that should not be suppressed, since these will become embodied and cause trouble;

preferring to precipitate conflict rather than precipitating stones; keeping the feminine and masculine forces in one's own game of life in a balanced state of (re)solution, and creating something new and qualitatively neutral from them, which unites both sides within itself; through offensive (painful) muscle contractions, bringing what has been held onto tightly, repressed and set in stone back into motion in order to get rid of it.

Resolution: Using concrete ideas about how to deal with the relevant issue as a means of preventing the formation of concretions in the corresponding organ.

Archetypal principle: Saturn-Pluto.

Strawberry marks

(haemangioma; benign blood vessel growth, occurring particularly in young children; usually disappears spontaneously, but can persist the whole life long)

Physical level: The whole body can be affected.

Symptom level: Amassed life force that has consolidated at the physical level; vitality blockage, life force that is brimming over and not getting enough room on the level of consciousness; being marked (with distinction) if the strawberry mark occurs at an exposed point (the mark of Cain).

Handling: (on the part of adults and children): vitality exercises in order to lure life energy to the surface; directing vitality into unusual channels: accepting the mark (of distinction) and facing up to the task.

Resolution: Vital life, brimming with liveliness; standing behind one's own vital strength; or if necessary, making transparent the double meaning of bearing a mark (of distinction).

Archetypal principle: Mars-Sun.

Stress symptoms

Physical level: Nerves (news service).

Symptom level: Stress overload and excessive demands lead to over-stimulation (→high blood pressure, →hyperactivity) and feelings of failure over no longer being able to manage it all (→depression); not being able to decide between "fight or flight".

Handling: Attuning the demands in accordance with one's own performance capability; either reducing the demands or enhancing one's capabilities; in other words, withdrawing from an exhausting situation or fighting resolutely for something; reconciling oneself to the rich and lean times of life.

Resolution: Creating a life situation for oneself which is supportive and fulfilling.

Archetypal principle: Uranus.

Striae

(see also Connective tissue weakness)

Physical level: Skin (border, contact, tenderness), connective tissue (connection, stability, binding commitment).

Symptom level: Rupture of the tissue structure, above all around the stomach area, following overstretching of the tissue, e.g. due to →obesity; weight gain that is too rapid for one's own tissue structures to be able to handle it; one's own limits become too tight; physical expression of having let things slide; often the result of a pregnancy that has overstretched one's limits: unrestrained, oppressive situation (stretching things to their tearing point); the centre is ripped apart ("one reaches the end of one's tether"); tearing oneself to pieces for the child (the next generation).

Handling: Consciously seeking tension release on the mental-spiritual level; tearing oneself to pieces in the figurative sense for one's own centre; taking on a great deal; calmly adjusting oneself to the new situation (pregnancy) and one's new needs; giving oneself loving attention also in the form of exercises for keeping fit and care of one's skin; yielding willingly and adapting oneself; making room for something new.

Resolution: Transforming the marks into marks of distinction; bearing the marks of excessive strain and sacrifice with dignity; granting inner room to the new life and taking it seriously; according womanhood the importance it deserves; letting go on the mental-spiritual level instead of on the level of the skin; trusting oneself to life and letting oneself be supported; being and showing oneself to be soft and yielding.

Archetypal principle: Venus/Saturn-Saturn/Uranus.

Stretch marks

see Striae (above)

Stroke

(apoplexy)

Physical level: Brain (communication, logistics), blood vessels (transport routes of the life force), nerves (news service).

Symptom level: First clarify and interpret the basic situation, frequently high blood pressure; a stroke strikes one to the very core and puts a violent end to one's accustomed life (as if hit and felled by a bolt of lightning); with a single stroke, a higher power strikes one down; a thrombus blocks a central blood vessel of the brain, which leads to blockage on the affected side of the body and all kinds of functional outages on the opposite side: not being able to bring together both of one's archetypal sides (the feminine left and the masculine right side), and by means of the stroke, (wanting to) shut down and later block

out the problematic sphere of life; tendency to turn away from the blocked side, as one has already done for a long time in the figurative sense (patients look at their lesion [in the right or left hemisphere of the brain]; the blocked side is on the opposite side of the body to that affected by the stroke [crossing of the nerve pathways]); switching off one side of life (the body) at the level of governance: blockage at the highest level; in the case of high blood pressure: gratefully taking up all other struggles in order not to have to face the decisive struggle in life.

Handling: Making oneself aware which (Archetypal) side of life one has been stripped of and which side one must now rely on; reconciling oneself with the still intact side in the archetypal (feminine – masculine) respect in such a way that all of its possibilities are exploited to their fullest; supported by the abilities of the remaining pole, turning one's loving attention towards the blocked side (of life) and bringing it back to life in the same way that a small child makes its first movements and steps; beginning once again to let this side be a part of one's life; consciously processing the experience that one needs both sides to live and be truly involved, just as one can only really take part in life with both spiritual sides developed (feminine and masculine); setting out in search of the lost half: integrating the shadow side, the opposite pole; venturing deeply into the feminine (Yin) side means finding in its depths the core of the masculine (Yang); venturing deeply into the masculine (Yang) side leads to the discovery of the core of the feminine (Yin), as represented in the Tai-Chi symbol; contemplation of the myth of the androgynous spherical man (Plato:"Symposium"), who has one side of the body chopped off, and from then on, seeks to find it again: to this extent, the stroke with hemiplegia becomes a re-enactment of the Fall of Man, and the deepest archetype which all people carry with them on their path.

Resolution: Making use of the blow to the supporting framework of one's own life dwelling as a chance for a completely new beginning; involving oneself with both sides of life in order to become a whole person.

Archetypal principle: Mars-Uranus.

Struma

see Goitre

Stunted growth

(see also Dwarfism)

Physical level: The whole body is affected in the full length of its "shortness".

Symptom level: Attracting attention through smallness; getting lost in the crowd; being limited to the level of a child and having the (clothing) size of a child.

Handling: Learning to stand up (admit) to one's small(-minded)ness; learning to be modest and to restrict oneself; learning to play a minor role: "Small but mighty", "Good things come in small packages"; learning to make the best out of one's small possibilities.

Resolution: Humility.

Archetypal principle: Saturn.

Stuttering

Physical level: Mouth (absorption, expression, maturity – ability to speak for oneself), neck (assimilation, connection, communication), tongue (expression, speech, weapon).

Symptom level: Failed attempt to control via speech what has been allowed to rise up from the unconscious into one's consciousness; inhibiting the flow in order to be able to control it better; not speaking out freely what

emerges; shifting of the belt-line to the neckline, respectively a shifting of sexuality into one's head; blockage in the speech centre of the intellect since the speech from the feminine hemisphere (e.g. in trance) and singing is usually freely possible; unconscious attempt to attract attention, to be the focus, to exercise power: one has to listen – as if spellbound, tense with excitement and mostly somewhat tormented; nobody can dare to interrupt one (exploitation of the general inhibition against kicking someone who is already down); in children: fear of blurting out something that is swelling up dangerously inside; being under pressure; being at the mercy of an overpowering authority; insecurity; wanting to say too much too quickly.

Handling: Confronting and making peace with such unconscious aspects in order to resolve the fear which they otherwise create; developing more courage in seizing the first thought that springs to mind: learning to stand up for one's own thoughts, and to trust one's inner imagery from the right hemisphere; owning up to one's desires for power and control over others and finding more resolved (redeeming) ways of realising it; learning other means of thought and voice control: e.g. pausing more often, repeating and reconsidering one's thoughts inwardly before expressing them instead of leaving this to the speech organs; wanting to be understood, wanting to share one's ideas: making efforts to find understanding; becoming self-assured: living as if in a trance, in which, as is the case when singing, the words usually flow without any problems.

Resolution: Entertaining others (stutterers are often secretly very witty); deriving enjoyment from the tension in order to then be able to let go of it again, e.g. within the stream of speech; trusting oneself to the flow of life and drawing strength from it in

order to also give oneself fully to the flow of the language.
Archetypal principle: Mercury-Saturn/Uranus.

Stye

(hordeolum)
Physical level: Eyes (perspective, insight, mirror and window of the soul).
Symptom level: Closing one's eyes hurts as does keeping them open: conflict over when to look on and when to look away, e.g. looking at something when one actually should not have looked, or looking away when keeping one's eyes open would have been required; aggression in one's eyes (the evil eye?); conflict between crying and being angry; the eye has a tendency to swell up and become gummed up overnight: "the beam in one's own eye" becomes visible to all; congealed tears: hardening of the spiritual.
Handling: Observing the world (self-) critically; allowing oneself to be stirred up by what is seen; developing an offensive point of view; learning to keep one's eyes open, but also to consciously turn a blind eye now and then; consciously taking visible conflicts for real (perceiving them); learning to withstand the gazes of others.
Resolution: Being able to change one's view(points); looking on and looking away at the right moment; in addition to the splinter in somebody else's eye, also being able to take "the beam in one's own eye" for real and to take it seriously.
Archetypal principle: Sun/Moon-Saturn.

Sudden infant death syndrome (SIDS)

Physical level: Lungs (contact, communication, freedom), breathing (exchange, law of polarity).

Symptom level: Breathing as the living expression of polarity stops: breaking off of communication with this world, which is seemingly not worth living in; bolting from it again straightaway: not risking life or letting oneself get involved with it.
Handling: (for jointly-affected parents, whose problems are often reflected by the children): recognising the role of parenthood in the sense of Khalil Gibran: "Your children are not your children. They are the sons and daughters of Life's longing for itself …"; addressing one's own mortality and and mortality in general: concerning oneself with Books of the Dead and spiritual philosophy; making clear to oneself that our perception is only limited, and that we therefore do not know what task this soul had to fulfil; learning to accept that death is a part of life; in fact, it is the natural opposite pole to it, which in the end draws in and reclaims all life; learning to see that it is always simply time which separates us from death and (re) solution: learning to see through the role of time.
Prevention: Getting to know and being mindful of the primary risk factors: smoking by the mother, a total lack of or only brief period of nursing, the child sleeping on its stomach – and the secondary risk factors: environmental contaminants, drug consumption, premature birth, electro-smog, being underweight, multiple pregnancies in short succession, alcohol consumption; doing without measures such as medications, vaccinations, etc. (unless absolutely necessary).
Resolution: (for the affected parents): reconciliation with one's own mortality, and that of children and all people; recognising and acknowledging death as also the (re)solution and unavoidable end point of all life; consciously preparing the most ideal nest

possible for the child in the physical, spiritual and social respect.
Archetypal principle: Moon-Saturn/ Uranus/Pluto.

Sudeck's syndrome

Physical level: Limbs (mobility, activity), bones (stability, strength).
Symptom level: Circulatory disorders, which (even in the view of traditionally-accepted medicine) are spiritually-based; these lead to pains, swellings and functional disorders in the area of a particular limb: cutting off the supply from the affected limb = cutting oneself off from the relevant domain of life; disruptions of the nutrition supply to bones and soft tissue: allowing the affected areas to die of starvation, taking their life, while the rest of the body lives on; bone atrophy and stiffening of the joints: the surrender of all structures and articulation possibilities in the strangulated domain.
Handling: Recognising the symbolic meaning of the relevant joint and admitting to oneself which domain of one's own life is being starved; including the corresponding feminine or masculine side of the body in one's observations; dissociating oneself from the issues that are symbolically associated with this area in their unresolved form in order to be able to take the load off the corresponding limb and thus keep hold of it; bidding farewell to these unresolved aspects, e.g. of one's own forward progress (in the case of the leg): first withdrawing the life energy from them, then blocking the possibilities for their expressive possibilities, and finally clearing up the inner structure.
Resolution: Doing justice to the spiritual-symbolic demands of the relevant affected region.
Archetypal principle: Mercury-Saturn.

Suicide (tendency/ attempt)

(see also Depression)
Physical level: Particularly frequent point of attack is the neck (assimilation, connection, communication), although all other systems can also be exposed to self-sabotage.
Symptom level: Openly lived out destructiveness towards oneself: 1. In an archetypally-masculine and active (Mars-driven) way as the clearest form of fleeing from responsibility: shooting oneself, jumping off a high building or slashing one's wrists;
2. In an archetypally-feminine and passive (Plutonic) way: taking poison, semi-conscious, slow wasting away right before the eyes of family members; giving up on oneself and giving oneself up to death, which takes its time; in general: wanting to simply steal away, fleeing from the demands of life; not coming to terms with the requirements imposed upon one or those which are perceived as being imposed; apparent way-out of a situation perceived as hopeless; falling victim to the illusion that death will put an end to everything; often as an act of defiance in order to punish others posthumously (even to the point of intending to get revenge); the so-called "appellative suicide" intends to send a signal: those concerned want to attract attention, and be rescued concretely, but above all, also in the figurative sense; this extends even to the point of hopeless blackmail attempts: "If you don't love me, then I'll kill myself."
Handling: Making oneself aware of the futility of suicide: the experiences of reincarnation therapy leave no doubt that those who commit suicide spare themselves nothing – on the contrary, Fate will simply keep on increasing the pressure until the still-to-be-completed learning tasks are accepted; admitting who the

deep aggression (killing oneself) is actually directed at; recognising and owning up to one's tendencies to flee; allowing oneself any possible past failures; resuming the search for a way out; psychotherapy for dealing with problems which do not seem to surmountable on one's own.

Resolution: Finding genuine solutions after it has become clear that one cannot get out of things so easily; using the aggressive energy for a more far-reaching transformation process; recognising the meaning in one's current life situation: "He who has a Why to live can bear almost any How" (Nietzsche).

Archetypal principle: Neptune-Pluto.

Sunburn

Physical level: Skin (border, contact, tenderness).

Symptom level: Damaging the skin: burning up and sacrificing the border, thereby leaving it in tatters; over-heating the body: letting the sun caress one with warmth and allowing oneself to be Sun-kissed (to a pathological degree); sure means of initiating →skin cancer: if one's skin is only allowed to get its required loving attention and tenderness via the sun, the resulting degeneration of the border and contact surfaces show how things really stand in relation to this issue; losing bodily fluids: risking one's soul for a (brown, vital) radiant aura; sacrificing the water of life in order to feel and look more lively; irrational hungering for sun: yearning for the Sun-principle (= vitality, strength, radiance, unity); confusion of the physical sun with this principle; worshipping the sun poses a threat (to life) in the concrete sense (skin cancer), but is life-promoting in the figurative sense in the form of turning towards the principle of unity; those "roasting" themselves in the sun end up getting burned (deceived) with

regard to vitality, since in the long term, they promote only the vitality of the cancer; belief that tanning improves one's own aura of health and overall tone; nowadays more a sign that one cannot let out (express) one's vitality in any other way and that one is not able to accurately assess the dangers.

Handling: Tearing open one's own outer borders, opening oneself up to (warming and maybe even) hot contacts; helping one's own contact surface to come into its own; exposing it to caresses and kisses; taking care of one's inner light: bringing spiritual aspects into play, allowing spiritual energies to flow, radiating one's aura through the soul; committing oneself to the Sun-principle instead of sacrificing one's skin and health on its altar; making oneself aware of the dangers of physical radiation from the sun.

Resolution: Flinging open the windows of the soul; looking for the sun in one's own heart and allowing it to shine.

Archetypal principle: Sun-Mars.

Sunstroke

see Heatstroke

Swallowing difficulties

see Sore throat, Tonsillitis

Swamp fever

see Malaria

Sweat gland abscess

Physical level: Sweat glands (floodgates), above all in the armpits and in the sexual and anal region (in the area of the secondary and primary genitalia).

Symptom level: Streptococci penetrate into the sweat gland duct and form a knotty node, which always also symbolises a knotty spiritual problem: inflammatory conflicts in the intimate areas of the body, which are related to the body's own odours and scent markings; wars over one's personal scent, one's intimate sphere in the domains of desire and love; unadmitted and unexpressed conflicts in the (confidential) area of attraction and seduction.

Handling: Allowing the volcano to erupt spiritually instead of physically; consciously opening oneself up to the matters that are causing a stir (above all in the area of sexuality) instead of opening the body up to stirring matters in the form of pathogens; allowing one's own alluring and enticing being to come out; learning to express oneself in this respect with offensive force; combative defence of one's own territory with one's scent marks; being aggressively committed to one's own personal essence; establishing one's own sphere in the intimate domain using one's own means; the patients must learn to let things out (ex-press them) for themselves; the letting out (squeezing) of the abscesses by doctors only leads to new volcanic eruptions (recurrence).

Resolution: Not accepting compromises in the intimate area; asserting one's own essence with open(ly offensive) force.

Archetypal principle: Venus/ Saturn/ Moon-Pluto/Mars.

Sweat secretion, increased

see Hyperhidrosis

Sweaty feet

(see also hyperhidrosis)
Physical level: Feet (steadfastness, deep-rootedness).

Symptom level: Stinking secretion of sweat via the roots; giving off the overflow via the roots; the inner stink vents itself externally; modern sports shoes as (sweat-inducing) standard shoewear promote the trend towards sweaty feet: always wanting to appear youthful and sporty, and thereby being left standing in deep water; detoxification via the roots; scent-marking of one's own territory; smelly feet repel others; also sending them the message that something smells fishy with regard to one's own deep-rootedness; fear that has been pushed deep down below (repressed): lack of (basic) trust with regard to whether one can stand up to life.

Handling: Strengthening detoxification measures: seeking out other ways, e.g. via the intestines and kidneys (by fasting), via the skin (sauna, sweating during sports), but above all, spiritually by letting go of all grudges that one is holding against others and giving up one's tendency towards being easily insulted; marking out one's own area of influence using more pleasant methods: with artificial scents, with one's own space-filling radiant aura, etc.; preferring to open one's mouth and make a stink rather than (unconsciously) stinking; keeping others at arm's length by more conscious methods: e,g. verbally through one's own energy field (radiant aura); the improvement produced by regularly going barefoot is easy to smell; ensuring healthier and undistorted contact with the ground.

Resolution: Inner purity and clarity; detoxification on all levels: "The healthy person smells of the last fruit enjoyed" (Indian proverb); strong radiant aura; reconciliation with the Earth.

Archetypal principle: Neptune.

Sweaty hands

(see also Hyperhidrosis)

Physical level: Hands (grasping, gripping, ability to act, expression).

Symptom level: Having sweaty hands through fear; wet, cold hands make one honest to the extent that they let out (express) the fear which their owners refuse to admit to themselves; fear of and defence against contact; according to Georg Groddeck, damp hands indicate displacement of the issue from the lower, sexual area into the supposedly clean upper area, in a similar way that blushing indicates the displacement of blood from down below to up top; favouring this analysis is the great shame which frequently accompanies these symptoms.

Handling: Getting to know one's own fear, standing up to it and standing behind it; finding forms of retreat in order to be protected; finding more conscious ways to let out (express) and address one's fear (consciously pushing through the restrictive domain which is constricting one).

Resolution: Via the confrontation with one's own absolute restrictiveness, experiencing the expansiveness which lies beyond and willingly opening oneself up for contact and communication.

Archetypal principle: Mercury-Saturn/Pluto.

Swine Erysipelas

see Erysipelas (more severe form of swine erysipelas)

Sympathicotonia

(permanent high tension/excitement of the sympathetic nervous system)

Physical level: The whole organism is affected.

Symptom level: Being bound to the masculine pole of activity; the sympathicus ensures dynamism, with symptoms such as a racing heart, outbreaks of sweating, dilation of the pupils, inhibition of gastric activity and mental-spiritual arousal: high tension and power surges in various systems, such as the vascular system (→high blood pressure).

Handling: Committing oneself to the resolved (redeeming) levels of masculine, active behaviour with energy and dynamism: getting straight to the point with one's whole heart pounding; wiping the sweat from one's brow as one wrestles for one's own masculinity; with one's eyes wide open, really looking closely at and confronting the full extent of the problem; in decisive situations, learning not to waste any energy on what is unimportant at that moment (such as digestion); tensing one's nerves and being ready for battle.

Resolution: Resolving (redeeming) the masculine pole: being man enough to stand one's ground at any time, but never having to (show it).

Archetypal principle: Mars.

Syphilis

(lues; see also Sexual diseases, Inflammation)

Physical level: Genitalia (sexuality, polarity, reproduction); in the advanced stage, the whole organism can be affected.

Symptom level: Creeping conflict which flares up in the area of sexuality; begins with small, painless ulcerations (conflict) in the genital area (the point of inflammation, respectively infection); in the second stage, syphilis can imitate almost all other disease patterns and attack all organs; typically shows itself in the form skin manifestations such as flecks, papular ulcers, pustules and nodules: the conflict spreads insidiously to the outer borders and contact surfaces; only the swollen lymph nodes in the groin area remain as a reminder of the origins (rosary-bead effect: one pearl is followed by the next); hair loss shows that the skin appendages are also affected and indicates the unconscious loss of freedom, independence and power; infertility, stillbirths or deformed children (→fetopathy) point to problematic sexuality, an unfruitful life; in the next stage, the conflict rests in hiding for years without visibly making its mark; in the advanced stage, coarse, degenerating tumours in ulcerous form (gummata) can occur in all possible organs and regions of the body; along with nerve and cardiovascular inflammations, aneurysms (bulging of the heart or aorta wall), and ultimately as diseases of the central nervous system, i.e. tabes dorsalis and progressive paralysis (neurolues); severe emotional and mental symptoms: extreme eruptions of feelings, stereotypical repetitions, violent reactions if contradicted, unpredictability, verbiage, weakness of memory (particularly with respect to numbers and calculation); rapid premature ageing; in the case of neurolues, the spirochetes (syphilis pathogens) can still lead to feelings of being in love and floating on air even after 70 years of latency, as Cupid's belated arrows, so to speak.

Handling: Taking small, harmless conflicts in the interpersonal domain for real and taking them seriously; fighting these out until they are cleared up; critical poison can get into the system through even the smallest conflicts; following the creeping spreading of the conflict to the border and contact areas, confronting these domains courageously and in an open(ly offensive) way; admitting to oneself that the subject matter for the conflicts actually originates from one's own inner being; courageously allowing oneself to get involved with the loin and groin domain; deploying one's own love energy effectively;

consciously foregoing external claims to freedom and power; voluntarily letting the fur fly and being upright about taking responsibility for outstanding accounts; struggling for a fruitful, creative life; making clear to oneself that conflicts, no matter how deeply suppressed they are, and confrontations that have been put off until later or temporarily settled by rotten compromises will eventually break out again at some point – even though this might be years later; in the advanced stage, the final, do-or-die battle is ready to be played out; learning to see through the problem of "love" without binding commitment (having everything [physically], not wanting to give anything [spiritually]); instead of sacrificing oneself physically (due to the syphilis), sacrificing oneself for one's partner in the figurative sense; making oneself the conscious victim of Cupid's arrows instead of drawing the poison arrows of the spirochetes into one's own being; developing willingness for intensive emotional involvement instead of suffering uncontrollable emotional outbreaks; forgetting oneself in love (selfless love) instead of provoking great forgetfulness in the late stage of syphilis.

Resolution: Facing up to impending conflicts from the very beginning; making oneself aware that even the smallest conflicts and impurities can result in the most serious complications when dealing with the sexual domain, which stands symbolically for one's involvement with polarity; reconciling oneself with polarity as early as possible.

Archetypal principle: Venus-Pluto.

T

Tachycardia

(see also Heart rhythm disorders)
Physical level: Heart (seat of the soul, love, feelings, energy centre).
Symptom level: Inner turmoil: one is almost torn apart by the pounding of one's heart; frantic fears: tendency to frantic escape; one's heart races like that of a hunted animal; not being up to the challenges/demands; the centre is not adequately prepared/ in condition for life; love that has not been lived (out freely); not being able (willing) to own up to the emotions that whip one into a frenzy.
Handling: Allowing oneself to be pounded awake; letting oneself be set in motion inwardly; tearing oneself to pieces for one's heartfelt needs; letting the heart run one off one's feet; clarifying one's own fears and tendencies to flee and allowing these into consciousness; facing up to challenges and giving the heart something to do for which it can work frenetically; preparing one's centre for life in all respects: training on all levels; bringing the emotions up to speed; sensing love in one's heart and allowing it to spill over into life; allowing one's wildly pounding heart to rattle one out of one's state of rest and make one more offbeat in one's standpoints: granting the blazing heart more opportunities than the cool head; turning one's attention to the voice of one's own heart; identifying the frenzied ambition that is driving one; owning up to conflicting individual interests.
Resolution: A courageous, alert and open heart which lets out emotions.
Archetypal principle: Sun-Mars.

Tachycardia, paroxysmal

(fit-like racing of the heart; see also Tachycardia)
Physical level: Heart (seat of the soul, love, feelings, energy centre).
Symptom level: Spiritual over-stimulation; emotions fail to reach one's consciousness; being compulsively driven, suppressed instinctive drives; something is inhibited and can go no further; having "feign"ting spells (dizziness due to self-deception), and then fleeing into another world.
Handling: Allowing oneself to be stirred up spontaneously by matters of the heart; allowing the issues behind the emotional stirrings to rise up into consciousness; letting oneself be driven by one's own instinctive drives, but not letting oneself drift (be driven) off.
Resolution: Not turning one's heart into a skeleton closet: not putting it under pressure.
Archetypal principle: Sun-Mars/ Uranus.

Tapeworm infestation

Physical level: Intestines (processing of material impressions).
Symptom level: Nourishing freeloaders, having uninvited guests and having to feed them; being exploited; granting oneself nothing, not allowing oneself to grow (expand) (nowadays also used as a deliberate therapy in order to avoid putting on weight, tapeworms as invited guests); "a can of worms": feeling that something is going wrong (one's nourishment is going into the wrong channel); feeling of impurity; fear of being eaten up inside.
Handling: Consciously nourishing dependent, weaker beings (creatures); clarifying the issue of "exploiting and being exploited": observing

the parasites and recognising one's own parasitic behaviour; consciously restricting oneself, fasting, for example, (also physically starves out the parasites); instead of artificial tapeworm implantation: paying attention to what has gone down the wrong way; consciously redirecting one's energies; not being afraid to get one's own hands dirty, concentration on the real hunger.

Resolution: Live and let live, love of others, charity; hospitality; patronage; reducing oneself to the essential, restriction, ascesis in the sense of the art of living; developing a feeling for one's own needs and those of other beings; co-operation and co-existence.

Archetypal principle: Jupiter-Pluto.

Tartar

Physical level: Teeth (aggression, vitality), gums (basic trust).

Symptom level: The independence of the teeth as individual living beings tends to be cancelled out to the extent that they merge together into a closed phalanx; threat to the gums due to →parodontitis and later →parodontosis; deposit of salts, which are precipitated from the saliva with the aid of oral bacteria; the teeth become walled in together = basis of →inflammation of the gums and →periodontium inflammation: the proud warriors (teeth) build up their armour with additional plates and thereby calcify; the "weapons become rusty" while they seemingly continue to be strengthened; hindrance of the individual existence of the teeth, which is important for the overall energetic situation of the organism; block formation, blocking something off; in the view of naturopathically-minded dentists, this also hinders cranial breathing.

Handling: Owning up to the tendential conflict at the foundations of one's own vitality; consciously creating a better basis for the capability of sinking one's teeth into things; developing a closed-formation (united) defensive strategy on the figurative level instead of making the weapons in one's mouth close ranks; preferring to close the gaps in one's defensive strategies (knowledge, rhetoric, etc.) instead of the gaps between one's teeth; processing conflicts at the roots (cleaning the root-level formation points of the tartar using appropriate oral hygiene); ensuring the cohesion of the defensive functions on the mental-spiritual level; calling into question any possible lone fighter positions.

Resolution: Recognising and acknowledging the unity of the mouth system in its energetic dimension; classifying the tartar as an early attack on it and preventing it; developing a healthy bite.

Archetypal principle: Mars-Saturn.

TBC

see Pulmonary consumption

Tear fracture

Physical level: Connection points of the bones (stability, strength) and tendons (binding cords that everything hinges on).

Symptom level: Demanding too much of the movement capabilities of the musculoskeletal system; overly vigorous and sudden movement tears the cords out of their anchoring point.

Handling: Exploring one's own expressive potential with great force and energy up to and beyond one's limits; questioning on which levels it is advisable to outdo oneself or develop beyond one's own capacities.

Resolution: Making peace with one's own capacities for articulation/expression; remaining within the framework of one's own possibilities.

Archetypal principle: Mars-Saturn, Jupiter-Saturn (excessiveness in movement).

473

Tear gland inflammation

Physical level: Tear glands (expression of emotions and feelings).
Symptom level: Conflict over the bringing to life and cleansing of the cornea; aggressive conflict over the production of the symbols of pain and joy: unconscious conflict over crying.
Handling: Involving oneself with pain and joy in a courageous and open(ly offensive) way.
Resolution: Allowing one's overflowing spiritual energy in the form of tears to wash the windows of the soul.
Archetypal principle: Moon-Mars.

Tear production, excessive

(epiphora)
Physical level: Tear glands (expression of emotions and feelings), eyes (insight, perspective, mirrors and windows of the soul), face (visiting card, individuality, perception, façade).
Symptom level: Blockage of the outflow in the tear duct or an overflow in the production of tears ("turning on the waterworks") results in continual unspectacular shedding of tears: unconscious crying, suppressed tears, unlived sorrow; one's spiritual water trickles away drop by drop; a life perceived as sad leaves its mark across one's face and becomes visible in the watery, teary-eyed, and ostensibly soft aura that one streams out; being softened up; in contrast, those who are constantly on the verge of tears are not able to master the emotions that force their way to the surface and overflow.
Handling: Allowing oneself to get involved with the soul; consciously crying, consciously allowing the unlived tears to flow: washing the windows of the soul so that they become clearer; identifying the inner source of the tears and devoting oneself to it; catching up on grief and consciously taking leave; deliberately allowing oneself to be softened up spiritually and making room for soft feelings and sensations; letting out (expressing) emotions as tears of joy, sorrow or also rage.
Resolution: Allowing the anima (the archetypally-feminine aspect of the soul) to come into its own in terms of feelings and emotions; bringing it (more) into the focal point of life; living up to one's overflowing spiritual energy in the form of tears on the level of the soul (renewed access to the relevant emotional level; allowing one's feelings to run their course).
Archetypal principle: Moon-Moon.

Tear sacs

(see also Connective tissue weakness, Eyes, rings under)
Physical level: Connective tissue (connection, stability, binding commitment), frames of the eyes (insight, perspective, mirrors and windows of the soul).
Symptom level: Emotions that have not been let go; clinging tightly to things for fear of otherwise losing everything; resigned, unlived sorrow: unshed tears (spiritual water), sitting on things, getting hung up; lacking inner hold: allowing oneself (and often also everything else) to slide; problems with processing things; not getting completely over and done with problems; build-up of congestion (connection with the kidneys and the lymph system).
Handling: Identifying pent-up, unlived sorrow and letting it out (expressing it); giving unshed tears another chance; letting the cat out of the bag, emptying the tear sacs, crying one's eyes out; consciously hanging loose and trusting oneself to the flow of life.
Resolution: Allowing one's emotions to flow.
Archetypal principle: Moon-Saturn.

Teeth, grinding overnight

(bruxism)
Physical level: Teeth (aggression, vitality).
Symptom level: The weapons of the upper world wage war with those of the lower world; day-to-day strain and tension discharge themselves in night-time orgies of teeth-grinding, ("being contrite" [= Latin: 'crushed']); essential, unprocessed aggressive situations of the day are repeated during the night (ruminating/re-hashing method); the teeth grind together, biting one's way through with difficulty, having to survive lean periods; night-time blunting of one's own weapons (ground-down teeth): powerless aggression; unacknowledged desires to "sink one's teeth into something"; valuable, vital energy disappears into thin air as a result of all the grinding, grating, gnashing and pounding to a pulp; great resistance to the existing situation: compliantly resigning oneself to one's life by simply gritting one's teeth.
Handling: Becoming aware of one's own aggressions and reconciling oneself with them; learning to defend oneself: baring one's teeth, sinking one's teeth into things; learning to rip into one's prey; recognising and acknowledging the dangerousness of one's own weapons and taking the edge off by getting to know them well; wearing them down through use; not allowing difficulties to get one down, but instead biting one's way through them; learning to consciously grit one's teeth, developing frustration tolerance.
Resolution: Ensuring a fruitful confrontation between one's own mental-spiritual world (upper jaw) and the physical world (lower jaw) which goes right down to the bone; recognising aggression as a principle of life and integrating it into one's own life.

Archetypal principle: Mars-Saturn/Pluto.

Teeth loss (in adults)

(see Adontia with congenital lack of teeth; see also Tooth gap)
Physical level: Teeth (aggression, vitality).
Symptom level: Avoidance of aggression; lack of vitality, powerlessness; regression into early childhood (toothless) domains: experiencing "turning around and becoming like a child again" on the physical level.
Handling: (Unresolved form): stop-gap, bridge, prosthesis = borrowed vitality and bite, store-bought weapons for decorative purposes; (Resolved form): showing one's teeth, biting one's way through life; reduction to the essential.
Resolution: Turning around and becoming like a child again in the figurative sense.
Archetypal principle: Mars-Saturn.

Tendon sheath inflammation

(tendovaginitis)
Physical level: Arms (force, strength, power).
Symptom level: Cramping, resistance, friction and doggedness in one's hand and arm movements; looseness, lightness and lubrication are lacking in the tendon sheath: becoming increasingly cramped in deeply-ingrained movements due to a constant conflict which is concealed behind rationalisations; combining something deadly boring and generally considered of little worth with a high level of expectation: e.g. "snagging" the beloved little ones with one's hand-knitted pullovers, "stitching up" a loved one with one's sewing; allowing unacknowledged additional aspects to flow into one's hand movements, e.g. when typing

475

the letters of one's highly-respected or deeply-hated boss; disappointments in one's attempt to cling on tightly to others.

Handling: Accepting and using the pause for thought ordained by Fate; going about one's handiwork with strenuous effort and concentration; discovering one's hard-bitten inner attitude and separating it from the activity so that one can once again turn one's hand to it in a more laid-back manner.

Resolution: Carrying out one's handiwork with deep commitment in the sense of handicraft and recognising that it is not the action itself, but rather the corresponding inner attitude which represents the problem.

Archetypal principle: Mercury-Mars.

Tendovaginitis

see Tendon sheath inflammation (above)

Tennis arm

(epicondylitis)

Physical level: Musculature (motor, strength), arm (power, strength), joints (mobility, articulation).

Symptom level: Conflict over one's ability to elbow one's way through life: not being able to defend oneself, feeling oneself at the mercy of others; using one's own elbows causes pain; repressed aggression, suppressed desire "really pounding one's fist on the table"; not applying one's whole strength when striking blows; problematic tendencies related to "setting all levers in motion", respectively the "levering out" of others; directing too much unconscious ambition into one's movements.

Handling: Concerning oneself aggressively and critically with the issue of one's own ability to push through one's will: learning to push through one's will where it is really important (instead of on the sports field, where

it is merely puffed-up exaggeration?), or using one's elbows more sparingly and with more restraint; in fact, doing without them as a whole in order to have them fully and whol(e)-ly available when it comes to essential matters; using the enforced pause for thought in order to address the meaning (of life) of the now hindered and slowed down movements; voluntarily slowing oneself down and becoming active inwardly instead of outwardly.

Resolution: Playing more playfully: seeing through one's own doggedness and the overloading of the game with issues that do not belong to it; playing like children again as the preliminary stage to "becoming like a child again".

Archetypal principle: Mars/Mercury-Saturn.

Tennis elbow

see Tennis arm (above)

Tension headaches

see Headaches, Migraine

Teratoma

(embryonic tumour)

Physical level: Various localisations, e.g. in the ovaries or testicles (fertility, creativity).

Symptom level: Cyst, which in addition to sebaceous tissue, contains all kinds of embryonic tissue structures, such as bones, teeth, skin and hair: reminder of the source, the origin; remains of a so-called "parasitic foetus", a twin present since birth, which has failed to develop: a dead sibling that one carries around with one; reference to the ever-present twin that is in the shadow – the opposite spiritual pole – which contains everything that we are not willing to own up to; a teratoma can begin to grow later in life and reach a considerable size (the so-called "pregnant

Captain of Passau" fell victim to an enormous teratoma, which resembled a pregnancy and eventually cost him his rank and career); the mixture of remaining tissue can be life-threatening due to the risk of degeneration: backwardness; being stuck in the past without realising it; testicular teratomas are always malignant (→cancer).

Handling: Being reminded that we are never alone, and that the dark sister/dark brother in the shadow is always hanging around us, waiting to be acknowledged; clarifying one's relationship to one's own dark past and the dark past that we all share so that they cannot end up proving to be our undoing.

Resolution: Reconciling oneself with one's shadow twin and the dangers (degeneration) which can result from disregarding it; admitting to oneself that it belongs to us just as much as our light side - our Ego - with which we are so firmly identified.

Archetypal principle: Pluto.

Tertian fever

see Malaria

Testicles, inflammation

(orchitis)

Physical level: Testicles (fertility, creativity).

Symptom level: Conflict and struggle in the area of fertility and creativity: e.g. not admitting to oneself that one wants (or does not want) to have a child; unconscious prevention of a pregnancy (due to bilateral orchitis); extremely painful conflict (because men react so much more sensitively to pain?) in the area of masculinity; murderous rage that one cannot live up to one's own creative demands; anger at falling short of one's potential, frequently because one has

stuck for too long and too slavishly to one's role patterns (e.g. looking after a family which has long since ceased to be one).

Handling: Courageous, open(ly offensive) involvement with one's own masculinity; aggressive application of creativity in the form of fertile ideas and projects.

Resolution: Reconciliation with being a man in a committed, open(ly offensive) way.

Archetypal principle: Pluto-Mars.

Testicular cancer

(see also Cancer)

Physical level: Testicles (fertility, creativity).

Symptom level: Wild proliferation in the area of fertility; rampant growth – without structure or order – in the area of creativity and fertility; having strayed so far off track from one's inherent development path with regard to fertility that the body has now had to leap in to help the subject express itself; the mental-spiritual growth in this area has been blocked for so long that it now forges a path in the body in an aggressive and ruthless way; the cancer realises physically in the area of creativity that (turnaround) which would be spiritually necessary in the corresponding area of consciousness.

Handling: Consciously, courageously and committedly opening up one's own borders (to the world); opening oneself up with love to the surrounding world and devoting one's own life to it; opening oneself up in the area of fertility and creativity to one's own wild ideas and bold fantasies; courageously and (sometimes) daringly allowing them to grow; growing beyond the boundaries imposed by oneself or others; thinking back to early dreams of a life of overflowing creativity and bringing these back to life with wild decisiveness; adopting all the measures mentioned under →cancer: since cancer affects the complete organism, it must also be met across-the-board.

Resolution: Discovering love for oneself and the world that transcends all boundaries, setting oneself above external rule and standards laid down by oneself or others, and living openly and communicatively solely in accordance with the obligations of one's own highest law; relying on one's own ideas and fantasies; recognising the necessity to switch from the physical and thus (life-)threatening level to the challenging, but life-saving mental-spiritual level, and relying in this realm on expansive development.

Archetypal principle: Mars-Pluto.

Testicular feminisation

(reversal of the →adrenogenital syndrome)

Physical level: Genitalia (sexuality, polarity, reproduction).

Symptom level: A genetically-male person with the appearance of an often strikingly-attractive woman; instead of female genitalia frequently testicles, which have remained lodged in the inguinal canal; a man who has unconsciously camouflaged himself as a woman.

Handling: Empathising with the feminine pole and giving in to it; reconciliation with the feminine aspect of the soul on the spiritual level as well; due to the fact that the disease pattern is usually only discovered after puberty and those affected are frequently very attractive, the identification with femininity on the physical level always takes place early.

Resolution: Living out the feminine aspect of the soul completely; consciously carrying the aspects of both sexes (anima and animus) within oneself.

Archetypal principle: Uranus.

Testicular torsion

Physical level: Testicles (fertility, creativity).

Symptom level: Physical twisting (manipulation) of the testicle (usually in young boys) by more than 180° results in interruption of the blood supply, the consequences being severe pain, swelling, discoloration from blue to black, and eventual dying off of the testicle (→necrosis): twisted ideas in the area of fertility and masculinity.

Handling: (also for jointly-affected parents, whose problems are often reflected by the children): operation within 24 hours, otherwise irreparable damage will occur; adjusting the twisted ideas about the affected area of masculinity; creating awareness of the danger of dying off in the area of creativity and fertility.

Resolution: Courageously bearing down hard on the subjects of masculinity and fertility in an open(ly offensive) way and understanding them in their essence.

Archetypal principle: Mars-Uranus.

Tetania

(see also Hyperventilation)

Physical level: Musculature (motor, strength), parathyroid glands (balance between ossification and instability), metabolism (dynamic equilibrium).

Symptom level: Tetania triggered by →hyperventilation or tetania occurring due to underactive parathyroid glands and a reduced blood calcium level, with accompanying muscle cramps, as is also the case in hyperventilation tetania (in contrast to the latter form, however, there is a genuine calcium deficiency in the alternative form, which must be treated); spontaneous adopting of the embryo posture (although admittedly in a highly cramped way if the birth trauma has yet not been properly processed: self-healing attempt by the organism that arises from a situation of restriction/fear; the cramping shows the highly-charged sensation that is still associated with the most basic fear of primordial restrictiveness (as in birth) or other comparable fear-inducing situations; being trapped like a prisoner in one's own body.

Handling: Giving in to the restrictiveness until the fear is at its greatest in order to experience how the fear then leads into its opposite pole - expansiveness; pushing ahead with one's own struggle for liberation/ deliverance from the primordial fear (often corresponding to the primordial restrictiveness during birth); tackling the struggle for liberation/deliverance from the fear of restrictiveness with strength and perseverance.

Resolution: Liberation/deliverance using one's own powers by venturing into the fear and beyond.

Archetypal principle: Mars-Saturn/ Uranus.

Tetanus

see Lockjaw (tetanus)

Thigh fracture

see Leg fracture

Threadworm infestation

(in small children, oxyuriasis)

Physical level: Digestive tract (Buddhism: Bhoga = " consuming and digesting the world"): the worms live here, but come out at night to lay their eggs in the folds of the anus; the resulting itching causes the children to scratch, with the consequence that the worms get under the fingernails, and from there into the mouth).

Symptom level: Small, medically quite harmless, but symbolically highly dangerous companions (because they originate from the underworld of the shadow kingdom) which

repeatedly succeed in being assimilated through the mouth (continual self-infection with the worm eggs via the above method); something is out of order – "full of worms".

Handling: (for jointly-affected parents, whose problems are often reflected by the children): cleanliness issue: keeping the upper and lower level apart; getting to know the inhabitants (subjects) of the shadow kingdom in a mental-spiritual way, thereby taking the load off the physical level (e.g. fairy stories, myths, sagas, legends); finding out what is out of order, what is full of worms (the digestive system!); voluntarily doing justice to parasites: learning to share.

Resolution: Reconciliation with one's own shadow world that the little beasts represent.

Archetypal principle: Pluto.

Three-month colic

Physical level: Small intestine (analysis, assimilation).

Symptom level: Refusal to digest so much, so quickly and at the wrong time; the child actually wants contact, loving care and attention, but is fed instead due to a misunderstanding; as a result, all stages of digested, pre-digested and semi-digested milk come together in the intestines, which puts too many demands on the intestines and forces them to go on strike: not yet being able to live up to the demands associated with the digestion of life; painful processing of the world: first having to learn how to digest; from the fourth month onwards, the child then has other means available of obtaining skin contact, resulting in the improvement of the situation.

Handling: (for the parents): feeding only at intervals of a few hours (not according to a rigid hourly system, but also not whenever the child cries, because this also leads to the impression that all problems can be

alleviated by eating); giving enough (skin) contact irrespective of feeding; nourishing and nurturing the child spiritually instead of overnourishing (overwhelming) it physically
Resolution: Approaching the child not with concepts (feeding on demand, feeding every four hours, etc.), but with one's own feeling.
Archetypal principle: Moon/Mercury-Pluto (colic).

Throat inflammation

see Sore throat

Throat, lump sensation

(Globus pharyngis, globus feeling, lump in one's throat, typical anxiety symptom; see also Anxiety)
Physical level: Neck (assimilation, connection, communication).
Symptom level: Rotten compromise between impulse and actual defence; "biting off more than one can chew" without taking the consequences on board; no inner openness for big-mouthed/full.mouthed demands; "having a frog in one's throat": sexual blockage; the neck swells up with anger instead of desire; the throat is choked shut with fear.
Handling: Making oneself aware of the blockage in the transfer passageway between the head and body, respectively the feeling of being "fed up to the gills"; actually filling the passage with content; making oneself aware of rotten compromises.
Resolution: Confronting the fear (fronting up to it), until it loosens up (resolves itself) into its opposite pole, expansiveness; clearing the way (of expression) for oneself; overcoming and loosening up (resolving) one's own restrictiveness.
Archetypal principle: Saturn/ Pluto.

Thrombocytopenia

(Werlhof's disease)
Physical level: Blood (life force).
Symptom level: Too few blood platelets (thrombocytes) are formed in the bone marrow; too little stability for the life force, the vitality flows away at every opportunity; every minor injury is life-threatening.
Handling: Making oneself aware of the vulnerability of one's own vitality; paying attention to one's own life energy: consciously preserving it physically, but letting it flow more spiritually.
Resolution: Living mindfully; allowing the life energy to flow, giving it away freely, allowing others to have a share of it.
Archetypal principle: Mars-Saturn.

Thrombophlebitis

see Vein inflammation

Thrombosis

(see also Blood coagulation, Pelvic vein thrombosis, Leg oedema, Vein inflammation)
Physical level: Blood (life force), blood vessels (transport routes of the life force), connective tissue (connection, stability, binding commitment).
Symptom level: The life energy comes to a standstill on its return path to the centre: not getting back what one has sent out; valuing stability and security more highly than the flowing of the life energy; lack of trust in the life flow and its dynamics, bringing it to a standstill by means of congealed, bogged down life energy; blockage of the life energy and one's inner sense of being-in-flow: being jammed, stuck in a rut, inhibited; outer flexibility is prevented: no further transformation, refusing to bend: rigid views/judgements; one's opinion of life has solidified into a fixed (pre-)judgement; non-living state in a living body.

Handling: Reducing the speed of life and pausing to reflect on the path taken, which has been characterised by many detours (→varicose veins) and excesses (overflows); learning to give without immediate reward in the sense of return flow: practising foregoing fruit (Buddhism: Phala varja); voluntarily and completely foregoing outward movement and inwardly coming to rest and reflection; developing consistency and clarity in order to loosen up deadlocks and congealment; learning to act by not acting, i.e. acting without becoming too dogged in one's actions and thereby inwardly making oneself dependent on them.

Resolution: Finding the calm amidst all the movement: experiencing the tranquillity of one's own centre; working from the opposite pole: understanding that, as far as polar life is concerned, everything flows (Heraclitus: "Panta rhei") and trusting oneself to the eternal process of transformation.

Archetypal principle: Mars-Saturn.

Thrush

see Candidamycosis

Thyroid cancer

(see also Cancer)

Physical level: Thyroid gland (development, maturity); neck (assimilation, connection, communication).

Symptom level: Suppressed, unrealised development impulses begin to go their own ways, to run riot in the physical domain and thus realise themselves in this way after all; having always only led a non-committal life, full of non-binding relationships and always full of unrest and in flight; in connection with maturity and development, having strayed so far from one's determination in life that the long-suppressed forces strike out on their own initiative and begin

their physical ego trip in the form of degeneration; the reversion to one's origin in the sense of re-ligio(n) (from Latin religāre 'to bind, tie again') turns up on the developmental level in the form of a reversion to primitive, primordial cellular life: allowing developmental possibilities to degenerate, misusing potentials.

Handling: Consciously allowing the long-suppressed mental-spiritual forces of maturity and development to come to the fore in order to relieve the body of the burden of this issue; whatever is allowed to be acted out on the stage of our consciousness becomes unimportant on the stage of our body; courageously ensuring relief in the area of development; courageously allowing suppressed, offensive maturational tendencies to run their course; aggressively letting out (expressing) one's own developmental strength; adopting all the measures mentioned under →cancer: since cancer affects the complete organism, it must also be met across-the-board.

Resolution: Finding the way back to one's own inherent development path; no longer allowing oneself to be prevented from self-realisation; recognising the necessity to switch from the physical and thus (life-)threatening level to the challenging, but life-saving mental-spiritual level and relying in this realm on expansive growth; discovering love that transcends all boundaries; setting oneself above external rule and standards laid down by oneself or others and living and developing oneself solely in accordance with the obligations of one's own highest law.

Archetypal principle: Mercury-Pluto/ Jupiter.

Thyroid gland hyperfunction

(hyperthyreosis)
Physical level: Thyroid gland (development, maturity); neck (assimilation, connection, communication).
Symptom level: Drive for growth and development, having the hots for expansion and development (being allergic to any form of constriction around one's neck), more or less insatiable appetite for life; burning ambition: inflated performance demands; demanding too much of oneself; greed for life, fear of missing out on something; being continually in a state of red alert; authority conflicts; self-denial; disappointed childish dependency desires; more often than not also chasing after the acknowledgement of the parents and later of the partner; constrictive situations are anxiously avoided; holding back of feelings, oppressive depression; suppressed fear of death.
Handling: Making oneself aware of one's partly unconscious desires for growth and expansion in order to make them a reality: bringing one's life into full swing, picking up the pace, allowing one's own heart to help one get a move on; being alert in order to seize every opportunity by the throat; risking the struggle to reach the cutting edge, declaring (competitive) war against authorities; learning to stand up for oneself and one's own ambitious aspirations; recognising the contradictions between the fear of death and the enormous desire to perform; psychotherapy; measuring high-flying dreams against reality; undoing spiritual knots which separate what is above and below from each other; owning up to one's panic over life, encountering Pan and prevailing in the struggle.
Resolution: Making independent decisions in life; facing up to the fullness of life with all its possibilities; causing the energy which runs riot as part of the disease pattern to flow into the struggle of life.
Archetypal principle: Mercury-Mars-Jupiter.

Thyroid gland hypofunction

(hypothyreosis; see also Myxoedema)
Physical level: Thyroid gland (development, maturity).
Symptom level: Shutting oneself off from the outside world, entrenching oneself behind thick walls (→myxoedema); lack of deep-rootedness; everything leaves one cold, playing dead, lack of interest in life; life lacks sweetness; often enormous disappointment in life, giving up on life (and oneself); deep-seated frustration.
Handling: Withdrawing into oneself, seeking refuge behind thick walls: considering retreat into a cloistered, meditative life situation; consciously allowing what must happen to happen; letting everything old die; involvement with death.
Resolution: Inwardly seeking and finding the meaning of one's own life.
Archetypal principle: Mercury-Saturn/Neptune.

Thyroid gland inflammation

(thyroiditis; see also Auto-aggressive/ Auto-immune diseases)
Physical level: Thyroid gland (development, maturity).
Symptom level: Conflict in the metabolic domain over the inner fire; conflict over development.
Handling: Active showdown over the volume of life energy available to burn; offensive clarification of one's own development wishes.
Resolution: Courageous development steps by making use of one's own inner fire.
Archetypal principle: Mercury-Mars.

Thyroiditis

see Thyroid gland inflammation (above)

Tick bite

see Meningitis, Borreliosis

Tics

see Muscle twitching, Tourette's syndrome, Twitching of the limbs

Tinnitus

see Ear noises

Tongue, burning

(classified as psychogenic even in the view of traditionally-accepted medicine; see also Tongue inflammation)
Physical level: Tongue (expression, speech, weapon).
Symptom level: A conflict "is on the tip of one's tongue" and is burning to be expressed; having to deal with a "red-hot iron"; "having inflamed controversy and been badly "burned"; blazing a path too quickly; naivety, credulity.
Handling: Owning up to the burning conflict: addressing the areas of expression and taste in an open(ly offensive) way; verbally tackling the red-hot irons in order to take the load off the physical tongue; carefully sampling and savouring/seasoning to taste before biting into anything; quenching the burning thirst for experiences.
Resolution: Learning to express oneself courageously and developing adventurous tastes.
Archetypal principle: Venus-Mars.

Tongue inflammation

(glossitis)
Physical level: Tongue (expression, speech, weapon).

Symptom level: Inflammatory conflict in the area of expression and taste; often on the basis of metal amalgams used in dentistry ([electrical] tensions in the mouth); conflicts related to taste: "something is not to one's taste", and one fails to own up to it; the tongue becomes the stage of the body in order to give this subject (a) space.
Handling: Critically addressing the issue of (one's own) taste; approaching questions of taste in an open(ly offensive) and combative way; courageously battling to help one's own taste to come into its own; fighting out verbal problems with a sharp, swift tongue and pointed arguments.
Resolution: Standing up for one's own taste and fighting for it (pushing it through assertively); finding one's own (level of) language and putting it into practice.
Archetypal principle: Venus/Mercury/Jupiter-Mars.

Tonsillitis

(Angina tonsillaris)
Physical level: Neck (assimilation, connection, communication), Waldeyer's tonsillar ring (defensive ring).
Symptom level: Aggressive struggle for access to the world of the body; pathogens stir up the defensive troops at the narrow entrance gates to the body; restriction, fear: shutting up, sealing things tight; no longer being able /willing to swallow everything; attempt to close oneself off against outside influences; anger at having to swallow far too much in order to please others because one is dependent on their love and devotion and continually chases after their love, thereby humiliating oneself.
Handling: Letting out (expressing) aggressions; learning to defend one's own skin; allowing oneself to be challenged and stirred up by new elements; learning to determine one's

limits off in an open(ly offensive) way, shutting oneself off and shutting things down when one has had enough.

Resolution: Offensively and courageously saying 'no'.

Archetypal principle: Venus (neck)-Mars (struggle)-Saturn (restriction).

Tooth gap

(see also Teeth loss)

Physical level: Teeth (aggression, vitality), gums (basic trust).

Symptom level: Lack of vitality; specific deficits depending on the position (→Part 1, Teeth, allocation to the meridians).

Handling: Learning to do without the corresponding energy.

Resolution: Replacing the lost energy in other ways; finding new ways to integrate this subject into one's life.

Archetypal principle: Mars-Saturn.

Tooth hygiene, lacking

Physical level: Teeth (aggression, vitality), gums (basic trust).

Symptom level: Uncultivated dealing with the subject of aggression, which is a little fishy or even stinks to high heaven; in the case of yellowish-brown teeth: red wine, coffee, black tea and tobacco corrode the impression of vitality in one's ability to put up a fight; rSun-down weapons, rSun-down vitality, blackening one's own image; lack of healthy aggression.

Handling: Consciously concerning oneself with the issue of aggression: less unconscious exercising of aggression, more conscious care of the weapons (teeth); clarifying the background motivations behind the consumption of "tainting" pleasures, such as coffee, alcohol and tobacco.

Resolution: Recognising the issue of aggression as one's own; cultivating

martial arts (combat sports such as archery); learning to enjoy life for itself.

Archetypal principle: Mars-Saturn.

Toothlessness (in adults)

See Teeth loss (in adults)

Tooth root granuloma

(tooth root inflammation, collection of pus at the base of the tooth; see also Inflammation, Lesion)

Physical level: Teeth (aggression, vitality), jaw (weapons store).

Symptom level: Conflict which extends to the roots of one's own existence; a powder keg threatening to explode.

Handling: getting to the roots of a problem in order to finally resolve old conflicts which have perhaps already become chronic; unresolved form: root canal treatment, covering with a crown, removal of the tooth = castration of the aggression or a dazzling cover-up.

Resolution: Allowing the deepest vital forces to come to light.

Archetypal principle: Mars-Mars/Pluto.

Tooth root inflammation/ suppuration

see Tooth root granuloma (above)

Torn ligament

Physical level: Ligaments/tendons (binding cords that everything hinges on), joints (mobility, articulation).

Symptom level: Being over-stretched: "over-extending oneself", "overdrawing one's bow", "losing one's grip on the reins", "cutting loose"; (mentally) no longer having a grip.

Handling: Going to the limits in the figurative sense; testing one's own powers (of consciousness); over-stretching the imagination/one's consciousness instead of the tendons: bending over backwards and pushing the limits; longing = wishing to extend one's life beyond the current possibilities; living out longings.

Resolution: getting a grip on the situation mentally; mentally growing beyond one's own limits (and thereby releasing the tension in the body).

Archetypal principle: Uranus-Saturn.

Torn tendon

see Torn ligament (above)

Torpor

Physical level: Head (capital city of the body), brain (communication, logistics).

Symptom level: Something is not right with oneself; not being completely oneself or in full possession of one's powers; rejecting responsibility; making oneself insensitive and unreceptive towards the outer world; plea for extenuating circumstances.

Handling: Conscious request for gentle treatment and special consideration.

Resolution: Extending the feelings over into transcendental worlds or even travelling to them.

Archetypal principle: Neptune.

Torticollis spasticus

see Cervical dystonia

Tourette's syndrome

(large number of →muscular twitches [tics] in rapid succession, combined with compulsive actions; see also Twitching of the limbs)

Physical level: Nerves (news service), musculature (motor, strength).

Symptom level: Stereotyped movements which occur totally free from the influence of one's will; they discharge themselves in machine-gSun-style bursts, particularly in situations of great inner tension; often triggered by confrontation with authorities; in the mild form: patterns of movement which originate from (foolish) habits and eventually develop their own uncontrollable independence; not being aware of one's own rigid, preformed modes of reaction; seeming to be helplessly at the mercy of foreign programs, just like a robot, and appearing to other people to be mad, since the movement patterns seem to be without sense; also compulsive mimicking of the movements of others (echopraxia); off-beat geniality: every thought leads to physical reactions: twitching to countless strings like a puppet (opposite pole to meditation and inner calm); lack of the filters which let only important information through: being defencelessly at the mercy of all external influences and reacting to them with movement impulses or other compulsive actions such as coprolalia (compulsive use of vulgar expressions), klazomania (compulsive bursts of shouting).

Handling: Learning to observe processes consciously, while at the same time remaining an uninvolved witness; tracing patterns back to their beginnings and symbolic sign-ificance; discovering the robotically-reacting machine in oneself and learning to accept it; based on this, making the decision to wake up (for Gurdjieff, all non-realised people were machines); consciously going haywire and thus sparing the syndrome the work: kicking over the traces, stepping out of line, finding the attraction in the most off-beat ideas, notions and flashes of inspiration; understanding life as an eccentric game, being eccentric (= off-centre) in a creative way and leaping out of the usual role; those afflicted only find peace after fulfilling sexual intercourse and deep sleep; drawing the right consequences from this and running riot: letting one's energies flow without control (sexual intercourse) or surrendering control in the world of imagery and letting oneself be carried through one's inner spiritual landscapes on the wings of dreams (sleep); integrating as many Uranian aspects as possible into one's life on resolved (redeeming) levels: seeking the explosions associated with orgiastic happenings; voluntarily exposing oneself to the flood of images on inner journeys; liberating oneself by dancing to the point of exhaustion and ecstasy and allowing oneself excursions into the shadow domain along with all the "bad words" that spontaneously spring to mind and roll off one's tongue.

Resolution: Putting into practice one of the basic formulae of psychosynthesis: while in the process of observing one's own ongoing behavioural patterns, saying to oneself inwardly: "That is not me who is doing that; I am the self within me that is at rest." Archetypal principle: Uranus.

Toxic shock syndrome

Physical level: Vagina (commitment, desire).

Symptom level: Explosive multiplication of bacteria (staphylococcus aureus) in the vagina due to using a tampon for too long; in women with extremely-weakened immune defence capacities, this causes potentially-fatal poisoning; something is rotten in the underworld; hindrance of the free flow of energy; conflict over the monthly bleeding; the female wound should be concealed and forgotten; suppression and neglect of the feminine underworld.

Handling: Using the shock in order to wake up and once again make oneself aware of the lower domain of life and desire and to thereby turn one's loving attention to it.

Resolution: Allowing one's own feminine river of life to flow, swinging into synch with one's own female rhythm. Archetypal principle: Pluto-Uranus.

Toxoplasmosis

Physical level: The whole organism is affected, particularly the liver (life, evaluation, reconnection), spleen (filter of the life force), lymph nodes (police stations), central nervous system (message centre), eyes (insight, perspective, mirrors and windows of the soul).

Symptom level: In the acute form: flu-like symptoms and corresponding progression including →headaches, →tonsillitis, swelling of the lymph nodes: acute conflicts, which have sunk down into the body and now precipitate at the corresponding, symbolically-meaningful places: see the individual symptoms for the corresponding interpretations; in the chronic form, the liver, spleen, lymph nodes, central nervous system and eyes are affected (with no treatment possibilities according to traditionally-accepted medicine): localised inflammation clusters, in which cysts form and in which the tissue tends to die off (necrosis); severe, chronic conflicts, which are not directed towards a solution, precipitate in the affected areas; in the foetus, this can result in severe deformities, in particular of the brain (fetopathy), if the mother is affected during pregnancy.

Handling: Having out conflicts in good time in consciousness and in the social sphere.

Resolution: Courageously facing up to all conceivable challenges, and if

needs be, also combatively; cultivating the aspects of the soul that are difficult to tame.
Archetypal principle: Mars-Pluto.

Traffic accident

(see also Accident, Work accident/ Domestic accident)
Physical level: All levels of the body can be affected.
Symptom level: Seeking more aggressive confrontations: "clashing with somebody", "hurtling into somebody"; depending on the relevant accompanying circumstances, making more offensive advances or allowing them to happen: "having a rSun-in with someone", "taking a beating"; bringing oneself to make erotic advances: "riding someone's tail", "getting too close", "bumper to bumper"; wanting to change one's direction in life: "being thrown off course", "deviating from one's (prescribed) path", "spinning out of control", "not managing to take the corner"; wanting to appear more relaxed and uncontrolled: "losing one's grip/control/mastery".
Handling/Resolution: General: Finding healthy outlets, respectively creative forms of expression for aggressive Mars-driven energy; transference of the accident event to one's current life situation; e.g. "not being able to brake in time" = call to slow down one's tempo (of life); making erotic contact instead of "riding the tail" of other cars; voluntarily following new routes instead of allowing oneself to be thrown off course.
Archetypal principle: Uranus.

Transverse presentation

see Birth complications: Transverse presentation

Trauma

(injury, effect of violence)
Physical level: Every part of the body and consciousness level can be affected, beginning from birth trauma (→birth complications) to whiplash or →accident.
Symptom level: Break in the general continuity, disturbance of the status quo.
Handling: Being thrown off course, consciously changing track, opening oneself up to the new.
Resolution: Consciously stepping out of line and finding new ways in a committed and intentional way; kicking over the traces and further pushing one's (consciousness) limits; opening oneself up to the transforming force of time, metamorphosis, metanoia.
Archetypal principle: Uranus-Mars.

Travel constipation

(see also Constipation)
Physical level: Large intestine (unconscious, underworld).
Symptom level: Fear of deviation from the norm, and from the norms and rules of life; fear of chaos, the ("unhygienic") foreign elements; fear of Archetypal feminine aspects, primal vitality, the swamp in one's own underworld, which for safety's sake is drained completely (in constipation, too much water is removed from the large intestine); insecurity with regard to the supply situation; the (new) food is unsafe, so the old, safe food is retained instead: rejection of the exchange with the new territory (unconscious strike); preferring to carry home the newly-acquired treasures instead; problem with giving and taking; caginess, lack of vitality.
Handling: Admitting to oneself that the strict adherence to norms and prescribed structures is simply fear; recognising and acknowledging one's own rejection of the deepest feminine

underworld level; next time, being totally honest in applying the "I'd rather have stayed at home" feeling: seeing through the senselessness of visiting a country simply to boycott it.
Resolution: Recognising and acknowledging one's own narrowness and putting down roots in one's own small world before one risks approaching the opposite pole: reconciling oneself with the world and resolving one's own fears; entering into lively exchange.
Archetypal principle: Moon-)Pluto.

Travel sickness

see Kinetoses, Balance disorders

Traveller's diarrhoea

(see also Diarrhoea)
Physical level: Small intestine (analysis, assimilation).
Symptom level: Agitated "busyness", being over-wound; inability to absorb and process things; fear of opening up to the world: "shitting oneself"; in reality, feeling drawn to the privacy and silence of the toilet /bathroom, where one can be alone and at peace; desire for rest/regeneration instead of conquest; an overblown stance of openness / boldness (like the youth in the Brothers Grimm fairytale who "went forth to learn to shudder with fear") is projected outwards; in (spiritual) reality, he has already been fearful for a long time.
Handling: Letting go of high-flying plans and ambitious intentions; admitting to oneself that one cannot absorb and process anything at all; drawing back into solitude and coming back to oneself in peace and quiet; becoming honest with oneself: discovering the boastful stirrer in oneself.
Resolution: Staying at home in all honesty and putting less on one's plate; beginning very slowly – depending on one's own digestion speed, practising Bhoga

(Buddhism:"consuming the world") and overcoming being shit-scared of the world and of life.
Archetypal principle:
Mercury-Uranus.

Trichinosis

Physical level: The whole organism is affected.
Symptom level: Eating infected pork results initially in nausea and gastric complaints, and later muscle pains, fever, diarrhoea, cramps, urticaria (hives) and haemorrhaging (up to 20% of those who eat pork are still being infected; in the greater majority, however, the disease remains more or less without symptoms, although if the symptoms do arise, the death rate is 5%); defensive struggle of the organism against the attack on its muscles: nausea, diarrhoea and the other gastric complaints signify that the organism cannot digest what has been swallowed, but instead would like to get rid of it; the muscle pains and cramps reveal the struggle of the muscles against the trichinae; the urticaria expresses the defensive struggle at the border; haemorrhaging indicates that the life force is flowing away.
Handling: Attuning oneself to and letting oneself get involved with difficult spiritual struggles, defending one's field of mobility and keeping it clean; getting rid of what is doing one damage; defending one's own borders and putting one's life energy into this conflict; weighing up whether the "enjoyment" of pork, which also has various other disadvantages, is worth the risk; questioning what one assimilates: "You are what you eat!"
Resolution: Courageously facing up to the conflicts one has brought on oneself and courageously defending one's own spiritual terrain.
Archetypal principle: Pluto.

Trichomoniasis

(see also Sexual diseases)

Physical level: Genitalia (sexuality, polarity, reproduction).

Symptom level: Triggered by the single-celled, flagellate parasite trichomonas vaginalis, which can be passed on by sexual intercourse or also unclean warm water (swimming pool! – in this respect, an exonerating diagnosis); greenish-yellow foamy efflux, which creates a decidedly impure and disgusting impression and points to impure affairs; unpleasant, difficult to define, but typical smell, which draws attention to the fishy nature of the situation; burning sensation, pain, and more rarely, also itching are limited to the vagina; the skin in the area of the genitals is irritated and reddened; burning, sore feeling, which can extend to light bleeding, corresponding to an unconscious burning desire to open oneself up; fear of contagious infection exacerbates the problem, since fear weakens the immune defence system in general.

Handling: Shifting one's sensibility and receptiveness to more resolved (redeeming) levels; recognising one's own restrictiveness in one's fear; perceiving in one's resistance to impure conditions one's resistance to one's own impure needs and fantasies.

Resolution: Opening oneself up more consciously in the mental-spiritual area to the issues related to sexuality (polarity) in order to be able to better set one's limits in the body and exclude what is dangerous.

Archetypal principle: Pluto.

Trichotillomania

(compulsive pulling out of one's own hair, usually from the head: scalp hair, eyebrows and eyelashes)

Physical level: Hair (freedom, vitality).

Symptom level: Act of desperation carried out in times of great tension ("tearing one's hair out"), which only eases off after successful tearing loose; living out the aggression leads to short-term relief; destroying the symbols of one's own strength, power and radiant charisma in an auto-aggressive way; not wanting to do oneself any good, rating and representing oneself as weak ("having nothing up top"); seeing oneself in a negative way, and tearing down anything which might radiate dignity and charisma ("leaving no hair unturned" when criticizing oneself); not allowing oneself any unbridled or loose living, but instead keeping oneself on a markedly short rein: cropping the proliferation of excesses in the form of hair; those affected banish all fluff from their heads by themselves, and consistently destroy their crowning glory until finally nothing remains but a spiky crown of thorns; in extreme cases, the bald head comes to resemble the typical convict's or monk's hairstyle: the former is not granted anything more by society, the latter does not want to grant himself anything more in the external world (the affected patients would belong to this second category); complication: →intestinal blockage, since this form of auto-aggression frequently also leads to the swallowing of the torn-out hair and even extends to the point of intestinal displacement.

Handling: Becoming aware of one's own aggression directed against one's personal radiant charisma; making the cutting back of one's own Ego claims with regard to radiant charisma and power into a conscious act: for instance, cutting off all one's hair as part of a ritual; recognising the coarseness and roughness in those who have been cropped short this way, but also the possibility of arriving at a higher awareness in the sense of the monk's tonsure; finding and living out more sensible outlets for one's own aggression and vitality.

Resolution: Forgiving oneself and letting oneself simply be in the sense of self-realisation and self-awareness; recognising, acknowledging and putting into practice the longing for inner realisation that is behind the aggressive destruction of the symbols of one's radiant charisma (changing from a "plucked chicken" into a "nun" or "monk").

Archetypal principle: Mars-Pluto.

Tricuspidal insufficiency

see Heart valve insufficiency

Tricuspidal stenosis

Physical level: Heart (seat of the soul, love, feelings, energy centre).

Symptom level: One's own centre is not opening itself up sufficiently to the life flow, but instead partially knocks it back.

Handling: Economy in dealing with one's life energies, prudent restriction to what is essential; seeking calm and solitude, being silent; posing oneself questions about the meaning of life (re-ligio[n] in the sense of reconnection).

Resolution: Finding a happy medium between withdrawal and openness; becoming clearer and more mature in matters of the heart.

Archetypal principle: Sun-Saturn.

Trigeminal neuralgia

(facial pains; see also Facial nerve paralysis)

Physical level: Face (visiting card, individuality, perception, façade).

Symptom level: Terrible pains which threaten to tear one's face apart; fear of losing face, respectively of showing one's true face; torture of having to grin and bear things; the effort required to "just keep smiling" becomes increasingly more of a strain and gets on one's nerves; threat of losing control: the poker face can no longer be upheld; blows/slaps that have been held back are reflected across one's own cheeks: unacknowledged aggressions; the rage (pain) attack behind the mask; frequently fear of showing one's own face in life; being trapped in the point of view of someone else (often a parent or other person of authority).

Handling: Discovering the terror behind the pain; consciously sensing the pains which one's efforts to keep a straight face or to grin and bear things are causing one; consciously letting the mask fall and screaming out the pain, giving vent to one's pent-up aggression; letting out (expressing) feelings openly; seeking confrontations; practising forceful self-assertion without the mask; developing "bite"; depending on which side is affected, addressing in a courageous and open(ly offensive) way the feminine (left) or masculine (right) side of one's life that is painful, i.e. calling for help.

Resolution: Making oneself aware once again of all the unstruck blows which are now striking back like a slap in the face, and applying the energies that were blocked back then and that have been tightly held onto ever since on more resolved (redeeming) levels.

Archetypal principle: Venus/Mercury-Mars.

Trismus

see Lockjaw

Trisomie 21

see Down's syndrome

Tubal pregnancy

see Ectopic pregnancy

Tuberculosis

see Pulmonary consumption

Twitching of the limbs

(jactitation; see also Muscle twitching)
Physical level: Limbs (mobility, activity).
Symptom level: Sudden, unexpected, spasmodic energy discharges of the limbs; involuntary, unintentional movements of the legs and arms: restrained movement energy discharges itself in an uncontrolled way.
Handling: Giving way to movement impulses; allowing the limbs to run riot through well-targeted actions: free dancing, shaking out the body; letting go of tensions; if the fingers twitch and jerk, also letting them have their turn.
Resolution: Allowing inwardly blocked actions and frozen patterns of movement to work themselves loose in a fun way.
Archetypal principle: Uranus.

Typhus abdominalis

Physical level: Digestive tract (Buddhism: Bhoga = "Consuming and digesting the world").
Symptom level: Neck aches and headaches result in a rising fever of up to 40 °C, stomach pains with alternating diarrhoea and constipation (the two forms of refusing to digest things), states of weakness to the point of non-responsiveness; complications include intestinal haemorrhaging, perforations, meningitis and psychoses: war in the underworld over the intestines and the digestion of nourishment and life; the fever shows the general mobilisation of one's own defences, the alternation between diarrhoea and constipation one's alternating deep fears; haemorrhaging and perforation in the

intestines indicate that the struggle is being waged to a bloody end and that the digestive area is being stretched to the limit, with corresponding loss of the life energy (blood); rejection of life: one refuses to digest anything more; either it "goes straight through one" or is boycotted (blocked); not being able/willing to hold onto anything more: be it nourishment or one's own life energy.
Handling: Waging massive conflicts over the processing and digestion of life which require one's whole strength; granting oneself a total time-out, doing nothing more, no longer taking part, existing completely for oneself, and also putting life energy to use for this purpose; making sacrifices and dealing with conflicts; working from the opposite pole: voluntarily getting involved with one's own fears; contributing one's own life energy to the struggle and also not shying away from trials which stretch one to the limit.
Resolution: Letting oneself get involved with conflicts in and over the underworld, the shadow kingdom – in a time-out period which is long enough to give one's life a new direction; clarifying the question: "How should I digest the world (practising Bhoga)?"; reconciling oneself with one's own dark side so that it cannot attack one behind one's back.
Archetypal principle: Pluto-Mars.

U

Ulceration

(see also Stomach ulcer)
Physical level: Skin (border, contact, tenderness) or mucous membranes (inner boundary, barrier).
Symptom level: Ulcerous breaking open of the skin; breakthrough of

sinister energy via one's own borders to the outside; something eats its way into the depths, gnaws away at one; destroying the surface, making the depths visible; tearing oneself apart: aggression is directed against one's own borders.

Handling: Consciously letting out the dark, disgusting juices (spiritual subjects); taking other, less harmful means of detoxification into consideration; being rigorous with oneself; allowing conflicts to touch one more deeply, letting oneself get involved with them; exploratory groundwork in one's own depths; approaching one's own depths; courageously applying one's own vital powers in breaking through self-imposed limits.

Resolution: Voluntarily looking at one's own shadow on the mental-spiritual level; confronting and tending to the dark shadow wounds; re-drawing one's own boundaries in lively areas of conflict.

Archetypal principle: Mars-Pluto.

Ulcus cruris

see Open leg ulcers

Ulcus duodeni

see Duodenal ulcer

Umbilical hernia

(see also Rupture)
Physical level: Stomach (feeling, instinct, enjoyment, centre).
Symptom level: Breaking open of the first wound of humankind; 1. In the newborn: when crying out, wanting to reach out beyond one's own limits; building up pressure against the former gateway to the world; tendency towards regression;
2. In the adult: coming under pressure in one's archaic worlds of emotion; not being able to satisfy basic needs; attempted retreat back to the good old days.

Handling: Tracing one's way back to one's beginnings; considering old ways in a new light; consciously allowing oneself to fall back into old domains of experience and processing any issues that are still open; making oneself aware of the pressure from one's archaic worlds of emotions and giving way to it.

Resolution: Going new ways, opening up new areas for oneself, but at the same time, falling back on old experiences; following one's instinct.

Archetypal principle: Moon-Uranus.

Underweight

(see also Anorexia)
Physical level: Stomach (feeling, receptiveness), figure (self-expression, self-portrayal).
Symptom level: Longing for the immaterial; being at war with the pleasure principle: not granting oneself anything, respectively burning everything up immediately; unconscious greed; not allowing oneself to become well-rounded and healthy; not wanting to make things cushy by putting on padding; unconscious ascetic ideals; making oneself scarce; being found wanting; not trusting oneself any weightiness (importance).

Handling: 1. Homeopathically: conquering the spiritual world and experiencing the weightlessness/lack of gravity there in order to trust oneself again to the material world (eating, gravity, etc.); finding enjoyment in less ("less is more"); 2. Allopathically: consciously venturing closer to the domain of enjoyment; allowing unconscious greed to become conscious and owning up to it; getting to know and accept the secret figure ideal living in one's spiritual depths; frequent short periods of fasting (2-4 days) in order to arrive at one's proper weight and also to gain weight in the spiritual sense; learning to trust oneself to deal with weight and enjoyment.

Resolution: Finding and taking on one's weight and individual figure.
Archetypal principle: Venus-Saturn.

Uraemia

see Kidney insufficiency

Ureteral constriction

(ureteral stenosis)
Physical level: Ureter (waste water channels).
Symptom level: A tight spot in the waste water-outflow system (first clarify and interpret the basic problem) leads to a back-up of the spiritual waste into the kidneys (balance, partnership); obstacle in the outflow area of the spiritual waste.
Handling: Tackling the spiritual waste more defensively, preferring to go through it once again (e.g. in the partnership) with the question of whether everything is really superfluous; proceeding more slowly with the disposal, the letting go of spiritual matters.
Resolution: Allowing oneself time when dealing with spiritual matters that have been worked through; letting their effects continue to be felt instead.
Archetypal principle: Moon-Saturn.

Ureteral papilloma

Physical level: Ureter (waste water channel which connects the kidneys and the bladder).
Symptom level: Benign growth with a pedicle (stalk) that can be up to 15cm long: similar to a club, which hangs about in the waste water without, however, completely laying itself across the outflow and threatening life; can result in metastases, but only in the ureter and bladder area: its subject is strictly limited to the discharge of outlived spiritual contents; the spiritual waste waters produce strange blossoms: original growth.

Handling: Allowing something original to grow from one's spiritual experiences.
Resolution: Acting in analogy to the folk wisdom of turning (liquid) waste into gold.
Archetypal principle: Mercury-Jupiter/Pluto.

Urethral distension

see Kidney distension

Urethral inflammation

(urethritis; see also Urinary bladder inflammation)
Physical level: Urethra (channel for waste water and the water of life).
Symptom level: Conflict in the waste water disposal system: letting go of (spiritual) waste water that has become superfluous becomes painful and difficult; burning need to let go, but painful difficulties in doing so, along with the experience that this is often only possible in small amounts; conflict between retaining and letting go (urgent need, which nevertheless causes pain).
Handling: Aggressive effort and struggle in letting out outlived spiritual energies; recognising what is paining to be let go of on other levels.
Resolution: Giving way to the burning need to let go in good time.
Archetypal principle: Pluto.

Urethritis

see Urethral inflammation

Urinary bladder cancer

(see also Cancer)
Physical level: Urinary bladder (withstanding and relieving pressure).
Symptom level: Wildly rampant growth in the area of the waste water

493

reservoir (spiritual waste); unresolved conflict with regard to the limits of one's spiritual scope of influence, which has been forced back into the shadows; having strayed so far off track from one's inherent line in dealing with the spiritual waste that the body has now had to take over the issue on its own initiative in order to give expression to it; the mental-spiritual growth in this area has been blocked for so long that it now realises itself in the body in an aggressive, ruthless way; the cancer realises physically in the waste water area that (turnaround) which would be necessary in a spiritual sense in the corresponding area of consciousness.

Handling: Devoting oneself coura- geously, consciously and dedicatedly to one's own spiritual waste; opening oneself up in the spiritual domain to one's own wild ideas and bold fantasies, courageously and daringly allowing them to grow: extending and defending one's own territory; thinking back to early life dreams with respect to spirituality and bringing them back to life in an open(ly of- fensive) and decisive way; adopting all the measures mentioned under →cancer: since cancer affects the complete organism, it must also be met across-the-board.

Resolution: Discovering love for oneself and the world that transcends all boundaries, setting oneself above external rule and standards laid down by oneself or others, and living with an attitude of openness towards everything spiritual and particularly towards spiritual waste (instead of holding on to grudges) and solely in accordance with the obligations of one's own highest law; recognising the necessity to switch from the phys- ical and thus (life-) threatening level to the challenging, but life-saving mental-spiritual level, and relying on expansive growth in this realm.

Archetypal principle: Moon-Pluto.

Urinary bladder fistula

Physical level: Urinary bladder (withstanding and relieving pressure), intestines (processing of material impressions), vagina (commitment, desire).

Symptom level: 1. Internal fistulas: connections between the urinary bladder and intestines or the urinary bladder and vagina;

2. External fistulas: waste water looks for another direct way out. Spreading of irritating matters (pathogens) into the sexual or digestive area; connec- tion between waste water channels and waste disposal or the vagina: spiritual waste takes roundabout routes and detours; escape routes lead astray.

Handling: Seeking spiritual outlets in order to get rid of old, outlived matters; courageously dealing with conflicts over letting go; departing from established paths in the disposal of the spiritual waste water.

Resolution: Creating connections; using new, unconventional ways of letting go; allowing and encouraging the mixing of previously-separated spiritual areas.

Archetypal principle: Uranus/ Neptune-Mercury.

Urinary bladder inflammation

(cystitis)

Physical level: Urinary bladder (with- standing and relieving pressure).

Symptom level: Conflict, war over letting go (passing water = letting go of the spiritual sewage or waste); burning pains drive one to the toilet: burning need to let go of the spiritual (waste water); painful, incomplete letting go of (spiritual) ballast; crying down below that is accompanied by pain; feeling oneself continually under painful pressure, holding back pressing feelings; unconsciously putting oneself under pressure (or allowing this to happen); making oneself aware of external pressure only via the bladder; exerting pressure/ exercising power with pain; conflict between retaining (holding out) and letting go; often being forced to sacrifice something that is spiritually essential "too early" (false sacrifice).

Handling: Making oneself aware of the spiritual pressure that one is under; recognising the urgency of letting go of spiritual waste; perceiving how much one is burning to put it all behind oneself; learning to re-apply the pressure in the mental-spiritual respect; practising letting off pressure when there is pain: practising letting go in the extended sense; sensing and doing justice to burning needs; letting (the water of) the soul flow on all levels, not allowing it to build up for too long.

Resolution: Being willing to deal with conflict with regard to spiritual pressure; giving way to spiritual needs, even if it hurts; having a burning interest in letting go of spiritual waste: turning letting go of the outlived into an approach to life; on the one hand, preserving the essence of one's spiritual nature, and on the other, sacrificing the spiritual waste (not the soul).

Archetypal principle: Moon/ Pluto-Mars.

Urinary bladder stones

(see also Stony concretions)

Physical level: Urinary bladder (withstanding and relieving pressure).

Symptom level: Spiritual overflow (excess) is held back; this then petrifies and remains stuck in the waste water reservoir instead of being excreted.

Handling: Continuing to pay attention to old spiritual matters and keeping them in flow; consciously listening

inwardly and sensing where matters want to become crystallised; addressing these with concentration and discipline; taking in enough new spiritual fluid; therapy with one's own urine in order to deal with what is superfluous (excessive) also on the physical level.

Resolution: Enabling spiritual matters to consolidate and settle down, instead of immediately wanting to get rid of these again (pearls grow from a particle of dirt in the oyster); letting the spiritual become concrete instead of forming concrement.

Archetypal principle: Saturn-Moon.

Urinary bladder weakness

see Incontinence

Urinary retention

(often accompanies →prostate enlargement)

Physical level: Urinary bladder (withstanding and relieving pressure).

Symptom level: Holding back of the spiritual (waste) water; extreme restraint in spiritual matters; complete holding back of water that is not compatible with life: complete blockage of the spiritual exchange with the world.

Handling: Keeping the spiritual (important) for oneself; return to and consideration of oneself: taking oneself out of circulation from time to time; in the extreme case of total blockage of the spiritual exchange with the world, recognising how important this is to (survival in) life.

Resolution: Retaining essential spiritual moments for oneself, and above and beyond this, walking the middle ground between retaining and letting go; setting feelings in one's heart in motion and clarifying these with oneself.

Archetypal principle: Moon-Saturn.

Urination, frequent

see Pollacisuria

Urination, involuntary

see Incontinence

Urticaria

(hives; see also Itching, Allergy)
Physical level: Skin (border, contact, tenderness).
Symptom level: Allergic skin reactions, which are named after the blisters and welts caused by stinging nettles (Urtica urens), reveal the burning needs of somebody who has already grasped the nettle and been badly stung; being challenged to have it out: "itching to do something", "stirred up and on edge"; lustfulness/lasciviousness; passion/inner fire/fury thrusting to the surface: "bristling with excitement"; reaction to an allergen, which stimulates/arouses and is experienced either as enticing or provocative; struggle against symbolic concepts of an enemy in the allergens (for interpretations: see →allergy); over-reaction, overblown concept of an enemy; strong unconscious aggressiveness; tyrannising one's environment through the avoidance of allergens and thereby living out aggressions: unconscious power games; pent-up aggression; suppressed vitality.
Handling: Making oneself aware of one's own (skin-)burning needs; scratching around in one's consciousness until one knows what is itching and stirring one up and what burning issue is ablaze in one's soul; voluntarily allowing oneself to be challenged to have it out: life with its stimuli and irritations is allowed to make one itch to act; consciously absorbing the many stimuli and allowing oneself to be lured out of one's shell; conscious confrontations with the avoided and rejected domains; becoming more responsive; granting oneself more and also taking the risk of grasping the nettle and being stung; allowing the borders (skin) to let more through in order to be able to let inner aspects out more easily; relieving the body once again of the task of exercising aggression and oneself becoming more aggressive and offensive: daring to live; consciously accepting challenges; acting offensively; (learning the) enjoyment of eroticism.
Resolution: Grasping the nettle and the red-hot irons in life; putting up a bold front to life (Latin frons, -tis – 'forehead').
Archetypal principle: Venus-Mars.

Uterine carcinoma

see Uterus, cancer of, Cervical cancer

Uterine polyps

(see also Cervical polyps)
Physical level: Womb (fertility, safety and security), mucous membranes (inner boundary, barrier).
Symptom level: Outgrowths of the mucous membrane in the interior of the womb, which can also lead to →infertility; multiple small polyps as materialised tears of the womb; a large polyp as a sign of a great pain in this area, possibly also physically-manifested, unfulfilled desire to have a child; lack of safety and security and creative impulses.
Handling: Looking after oneself in a creative way, creating a comfortable nest for oneself, spoiling oneself; warming to the thought of having one's own child.
Resolution: Nurturing one's inner child; living out intimacy creatively.
Archetypal principle: Moon-Jupiter.

Uterine prolapse

(Prolapsus uteri; see also Connective tissue weakness)

Physical level: Womb (fertility, safety and security), urinary bladder (withstanding and letting go of pressure), rectum (underworld) and vagina (commitment, desire) sag downwards.

Symptom level: Due to the slackening of the surrounding area, the womb (fertility) droops down and presses on the vagina, urinary bladder and rectum; the urinary bladder pressure often leads to it overflowing under physical stress: the subject of fertility creates pressure; letting go takes place as soon as the control is lessened slightly or the pressure increases slightly (when laughing, running, lifting); tendency to want to leave all organs of femininity to themselves (in homeopathy - Sepia: everything pushes its way downwards and out); occurs more frequently when having children comes about more out of sticking to tradition rather than personal wishes.

Handling: Lowering, loosening up and letting go of one's fertility ambitions; letting go on the mental-spiritual level instead of in the body; letting things slide, and for once, really loosening up; deep rest and relaxation; making oneself aware of the pressure being exerted by the issue of fertility; making conscious decisions; consciously confronting the unconscious and now physically-manifested wish: she would prefer to push the subject of (womb)anly motherhood far down and get rid of it completely; reconciling oneself with tradition or totally leaving it behind oneself.

Resolution: Consciously and openly letting oneself get involved with the mother issue; surrendering oneself to the pressure of the (womb)anly motherhood role; relaxing spiritually and allowing the body to regain its strength.

Archetypal principle: Moon-Pluto.

Uterine rupture

(occurs in pregnancy or during the birth process, almost solely following Caesarean section and other operations involving the uterus [e.g. because of myomas] or in the case of a scarred cervix, or due to too much external assistance during the birth [Kristeller method], for instance, in the case of a transverse presentation of the child)

Physical level: Womb (fertility, safety and security).

Symptom level: Struggle for deliverance; situation that is tense to the point of bursting; imbalance between the mother's power and that of the child (→birth complications); threat to the life of the mother due to bleeding to death, and to the life of the child due to asphyxiation: the mother is in danger of losing too much life energy, and the child of discontinuing its exchange with the world before it has really begun;

1. The child makes too many demands on the strength of the mother; forces its way through regardless of adverse consequences; has to tear a hole in its own nest in order to free itself; irrepressibility;

2. The mother can no longer carry (bear) the load of the child, can no longer measure up to the increasing inner pressure, can only let go of the child under duress; not opening oneself quickly enough; overload in the creative domain (when one is at the end of one's tether, it is already overdue; when such a strong muscle tears, it is high time).

Handling: allopathically and as an immediate measure: provide relief and operate to remove the child; 1. (On the part of the later adult) learning to estimate one's own strength,

497

and applying it moderately; 2. (On the part of the mother) Admission of having overdone things and asked too much of oneself; opening oneself at the right time to outside assistance; learning to accept it willingly; releasing the child into independence, letting it free in time; giving support. Resolution: Finding one's own middle ground between being demanding too much or too little of oneself.
Archetypal principle: Moon-Uranus.

Uterus, cancer of

(carcinoma of the uterus; see also Cancer)
Physical level: Mucous membranes (inner boundary, barrier) of the womb (fertility, safety and security).
Symptom level: Cancer of the second half of life, occurs more predominantly with →high blood pressure, →diabetes mellitus and →adipositas; chronic unresolved sexual conflict that has been pushed down into the shadow realm accompanied by high frustration; the high blood pressure indicates the pressure one is under, the diabetes indicates problems with love, and the obesity that the subject of fulfilment has sunk down into the body; particularly frequent in women whose longing for sexual fulfilment has never been satisfied, or who have even swung over to the opposite extreme: unwillingness in intercourse ("lie back and think of England"; "just shut your eyes tight and get through it") or even the feeling of being used and sexually abused; wild and ruthlessly proliferating growth without structure and order in the field of fertility and creativity; having strayed so far off track from one's inherent development paths with regard to the feminine-motherly domain that one's own development takes over the issues related to this area on the physical level; the mental-spiritual growth in this area has been blocked

so long that it now forges a path in the body and strikes out in an aggressive and ruthless way; the cancer realises physically in the womb area that (turnaround) which would be spiritually necessary in the corresponding area of consciousness; often on the basis of too much oestrogen (the "love hormone") following menopause: instead of preparation for the nesting (embedding) of the egg, there is rampant degeneration of the cells of the mucous membrane (tumours); unlived (degenerated) motherhood or also unlived longings for love (predominantly in childless women, nuns, prostitutes), unfulfilled desire to have a child; being under great pressure as a woman and living the masculine pole.
Handling: Finding fulfilment on levels other than the sexual; in the area of fertility and creativity, throwing open the doors to one's own (even wild) ideas and offensive boldness; giving way to courageous and daring growth impulses; once again remembering and reliving one's life dreams with regard to the issue of having children and fertility; following one's own path, avoiding rejuvenation cures (with oestrogen); adopting all the measures mentioned under →cancer: since cancer affects the complete organism, it must also be met across-the-board.
Resolution: Discovering where one's own creativity and identity lie; recognising the necessity to switch from the physical and thus (life-) threatening level to the challenging, but life-saving mental-spiritual level, and relying in this realm on expansive growth; consciously experiencing and living out motherhood: before menopause in the concrete sense, and after that, in the sense of being the "grand"mother.
Archetypal principle: Moon-Pluto.

V

Vaccination damage

Physical level: Immune system (defence), all other areas can also be affected.

Symptom level: The process of getting over and done with inherited disease potentials (= task of childhood diseases from the homeopathic and holistic point of view) is boycotted by vaccinations, resulting in inherited diseases being dragged along from further back and general immune deficiency; in consequence, there is a tendency towards chronification, or at best, deferment of childhood diseases into adulthood, where they do not belong and can also cause corresponding problems; confusion of the combat strength (→allergy), suppression of the potential for aggression that is let out (expressed), for example, in childhood diseases or infections (→inflammation); (collective) hostility towards conflict (→depression); dragging around the legacy of disease of one's forebears.

Handling: Sparing oneself nothing; facing up to the struggle; freeing oneself from the unwanted family legacy; cutting the umbilical cord; healing old wounds.

Resolution: Willingness to face conflict; appreciating the value of aggression as an expression of the life force; familiarising oneself with challenges (which in principle also includes vaccinations).

Archetypal principle: Pluto-Mars.

Vaginal cramps

see Vaginism

Vaginal dryness

(mucous membrane dryness; see also Frigidity, Climacteric complaints, Bartholinitis)

Physical level: Vagina (commitment, desire).

Symptom level: Enflamed emotions, great heat, (unconscious) burning wishes and desires, which are, however, hindered by dryness; the libido wants to be lived out on another level other than the sexual; having a burning interest in a particular issue; seeking out a partner who will clear up the issue for one in order to learn from him and with him (see also →Prostate enlargement); dryness as a general issue associated with old age.

Handling: First assigning love a more sophisticated level than is the case at just the physical level; being fired up with passion for one's own task in life; exploring the burning need for deeper communication and spiritual development; looking after one's brainchildren (i.e. mental-spiritual conceptions).

Resolution: Concentration on the essential and deep exchange.

Archetypal principle: Venus-Pluto/Saturn.

Vaginal inflammation

(colpitis; see also Inflammation, Efflux, Vaginal mycosis)

Physical level: Vagina (commitment, desire).

Symptom level: The basis is formed by conflicts with trichomonads, fungi, etc. and/or lack of the female (oestrogen hormone): inflammation of a conflict over (the point of) access to feminine receptive desire and love; open(ly offensive) conflict over the site of sheltering receptiveness and giving oneself completely; possibility of taking oneself out of circulation (intercourse).

Handling: Facing up to one's conflict over (the point of) access to desire

499

and love; struggle over the issues of willingness for being receptive and giving oneself completely; preferring to let the burning conflict flare up in the battle of the sexes rather than as burning infections; also fighting back against masculine assaults in an open(ly offensive) way instead of directing this energy against oneself; making oneself aware of any deficiencies with regard to femininity; developing more conscious possibilities of keeping the partner or men away from one's (lower) body.

Resolution: Becoming "mistress" over one's own underworld.

Archetypal principle: Venus-Mars.

Vaginal mycosis

(see also Efflux, Vaginal inflammation, Candidamycosis)

Physical level: Vagina (commitment, desire).

Symptom level: Conflict over the selection of one's intimate partner and/or conflict with one's partner in the domain of intimacy; the entrance to one's most intimate area is not being adequately supplied with life force and is not being guarded alertly enough; (unconscious) detachment from issues related to the lower body, sexuality without love; auto-aggression.

Handling: Bringing the underworld back to life through pleasurable sexuality; discovering the lower part of the body as a playground for experiencing joy for life; ensuring clean relationships; making a new choice.

Resolution: Striving for harmonious and fulfilling relationships full of liveliness; swinging in synch with one's own feminine rhythm; offensively defending one's own femininity.

Archetypal principle: Venus-Pluto.

Vaginal prolapse

(prolapsus vaginae; see also Uterine prolapse)

Physical level: Vagina (commitment, desire).

Symptom level: The vagina pushes towards the outside (→connective tissue weakness as the physical basis, weakness in binding sexual connections as the spiritual basis); the issues of giving way (yielding) and desire force themselves into the foreground on the physical level, thereby thrusting themselves forward as the central focal point of interest.

Handling: Consciously taking the task of portraying this issue away from the body, and once again, giving erotic-sexual and genital aspects sufficient space.

Resolution: Making polarity the central focal point of life and consciously reconciling oneself with it.

Archetypal principle: Venus-Pluto-Uranus.

Vaginism

Physical level: Vulva (protective wall), vagina (commitment, desire).

Symptom level: Vaginal cramping which accompanies penetration by a thrusting member: more an expression of masculine castration anxiety than an important female disease pattern; man's fear of getting stuck; the vulva as a symbol of the grave, fear of dying, vagina dentata: classic symbol of the masculine fear of sexual intercourse, more exactly: of being bitten, devoured; nowadays, however, there is more the phenomenon of vaginal cramping in order to prevent masculine penetration; unwillingness to be receptive; fear of the man, of pregnancy and subsequent abandonment (both the prevention of his penetration and his "capture" after it has happened fit in well with this fear); scars on the physical and spiritual level which create restriction and fear, also after violation due to rape or abuse.

Handling: Consciously learning to better secure the narrow gateway; shutting oneself off if there is no willingness/readiness for intimacy; owning up to one's own need to cling on tightly; making oneself aware of one's tenseness with regard to the issue.
Resolution: Opening oneself up spiritually and shutting oneself off again at the appropriate time; taking over conscious discretionary power over the narrow gateway.
Archetypal principle: Venus-Pluto/Uranus.

Vaginitis

see Vaginal inflammation

Varices

see Varicose veins in the legs, Oesophageal varices, Vulval varices

Varicose veins in the legs

(see also Low blood pressure, Connective tissue weakness)
Physical level: Blood vessels (transport routes of the life force), connective tissue (connection, stability, binding commitment).
Symptom level: Contrast between gently winding vessels and spasms (cramps): the feminine (meandering flow) and masculine pole ([spasm] odic struggle) fail to come into harmony; one does not receive one's due reward for one's efforts; the life energy that one sends out has the tendency not to come back: disappointed expectations; frequent tendency to talk up one's self-sacrifice and to experience and present oneself as the poor victim; vitality slowly sinks down and becomes stuck in the lower half of the body: standing still, becoming bogged down; more and more spiritual energy leaks out and puts emphasis (weight) on the lower

pole (tendency to oedema); strong, enforced connection to the Earth; sluggishness, being heavy-footed; insecure footing, tendency to give way, lack of inner resilience (tensioning force) and elasticity, living life on a low flame: situation without pressure; standstill (of the life energy): a lot of standing still at places one does not like; lack of capability in bonding and connecting; non-binding commitment, low dependability; playing the victim but being highly demanding at the same time: belief that one has done everything necessary, and that now others should pull the chestnuts out of the fire (for one); reacting in an easily hurt way and bearing a grudge (black marks [bruises] form at the slightest prodding/provocation and remain for a long time).
Handling: Expending one's life energy and letting it flow without expectation of reward (resolved parent situation); directing one's energy and attention to the lower feminine pole of the body; voluntarily letting it carry weight (importance); readily giving recognition and loving attention to the earth element and one's own roots; consciously learning to go with the flow of life, giving way consciously: Tai-Chi exercises; using the life energy that is saved externally for inner processes; putting sensibility to use in a constructive way (e.g. as an intuitive, empathetic educator, therapist, etc.); consciously applying the attitude to life of "Panta rhei" ("everything flows"), getting things moving, allowing development; going about inner tasks with feeling and commitment; sacrificing oneself instead of making oneself a victim; relinquishing speculative thought; practising Phala varja (Buddhist: "foregoing fruit"): doing things because they have to be done and not in order to get thanks.
Resolution: Yielding freely instead of becoming slack and losing one's stability; trusting oneself to the flow

of life and all its winding paths, free of particular expectations; softness of one's disposition instead of one's tissue.
Archetypal principle: Moon-Pluto.

Variola major

see Smallpox

Vascular blockage

(see also Thrombosis)
Physical level: Blood (life force), blood vessels (transport routes of the life force).
Symptom level: Blockage of a channel of the life energy; obstruction of the life (flow). 1. In the case of arterial blockage: the life energy has run into a dead-end, a situation with no way out; vitality which has become sluggish, congeals and forms a blockage; danger of necrotic degeneration in the dependent areas;
2. In the case of venous blockage: blockage of the return flow vessel, one no longer gets back the vitality expended; giving more than receiving; spiritual (water) blockage throughout the whole area: →oedema; flooding of the surrounding part of the body with (spiritual) water.
Handling: Allowing oneself more time; slowing down the tempo of life; taking care of these regions in a different way and with more attention; going new ways with the life energy, building bridges, taking small steps, coming to a standstill now and again and determining where one stands; redefining the energy expenditure; beginning again. 1. Reducing the energy supply to the organs/life themes (affected by the embolisms) to a new, more economical level; 2. Consciously and voluntarily giving more than one expects to receive in return; distributing spiritual energy over the whole spectrum of the theme concerned (e.g. in the case of the leg, the domain of progress).

Resolution: Letting life flow at a more leisurely pace.
Archetypal principle: Mercury-Mars/Saturn.

Vascular calcification

see Arteriosclerosis

Vascular cramps

(angiospasm)
Physical level: All vessels can be affected; particularly dangerous in relation to the heart (danger of →cardiac infarction).
Symptom level: Struggle for vitality; the free flow of the life energy is convulsively hindered.
Handling: Consciously battling for one's own vitality; pitching oneself headlong into real life; becoming aware of the overly tense (cramped) domains of one's own life.
Resolution: Flowing with the energy of the life flow, entrusting oneself to it; enjoying the freeflow of vitality; allowing suspense to build up in the earnest domain of the world of feelings.
Archetypal principle: Mercury-Uranus.

Vegetative dystonia

(see also Sympathicotonia, High blood pressure)
Physical level: Visceral nervous system (nerves = news service).
Symptom level: Vegetative distension, psycho-vegetative syndrome: displacement of the natural balance between sympathicotonous (masculine) and parasympathicotonous (feminine) energies in favour of the masculine, active energies; these hustle the organism into a state of permanent tension to the point of being highly strung and completely over-wound and are accompanied by an incalculable number of symptoms

for which traditional science has been unable to uncover any substantial physical findings; imbalance between the accelerator (sympathicus) and brake (parasympathicus): being continually on the move at full speed without properly-functioning brakes; symptoms extend from high blood pressure to headaches and back pains, feelings of dizziness, fatigue, outbreaks of sweating, fearfulness and disturbed sexual functioning, as well as respiratory and heart complaints (galloping/racing heartbeat, heart pains).

Handling/Resolution: Letting oneself get involved with the tensions of life, leading an exciting life ("Be hot or cold, the lukewarm I will spit out of My mouth"); once the masculine pole (the hot side of life) has been exhausted, and it has become clear that this one-sidedness offers no solution, re-discovering the brake and learning to make use of it again; finding the centre, respectively the balance, between forward-thrusting masculine forces and regenerating feminine powers; in interpreting the individual symptoms, taking into account the issue of "finding the centre".

Archetypal principle: Sun/ Moon-Uranus.

Vein inflammation

(Thrombophlebitis; see also Thrombosis, Varicose veins)

Physical level: Connective tissue (connection, stability, binding commitment), blood vessels (transport routes of the life force).

Symptom level: Aggressive confrontation and violently painful conflicts over blockages along the return paths of the life energy; overloading in the energy transport system; restricted flexibility: being jammed, stuck in a rut, inhibited; non-living state in a living body.

Handling: Battling over the return paths of the life energy: wanting to get back what one has sent out; accepting the enforced rest in order to come to terms with the pain caused by the energy blockages in one's system.

Resolution: Having out the conflicts which result from the blockages and delays in the flow of one's life energy.

Archetypal principle: Venus/ Mars-Saturn.

Venereal diseases

see Sexual diseases

Vertigo

(fear of heights, see also Phobia)

Symptom level: Dizziness and fear of heights and ultimately of falling; the primordial fear held by humankind of the Fall; every rise makes the fall more likely; the more dubious the rise, the greater the fear of falling.

Handling: Making oneself aware of one's own position and the dependability of one's own standpoints; making insecure and unjustified rises secure after the fact, assuring oneself of the necessary firm bases; recognising that ultimately every position reached is unstable and insecure.

Resolution: Reconciliation with the Archetypal subject of the Fall from Grace; acknowledging rising and falling as unavoidable stations in the cycle of life.

Archetypal principle: Uranus-Saturn.

Virus infection

see Inflammation

Vitiligo

(skin depigmentation; pigment disorder of unknown cause)

Physical level: Skin (border, contact, tenderness).

Symptom level: The colour is missing in places in life; blind spots on the map of the soul which are mirrored outwardly on the surface of the body; being marked (with distinction).
Handling: Bringing colour into the marked areas; getting to know the white spots (uncharted territory) on the map of the soul; accepting being marked (with distinction) and allowing oneself to be stirred to action by it.
Resolution: Proving oneself worthy of being marked (with distinction): seeking the special distinctiveness that this sign-ifies: marking oneself with distinction.
Archetypal principle: Venus/ Saturn-Pluto.

Voice problems

(see also Hoarseness, Spitting)
Physical level: Larynx (expression, tone [mood]), vocal cords (expression, speech).
Symptom level: Problem of the resonance base; our voice shows how strongly we are in resonance with our body and our inner voice; heady voice: only being in resonance with the head; squeaky, shaky voice: not trusting oneself to stand up for one's capabilities and make use of them; fear of one's own strength; hoarse voice: irritation, not standing behind one's utterances; soft, wishy-washy voice: not wanting to pin oneself down, undifferentiated thoughts; stifled voice: suppressed tears, suppressed anger; rough voice: struggling strenuously against inner resistances, not committing oneself; booming voice, life of the party - a real blast: discordant, inability to attune oneself to new, changing situations; hissing voice: wanting to be seductive and to share something hidden/forbidden, suppressed aggression; shrill voice: struggling for recognition and attention; →compulsive coughing: remaining stuck in the very beginnings of self-expression, trying in vain to gain an audience, not expressing criticism openly.
Handling: Making oneself aware of one's limitations in the overall tone of one's voice and mood: bringing to life those regions that are currently not resonating and also giving them their voice (voting rights).
Resolution: Integrating inactive regions of the body into life more fully and drawing on every cadence in order to make oneself heard as a harmonious whole.
Archetypal principle: Mercury-Saturn/Moon.

Vomiting and diarrhoea (combined)

(see also Vomiting and Diarrhoea separately)
Physical level: Stomach (feeling, receptiveness), intestines (processing of material impressions).
Symptom level: Not being able to digest and process the acute life situation; simply wanting to be rid of everything again somehow, but not wanting to take anything in; opening all the floodgates in order to get rid of the indigestible by every possible channel.
Handling: Letting go in a comprehensive sense of what one cannot and does not want to process.
Resolution: Letting everything simply pass through oneself, without letting oneself get entangled in it: Buddhist Bhoga = consuming the world without losing oneself in the world.
Archetypal principle: Moon-Mercury-Pluto.

Vomiting/Nausea

(Emesis, see also Vomiting and diarrhoea, Faecal vomiting, Pregnancy complaints, Kinetoses [travel and movement sickness])

Physical level: Gullet (assimilation, defence), stomach (feeling, receptiveness).

Symptom level: Something spews forth; having stuffed oneself with too much that is unsuitable/indigestible; getting rid of things and impressions which one does not want to have/ to digest; defence, rejection, non-acceptance: "my stomach is turning", "something is coming back up"; acute uprising: "the situation makes me sick"; a problem lies in the pit of one's stomach like a stone and spoils one's appetite; boiling with rage and blurting out venomous aggression: "spitting poison and bile"; seeking relief, liberation, wanting to let go of something oppressive.

Handling: Consciously owning up to one's resistance; learning to rise up (rebel), not simply accepting everything; owning up to one's own rage and venomous nature; exercises in letting go of pent-up, "quashed" aggression; accepting that one cannot digest everything under all circumstances; consciously lightening one's load (vomiting as a method used in older forms of naturopathy).

Resolution: Liberation from things which one has been deceived in, which one cannot come to terms with, which one does not want to and cannot digest; spitting out what is pressing down on one.

Archetypal principle: Moon-Mars/ Uranus.

Vulval carcinoma

(cancer of the outer female genitalia; see also Lichen sclerosus et atrophicus as the preliminary stage of this disease)

Physical level: Vulva (protective wall).

Symptom level: Rare type of skin cancer in older women; sexuality has been experienced as a burden and shows itself to be an unresolved issue by means of the malignant growth; the lovelessness and unwanted advances by the partner that one has borne over the years materialise as malignant growths, which stink to high heaven; loathing of the dirty partner and his lustful desires.

Handling: Offensively tackling the confrontation and processing of issues such as "sexual desire" and "sexual exploitation"; recognising the rejection of one's own sexuality; learning to protect oneself against assaults and attacks from foreign interests; considering all the measures mentioned under →cancer: since cancer affects the complete organism, it must also be met across-the-board.

Resolution: Safeguarding one's own interests in conflicts over love and sexuality; recognising the necessity to switch from the physical and thus (life-)threatening level to the challenging, but life-saving mental-spiritual level, and relying in this realm on expansive growth; discovering love that transcends all boundaries; setting oneself above external rule and standards laid down by oneself or others, and living and developing oneself solely in accordance with the obligations of one's own highest law; finding and offensively living out one's own feminine strength

Archetypal principle: Pluto-Saturn.

Vulval varices

(varicose veins of the vagina, rare disease pattern during pregnancy)

Physical level: Vulva (protective wall), blood vessels (transport routes of the life force), vagina (commitment, desire), labia (entrance gates to the sexual underworld).

Symptom level: In the form of large, swollen labia, the lakes of blood (varicose veins) convey the feeling that everything is forcing its way out through the lower (vaginal) channel;

feeling of fullness to the point of restricting physical movement; prevention of sex life; backup of energy in front of the sexual entrance; sinking life force; rejection of the partner.

Handling: Concerning oneself with one's own shame; considering oneself to be important sexually, and carefully but firmly, ensuring one's own right of self-determination; ensuring that, in the domain of sexuality, she also gets back what she puts into it in terms of life energy (allopathic approach).

Resolution: Giving everything without expectation of reward; expending oneself and letting the energy flow.

Archetypal principle: Moon-Venus.

Vulvitis

(see also Pruritus vulvae, Lichen sclerosus et atrophicus)

Physical level: Vulva (protective wall).

Symptom level: Conflict at the forefront of sexuality.

Handling: Concerning oneself actively and offensively with one's own wishes and longings in the erotic-genital respect; conspicuously accentuating one's own sensuality on other levels (clothing, attitude, make-up, etc.).

Resolution: Reconciliation with polarity in the form of one's own sexuality.

Archetypal principle: Venus-Mars-Pluto.

W

Waldenström's disease

(Waldenström macroglobulinemia [WM])

Physical level: Immune system (defence).

Symptom level: Increase of the IgM (immunglobulines fraction M) above the normal value of 250 mg/dl up to over 6,000; in traditionally-accepted medicine, this is treated with cytostatics; overblown, one-sided physical immune defence measures: need to defend oneself, to put up resistance.

Handling: Learning to defend oneself on other levels than the physical immunological level: nevertheless, this must penetrate to the core, right down to and into the bones.

Resolution: Finding the way to one's own mental-spiritual strength.

Archetypal principle: Mars-Jupiter.

Warts

(see also Foot-sole warts, Plantar warts, Genital warts)

Physical level: Skin (border, contact, tenderness).

Symptom level: (Unattractive) outgrowths from the inside: message from the shadow kingdom (the warts of the witch, the warthog); confrontation with one's own dark sides; attacks against one's own flawlessness; reminder of the magical roots of childhood.

Handling: Asking oneself where the warts bother one, what they prevent one doing, what was hidden away when the warts developed; checking which reflex zones and meridians they lie on: what subjects do they want to put one in contact with?; admitting one's own magical roots in the past: spiriting the warts away (wart-charmer: change of mind = metanoia).

Resolution: Acknowledgement of the shadow sides: treating the outgrowth of the dark inner world with dark (occult) methods (homeopathically).

Archetypal principle: Pluto.

Weather sensitivity

(see also Foehn disorder)

Symptom level: Resistance against the divine force of the weather;

physical immune defence reactions against "atmospheric" changes; a life situation characterised by unstable moods: the dynamism generated by the weather is already in itself too much movement and clashes with one's own stagnation.
Handling: Transforming increased sensibility into the positive opportunity of foresight; learning to understand sensitivity as an opportunity: instead of allowing oneself to be disturbed, directing one's conscious attention to changes; working from the opposite pole: grounding oneself in order to achieve harmony with the forces of Heaven and Earth: raising one's head to the Father in Heaven, with one's feet firmly rooted in Mother Earth (Indian proverb).
Resolution: Opening oneself up to Heaven and its messages; consciously learning to believe the upper worlds: developing faith in God.
Archetypal principle: Moon-Uranus/Neptune.

Werlhof's disease

see Thrombocytopenia

Whiplash

(catapult trauma; see also Traffic accident)
Physical level: Cervical vertebra (column) (being easily swayed, flexibility of the head).
Symptom level: Most commonly caused by car-crash accidents which result in the neck being thrown forward and back, with resulting damage to the spinal column, and in extreme cases, to the point of →paraplegia (→neck fracture) and vascular injuries: being thrown/catapulted off course; sensory deficiencies and pain in the shoulders and arms (→shoulder-arm syndrome): no longer having a grip on anything; failing to recognise the signs of the times until one receives an impetus (impact) from

behind; being rammed into something that is right under one's nose.
Handling: Using the compulsion to rest as a result of being mechanically brought to rest as a chance to gain a rested and unobstructed overview of one's own life; developing the awareness that one was going through life too quickly and with too little foresight; increasing the mobility of the head in the long term, however, in order to get through life with more foresight and greater flexibility; increasing the ability to bend one's neck and reducing its rigidity - only offering resistance where it makes sense.
Resolution: Finding the happy medium between being a dynamic whirlwind (vertrebrae from Latin: vert(ere) 'to turn') and (having) backbone: creating a perfect and harmonious interplay of dynamic and static abilities.
Archetypal principle: Venus-Saturn/Uranus.

Whitlow

(panaritium)
Physical level: Finger- and toenails (claws, aggression).
Symptom level: Conflict over vitality and basic trust; too little room for stimulating subjects.
Handling: Creating a basis for vitality and aggression; living out conflicts in the area of the claws more consciously: learning to show one's claws; using one's claws in an aggressive and open(ly offensive) way to get what one needs in life.
Resolution: First ensuring inner safety and security (basic trust) so that, working from a state of inner calm, one can step up to one's challenges powerfully and courageously.
Archetypal principle: Mars (claws)/Moon (nail bed/basic trust)-Mars (inflammation).

Whooping cough

(pertussis; see also Childhood diseases, Coughing)

Physical level: Lungs (contact, communication, freedom).

Symptom level: Dry, non-(mucous)-dissolving and therefore non-resolving coughing occurring mainly at night: often desperate struggle; violent, almost unquenchable outbreak of aggressions; several barking, exhausting coughing fits with the typical wheezing intake of breath combine into volleys of coughing that have the character of an attack: causing a fuss, "coughing up" what one really thinks to the surrounding world; showing who one is and what aggressions one has built up; combatively placing oneself in the central focus of attention, and occupying a great deal of time for this; attacks extend to the point of severe respiratory distress, cramps, cerebral haemorrhages and damage; most common subsequent disease pattern: →bronchiectases (enlargement of the bronchia); often with a typical progression curve: three weeks rising, then three weeks declining development; breakthrough of aggression in childhood in order to reach a new development stage; taking a step towards oneself in order to win the battle to carve out a new position in one's family and in life.

Handling: (for parents): Recognising aggression as a vitally important principle in life and actively helping it to break through: educating children to show courage and civil courage - an attitude which takes life firmly in hand and promotes the will to act; making clear to oneself that hindering the development of aggression (cramping) can become dangerous (to life); expansion of the field of communication (bronchiectases).

Resolution: Accepting aggression in both its dark (night-time) and light, everyday sides: recognising and acknowledging the Mars principle in the power to push through one's will and hold one's ground as evident in the spring (rising juices [sap], trees catapulting their seeds and erupting with blossoms, buds bursting their seed cases, vegetables shooting out of the ground); granting the child more independence; welcoming and supporting its forthcoming leap in development.

Archetypal principle: Mars-Uranus-Mercury.

Winter depression

(see also Depression)

Symptom level: The winter, the darkness and the dying off of nature remind one of the suppressed issue of death.

Handling: As is the case for →depression: reconciling oneself with one's own mortality; acknowledging stillness and darkness as necessary regeneration periods.

Resolution: Arising from the ashes like the Phoenix: experiencing that true life begins beyond death, and that out of the deepest darkness, light is born (compare Christmas).

Archetypal principle: Saturn.

Work accident/ Domestic accident

(see also Accident, Traffic accident)

Physical level: All levels of the body can be affected.

Symptom level: "having something explode in one's face", "getting one's fingers burnt"; "taking a tumble"; "cutting off one's nose to spite one's face"; allowing oneself a "slip-up", "being tripped up by something", "taking a bruising", "making a crash landing" or "taking a bad fall" (from the career ladder); "being bled dry by something", "losing fur in the fray"; "stabbing someone in the back"; "being down for the count" or "K.O."

(in business), suffering "burn out", "a setback"; "dealing someone a blow", "pulling the carpet out from under someone"; "failing to get a grip on something", "missing the mark"; "having gone wrong", "gone astray", "lost one's way"; "getting a warning shot across the bows", "shooting at someone", "kicking someone in the shin", "knocking someone over" or "pushing them out of the way", "backing someone up against the wall", "pushing someone aside", "letting something slide", "setting a trap for someone", "getting a resounding slap across the face"; "biting off more than one can chew" (doing oneself an injury), "overstretching oneself (physically and financially)" (overbearingness); "pride comes before a fall (accident)"

Handling: Reconstruction of the circumstances of the accident and transferral of these to the current life situation in mental-spiritual terms, e.g. allowing oneself to be thrown off track (in life) = breaking new ground instead of being violently compelled in a new direction; alternatively: concerning oneself with the theme of the Fall from unity (from Paradise) and addressing one's own pride, which comes before a fall, instead of repeatedly falling flat on one's face.

Resolution: Comprehending the circumstances of the accident at a higher level in the mental-spiritual respect; finding healthy outlets or creative forms of expression for aggressive Mars-driven energy, e.g. breaking new ground instead of repeatedly losing one's way or getting lost; stepping out of line and kicking over the traces instead of stumbling; following explosive trains of thought instead of having things blow up in one's face; coming to grips with red-hot irons (hot topics) instead of getting one's fingers burnt; thinking in-depth thoughts instead of sustaining surface wounds; making one's mark instead of cutting off one's nose to spite one's face; living flexibly in all directions instead of slipping up and tripping; developing a conflict culture instead of clashing with others; lowering one's sights in good time and fortifying the foundations instead of coming crashing down; deploying one's life energy voluntarily and in good time instead of bleeding dry; paying in good time (ideally with cash) instead of later being bled dry or losing fur in the fray; always looking at both sides, instead of stabbing someone in the back; coming back down to Earth in good time instead of going down for the count with a thud; being fired up for solutions instead of burning out; fanning the flames of enthusiasm and inspiration; considering the other side of things instead of suffering a blow from behind; putting up a good fight and practising being able to take the blows instead of dealing others a blow; ensuring a sound footing instead of allowing the carpet to be pulled out from under one's feet; preferring to exhaust all possibilities and paths thoroughly in one's mind before failing to get a grip on something or missing the mark or before something else goes wrong (exercising creativity); losing oneself in one's task/purpose instead of losing oneself in general; being ready for everything long before one gets a warning shot across the bows; shooting down fleeting thoughts instead of people (from their posts); offensively standing up to others in good time in order not to have to open fire on them or shoot them down later; meditating on one's own mortality instead of executing others (verbally); seizing things with all one's strength and in good time instead of later becoming overbearing.

Archetypal principle: Uranus.

Worm diseases

(see also Tapeworm infestation, Threadworm infestation)

Physical level: Digestive tract (Buddhism: Bhoga = "consuming and digesting the world") is the preferred living space for the worms, although they may also migrate to other areas, e.g. the liver.

Symptom level: Even though they are sometimes harmless in a medical sense (such as threadworm in children), in symbolic terms, they still always remain highly dangerous because they come from the underworld of the shadow kingdom (the lindworm): being possessed on a physical level; something is not correctly attuned; something is running the wrong way (for example, in the case of a tapeworm infestation, in concrete terms, the nutrients end up in the wrong channel): "a can of worms"; sense of uncleanliness: being internally infested with vermin ("a wretched worm"); being full of worms, worm-ridden; fear of being eaten up from inside: "the worm gnaws and eats away at one", "something rankles one" (derived from Latin dracunculus 'a small serpent'); nurturing parasites, hosting uninvited guests and having to feed them; being a victim of exploitation; worms, which are (close to) dead (they also prefer to settle in the intestines, the kingdom of the dead of the body), eat one alive; the worm as a harmless, small snake.

Handling: Issue of cleanliness: keeping the upper and lower levels apart; getting to know the inhabitants (subjects) of the shadow kingdom in a mental-spiritual way, and thus relieving the physical level of this load; using the related issue(s) of the affected organ to find out what is not correctly attuned, what has wormed its way in; consciously sharing nourishment with weaker, dependent beings (creatures); inviting guests; becoming a patron; in the case of children: learning to share; clarifying the issues of exploitation and being exploited; observing the parasites; reconciling oneself with death and its foreshadowing signs; consciously restricting oneself, e.g. fasting (also physically starves out the parasites); paying attention to what one has swallowed down the wrong way; consciously re-directing energies.

Resolution: "Live and let live", cultivating love of others; developing a sense one's own needs and those of other beings; reconciliation with one's own shadow world: tackling one's own battle with the dragon (the mythical lindworm).

Archetypal principle: Pluto.

Wrist joint inflammation

see Rheumatism

Writer's cramp

Physical level: Hands (grasping, gripping, ability to act, expression).

Symptom level: Security/insecurity problem: extreme ambition, overblown level of expectation; desire for social advancement with modesty that is merely put on for show; efforts of a cramped nature, in reality, having nothing to say (= write).

Handling: Making oneself aware of all the additional expectations which are also flowing into one's writing; bringing one's wishes and expectations into harmony with one's behaviour: all behaviour that is simply put on for show ultimately leads to cramping in the long run; honestly admitting to oneself whether what has been written really needs to be written, whether what has been said is really worth mentioning.

Resolution: Standing behind one's form and style of writing; reconciling

oneself with one's own words; allowing thoughts to flow: making oneself
aware that one must always make
compromises and that the complete
truth is not easy to put down on
paper.
Archetypal principle: **Mercury-Pluto.**

Y

Yeast infection

see Pityriasis versicolor

About the Author

Ruediger Dahlke, M.D.

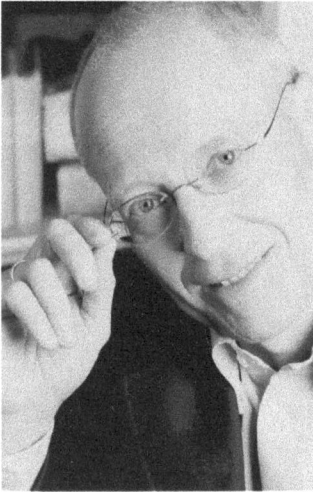

A doctor and psychotherapist since 1979, he completed additional qualifications in naturopathic medicine, as well as furthering his training in homeopathy during the course of his medical studies.

In the meantime, he has become well-known to a broader public above all as the author of books such as *Krankheit als Symbol (*Disease as a Symbol), Krankheit als Sprache der Seele (Illness As a Language of the Soul), Krankheit als Weg (*The Healing Power of Illness), Lebenskrisen als Entwicklungschancen (Life Crises as an Opportunity for Development), Frauen-Heil-Kunde (The Female Healing Arts), Aggression als Chance (Aggression as an Opportunity)* and *Die Schicksalsgesetze – Spielregeln fürs Leben (The Laws of Fate – Rules For the Game of Life)* as well as through numerous TV and radio appearances.

As a complement to the interpretation of disease patterns, he has also developed the use of guided meditations into an effective method of self-help. In keeping with this, audio programs (on CD) have been created to accompany many of the disease patterns as well as various health topics in general, which, together with the interpretations themselves, allow people more "response-ability" in dealing with health-related challenges.

In 1989, after a 12 year period spent working in Munich, during which time he laid the foundations for his holistic approach to psychosomatic medicine and (together with Thorwald Dethlefsen) produced the book

Krankheit als Weg (The Healing Power of Illness), he established, along with Margit Dahlke – his wife in the first half of his life - the Heil-Kunde-Ze-ntrum Johanniskirchen in Niederbayern, which has since developed into a key location for treatment in line with his spiritual psychotherapy ap-proach. Since 2010, he and Rita Fasel - his partner and co-author of *Die Spuren der Seele – was Hand und Fuß über uns verraten (Traces of the Soul – What Our Hands and Feet Reveal About Us)* have been involved in the planning and construction of the TamanGa centre, which is sched-uled to begin its operations as a seminar venue by the end of 2011.

In Germany, Austria, Switzerland and Italy, Ruediger Dahlke regu-larly gives presentations and (training) seminars to the general public on topics such as the spiritual significance of different disease patterns, conscious fasting, connected breathing, meditation, and the further de-velopment of spiritual awareness, as well as providing corporate training seminars in companies. In addition, he has presented his ideas on ho-listic medicine and spiritual philosophy, not only in the many books men-tioned above, but also in numerous newspaper and journal articles, and in TV and radio appearances. The ultimate aim of all of these activities is to support patients along their path towards greater self-responsibility, self-determination and optimal health.

In the German-speaking world, Ruediger Dahlke's books have al-ready attracted a following of millions and have thus contributed to cre-ating an ever-expanding consciousness for psychosomatic correlations and a holistic approach to medicine. In addition, there are currently over 200 translations available in 24 different languages – a number that is expected to steadily increase as interest in these topics continues to grow. Further information can be found at: www.dahlke.at (under "Dahlke International").

Further Addresses

Information about seminars, courses of study, management training sessions and presentations

Heilkundeinstitut GmbH
Oberberg 92
A-8151 Hitzendorf
Tel: +43-316-7198885
Fax: +43-316-7198886
Internet: www.dahlke.at
Email: info@dahlke.at

Information about therapy

Heil-Kunde-Zentrum Johanniskirchen
Schornbach 22
D-84381 Johanniskirchen
Tel: 08564-819
Fax: 08564-1429
Internet: www.dahlke-heilkundezentrum.de
Email: hkz-dahlke@t-online.de

www.ingramcontent.com/pod-product-compliance
Lightning Source LLC
Chambersburg PA
CBHW011743020426
42333CB00022B/2710